T0362101

Fundamentals of Optical Waveguides

Fundamentals of Optical Waveguides

Second Edition

KATSUNARI OKAMOTO

Okamoto Laboratory Ltd Ibaraki, Japan

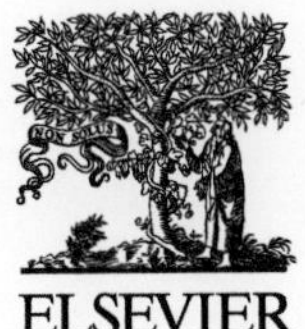

ELSEVIER

AMSTERDAM • BOSTON • HEIDELBERG • LONDON
NEW YORK • OXFORD • PARIS • SAN DIEGO
SAN FRANCISCO • SINGAPORE • SYDNEY • TOKYO

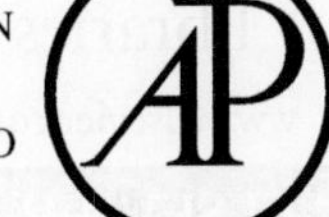

Academic Press is an imprint of Elsevier

Academic Press is an imprint of Elsevier
30 Corporate Drive, Suite 400, Burlington, MA 01803, USA
525 B Street, Suite 1900, San Diego, California 92101-4495, USA
84 Theobald's Road, London WC1X 8RR, UK

This book is printed on acid-free paper. ♾

Library of Congress Cataloging-in-Publication Data
Application Submitted

British Library Cataloguing in Publication Data
A catalogue record for this book is available from the British Library

ISBN 13: 978-0-12-525096-2
ISBN 10: 0-12-525096-7

For information on all Elsevier Academic Press publications
visit our Web site at www.books.elsevier.com

Printed in the United States of America
05 06 07 08 09 10 9 8 7 6 5 4 3 2 1

To Kuniko, Hiroaki and Masaaki

Contents

Preface to the First Edition

This book is intended to describe the theoretical basis of optical waveguides with particular emphasis on the transmission theory. In order to investigate and develop optical fiber communication systems and planar lightwave circuits thorough understanding of the principle of lightwave propagation and its application to the design of practical optical devices are required. To answer these purposes, the book explains important knowledge and analysis methods in detail.

The book consists of ten chapters. In Chapter 1 fundamental wave theories of optical waveguides, which are necessary to understand the lightwave propagation phenomena in the waveguides, are described. Chapters 2 and 3 deal with the transmission characteristics in planar optical waveguides and optical fibers, respectively. The analytical treatments in Chapters 2 and 3 are quite important to understand the basic subjects of waveguides such as (1) mode concepts and electromagnetic field distributions, (2) dispersion equation and propagation constants, and (3) chromatic dispersion and transmission bandwidths. Directional couplers and Bragg gratings are indispensable to construct practical lightwave circuits. In Chapter 4 coupled mode theory to deal with these devices is explained in detail and concrete derivation techniques of the coupling coefficients for several practical devices are presented. Chapter 5 treats nonlinear optical effects in optical fibers such as optical solitons, stimulated Raman scattering, stimulated Brillouin scattering and second-harmonic generation. Though the nonlinearity of silica-based fiber is quite small, several nonlinear optical effects manifest themselves conspicuously owing to the high power density and long interaction length in fibers. Generally nonlinear optical effects are thought to be harmful to communication systems. But, if we fully understand nonlinear optical effects and make good use of them we can construct much more versatile communication systems and information processing devices. From Chapter 6 to 8 various numerical analysis methods are presented; they are, the finite element method (FEM) waveguide and stress analyses, beam propagation methods (BPM) based on the fast Fourier transform (FFT) and finite difference methods (FDM), and the staircase concatenation method. In the analysis and design of practical lightwave circuits, we often encounter problems to which analytical methods cannot be applied due to the complex waveguide structure and insufficient accuracy in the results. We should rely on numerical techniques in such cases. The finite element method is suitable for the mode analysis and stress analysis of optical waveguides having arbitrary and complicated cross-sectional geometries.

The beam propagation method is the most powerful technique for investigating linear and nonlinear lightwave propagation phenomena in axially varying waveguides such as curvilinear directional couplers, branching and combining waveguides and tapered waveguides. BPM is also quite important for the analysis of ultrashort light pulse propagation in optical fibers. Since FEM and BPM are general-purpose numerical methods they will become indispensable tools for the research and development of optical fiber communication systems and planar lightwave circuits. In Chapters 6 to 8, many examples of numerical analyses are presented for practically important waveguide devices. The staircase concatenation method is a classical technique for the analysis of axially varying waveguides. Although FEM and BPM are suitable for the majority of cases and the staircase concatenation method is not widely used in lightwave problems, the author believes it is important to understand the basic concepts of these numerical methods. In Chapter 9, various important planar lightwave circuit (PLC) devices are described in detail. Arrayed-waveguide grating multiplexers (AWGs) are quite important wavelength filters for wavelength division multiplexing (WDM) systems. Therefore the basic operational principles, design procedures of AWGs, as well as their performances and applications, are extensively explained. Finally Chapter 10 serves to describe several important theorems and formulas which are the bases for the derivation of various equations throughout the book.

A large number of individuals have contributed, either directly or indirectly, to the completion of this book. Thanks are expressed particularly to the late Professor Takanori Okoshi of the University of Tokyo for his continuous encouragement and support. I also owe a great deal of technical support to my colleagues in NTT Photonics Laboratories. I am thankful to Professor Un-Chul Paek of Kwangju Institute of Science & Technology, Korea, and Dr. Ivan P. Kaminow of Bell Labs, Lucent Technologies, who gave me the opportunity to publish this book. I would like to express my gratitude to Prof. Gambling of City University of Hong Kong who reviewed most of the theoretical sections and made extensive suggestions. I am also thankful to Professor Ryouichi Itoh of the University of Tokyo, who suggested writing the original Japanese edition of this book.

May 1999
Katsunari Okamoto

Preface to the Second Edition

Since the publication of the first edition of this book in 1999, dramatic advancement has occurred in the field of optical fibers and planar lightwave circuits (PLCs). Photonic crystal fibers (PCFs) or holey fibers (HFs) are a completely new class of fibers. Light confinement to the core is achieved by the Bragg reflection in a hollow-core PCF. To the contrary, light is confined to the core by the effective refractive-index difference between the solid core and holey cladding in the solid-core HF. One of the most striking features of PCFs is that zero-dispersion wavelength can be shifted down to visible wavelength region. This makes it possible to generate coherent and broadband supercontinuum light from visible wavelength to near infrared wavelength region. Coherent and ultra broadband light is very important not only to telecommunications but also to applications such as optical coherence tomography and frequency metrology.

The research on PLCs has been done for more than 30 years. However, PLC and arrayed-waveguide grating (AWG) began to be practically used in optical fiber systems from the middle of 1990s. Therefore, PLCs and AWGs were in their progress when the first edition of this book was published. Performances and functionalities of AWGs have advanced dramatically after the first edition. As an example, 4200-ch AWG with 5-GHz channel spacing has been fabricated in the laboratory. Narrow-channel and large channel-count AWGs will be important not only in telecommunications but also in spectroscopy.

Based on these rapid advances in optical waveguide devices over the last six years, the publisher and I deemed it necessary to bring out this second edition in order to continue to provide a comprehensive knowledge to the readers.

New subjects have been brought into Chapters 2, 3, 5, 6, 7 and 9. Multimode interference (MMI) devices, which have been added to Chapter 2, are very important integrated optical components which can perform unique splitting and combining functions. In Chapter 3, detailed discussion of the polarization mode dispersion (PMD) and dispersion control in single-mode fibers are added together with the comprehensive treatment of the PCFs. Four-wave mixing (FWM) that has been added to Chapter 5 is an important nonlinear effect especially in wavelength division multiplexing (WDM) systems.

High-index contrast PLCs such as Silicon-on-Insulator (SOI) waveguides are becoming increasingly important to construct optoelectronics integrated circuits. In order to deal with high-index contrast waveguides, semi-vector analysis becomes prerequisite. In Chapters 6 and 7, semi-vector finite element method

(FEM) analysis and beam propagation method (BPM) analysis have been newly added. Moreover, comprehensive treatment of the finite difference time domain (FDTD) method is introduced in Chapter 7.

Almost all of the material in Chapter 9 is new because of recent advances in PLCs and AWGs. Readers will acquire comprehensive understanding of the operational principles in various kinds of flat spectral-response AWGs. Origin of crosstalk and dispersion in AWGs are described thoroughly. Various kinds of optical-layer signal processing devices, such as reconfigurable optical add/drop multiplexers (ROADM), dispersion slope equalizers, PMD equalizers, etc., have been described.

I am indebted to a large number of people for the work on which this second edition of the book is based. First, I should like to thank the late Professor Takanori Okoshi of the University of Tokyo for his continuous encouragement and support. I owe a great deal of technical support to my colleagues in NTT Photonics Laboratories. I am thankful to Professor Un-Chul Paek of Gwangju Institute of Science and Technology, Korea, and Dr Ivan P. Kaminow of Kaminow Lightwave Technology, USA, who gave me the opportunity to publish the book. I am also grateful to Prof. Gambling of LTK Industries Ltd, Hong Kong, who made extensive suggestions to the first edition of the book.

Finally, I wish to express my hearty thanks to my wife, Kuniko, and my sons, Hiroaki and Masaaki, for their warm support in completing the book.

June 2005

Katsunari Okamoto

Chapter 1

Wave Theory of Optical Waveguides

The basic concepts and equations of electromagnetic wave theory required for the comprehension of lightwave propagation in optical waveguides are presented. The light confinement and formation of modes in the waveguide are qualitatively explained, taking the case of a slab waveguide. Maxwell's equations, boundary conditions, and the complex Poynting vector are described as they form the basis for the following chapters.

1.1. WAVEGUIDE STRUCTURE

Optical fibers and optical waveguides consist of a core, in which light is confined, and a cladding, or substrate surrounding the core, as shown in Fig. 1.1. The refractive index of the core n_1 is higher than that of the cladding n_0. Therefore the light beam that is coupled to the end face of the waveguide is confined in the core by total internal reflection. The condition for total internal reflection at the core–cladding interface is given by $n_1 \sin(\pi/2 - \phi) \geqslant n_0$. Since the angle ϕ is related with the incident angle θ by $\sin\theta = n_1 \sin\phi \leqslant \sqrt{n_1^2 - n_0^2}$, we obtain the critical condition for the total internal reflection as

$$\theta \leqslant \sin^{-1}\sqrt{n_1^2 - n_0^2} \equiv \theta_{max}. \tag{1.1}$$

The refractive-index difference between core and cladding is of the order of $n_1 - n_0 = 0.01$. Then θ_{max} in Eq. (1.1) can be approximated by

$$\theta_{max} \cong \sqrt{n_1^2 - n_0^2}. \tag{1.2}$$

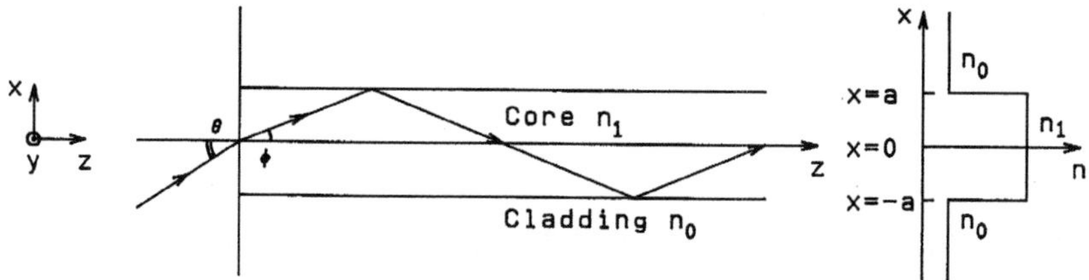

Figure 1.1 Basic structure and refractive-index profile of the optical waveguide.

θ_{max} denotes the maximum light acceptance angle of the waveguide and is known as the *numerical aperture (NA)*.

The relative refractive-index difference between n_1 and n_0 is defined as

$$\Delta = \frac{n_1^2 - n_0^2}{2n_1^2} \cong \frac{n_1 - n_0}{n_1}. \tag{1.3}$$

Δ is commonly expressed as a percentage. The numerical aperture NA is related to the relative refractive-index difference Δ by

$$\mathrm{NA} = \theta_{max} \cong n_1\sqrt{2\Delta}. \tag{1.4}$$

The maximum angle for the propagating light within the core is given by $\phi_{max} \cong \theta_{max}/n_1 \cong \sqrt{2\Delta}$. For typical optical waveguides, $\mathrm{NA} = 0.21$ and $\theta_{max} = 12°(\phi_{max} = 8.1°)$ when $n_1 = 1.47, \Delta = 1\%$ (for $n_0 = 1.455$).

1.2. FORMATION OF GUIDED MODES

We have accounted for the mechanism of mode confinement and have indicated that the angle ϕ must not exceed the critical angle. Even though the angle ϕ is smaller than the critical angle, light rays with arbitrary angles are not able to propagate in the waveguide. Each mode is associated with light rays at a discrete angle of propagation, as given by electromagnetic wave analysis. Here we describe the formation of modes with the ray picture in the slab waveguide [1], as shown in Fig. 1.2. Let us consider a plane wave propagating along the z-direction with inclination angle ϕ. The phase fronts of the plane waves are perpendicular to the light rays. The wavelength and the wavenumber of light in the core are λ/n_1 and $kn_1(k = 2\pi/\lambda)$, respectively, where λ is the wavelength of light in vacuum. The propagation constants along z and x (lateral direction) are expressed by

$$\beta = kn_1 \cos\phi, \tag{1.5}$$

$$\kappa = kn_1 \sin\phi. \tag{1.6}$$

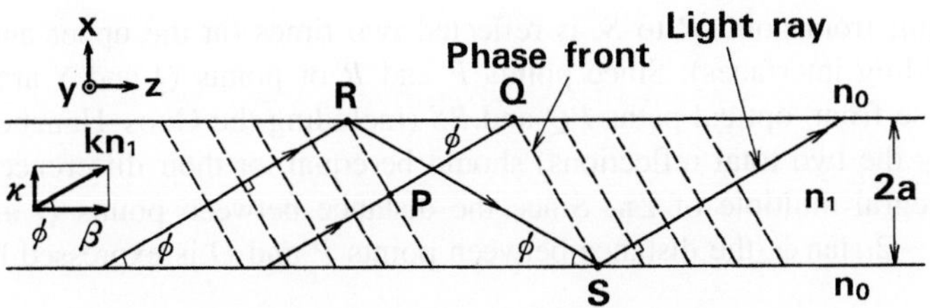

Figure 1.2 Light rays and their phase fronts in the waveguide.

Before describing the formation of modes in detail, we must explain the phase shift of a light ray that suffers total reflection. The reflection coefficient of the totally reflected light, which is polarized perpendicular to the incident plane (plane formed by the incident and reflected rays), as shown in Fig. 1.3, is given by [2]

$$r = \frac{A_r}{A_i} = \frac{n_1 \sin\phi + j\sqrt{n_1^2 \cos^2\phi - n_0^2}}{n_1 \sin\phi - j\sqrt{n_1^2 \cos^2\phi - n_0^2}}. \tag{1.7}$$

When we express the complex reflection coefficient r as $r = \exp(-j\Phi)$, the amount of phase shift Φ is obtained as

$$\Phi = -2\tan^{-1}\frac{\sqrt{n_1^2\cos^2\phi - n_0^2}}{n_1 \sin\phi} = -2\tan^{-1}\sqrt{\frac{2\Delta}{\sin^2\phi} - 1}. \tag{1.8}$$

where Eq. (1.3) has been used. The foregoing phase shift for the totally reflected light is called the Goos–Hänchen shift [1, 3].

Let us consider the phase difference between the two light rays belonging to the same plane wave in Fig. 1.2. Light ray PQ, which propagates from point P to Q, does not suffer the influence of reflection. On the other hand, light ray RS,

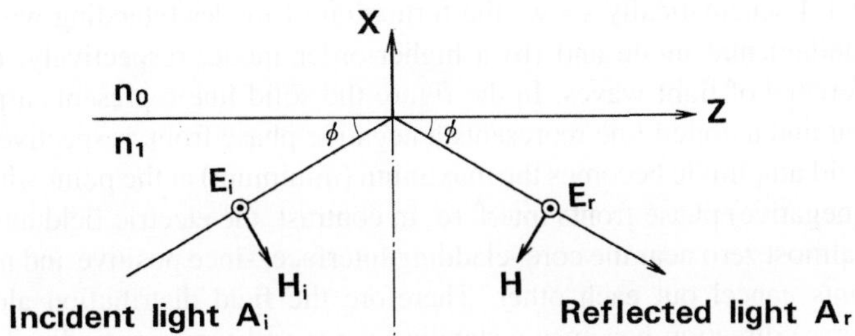

Figure 1.3 Total reflection of a plane wave at a dielectric interface.

propagating from point R to S, is reflected two times (at the upper and lower core–cladding interfaces). Since points P and R or points Q and S are on the same phase front, optical paths PQ and RS (including the Goos–Hänchen shifts caused by the two total reflections) should be equal, or their difference should be an integral multiple of 2π. Since the distance between points Q and R is $2a/\tan\phi - 2a\tan\phi$, the distance between points P and Q is expressed by

$$\ell_1 = \left(\frac{2a}{\tan\phi} - 2a\tan\phi\right)\cos\phi = 2a\left(\frac{1}{\sin\phi} - 2\sin\phi\right). \tag{1.9}$$

Also, the distance between points R and S is given by

$$\ell_2 = \frac{2a}{\sin\phi}. \tag{1.10}$$

The phase-matching condition for the optical paths PQ and RS then becomes

$$(kn_1\ell_2 + 2\Phi) - kn_1\ell_1 = 2m\pi, \tag{1.11}$$

where m is an integer. Substituting Eqs. (1.8)–(1.10) into Eq. (1.11) we obtain the condition for the propagation angle ϕ as

$$\tan\left(kn_1 a\sin\phi - \frac{m\pi}{2}\right) = \sqrt{\frac{2\Delta}{\sin^2\phi} - 1}. \tag{1.12}$$

Equation (1.12) shows that the propagation angle of a light ray is discrete and is determined by the waveguide structure (core radius a, refractive index n_1, refractive-index difference Δ) and the wavelength λ of the light source (wavenumber is $k = 2\pi/\lambda$) [4]. The optical field distribution that satisfies the phase-matching condition of Eq. (1.12) is called the *mode*. The allowed value of propagation constant β [Eq. (1.5)] is also discrete and is denoted as an eigenvalue. The mode that has the minimum angle ϕ in Eq. (1.12) ($m = 0$) is the fundamental mode; the other modes, having larger angles, are higher-order modes ($m \geqslant 1$).

Figure 1.4 schematically shows the formation of modes (standing waves) for (a) the fundamental mode and (b) a higher-order mode, respectively, through the interference of light waves. In the figure the solid line represents a positive phase front and a dotted line represents a negative phase front, respectively. The electric field amplitude becomes the maximum (minimum) at the point where two positive (negative) phase fronts interfere. In contrast, the electric field amplitude becomes almost zero near the core–cladding interface, since positive and negative phase fronts cancel out each other. Therefore the field distribution along the x-(transverse) direction becomes a standing wave and varies periodically along the z direction with the period $\lambda_p = (\lambda/n_1)/\cos\phi = 2\pi/\beta$.

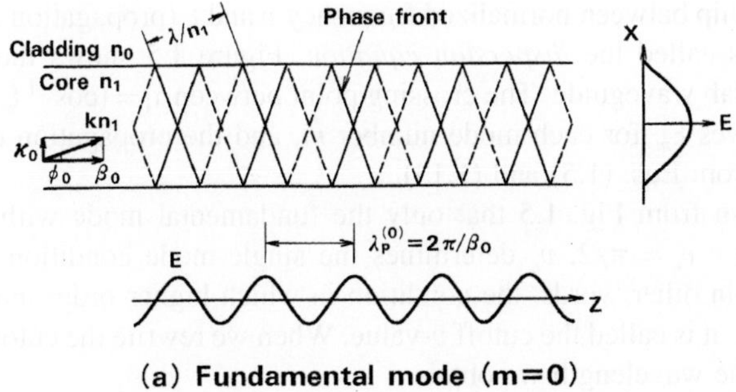

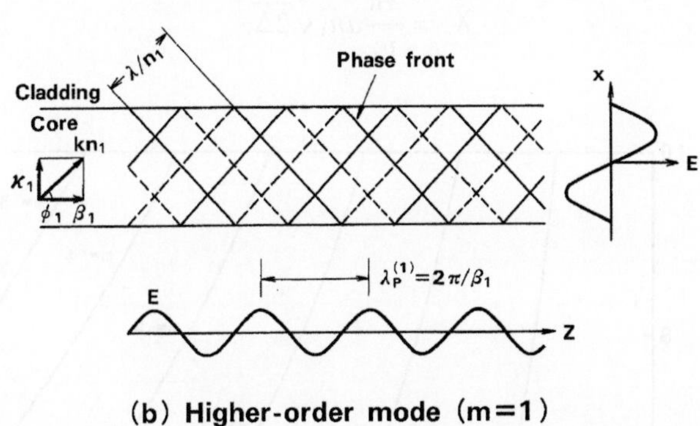

Figure 1.4 Formation of modes: (a) Fundamental mode, (b) higher-order mode.

Since $n_1 \sin\phi = \sin\theta \leqslant \sqrt{n_1^2 - n_0^2}$ from Fig. 1.1, Eqs. (1.1) and (1.3) give the propagation angle as $\sin\phi \leqslant \sqrt{2\Delta}$. When we introduce the parameter

$$\xi = \frac{\sin\phi}{\sqrt{2\Delta}}, \tag{1.13}$$

which is normalized to 1, the phase-matching Eq. (1.12) can be rewritten as

$$kn_1 a\sqrt{2\Delta} = \frac{\cos^{-1}\xi + m\pi/2}{\xi}. \tag{1.14}$$

The term on the left-hand side of Eq. (1.14) is known as the *normalized frequency*, and it is expressed by

$$v = kn_1 a\sqrt{2\Delta}. \tag{1.15}$$

When we use the normalized frequency v, the propagation characteristics of the waveguides can be treated generally (independent of each waveguide structure).

The relationship between normalized frequency v and ξ (propagation constant β), Eq. (1.14), is called the *dispersion equation*. Figure 1.5 shows the dispersion curves of a slab waveguide. The crossing point between $\eta=(\cos^{-1}\xi+m\pi/2)/\xi$ and $\eta=v$ gives ξ_m for each mode number m, and the propagation constant β_m is obtained from Eqs. (1.5) and (1.13).

It is known from Fig. 1.5 that only the fundamental mode with $m=0$ can exist when $v<v_c=\pi/2$. v_c determines the single-mode condition of the slab waveguide—in other words, the condition in which higher-order modes are cut off. Therefore it is called the cutoff v-value. When we rewrite the cutoff condition in terms of the wavelength we obtain

$$\lambda_c=\frac{2\pi}{v_c}an_1\sqrt{2\Delta}. \tag{1.16}$$

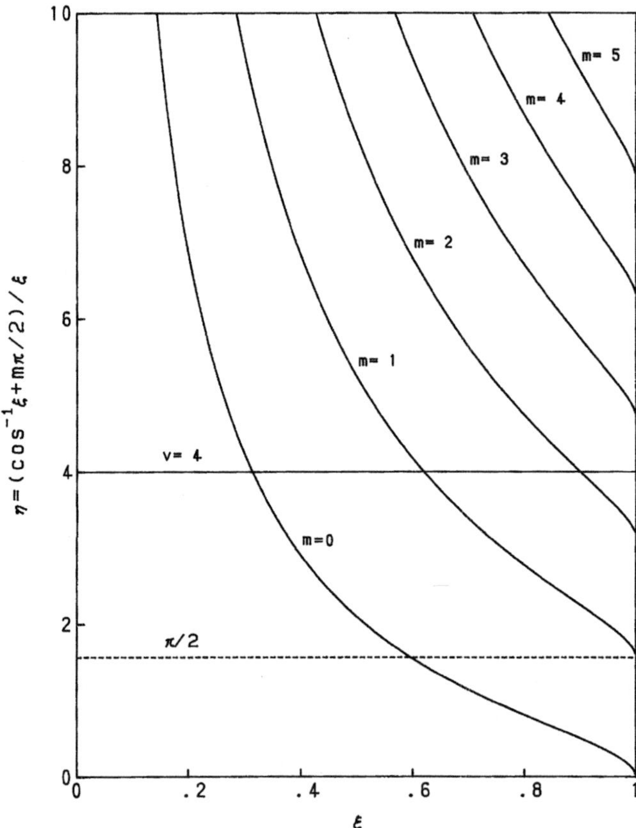

Figure 1.5 Dispersion curves of a slab waveguide.

λ_c is called the *cutoff* (free-space) *wavelength*. The waveguide operates in a single mode for wavelengths longer than λ_c. For example, $\lambda_c = 0.8\,\mu\text{m}$ when the core width $2a = 3.54\,\mu\text{m}$ for the slab waveguide of $n_1 = 1.46$, $\Delta = 0.3\%(n_0 = 1.455)$.

1.3. MAXWELL'S EQUATIONS

Maxwell's equations in a homogeneous and lossless dielectric medium are written in terms of the electric field **e** and magnetic field **h** as [5]

$$\nabla \times \mathbf{e} = -\mu \frac{\partial \mathbf{h}}{\partial t}, \tag{1.17}$$

$$\nabla \times \mathbf{h} = \varepsilon \frac{\partial \mathbf{e}}{\partial t}, \tag{1.18}$$

where ε and μ denote the permittivity and permeability of the medium, respectively. ε and μ are related to their respective values in a vacuum of $\varepsilon_0 = 8.854 \times 10^{-12}[\text{F/m}]$ and $\mu_0 = 4\pi \times 10^{-7}[\text{H/m}]$ by

$$\varepsilon = \varepsilon_0 n^2, \tag{1.19a}$$

$$\mu = \mu_0, \tag{1.19b}$$

where n is the refractive index. The wavenumber of light in the medium is then expressed as [5]

$$\Gamma = \omega\sqrt{\varepsilon\mu} = \omega n \sqrt{\varepsilon_0 \mu_0} = kn. \tag{1.20}$$

In Eq. (1.20), ω is an angular frequency of the sinusoidally varying electromagnetic fields with respect to time; k is the wavenumber in a vacuum, which is related to the angular frequency ω by

$$k = \omega\sqrt{\varepsilon_0 \mu_0} = \frac{\omega}{c}. \tag{1.21}$$

In Eq. (1.21), c is the light velocity in a vacuum, given by

$$c = \frac{1}{\sqrt{\varepsilon_0 \mu_0}} = 2.998 \times 10^8[\text{m/s}]. \tag{1.22}$$

The fact that the units for light velocity c are m/s is confirmed from the units of the permittivity ε_0 [F/m] and permeability μ_0 [H/m] as

$$\frac{1}{\sqrt{[\text{F/m}][\text{H/m}]}} = \frac{\text{m}}{\sqrt{\text{F} \cdot \text{H}}} = \frac{\text{m}}{\sqrt{[\text{A} \cdot \text{s/V}][\text{V} \cdot \text{s/A}]}} = \frac{\text{m}}{\text{s}}.$$

When the frequency of the electromagnetic wave is f[Hz], it propagates c/f[m] in one period of sinusoidal variation. Then the wavelength of electromagnetic wave is obtained by

$$\lambda = \frac{c}{f} = \frac{\omega/k}{f} = \frac{2\pi}{k}, \tag{1.23}$$

where $\omega = 2\pi f$.

When the electromagnetic fields **e** and **h** are sinusoidal functions of time, they are usually represented by complex amplitudes, i.e., the so-called phasors. As an example consider the electric field vector

$$\mathbf{e}(t) = |\mathbf{E}| \cos(\omega t + \phi), \tag{1.24}$$

where $|\mathbf{E}|$ is the amplitude and ϕ is the phase. Defining the complex amplitude of $\mathbf{e}(t)$ by

$$\mathbf{E} = |\mathbf{E}| e^{j\phi}, \tag{1.25}$$

Eq. (1.24) can be written as

$$\mathbf{e}(t) = \mathrm{Re}\{\mathbf{E} e^{j\omega t}\}. \tag{1.26}$$

We will often represent $\mathbf{e}(t)$ by

$$\mathbf{e}(t) = \mathbf{E} e^{j\omega t} \tag{1.27}$$

instead of by Eq. (1.24) or (1.26). This expression is not strictly correct, so when we use this phasor expression we should keep in mind that what is meant by Eq. (1.27) is the real part of $\mathbf{E}e^{j\omega t}$. In most mathematical manipulations, such as addition, subtraction, differentiation and integration, the replacement of Eq. (1.26) by the complex form (1.27) poses no problems. However, we should be careful in the manipulations that involve the product of sinusoidal functions. In these cases we must use the real form of the function (1.24) or complex conjugates [see Eqs. (1.42)].

When we consider an electromagnetic wave having angular frequency ω and propagating in the z direction with propagation constant β, the electric and magnetic fields can be expressed as

$$\mathbf{e} = \mathbf{E}(\mathbf{r}) e^{j(\omega t - \beta z)}, \tag{1.28}$$

$$\mathbf{h} = \mathbf{H}(\mathbf{r}) e^{j(\omega t - \beta z)}. \tag{1.29}$$

where **r** denotes the position in the plane transverse to the z-axis. Substituting Eqs. (1.28) and (1.29) into Eqs. (1.17) and (1.18), the following set of equations are obtained in Cartesian coordinates:

$$\left\{\begin{aligned} &\frac{\partial E_z}{\partial y} + j\beta E_y = -j\omega\mu_0 H_x \\ &-j\beta E_x - \frac{\partial E_z}{\partial x} = -j\omega\mu_0 H_y \\ &\frac{\partial E_y}{\partial x} - \frac{\partial E_x}{\partial y} = -j\omega\mu_0 H_z \\ &\frac{\partial H_z}{\partial y} + j\beta H_y = j\omega\varepsilon_0 n^2 E_x \\ &-j\beta H_x - \frac{\partial H_z}{\partial x} = j\omega\varepsilon_0 n^2 E_y \\ &\frac{\partial H_y}{\partial x} - \frac{\partial H_x}{\partial y} = j\omega\varepsilon_0 n^2 E_z. \end{aligned}\right. \tag{1.30}$$

The foregoing equations are the bases for the analysis of slab and rectangular waveguides.

For the analysis of wave propagation in optical fibers, which are axially symmetric, Maxwell's equations are written in terms of cylindrical coordinates:

$$\left\{\begin{aligned} &\frac{1}{r}\frac{\partial E_z}{\partial \theta} + j\beta E_\theta = -j\omega\mu_0 H_r \\ &-j\beta E_r - \frac{\partial E_z}{\partial r} = -j\omega\mu_0 H_\theta \\ &\frac{1}{r}\frac{\partial}{\partial r}(rE_\theta) - \frac{1}{r}\frac{\partial E_r}{\partial \theta} = -j\omega\mu_0 H_z \\ &\frac{1}{r}\frac{\partial H_z}{\partial \theta} + j\beta H_\theta = j\omega\varepsilon_0 n^2 E_r \\ &-j\beta H_r - \frac{\partial H_z}{\partial r} = j\omega\varepsilon_0 n^2 E_\theta \\ &\frac{1}{r}\frac{\partial}{\partial r}(rH_\theta) - \frac{1}{r}\frac{\partial H_r}{\partial \theta} = j\omega\varepsilon_0 n^2 E_z. \end{aligned}\right. \tag{1.31}$$

Maxwell's Eqs. (1.30) or (1.31) do not determine the electromagnetic field completely. Out of the infinite possibilities of solutions of Maxwell's equations, we must select those that also satisfy the boundary conditions of the respective problem. The most common type of boundary condition occurs when there are discontinuities in the dielectric constant (refractive index), as shown in Fig. 1.1.

At the boundary the tangential components of the electric field and magnetic field should satisfy the conditions

$$E_t^{(1)} = E_t^{(2)} \tag{1.32}$$

$$H_t^{(1)} = H_t^{(2)}, \tag{1.33}$$

where the subscript t denotes the tangential components to the boundary and the superscripts (1) and (2) indicate the medium, respectively. Equations (1.32) and (1.33) mean that the tangential components of the electromagnetic fields must be continuous at the boundary. There are also natural boundary conditions that require the electromagnetic fields to be zero at infinity.

1.4. PROPAGATING POWER

Consider Gauss's theorem (see Section 10.1) for vector $\mathbf{A}$ in an arbitrary volume V

$$\iiint_V \nabla \cdot \mathbf{A}\, dv = \iint_S \mathbf{A} \cdot \mathbf{n}\, ds, \tag{1.34}$$

where $\mathbf{n}$ is the outward-directed unit vector normal to the surface S enclosing V and dv and ds are the differential volume and surface elements, respectively. When we set $\mathbf{A} = \mathbf{e} \times \mathbf{h}$ in Eq. (1.34) and use the vector identity

$$\nabla \cdot (\mathbf{e} \times \mathbf{h}) = \mathbf{h} \cdot \nabla \times \mathbf{e} - \mathbf{e} \cdot \nabla \times \mathbf{h}, \tag{1.35}$$

we obtain the following equation for electromagnetic fields:

$$\iiint_V (\mathbf{h} \cdot \nabla \times \mathbf{e} - \mathbf{e} \cdot \nabla \times \mathbf{h}) dv = \iint_S (\mathbf{e} \times \mathbf{h}) \cdot \mathbf{n}\, ds. \tag{1.36}$$

Substituting Eqs. (1.17) and (1.18) into Eq. (1.36) results in

$$\iiint_V \left(\varepsilon \mathbf{e} \cdot \frac{\partial \mathbf{e}}{\partial t} + \mu \mathbf{h} \cdot \frac{\partial \mathbf{h}}{\partial t} \right) dv = -\iint_S (\mathbf{e} \times \mathbf{h}) \cdot \mathbf{n}\, ds. \tag{1.37}$$

The first term in Eq. (1.37)

$$\varepsilon \mathbf{e} \cdot \frac{\partial \mathbf{e}}{\partial t} = \frac{\partial}{\partial t} \left(\frac{\varepsilon}{2} \mathbf{e} \cdot \mathbf{e} \right) \equiv \frac{\partial W_e}{\partial t}, \tag{1.38}$$

represents the rate of increase of the electric stored energy W_e and the second term

$$\mu\mathbf{h}\cdot\frac{\partial\mathbf{h}}{\partial t}=\frac{\partial}{\partial t}\left(\frac{\mu}{2}\mathbf{h}\cdot\mathbf{h}\right)\equiv\frac{\partial W_h}{\partial t}, \tag{1.39}$$

represents the rate of increase of the magnetic stored energy W_h, respectively. Therefore, the left-hand side of Eq. (1.37) gives the rate of increase of the electromagnetic stored energy in the whole volume V; in other words, it represents the total power flow into the volume bounded by S. When we replace the outward-directed unit vector $\mathbf{n}$ by the inward-directed unit vector $\mathbf{u}_z(=-\mathbf{n})$, the total power flowing into the volume through surface S is expressed by

$$P=\iint_S -(\mathbf{e}\times\mathbf{h})\cdot\mathbf{n}\,ds=\iint_S(\mathbf{e}\times\mathbf{h})\cdot\mathbf{u}_z\,ds. \tag{1.40}$$

Equation (1.40) means that $\mathbf{e}\times\mathbf{h}$ is the vector representing the power flow, and its normal component to the surface $(\mathbf{e}\times\mathbf{h})\cdot\mathbf{u}_z$ gives the amount of power flowing through unit surface area. Therefore, vector $\mathbf{e}\times\mathbf{h}$ represents the power-flow density, and

$$\mathbf{S}=\mathbf{e}\times\mathbf{h}[\mathrm{W/m^2}] \tag{1.41}$$

is called the *Poynting vector*. In this equation, $\mathbf{e}$ and $\mathbf{h}$ denote instantaneous fields as functions of time t. Let us obtain the average power-flow density in an alternating field. The complex electric and magnetic fields can be expressed by

$$\mathbf{e}(t)=\mathrm{Re}\{\mathbf{E}e^{j\omega t}\}=\frac{1}{2}\{\mathbf{E}e^{j\omega t}+\mathbf{E}^*e^{-j\omega t}\}, \tag{1.42a}$$

$$\mathbf{h}(t)=\mathrm{Re}\{\mathbf{H}e^{j\omega t}\}=\frac{1}{2}\{\mathbf{H}e^{j\omega t}+\mathbf{H}^*e^{-j\omega t}\}, \tag{1.42b}$$

where * denotes the complex conjugate. The time average of the normal component of the Poynting vector is then obtained as

$$\begin{aligned}\langle\mathbf{S}\cdot\mathbf{u}_z\rangle&=\langle(\mathbf{e}\times\mathbf{h})\cdot\mathbf{u}_z\rangle\\&=\frac{1}{4}\langle[(\mathbf{E}e^{j\omega t}+\mathbf{E}^*e^{-j\omega t})\times(\mathbf{H}e^{j\omega t}+\mathbf{H}^*e^{-j\omega t})]\cdot\mathbf{u}_z\rangle\\&=\frac{1}{4}(\mathbf{E}\times\mathbf{H}^*+\mathbf{E}^*\times\mathbf{H})\cdot\mathbf{u}_z=\frac{1}{2}\,\mathrm{Re}\{(\mathbf{E}\times\mathbf{H}^*)\cdot\mathbf{u}_z\},\end{aligned} \tag{1.43}$$

where $\langle\rangle$ denotes a time average. Then the time average of the power flow is given by

$$P=\iint_S\frac{1}{2}\mathrm{Re}\{(\mathbf{E}\times\mathbf{H}^*)\cdot\mathbf{u}_z\}\,ds. \tag{1.44}$$

Since $\mathbf{E} \times \mathbf{H}^*$ often becomes real in the analysis of optical waveguides, the time average propagation power in Eq. (1.44) is expressed by

$$P = \iint_S \frac{1}{2}(\mathbf{E} \times \mathbf{H}^*) \cdot \mathbf{u}_z \, ds. \tag{1.45}$$

REFERENCES

[1] Marcuse, D. 1974. *Theory of Dielectric Optical Waveguides*. New York: Academic Press.
[2] Born, M. and E. Wolf. 1970. *Principles of Optics*. Oxford: Pergamon Press.
[3] Tamir, T. 1975. *Integrated Optics*. Berlin: Springer-Verlag.
[4] Marcuse, D. 1972. *Light Transmission Optics*. New York: Van Nostrand Rein-hold.
[5] Stratton, J. A. 1941. *Electromagnetic Theory*. New York: McGraw-Hill.

Chapter 2

Planar Optical Waveguides

Planar optical waveguides are the key devices to construct integrated optical circuits and semiconductor lasers. Generally, rectangular waveguides consist of a square or rectangular core surrounded by a cladding with lower refractive index than that of the core. Three-dimensional analysis is necessary to investigate the transmission characteristics of rectangular waveguides. However, rigorous three-dimensional analysis usually requires numerical calculations and does not always give a clear insight into the problem. Therefore, this chapter first describes two-dimensional slab waveguides to acquire a fundamental understanding of optical waveguides. Then several analytical approximations are presented to analyze the three-dimensional rectangular waveguides. Although these are approximate methods, the essential lightwave transmission mechanism in rectangular waveguides can be fully investigated. The rigorous treatment of three-dimensional rectangular waveguides by the finite element method will be presented in Chapter 6.

2.1. SLAB WAVEGUIDES

2.1.1. Derivation of Basic Equations

In this section, the wave analysis is described for the slab waveguide (Fig. 2.1) whose propagation characteristics have been explained [1–3]. Taking into account the fact that we treat dielectric optical waveguides, we set permittivity and permeability as $\varepsilon = \varepsilon_0 n^2$ and $\mu = \mu_0$ in the Maxwell's Eq. (1.17) and (1.18) as

$$\nabla \times \tilde{\mathbf{E}} = -\mu_0 \frac{\partial \tilde{\mathbf{H}}}{\partial t}, \tag{2.1a}$$

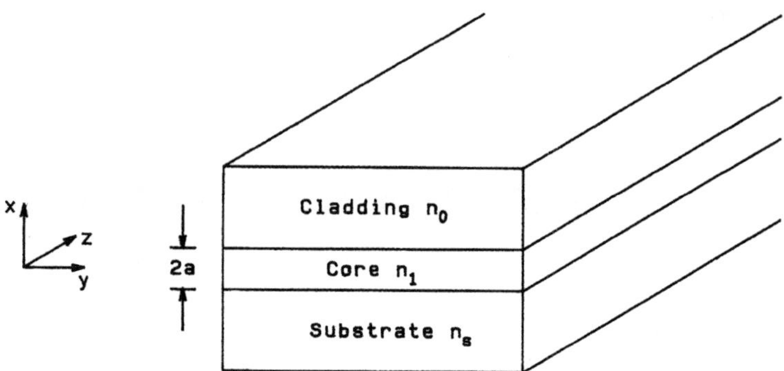

Figure 2.1 Slab optical waveguide.

$$\nabla \times \tilde{\mathbf{H}} = \varepsilon_0 n^2 \frac{\partial \tilde{\mathbf{E}}}{\partial t}, \tag{2.1b}$$

where n is the refractive index. We are interested in plane-wave propagation in the form of

$$\tilde{\mathbf{E}} = \mathbf{E}(x, y) e^{j(\omega t - \beta z)}, \tag{2.2a}$$

$$\tilde{\mathbf{H}} = \mathbf{H}(x, y) e^{j(\omega t - \beta z)}. \tag{2.2b}$$

Substituting Eqs. (2.2a) and (2.2b) into Eqs. (2.1a) and (2.1b), we obtain the following set of equations for the electromagnetic field components:

$$\left\{ \begin{array}{l} \dfrac{\partial E_z}{\partial y} + j\beta E_y = -j\omega\mu_0 H_x \\ -j\beta E_x - \dfrac{\partial E_z}{\partial x} = -j\omega\mu_0 H_y \\ \dfrac{\partial E_y}{\partial x} - \dfrac{\partial E_x}{\partial y} = -j\omega\mu_0 H_z \end{array} \right. \tag{2.3}$$

$$\left\{ \begin{array}{l} \dfrac{\partial H_z}{\partial y} + j\beta H_y = j\omega\varepsilon_0 n^2 E_x \\ -j\beta H_x - \dfrac{\partial H_z}{\partial x} = j\omega\varepsilon_0 n^2 E_y \\ \dfrac{\partial H_y}{\partial x} - \dfrac{\partial H_x}{\partial y} = j\omega\varepsilon_0 n^2 E_z. \end{array} \right. \tag{2.4}$$

In the slab waveguide, as shown in Fig. 2.1, electromagnetic fields **E** and **H** do not have y-axis dependency. Therefore, we set $\partial \mathbf{E}/\partial y = 0$ and $\partial \mathbf{H}/\partial y = 0$. Putting

these relations into Eqs. (2.3) and (2.4), two independent electromagnetic modes are obtained, which are denoted as TE mode and TM mode, respectively.
TE mode satisfies the following wave equation:

$$\frac{d^2E_y}{dx^2} + (k^2n^2 - \beta^2)E_y = 0, \tag{2.5a}$$

where

$$H_x = -\frac{\beta}{\omega\mu_0}E_y, \tag{2.5b}$$

$$H_z = \frac{j}{\omega\mu_0}\frac{dE_y}{dx}, \tag{2.5c}$$

and

$$E_x = E_z = H_y = 0. \tag{2.5d}$$

Also the tangential components E_y and H_z should be continuous at the boundaries of two different media. As shown in Eq. (2.5d) the electric field component along the z-axis is zero ($E_z = 0$). Since the electric field lies in the plane that is perpendicular to the z-axis, this electromagnetic field distribution is called transverse electric (TE) mode.

The TM mode satisfies the following wave equation:

$$\frac{d}{dx}\left(\frac{1}{n^2}\frac{dH_y}{dx}\right) + \left(k^2 - \frac{\beta^2}{n^2}\right)H_y = 0, \tag{2.6a}$$

where

$$E_x = \frac{\beta}{\omega\varepsilon_0 n^2}H_y, \tag{2.6b}$$

$$E_z = -\frac{j}{\omega\varepsilon_0 n^2}\frac{dH_y}{dx}, \tag{2.6c}$$

$$E_y = H_x = H_z = 0. \tag{2.6d}$$

As shown in Eq. (2.6d) the magnetic field component along the z-axis is zero ($H_z = 0$). Since the magnetic field lies in the plane that is perpendicular to the z-axis, this electromagnetic field distribution is called transverse magnetic (TM) mode.

2.1.2. Dispersion Equations for TE and TM Modes

Propagation constants and electromagnetic fields for TE and TM modes can be obtained by solving Eq. (2.5) or (2.6). Here the derivation method to calculate the dispersion equation (also called the eigenvalue equation) and the electromagnetic field distributions is given. We consider the slab waveguide with uniform refractive-index profile in the core, as shown in Fig. 2.2. Considering the fact that the guided electromagnetic fields are confined in the core and exponentially decay in the cladding, the electric field distribution is expressed as

$$E_y = \begin{cases} A\cos(\kappa a - \phi)e^{-\sigma(x-a)} & (x > a) \\ A\cos(\kappa x - \phi) & (-a \leqslant x \leqslant a) \\ A\cos(\kappa a + \phi)e^{\xi(x+a)} & (x < -a), \end{cases} \tag{2.7}$$

where κ, σ, and ξ are wavenumbers along the x-axis in the core and cladding regions and are given by

$$\begin{cases} \kappa = \sqrt{k^2 n_1^2 - \beta^2} \\ \sigma = \sqrt{\beta^2 - k^2 n_0^2} \\ \xi = \sqrt{\beta^2 - k^2 n_s^2}. \end{cases} \tag{2.8}$$

The electric field component E_y in Eq. (2.7) is continuous at the boundaries of core–cladding interfaces ($x = \pm a$). There is another boundary condition, that the magnetic field component H_z should be continuous at the boundaries. H_z is given by Eq. (2.5c). Neglecting the terms independent of x, the boundary

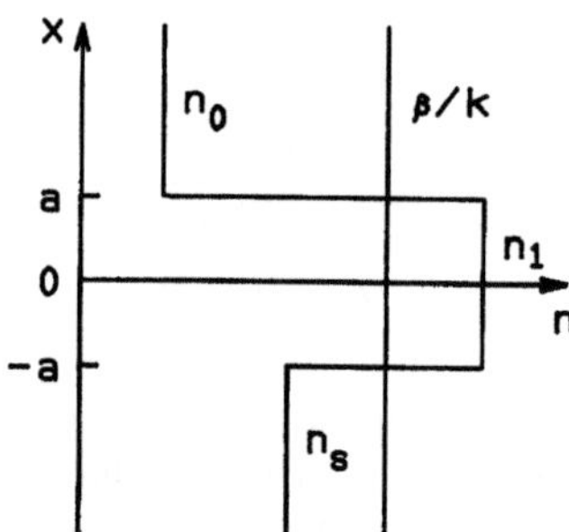

Figure 2.2 Refractive-index profile of slab waveguide.

condition for H_z is treated by the continuity condition of dE_y/dx as

$$\frac{dE_y}{dx} = \begin{cases} -\sigma A\cos(\kappa a - \phi)e^{-\sigma(x-a)} & (x > a) \\ -\kappa A\sin(\kappa x - \phi) & (-a \leqslant x \leqslant a) \\ \xi A\cos(\kappa a + \phi)e^{\xi(x+a)} & (x < -a). \end{cases} \tag{2.9}$$

From the conditions that dE_y/dx are continuous at $x = \pm a$, the following equations are obtained:

$$\begin{cases} \kappa A\sin(\kappa a + \phi) = \xi A\cos(\kappa a + \phi) \\ \sigma A\cos(\kappa a - \phi) = \kappa A\sin(\kappa a - \phi). \end{cases}$$

Eliminating the constant A, we have

$$\tan(u + \phi) = \frac{w}{u}, \tag{2.10a}$$

$$\tan(u - \phi) = \frac{w'}{u}, \tag{2.10b}$$

where

$$\begin{cases} u = \kappa a \\ w = \xi a \\ w' = \sigma a. \end{cases} \tag{2.11}$$

From Eqs. (2.10) we obtain the eigenvalue equations as

$$u = \frac{m\pi}{2} + \frac{1}{2}\tan^{-1}\left(\frac{w}{u}\right) + \frac{1}{2}\tan^{-1}\left(\frac{w'}{u}\right) \quad (m = 0, 1, 2, \ldots) \tag{2.12}$$

$$\phi = \frac{m\pi}{2} + \frac{1}{2}\tan^{-1}\left(\frac{w}{u}\right) - \frac{1}{2}\tan^{-1}\left(\frac{w'}{u}\right). \tag{2.13}$$

The normalized transverse wavenumbers u, w and w' are not independent. Using Eqs. (2.8) and (2.11) it is known that they are related by the following equations:

$$u^2 + w^2 = k^2a^2(n_1^2 - n_s^2) \equiv v^2, \tag{2.14}$$

$$w' = \sqrt{\gamma v^2 + w^2}, \tag{2.15a}$$

$$\gamma = \frac{n_s^2 - n_0^2}{n_1^2 - n_s^2} \tag{2.15b}$$

where v is the normalized frequency, defined as Eq. (1.15) and γ is a measure of the asymmetry of the cladding refractive indices. Once the wavelength of the light signal and the geometrical parameters of the waveguide are determined, the normalized frequency v and γ are determined. Therefore u, w, w' and ϕ are given by solving the eigenvalue equations Eqs. (2.12) and (2.13) under the constraints of Eqs. (2.14)–(2.15). In the asymmetrical waveguide ($n_s > n_0$) as shown in Fig. 2.2, the higher refractive index n_s is used as the cladding refractive index, which is adopted for the definition of the normalized frequency v. It is preferable to use the higher refractive index n_s because the cutoff conditions are determined when the normalized propagation constant β/k coincides with the higher cladding refractive index. Equations (2.12), (2.14) and (2.15) are the dispersion equations or eigenvalue equations for the TE_m modes. When the wavelength of the light signal and the geometrical parameters of the waveguide are determined—in other words, when the normalized frequency v and asymmetrical parameter γ are determined—the propagation constant β can be determined from these equations. As is known from Fig. 2.2 or Eqs. (2.7) and (2.8), the transverse wavenumber κ should be a real number for the main part of the optical field to be confined in the core region. Then the following condition should be satisfied:

$$n_s \leqslant \frac{\beta}{k} \leqslant n_1, \tag{2.16}$$

β/k is a dimensionless value and is a refractive index itself for the plane wave. Therefore it is called the *effective index* and is usually expressed as

$$n_e = \frac{\beta}{k}. \tag{2.17}$$

When $n_e < n_s$, the electromagnetic field in the cladding becomes oscillatory along the transverse direction; that is, the field is dissipated as the radiation mode. Since the condition $\beta = kn_s$ represents the critical condition under which the field is cut off and becomes the nonguided mode (radiation mode), it is called as *cutoff* condition. Here we introduce a new parameter, which is defined by

$$b = \frac{n_e^2 - n_s^2}{n_1^2 - n_s^2}. \tag{2.18}$$

Then the conditions for the guided modes are expressed, from Eqs. (2.16) and (2.17), by

$$0 \leqslant b \leqslant 1, \tag{2.19}$$

and the cutoff condition is expressed as

$$b = 0. \tag{2.20}$$

b is called the *normalized* propagation constant. Rewriting the dispersion Eq. (2.12) by using the normalized frequency v and the normalized propagation constant b, we obtain

$$2v\sqrt{1-b} = m\pi + \tan^{-1}\sqrt{\frac{b}{1-b}} + \tan^{-1}\sqrt{\frac{b+\gamma}{1-b}}. \tag{2.21}$$

Also Eq. (2.8) is rewritten as

$$\begin{cases} u = v\sqrt{1-b} \\ w = v\sqrt{b} \\ w' = v\sqrt{b+\gamma}. \end{cases} \tag{2.22}$$

For the symmetrical waveguides with $n_0 = n_s$, we have $\gamma = 0$ and the dispersion Eqs. (2.12) and (2.13) are reduced to

$$u = \frac{m\pi}{2} + \tan^{-1}\left(\frac{w}{u}\right), \tag{2.23a}$$

$$\phi = \frac{m\pi}{2}. \tag{2.23b}$$

Equation (2.23a) is also expressed by

$$w = u \tan\left(u - \frac{m\pi}{2}\right), \tag{2.24}$$

or

$$v\sqrt{1-b} = \frac{m\pi}{2} + \tan^{-1}\sqrt{\frac{b}{1-b}}. \tag{2.25}$$

If we notice that the transverse wavenumber $kn_1 a \sin\phi$ in Eq. (1.12) can be expressed by using the present parameters as $u = \kappa a = kn_1 a \sin\phi$, then Eq. (1.12) coincides completely with Eq. (2.24).

2.1.3. Computation of Propagation Constant

First the graphical method to obtain qualitatively obtain the propagation constant of the symmetrical slab waveguide is shown, and then the quantitative numerical method to calculate accurately the propagation constant is described. The relationship between u and w for the symmetrical slab waveguide, which is shown in Eq. (2.24), is plotted in Fig. 2.3. Transverse wavenumbers u and w should satisfy Eq. (2.14) for a given normalized frequency v. This relation is

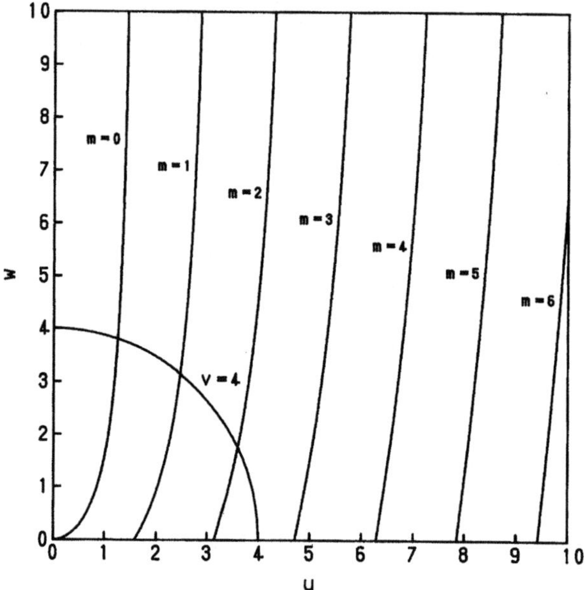

Figure 2.3 u–w relationship in slab waveguide.

also plotted in Fig. 2.3 for the case of $v = 4$ as the semicircle with the radius of 4. The solutions of the dispersion equation are then given as the crossing points in Fig. 2.3. For example, the transverse wavenumbers u and w for the fundamental mode are given by the crossing point of the curve tangential with $m = 0$ and the semicircle. The propagation constant (or eigenvalue) β is then obtained by using Eqs. (2.8) and (2.11). In Fig. 2.3, there is only one crossing point for the case of $v < \pi/2$. This means that the propagation mode is the only one when the waveguide structure and the wavelength of light satisfy the inequality $v < \pi/2$. The value of $v_c = \pi/2$ then gives the critical point at which the higher-order modes are cut off in the symmetrical slab waveguide. v_c is called the *cutoff normalized frequency*, which is obtained from the cutoff condition for the $m = 1$ mode,

$$\begin{cases} b = w = 0 & (2.26a) \\ u = v = \dfrac{\pi}{2}, & (2.26b) \end{cases}$$

where Eqs. (2.20) and (2.22) have been used. Generally, the cutoff v-value for the TE mode is given by Eq. (2.21) as

$$v_{c,\mathrm{TE}} = \frac{m\pi}{2} + \frac{1}{2}\tan^{-1}\sqrt{\gamma}, \tag{2.27}$$

and that for the TM mode is given by Eq. (2.38) (explained in Section 2.1.5) as

$$v_{c,\mathrm{TM}} = \frac{m\pi}{2} + \frac{1}{2}\tan^{-1}\left(\frac{n_1^2}{n_0^2}\sqrt{\gamma}\right). \tag{2.28}$$

A qualitative value can be obtained by this graphical solution for the dispersion equation. However, in order to obtain accurate solution of the dispersion equation, we should rely on the numerical method. Here, we show the numerical treatment for the symmetrical slab waveguide so as to compare with the previous graphical method. We first rewrite the dispersion Eq. (2.25) in the following form:

$$f(v, m, b) = v\sqrt{1-b} - \frac{m\pi}{2} - \tan^{-1}\sqrt{\frac{b}{1-b}} = 0. \tag{2.29}$$

Figure 2.4 shows the plot of $f(v, m, b)$ for $v = 4$. The b-value at which $f = 0$ gives the normalized propagation constant b for the given v-value. The solution of Eq. (2.29) is obtained by the Newton–Raphson method or the bisection method or the like. Here, the subroutine program of the most simple bisection method is shown in Fig. 2.5.

The normalized propagation constant b is calculated for each normalized frequency v. Figure 2.6 shows the v–b relationship, which is called *dispersion*

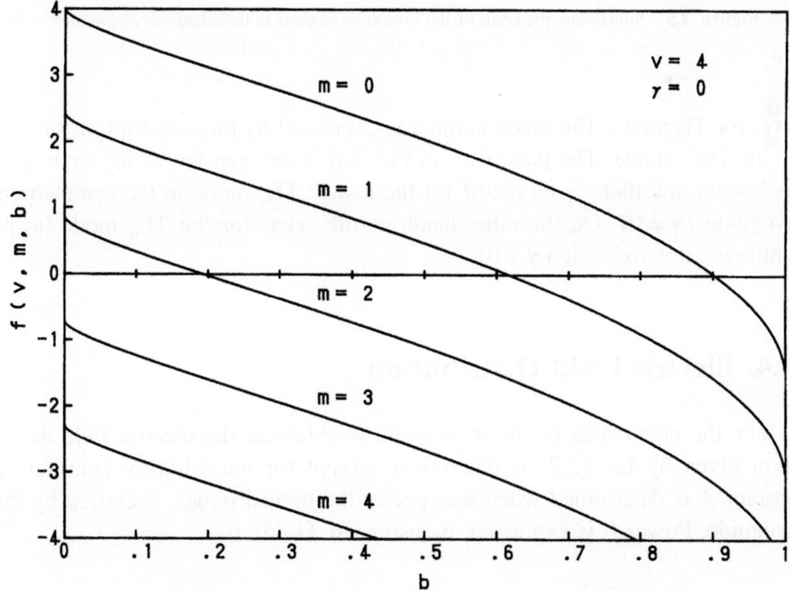

Figure 2.4 Plot of $f(v, m, b)$ for the calculation of the eigenvalue.

```
C      ********************** EIGEN *********************
C      *                                                 *
C      *          Eigen Value of Single Waveguide        *
C      *                                                 *
C      ***************************************************
       SUBROUTINE EIGEN(V,M,B)
C
       IMPLICIT INTEGER(I-N),REAL(A-H,O-Z)
       PAI=3.141592653589793
C
       EPS=1.0E-6
       B0=1.0-EPS
       DIVSN=0.01
       B1=B0
       B2=B1-DIVSN
       F1=V*SQRT(1.0-B1)-FLOAT(M)*PAI/2.0-ATAN(SQRT(B1/(1.0-B1)))
C
    10 F2=V*SQRT(1.0-B2)-FLOAT(M)*PAI/2.0-ATAN(SQRT(B2/(1.0-B2)))
        IF(F1*F2.LE.0.0) GO TO 20
       B1=B2
       B2=B1-DIVSN
       F1=F2
        GO TO 10
    20  IF(DIVSN.LE.EPS) GO TO 30
       B2=(B1+B2)/2.0
       DIVSN=DIVSN/2.0
        GO TO 10
C
    30 B=(B1+B2)/2.0
       RETURN
       END
```

Figure 2.5 Subroutine program of the bisection method to calculate the eigenvalue.

curve, for TE mode. The mode number is expressed by the subscript m, such as TE_m or TM_m mode. The parameter in Fig. 2.6 is the measure of asymmetry γ. It is known that there is no cutoff for the lowest TE_0 mode in the symmetrical waveguide ($\gamma = 0$). On the other hand, cutoff exists for the TE_0 mode in the asymmetrical waveguide ($\gamma \neq 0$).

2.1.4. Electric Field Distribution

Once the eigenvalue of the waveguide is obtained, the electric field distribution given by Eq. (2.7) is determined except for the arbitrary constant A. Constant A is determined when we specify the optical power P carried by the waveguide. Power P is expressed, by using Eq. (1.45) as

$$P = \int_0^1 dy \int_{-\infty}^{\infty} \frac{1}{2}(\mathbf{E} \times \mathbf{H}^*) \cdot \mathrm{u}_z \, dx = \int_{-\infty}^{\infty} \frac{1}{2}(E_x H_y^* - E_y H_x^*) \, dx. \tag{2.30}$$

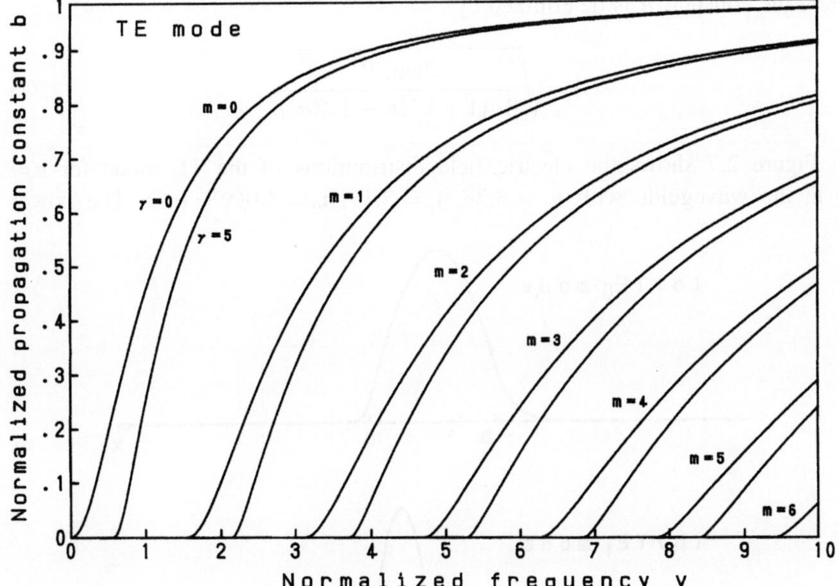

Figure 2.6 Dispersion curves for the TE modes in the slab waveguide.

For the TE mode we can rewrite Eq. (2.30), by using Eqs. (2.5) as

$$P = \frac{\beta}{2\omega\mu_0} \int_{-\infty}^{\infty} |E_y|^2 \, dx. \tag{2.31}$$

Substituting Eq. (2.7) into (2.31) we obtain power fraction in core, substrate, and cladding regions, respectively, as

$$P_{\text{core}} = \frac{\beta a A^2}{2\omega\mu_0} \left\{ 1 + \frac{\sin^2(u+\phi)}{2w} + \frac{\sin^2(u-\phi)}{2w'} \right\} \qquad (-a \leqslant x \leqslant a) \tag{2.32a}$$

$$P_{\text{sub}} = \frac{\beta a A^2}{2\omega\mu_0} \frac{\cos^2(u+\phi)}{2w} \qquad (x \leqslant -a) \tag{2.32b}$$

$$P_{\text{clad}} = \frac{\beta a A^2}{2\omega\mu_0} \frac{\cos^2(u-\phi)}{2w'} \qquad (x > a). \tag{2.32c}$$

For the calculation of Eq. (2.32a) we use Eq. (2.10). The total power P is then given by

$$P = P_{\text{core}} + P_{\text{sub}} + P_{\text{clad}} = \frac{\beta a A^2}{2\omega\mu_0} \left\{ 1 + \frac{1}{2w} + \frac{1}{2w'} \right\}. \tag{2.33}$$

Here the constant A is determined by

$$A = \sqrt{\frac{2\omega\mu_0 P}{\beta a(1 + 1/2w + 1/2w')}}. \tag{2.34}$$

Figure 2.7 shows the electric field distributions of the TE mode for $v = 4$ in the waveguide with $n_1 = 3.38, n_s = 3.17, n_0 = 1.0 (\gamma = 6.6)$. The power

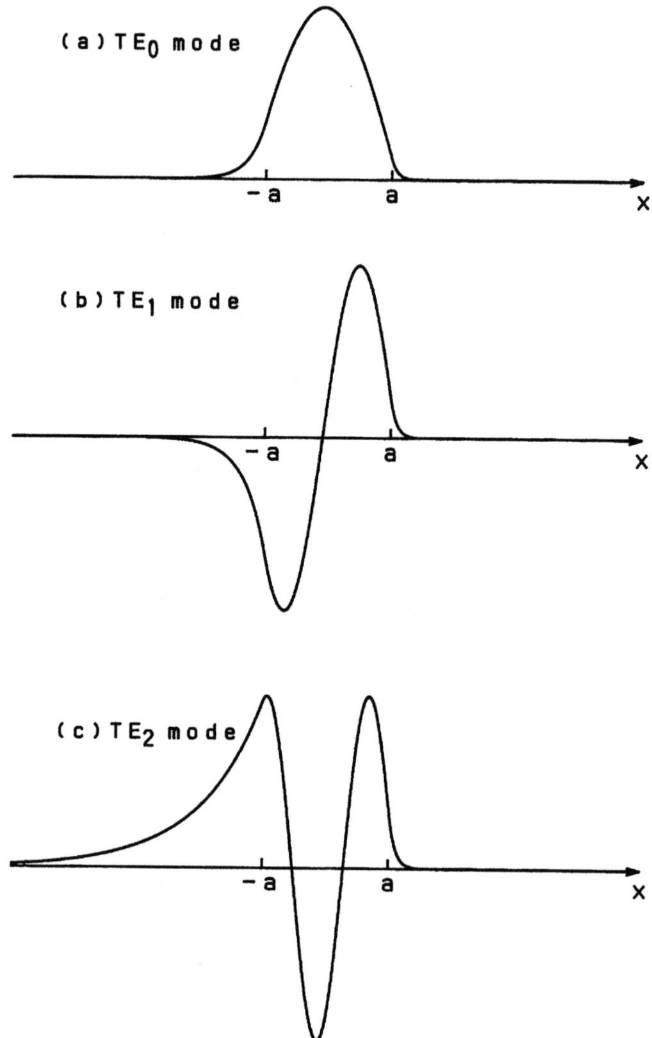

Figure 2.7 Electric field distributions in the slab waveguide.

confinement factor in the core is important to calculate the threshold current density J_{th} of semiconductor lasers [4]. The confinement factor is calculated by using Eqs. (2.32) and (2.33) as

$$\Gamma = \frac{P_{core}}{P} = \frac{1 + \dfrac{\sin^2(u+\phi)}{2w} + \dfrac{\sin^2(u-\phi)}{2w'}}{1 + \dfrac{1}{2w} + \dfrac{1}{2w'}}. \tag{2.35}$$

The power-confinement factor Γ and the ratio to the core width $2a/\Gamma$ for the fundamental mode are shown in Fig. 2.8. The vertical lines in the figure express the single mode core width.

2.1.5. Dispersion Equation for TM Mode

Based on Eq. (2.6), the dispersion equation for the TM mode is obtained in a similar manner to that of the TE mode. We first express the magnetic field

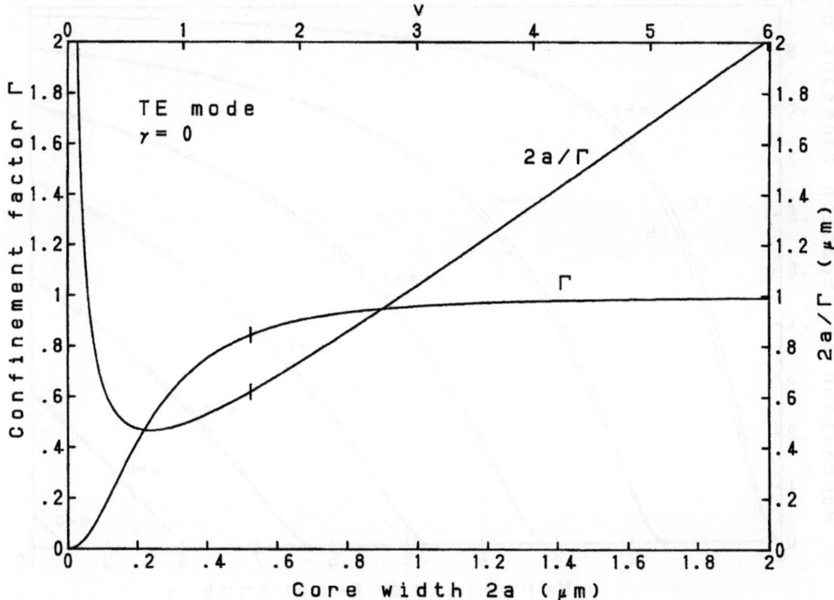

Figure 2.8 Power-confinement factor of the symmetrical slab waveguide.

distribution H_y as

$$H_y = \begin{cases} A\cos(\kappa a - \phi)e^{-\sigma(x-a)} & (x > a) \\ A\cos(\kappa x - \phi) & (-a \leqslant x \leqslant a) \\ A\cos(\kappa a + \phi)e^{\xi(x+a)} & (x < -a). \end{cases} \tag{2.36}$$

Applying the boundary conditions that H_y and E_z should be continuous at $x = \pm a$, the following dispersion equation is obtained:

$$u = \frac{m\pi}{2} + \frac{1}{2}\tan^{-1}\left(\frac{n_1^2 w}{n_s^2 u}\right) + \frac{1}{2}\tan^{-1}\left(\frac{n_1^2 w'}{n_0^2 u}\right). \tag{2.37}$$

Rewriting the above equation by using the normalized frequency v and the normalized propagation constant b, it reduces to

$$2v\sqrt{1-b} = m\pi + \tan^{-1}\left(\frac{n_1^2}{n_s^2}\sqrt{\frac{b}{1-b}}\right) + \tan^{-1}\left(\frac{n_1^2}{n_0^2}\sqrt{\frac{b+\gamma}{1-b}}\right). \tag{2.38}$$

The dispersion curve of the TM modes in the waveguide with $n_1 = 3.38$, $n_s = n_0 = 3.17 (\gamma = 0)$ are shown in Fig. 2.9 and compared with those for the TE

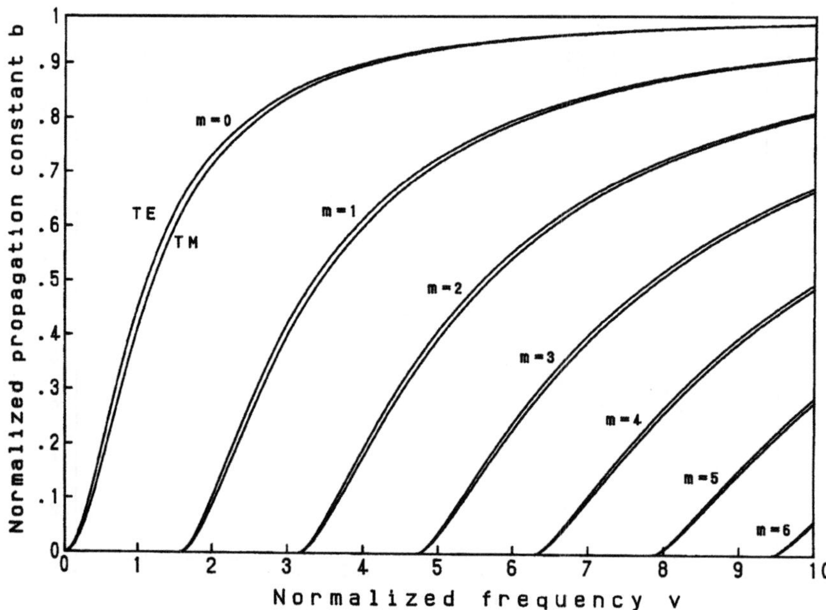

Figure 2.9 Dispersion curves of TE and TM modes in the slab waveguide.

modes. It is known that the normalized propagation constant b for the TM mode is smaller than that for the TE mode with respect to the same v. That means the TE mode is slightly better confined in the core than the TM mode. The power carried by the TM mode is obtained, from Eqs. (2.6) and (2.30) by

$$P = \frac{\beta}{2\omega\varepsilon_0} \int_{-\infty}^{\infty} \frac{1}{n^2} |H_y|^2 \, dx. \tag{2.39}$$

2.2. RECTANGULAR WAVEGUIDES

2.2.1. Basic Equations

In this section the analytical method, which was proposed by Marcatili [5], to deal with the three-dimensional optical waveguide, as shown in Fig. 2.10, is described. The important assumption of this method is that the electromagnetic field in the shaded area in Fig. 2.10 can be neglected since the electromagnetic field of the well-guided mode decays quite rapidly in the cladding region. Then we do not impose the boundary conditions for the electromagnetic field in the shaded area.

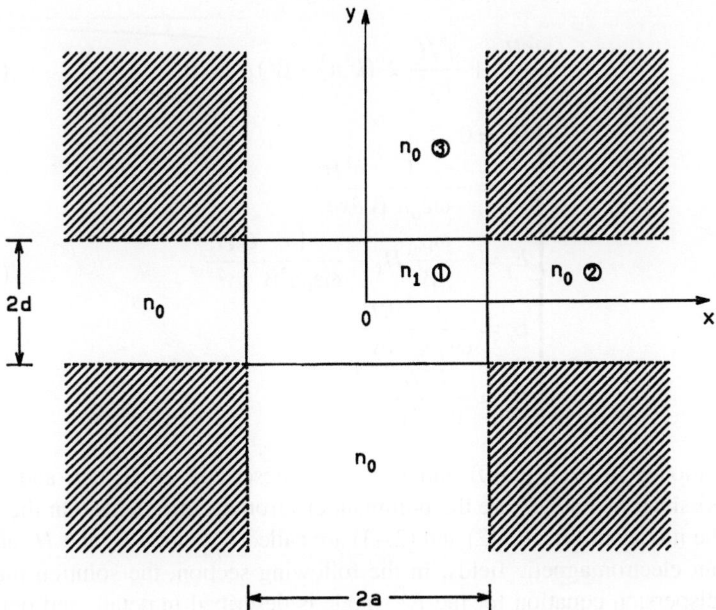

Figure 2.10 Three-dimensional rectangular waveguide.

We first consider the electromagnetic mode in which E_x and H_y are predominant. According to Marcatili's treatment, we set $H_x = 0$ in Eqs. (2.3) and (2.4). Then the wave equation and electromagnetic field representation are obtained as

$$\frac{\partial^2 H_y}{\partial x^2} + \frac{\partial^2 H_y}{\partial y^2} + (k^2 n^2 - \beta^2) H_y = 0, \tag{2.40}$$

$$\begin{cases} H_x = 0 \\ E_x = \dfrac{\omega\mu_0}{\beta} H_y + \dfrac{1}{\omega\varepsilon_0 n^2 \beta} \dfrac{\partial^2 H_y}{\partial x^2} \\ E_y = \dfrac{1}{\omega\varepsilon_0 n^2 \beta} \dfrac{\partial^2 H_y}{\partial x \partial y} \\ E_z = \dfrac{-j}{\omega\varepsilon_0 n^2} \dfrac{\partial H_y}{\partial x} \\ H_z = \dfrac{-j}{\beta} \dfrac{\partial H_y}{\partial y}. \end{cases} \tag{2.41}$$

On the other hand, we set $H_y = 0$ in Eqs. (2.3) and (2.4) to consider the electromagnetic field in which E_y and H_x are predominant. The wave equation and electromagnetic field representation are given by

$$\frac{\partial^2 H_x}{\partial x^2} + \frac{\partial^2 H_x}{\partial y^2} + (k^2 n^2 - \beta^2) H_x = 0, \tag{2.42}$$

$$\begin{cases} H_y = 0 \\ E_x = -\dfrac{1}{\omega\varepsilon_0 n^2 \beta} \dfrac{\partial^2 H_x}{\partial x \partial y} \\ E_y = -\dfrac{\omega\mu_0}{\beta} H_x - \dfrac{1}{\omega\varepsilon_0 n^2 \beta} \dfrac{\partial^2 H_x}{\partial y^2} \\ E_z = \dfrac{j}{\omega\varepsilon_0 n^2} \dfrac{\partial H_x}{\partial y} \\ H_z = \dfrac{-j}{\beta} \dfrac{\partial H_x}{\partial x}. \end{cases} \tag{2.43}$$

The modes in Eqs. (2.40) and (2.41) are described as E^x_{pq} (p and q are integers) since E_x and H_y are the dominant electromagnetic fields. On the other hand, the modes in Eqs. (2.42) and (2.43) are called E^y_{pq} since E_y and H_x are the dominant electromagnetic fields. In the following section, the solution method of the dispersion equation for the E^x_{pq} mode is described in detail, and only the results are shown for the E^y_{pq} mode.

2.2.2. Dispersion Equations for E^x_{pq} and E^y_{pq} Modes

Since the rectangular waveguide shown in Fig. 2.10 is symmetrical with respect to the x- and y-axes, we analyze only regions ①–③. We first express the solution fields, which satisfy the wave equation (2.40), as

$$H_y = \begin{cases} A\cos(k_x x - \phi)\cos(k_y y - \psi) & \text{region ①} \\ A\cos(k_x a - \phi)e^{-\gamma_x(x-a)}\cos(k_y y - \psi) & \text{region ②} \\ A\cos(k_x x - \phi)e^{-\gamma_y(y-d)}\cos(k_y d - \psi) & \text{region ③} \end{cases} \tag{2.44}$$

where the transverse wavenumbers k_x, k_y, γ_x, and γ_y and the optical phases ϕ and ψ are given by

$$\begin{cases} -k_x^2 - k_y^2 + k^2 n_1^2 - \beta^2 = 0 & \text{region ①} \\ \gamma_x^2 - k_y^2 + k^2 n_0^2 - \beta^2 = 0 & \text{region ②} \\ -k_x^2 + \gamma_y^2 + k^2 n_0^2 - \beta^2 = 0 & \text{region ③} \end{cases} \tag{2.45}$$

and

$$\begin{cases} \phi = (p-1)\dfrac{\pi}{2} & (p = 1, 2, \ldots) \\ \psi = (q-1)\dfrac{\pi}{2} & (q = 1, 2, \ldots). \end{cases} \tag{2.46}$$

We should note here that the integers p and q start from 1 because we follow the mode definition by Marcatili. To the contrary the mode number m in Eq. (2.12) for the slab waveguides starts from zero. By the conventional mode definition, the lowest mode in the slab waveguide is the $\mathrm{TE}_{m=0}$ mode (Fig. 2.7(a)) which has one electric field peak. On the other hand, the lowest mode in the rectangular waveguides is $E^x_{p=1,q=1}$ or $E^y_{p=1,q=1}$ mode (Fig. 2.11) which has only one electric field peak along both x- and y-axis directions. Therefore in the mode definition by Marcatili, integers p and q represent the number of local electric field peaks along the x- and y-axis directions.

When we apply the boundary conditions that the electric field $E_z \propto (1/n^2)\partial H_y/\partial x$ should be continuous at $x = a$ and the magnetic field $H_z \propto \partial H_y/\partial y$ should be continuous at $y = d$, we obtain the following dispersion equations:

$$k_x a = (p-1)\frac{\pi}{2} + \tan^{-1}\left(\frac{n_1^2 \gamma_x}{n_0^2 k_x}\right), \tag{2.47a}$$

$$k_y d = (q-1)\frac{\pi}{2} + \tan^{-1}\left(\frac{\gamma_y}{k_y}\right). \tag{2.47b}$$

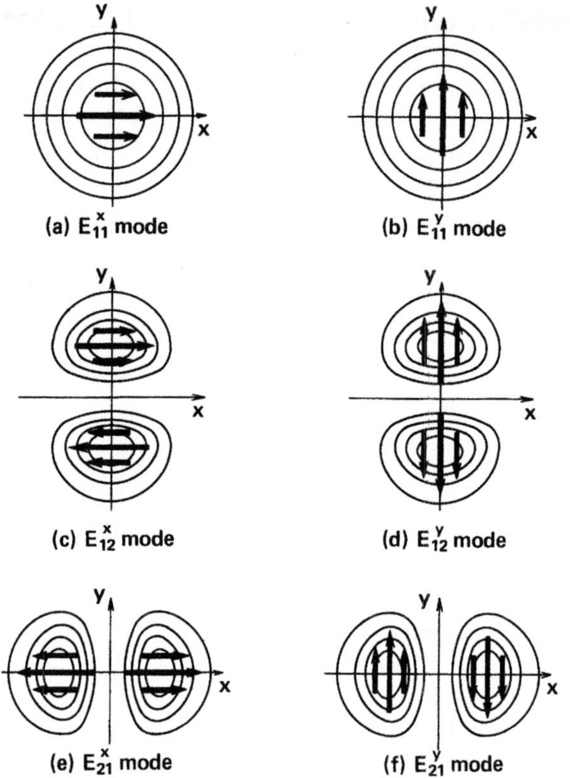

Figure 2.11 Mode definitions and electric field distributions in Marcatili's method.

Transversal wavenumbers k_x, k_y, γ_x, and γ_y are related, by Eq. (2.45) as

$$\gamma_x^2 = k^2(n_1^2 - n_0^2) - k_x^2, \tag{2.48}$$

$$\gamma_y^2 = k^2(n_1^2 - n_0^2) - k_y^2. \tag{2.49}$$

k_x is obtained from Eqs. (2.47a) and (2.48), and k_y is determined from Eqs. (2.47b) and (2.49), respectively. The propagation constant β is then obtained from

$$\beta^2 = k^2 n_1^2 - (k_x^2 + k_y^2). \tag{2.50}$$

In order to calculate the dispersion equation for the E_{pq}^y mode, we express the magnetic field H_x as

$$H_x = \begin{cases} A\cos(k_x x - \phi)\cos(k_y y - \psi) & \text{region ①} \\ A\cos(k_x a - \phi)e^{-\gamma_x(x-a)}\cos(k_y y - \psi) & \text{region ②} \\ A\cos(k_x x - \phi)e^{-\gamma_y(y-d)}\cos(k_y d - \psi) & \text{region ③} \end{cases} \tag{2.51}$$

Applying the boundary conditions that the magnetic field $H_z \propto \partial H_x/\partial x$ should be continuous at $x=a$ and the electric field $E_z \propto (1/n^2)\partial H_x/\partial y$ should be continuous at $y=d$, we obtain the following dispersion equations

$$k_x a = (p-1)\frac{\pi}{2} + \tan^{-1}\left(\frac{\gamma_x}{k_x}\right), \tag{2.52}$$

$$k_y d = (q-1)\frac{\pi}{2} + \tan^{-1}\left(\frac{n_1^2\gamma_y}{n_0^2 k_y}\right). \tag{2.53}$$

2.2.3. Kumar's Method

In Marcatili's method, electromagnetic fields and the boundary conditions in the shaded area in Fig. 2.10 are not strictly satisfied. In other words, the hybrid modes in the rectangular waveguides are approximately analyzed by separating into two independent slab waveguides as shown in Fig. 2.12. It is well understood when we compare the dispersion Eqs. (2.47a) and (2.47b) for the E_{pq}^x mode with the slab dispersion Eqs. (2.12) and (2.37). Equation (2.47a) corresponds to the TM mode dispersion equation of the symmetric slab waveguide [Fig. 2.12(b)], and Eq. (2.47b) corresponds to the TE mode dispersion equation [Fig. 2.12(c)], respectively.

Kumar et al. proposed an improvement of accuracy for the Marcatili's method by taking into account the contribution of the fields in the shaded area in Fig. 2.10 [6]. We call this method this *Kumar's method* and describe an example of it by analyzing the E_{pq}^x mode in rectangular waveguides.

In Kumar's method, the refractive-index distribution of the rectangular waveguide is expressed by

$$n^2(x, y) = N_x^2(x) + N_y^2(y) + O(n_1^2 - n_0^2), \tag{2.54}$$

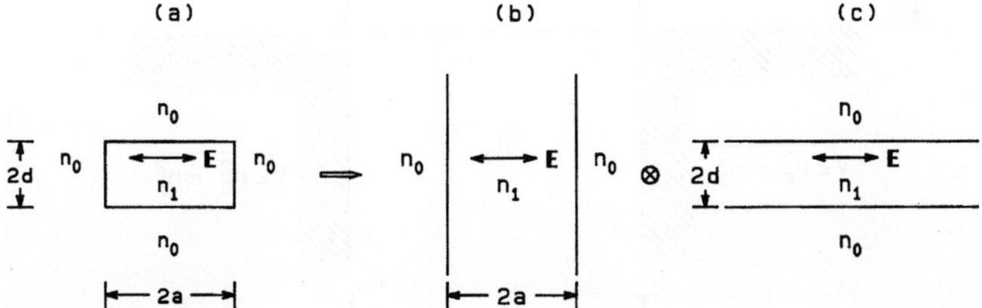

Figure 2.12 Rectangular waveguide and its equivalent, two independent slab waveguides, in Marcatili's method.

where

$$N_x^2(x) = \begin{cases} n_1^2/2 & |x| \leqslant a \\ n_0^2 - n_1^2/2 & |x| > a \end{cases} \tag{2.55a}$$

$$N_y^2(y) = \begin{cases} n_1^2/2 & |y| \leqslant d \\ n_0^2 - n_1^2/2 & |y| > d. \end{cases} \tag{2.55b}$$

The refractive-index distribution that is expressed by Eqs. (2.54) and (2.55) is shown in Fig. 2.13. Generally, the refractive-index difference between core and cladding is quite small ($n_1 \approx n_0$) and then we have $O(n_1^2 - n_0^2) \approx 0$ in Eq. (2.54). Also the refractive index in the shaded area is approximated as

$$\sqrt{2n_0^2 - n_1^2} \approx n_0. \tag{2.56}$$

Therefore it is known that the refractive index expressed by Eqs. (2.54) and (2.55) approximates quite well the actual refractive-index distribution of the rectangular waveguide. Although the approximation is good, there still remains the small difference in the refractive-index expression of Eq. (2.54) for the shaded area

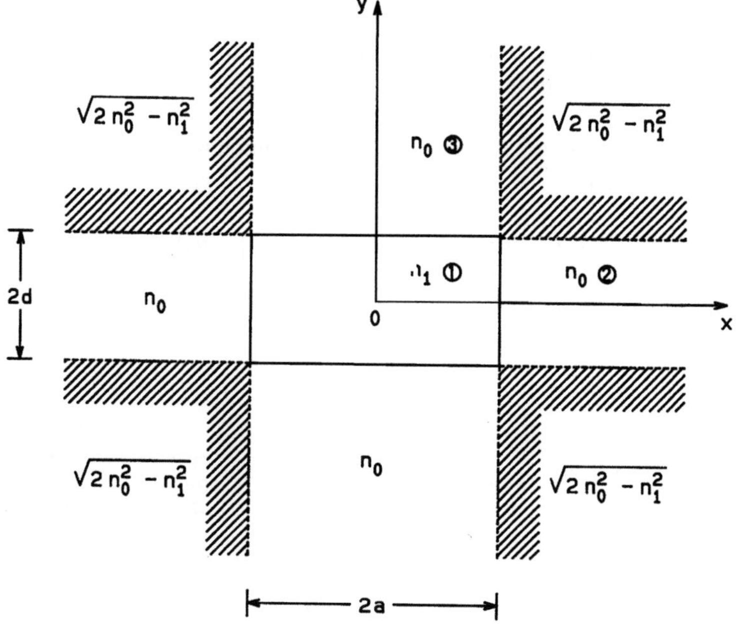

Figure 2.13 Refractive-index profile in Kumar's method.

from the actual value. In the present method, the correction is made by using the perturbation method as shown in the following.

We first express the solution of the wave Eq. (2.40) for the E^x_{pq} mode, by using the separation of variables, as

$$H_y(x, y) = X(x)Y(y). \tag{2.57}$$

Substituting Eqs. (2.54) and (2.57) into (2.40), the wave equation reduces to

$$\frac{d^2X}{dx^2}Y + X\frac{d^2Y}{dy^2} + \left[k^2(N_x^2 + N_y^2) - \beta^2\right]XY = 0, \tag{2.58}$$

where small quantities of the order of $O(n_1^2 - n_0^2)$ have been neglected. Dividing Eq. (2.58) by XY, it can be separated into two terms: one is dependent on variable x and the other is dependent on variable y, respectively, as

$$\frac{1}{X}\frac{d^2X}{dx^2} + k^2N_x^2(x) + \frac{1}{Y}\frac{d^2Y}{dy^2} + k^2N_y^2(x) = \beta^2. \tag{2.59}$$

The necessary conditions for Eq. (2.59) to be satisfied for arbitrary values of x and y are

$$\frac{1}{X}\frac{d^2X}{dx^2} + k^2N_x^2(x) = \beta_x^2, \tag{2.60a}$$

$$\frac{1}{Y}\frac{d^2Y}{dy^2} + k^2N_y^2(y) = \beta_y^2, \tag{2.60b}$$

where β_x and β_y are constants that are independent from x and y. We then have two independent wave equations as

$$\frac{d^2X}{dx^2} + \left[k^2N_x^2(x) - \beta_x^2\right]X(x) = 0, \tag{2.61a}$$

$$\frac{d^2Y}{dy^2} + \left[k^2N_y^2(y) - \beta_y^2\right]Y(y) = 0. \tag{2.61b}$$

From Eqs. (2.59) and (2.60) we can derive an equation to determine the propagation constant:

$$\beta^2 = \beta_x^2 + \beta_y^2. \tag{2.62}$$

The solution fields of Eqs. (2.61a) and (2.61b) are expressed in a similar manner as previously in Section 2.2.2 by

$$X(x) = \begin{cases} A\cos(k_x x - \phi) & (0 \leqslant x \leqslant a) \\ A\cos(k_x a - \phi)e^{-\gamma_x(x-a)} & (x > a) \end{cases} \tag{2.63}$$

$$Y(y) = \begin{cases} B\cos(k_y y - \psi) & (0 \leqslant y \leqslant d) \\ B\cos(k_y d - \psi)e^{-\gamma_y(y-d)} & (y > d), \end{cases} \tag{2.64}$$

where only the first quadrant is considered due to the symmetry of the waveguide, and transverse wavenumbers k_x, γ_x, k_y, and γ_y are related with β_x and β_y by

$$\gamma_x^2 = k^2(n_1^2 - n_0^2) - k_x^2, \tag{2.65a}$$

$$\gamma_y^2 = k^2(n_1^2 - n_0^2) - k_y^2, \tag{2.65b}$$

$$\beta_x^2 = \frac{k^2 n_1^2}{2} - k_x^2, \tag{2.66a}$$

$$\beta_y^2 = \frac{k^2 n_1^2}{2} - k_y^2, \tag{2.66b}$$

and optical phases are expressed by

$$\begin{cases} \phi = (p-1)\dfrac{\pi}{2} & (p = 1, 2, \ldots) \\ \psi = (q-1)\dfrac{\pi}{2} & (1 = 1, 2, \ldots). \end{cases} \tag{2.67}$$

When we apply the boundary conditions that the electric field

$$E_z \propto (1/n^2)\partial H_y/\partial x = (Y/n^2)dX/dx$$

should be continuous at $x = a$ and the magnetic field $H_z \propto \partial H_y/\partial y = XdY/dy$ should be continuous at $y = d$, we obtain the following dispersion equations:

$$k_x a = (p-1)\frac{\pi}{2} + \tan^{-1}\left(\frac{n_1^2\gamma_x}{n_0^2 k_x}\right), \tag{2.68}$$

$$k_y d = (q-1)\frac{\pi}{2} + \tan^{-1}\left(\frac{\gamma_y}{k_y}\right). \tag{2.69}$$

The propagation constant is obtained from Eqs. (2.62) and (2.66a), by

$$\beta^2 = k^2 n_1^2 - (k_x^2 + k_y^2). \tag{2.70}$$

Equation (2.68)–(2.70) for the dispersion and the propagation constant are known to be the same as the Eqs. (2.47a), (2.47b) and (2.50) by the Marcatili's method. But in the present Kumar's method, an improvement of the accuracy of the propagation constant can be obtained by the perturbation method with respect to the shaded area in Fig. 2.13. We rewrite the refractive-index distribution for the rectangular waveguide as

$$n^2(x, y) = N_x^2(x) + N_y^2(y) + \delta \cdot \eta(x, y), \tag{2.71}$$

where δ is a small quantity and $\delta \cdot \eta(x, y)$ denotes the perturbation term which is expressed by

$$\delta \cdot \eta(x, y) = \begin{cases} (n_1^2 - n_0^2) & |x| > a \quad \text{and} \quad |y| > d \\ 0 & |x| \leqslant a \quad \text{or} \quad |y| \leqslant d. \end{cases} \tag{2.72}$$

Generally the wave equation is expressed by

$$\nabla^2 f + (k^2 n^2 - \beta^2) f = 0, \tag{2.73}$$

where $\nabla^2 = \partial^2/\partial x^2 + \partial^2/\partial y^2$. The solution field f and the eigenvalue β^2 of the above equation are expressed in the first-order perturbation form as

$$f = f_0 + \delta \cdot f_1 \tag{2.74}$$

$$\beta^2 = \beta_0^2 + \delta \cdot \beta_1^2. \tag{2.75}$$

Substituting Eqs. (2.74) and (2.75) into (2.73) and comparing the terms for each order of δ, the following equations are obtained:

$$\nabla^2 f_0 + [k^2(N_x^2 + N_y^2) - \beta_0^2] f_0 = 0, \tag{2.76}$$

$$\nabla^2 f_1 + [k^2(N_x^2 + N_y^2) - \beta_0^2] f_1 + k^2 \eta f_0 - \beta_1^2 f_0 = 0. \tag{2.77}$$

Here we consider the integral

$$\iint [\text{Eq. } (2.76)^* \cdot f_1 - \text{Eq. } (2.77) \cdot f_0^*] \, dx \, dy$$

in the region D. Then we have

$$\beta_1^2 \iint_D \left| f_0 \right|^2 dx \, dy = \iint_D [f_0^* \nabla^2 f_1 - f_1 \nabla^2 f_0^*] dx \, dy + k^2 \iint_D \eta |f_0|^2 \, dx \, dy. \tag{2.78}$$

The first term in the right-hand side of the above equation is rewritten, by using Green's theorem (refer to Chapter 10), as

$$\iint_D [f_0^* \nabla^2 f_1 - f_1 \nabla^2 f_0^*] \, dx \, dy = \oint \left[f_0^* \frac{\partial f_1}{\partial n} - f_1 \frac{\partial f_0^*}{\partial n} \right] d\ell, \tag{2.79}$$

where $\partial/\partial n$ represent the differentiation along the outside normal direction on the periphery of the integration region, and $\oint d\ell$ represents the line integral along the periphery. The line integral of Eq. (2.79) becomes zero when region D is enlarged to infinity. Therefore we have

$$\beta_1^2 = \frac{k^2 \int_{-\infty}^{\infty}\int_{-\infty}^{\infty} \eta(x, y)|f_0|^2\,dx\,dy}{\int_{-\infty}^{\infty}\int_{-\infty}^{\infty} |f_0|^2\,dx\,dy}. \tag{2.80}$$

Equation (2.73) corresponds to (2.40) and Eq. (2.76) corresponds to (2.58). Then β_0 is the eigenvalue for the dispersion Eqs. (2.68)–(2.70) and $f_0(x, y)$ is the field distribution given by Eqs. (2.57), (2.63) and (2.64). The eigenvalue which is given by the first-order perturbation is therefore expressed from Eqs. (2.72), (2.75) and (2.80) by

$$\begin{aligned}
\beta^2 &= \beta_0^2 + \frac{k^2 \int_{-\infty}^{\infty}\int_{-\infty}^{\infty} \delta\cdot\eta(x, y)|X(x)Y(y)|^2\,dx\,dy}{\int_{-\infty}^{\infty}\int_{-\infty}^{\infty} |X(x)Y(y)|^2\,dx\,dy} \\
&= (k^2 n_1^2 - k_x^2 - k_y^2) + \frac{k^2(n_1^2 - n_0^2)\int_a^{\infty} |X(x)|^2 dx \int_d^{\infty} |Y(y)|^2\,dy}{\int_0^{\infty} |X(x)|^2\,dx \int_0^{\infty} |Y(y)|^2\,dy} \\
&= (k^2 n_1^2 - k_x^2 - k_y^2) + \frac{k^2(n_1^2 - n_0^2)\cos^2(k_x a - \phi)\cos^2(k_y d - \psi)}{(1+\gamma_x a)(1+\gamma_y d)}.
\end{aligned} \tag{2.81}$$

In the second term of Eq. (2.81), we approximated $n_0^2/n_1^2 \approx 1$. The normalized propagation constant is obtained from Eqs. (2.17), (2.18) and (2.81) as

$$b = 1 - \frac{k_x^2 + k_y^2}{k^2(n_1^2 - n_0^2)} + \frac{\cos^2(k_x a - \phi)\cos^2(k_y d - \psi)}{(1+\gamma_x a)(1+\gamma_y d)}. \tag{2.82}$$

Figure 2.14 shows the dispersion curves for the rectangular waveguides with core aspect ratios $a/d = 1$ and $a/d = 2$, which are calculated by using different analysis methods for the scalar wave equations [6]. Analysis by the point matching method [7] gives the most accurate value among four of the analyses and is used as the standard for the comparison of accuracy. The effective index method will be described in the following section. It is known from Fig. 2.14 that Kumar's method gives the more accurate results than Marcatili's method. The accuracy of the effective index method is almost the same as that of Marcatili's method; but the effective index method gives the larger estimation than the accurate solution, whereas, Marcatili's method gives the lower estimation than the accurate solution, respectively. For practicality, however, the effective index method is a very important method to analyze, for example, ridge waveguides which require a numerical method such as the finite element method.

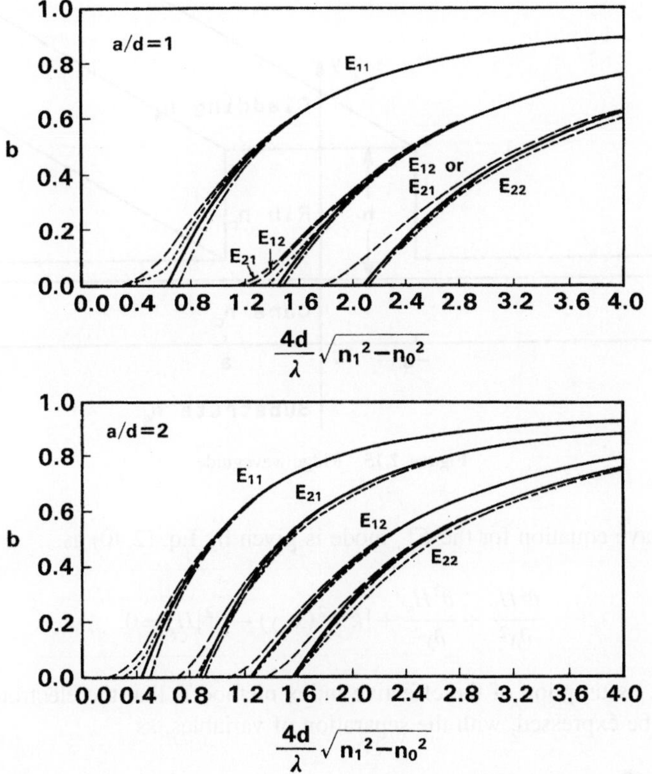

Figure 2.14 Comparison of the dispersion curves calculated with different analytical methods.——Marcatili's method [6];———Kumar's method,. . . . . .point matching method [7];——— effective index method. (After Ref. [6]).

2.2.4. Effective Index Method

The ridge waveguide, such as shown in Fig. 2.15, is difficult to analyze by Marcatili's method or Kumar's method since the waveguide structure is too complicated to deal with by the division of waveguide. In order to analyze ridge waveguides, we should use numerical methods, such as the finite element method and finite difference method. The effective index method [8]–[9] is an analytical method applicable to complicated waveguides such as ridge waveguides and diffused waveguides in $LiNbO_3$. In the following, the effective index method of analysis is described, taking as example the E^x_{pq} mode in the ridge waveguide.

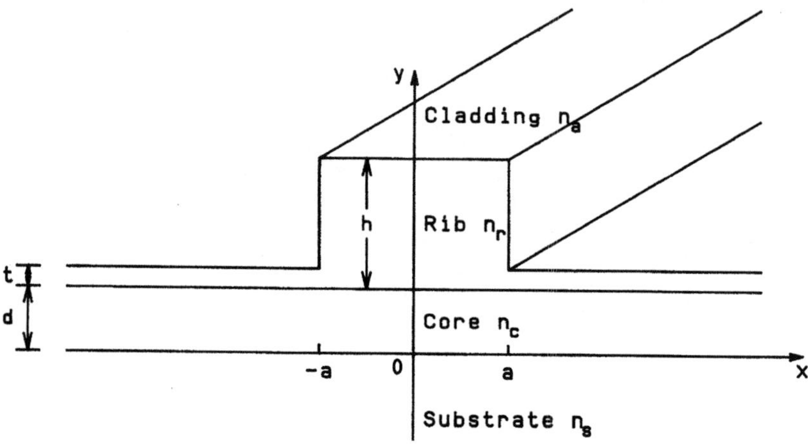

Figure 2.15 Ridge waveguide.

The wave equation for the E^x_{pq} mode is given by Eq. (2.40) as

$$\frac{\partial^2 H_y}{\partial x^2} + \frac{\partial^2 H_y}{\partial y^2} + [k^2 n^2(x, y) - \beta^2]H_y = 0. \tag{2.83}$$

The basic assumption of the effective index method is that the electromagnetic field can be expressed, with the separation of variables, as

$$H_y(x, y) = X(x)Y(y). \tag{2.84}$$

Therefore if the assumption of separation of variables are not accurate, due to the waveguide structure or the wavelength of light, the accuracy of the method itself becomes very poor. Substituting Eq. (2.84) into Eq. (2.83) and dividing it by XY, we obtain

$$\frac{1}{X}\frac{d^2 X}{dx^2} + \frac{1}{Y}\frac{d^2 Y}{dy^2} + [k^2 n^2(x, y) - \beta^2] = 0. \tag{2.85}$$

Here we add to, and subtract from, Eq. (2.85) the y-independent value of $k^2 n^2_{\text{eff}}(x)$ and separate the equation into two independent equations:

$$\frac{1}{Y}\frac{d^2 Y}{dy^2} + [k^2 n^2(x, y) - k^2 n^2_{\text{eff}}(x)] = 0, \tag{2.86a}$$

$$\frac{1}{X}\frac{d^2 X}{dx^2} + [k^2 n^2_{\text{eff}}(x) - \beta^2] = 0. \tag{2.86b}$$

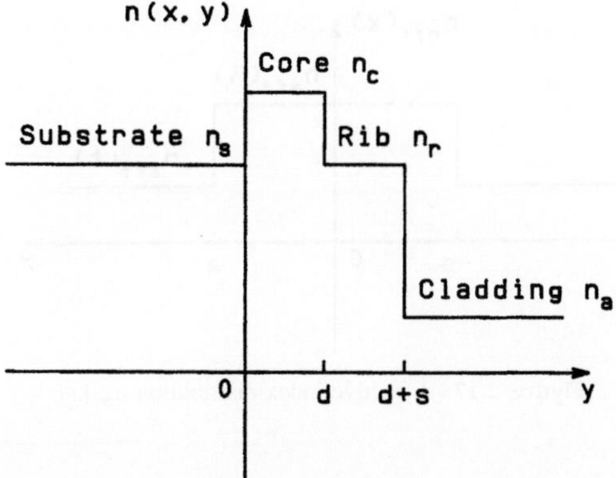

Figure 2.16 Variation of the actual refractive-index profile $n(x, y)$.

$n_{\text{eff}}(x)$ is called the *effective index distribution.* We first solve Eq. (2.86) and determine the effective index distribution $n_{\text{eff}}(x)$. The variation of the actual refractive-index profile $n(x, y)$ is depicted in Fig. 2.16 where $n_r = n_s$ and s is the height of the rib, which takes the following values, depending on the position x:

$$s = \begin{cases} h & 0 \leqslant |x| \leqslant a \\ t & |x| > a. \end{cases} \tag{2.87}$$

From the boundary condition that $H_z \propto \partial H_y/\partial y$ should be continuous at $y = 0$, d and $d + s$, we have the continuity condition for dY/dy at the foregoing boundaries. The dispersion equations for the four-layer slab waveguide shown in Fig. 2.16 is given by

$$\sin(\kappa d - 2\phi) = \sin(\kappa d) e^{-2(\sigma s + \psi)}, \tag{2.88}$$

where the parameters are

$$\phi = \tan^{-1}\left(\frac{\sigma}{\kappa}\right), \tag{2.89a}$$

$$\psi = \tanh^{-1}\left(\frac{\sigma}{\gamma}\right), \tag{2.89b}$$

$$\kappa = k\sqrt{n_c^2 - n_{\text{eff}}^2}, \tag{2.89c}$$

$$\sigma = k\sqrt{n_{\text{eff}}^2 - n_s^2}, \tag{2.89d}$$

$$\gamma = k\sqrt{n_{\text{eff}}^2 - n_a^2}. \tag{2.89e}$$

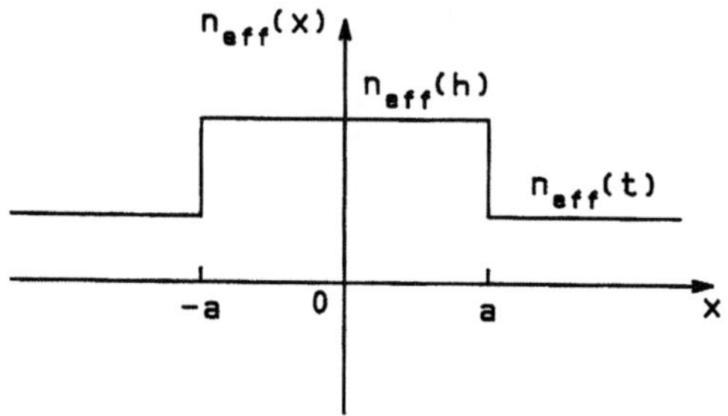

Figure 2.17 Effective index distribution $n_{\text{eff}}(x)$.

The solution of Eq. (2.88) with $s = h(0 \leqslant |x| \leqslant a)$ gives the effective index $n_{\text{eff}}(h)$ for $0 \leqslant |x| \leqslant a$, and the solution of Eq. (2.88) with $s = t(|x| > a)$ gives the effective index $n_{\text{eff}}(t)$ for $|x| > a$, respectively. Then the effective index distribution $n_{\text{eff}}(x)$ is obtained see Fig. 2.17. The solution of the wave equation (2.86b) is calculated by solving the three-layer symmetrical slab waveguide. The boundary condition is that $E_z \propto (1/n^2)\partial H_y/\partial x$ should be continuous at $x = \pm a$. Therefore $(1/n^2)X$ should be continuous at $x = \pm a$. Under the above boundary condition, the dispersion equation is obtained as

$$u \tan(u) = \frac{n_{\text{eff}}^2(h)}{n_{\text{eff}}^2(t)} w, \tag{2.90}$$

where

$$u = ka\sqrt{n_{\text{eff}}^2(h) - \left(\frac{\beta}{k}\right)^2}, \tag{2.91a}$$

$$w = ka\sqrt{\left(\frac{\beta}{k}\right)^2 - n_{\text{eff}}^2(t)}. \tag{2.91b}$$

The dispersion equations for the E_{pq}^y mode are obtained in the similar manner:

$$\sin(\kappa d - 2\phi) = \sin(\kappa d)e^{-2(\sigma s + \psi)}, \tag{2.92}$$

$$u \tan(u) = w, \tag{2.93}$$

where

$$\phi = \tan^{-1}\left(\frac{\sigma n_c^2}{\kappa n_s^2}\right), \tag{2.94a}$$

$$\psi = \tanh^{-1}\left(\frac{\sigma n_a^2}{\gamma n_s^2}\right). \tag{2.94b}$$

2.3. RADIATION FIELD FROM WAVEGUIDE

The radiation field from an optical waveguide into free space propagates divergently. The radiation field is different from the field in the waveguide. Therefore it is important to know the profile of the radiation field for efficiently coupling the light between two waveguides or between a waveguide and an optical fiber. In this section, we describe the derivation of the radiation field pattern from the rectangular waveguide.

2.3.1. Fresnel and Fraunhofer Regions

We consider the coordinate system shown in Fig. 2.18, where the endface of the waveguide is located at $z = 0$ and the electromagnetic field is radiated into the free space with refractive index n. The electric field at the endface of the waveguide is denoted by $g(x_0, y_0, 0)$ and the electric field distribution on the observation plane at distance z is expressed as $f(x, y, z)$. By the Fresnel–Kirchhoff diffraction formula [10] (see Chapter 10), the radiation pattern $f(x, y, z)$ is related to the endface field $g(x_0, y_0, 0)$ as

$$f(x, y, z) = \frac{jkn}{2\pi} \int_{-\infty}^{\infty} \int_{-\infty}^{\infty} g(x_0, y_0, 0) \frac{1}{r} e^{-jknr} \, dx_0 \, dy_0, \qquad (2.95)$$

where k is the free-space wavenumber $k = 2\pi/\lambda$ and the distance r between Q and P is given by

$$r = \left[(x - x_0)^2 + (y - y_0)^2 + z^2 \right]^{1/2}. \qquad (2.96)$$

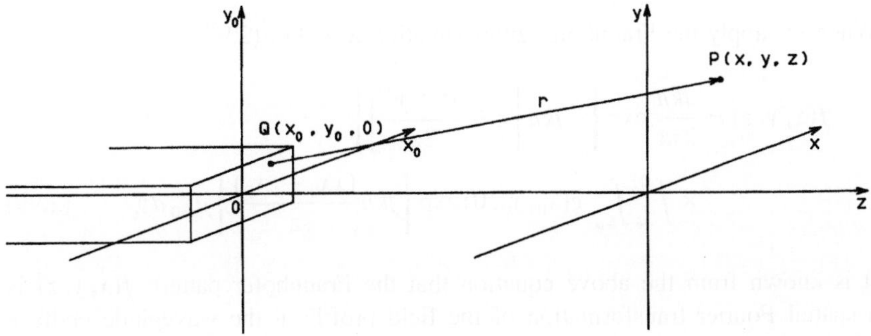

Figure 2.18 Coordinate system for the waveguide endface ($z = 0$) and obsevation plane ($z = z$).

When the distance of the observation plane z is very large compared with $|x-x_0|$ and $|y-y_0|$, Eq. (2.96) is approximated by

$$r = z\left[1+\frac{(x-x_0)^2+(y-y_0)^2}{z^2}\right]^{1/2} = z+\frac{(x-x_0)^2+(y-y_0)^2}{2z}+\cdots$$
$$= z+\frac{x^2+y^2}{2z}-\frac{xx_0+yy_0}{z}+\frac{{x_0}^2+{y_0}^2}{2z}+\cdots. \tag{2.97}$$

The number of expansion terms to approximate r accurately depends on the distance z between the endface of the waveguide and the observation plane. Generally, the electromagnetic field in the waveguide is confined in a small area of the order of 10 μm. Therefore if z is larger than, for example, 1 mm, any term higher than the fourth term in the right-hand side of Eq. (2.97) can be neglected. The radiation field where this condition is satisfied is called the far-field region or Fraunhofer region. On the other hand, when z is not so large, we should take into account up to the fourth term in Eq. (2.97). The radiation field in which this condition holds is called the near-field region or Fresnel region. However, we should note that even the Fresnel approximation is not satisfied in the region close to the waveguide endface. The fourth term in the extreme right of Eq. (2.97) determines which approximation we should adopt. Generally the contribution to knr by the fourth term, $kn(x_0^2+y_0^2)/2z$ determines whether the Fresnel or Fraunhofer approximation should be used. The measure for the judgment is $kn({x_0}^2+{y_0}^2)/2z=\pi/2$. If, for example, the optical field is confined in the rectangular region with square core area D^2, then $kn({x_0}^2+{y_0}^2)/2z=\pi/2$ at $z=nD^2/\lambda$ and we have the criteria:

$$\begin{cases} z > n\dfrac{D^2}{\lambda} & \text{Fraunhofer region} \\ z < n\dfrac{D^2}{\lambda} & \text{Fresnel region.} \end{cases} \tag{2.98}$$

When we apply the Fraunhofer approximation to r, Eq. (2.95) reduces to

$$f(x,y,z) = \frac{jkn}{2\pi z}\exp\left\{-jkn\left[z+\frac{x^2+y^2}{2z}\right]\right\}$$
$$\times\int_{-\infty}^{\infty}\int_{-\infty}^{\infty} g(x_0,y_0,0)\exp\left\{jkn\frac{(xx_0+yy_0)}{z}\right\}dx_0\,dy_0. \tag{2.99}$$

It is known from the above equation that the Fraunhofer pattern $f(x,y,z)$ is a spatial Fourier transformation of the field profile at the waveguide endface $g(x_0,y_0,0)$.

2.3.2. Radiation Pattern of Gaussian Beam

It has been described that the radiation pattern from the waveguide is expressed by Eq. (2.95) or (2.99). The accurate electromagnetic field distribution in the rectangular waveguide $g(x_0, y_0, 0)$ is determined numerically by, for example, the finite element method, as described in Chapter 6. An analytical method such as Marcatili's method does not give the accurate field distribution, especially for the cladding region. Even though the accuracy of the eigenvalue is improved by Kumar's method, the field distribution is not accurate since Eq. (2.77) is difficult to solve to obtain the perturbation field f_1. Therefore it is not easy to calculate the radiation pattern from the rectangular waveguide analytically. Here we approximate the electric field distribution in the rectangular waveguide by a Gaussian profile to obtain the radiation pattern analytically. The Gaussian electric field profile in the waveguide is expressed by

$$g(x_0, y_0, 0) = A \exp\left\{-\left[\frac{x_0^2}{w_1^2} + \frac{y_0^2}{w_2^2}\right]\right\}, \tag{2.100}$$

where w_1 and w_2 are the spot size of the field (the position at which electric field $|g|$ becomes $1/e$ to the peak value) along the x_0- and y_0-axis directions, respectively, and A is a constant. Substituting Eq. (2.97) and (2.100) into (2.95) we obtain

$$\begin{aligned} f(x, y, z) &= \frac{jkn}{2\pi z}\int_{-\infty}^{\infty}\int_{-\infty}^{\infty} g(x_0, y_0, 0) \\ &\quad \times \exp\left\{-jkn\left[z + \frac{(x-x_0)^2 + (y-y_0)^2}{2z}\right]\right\} dx_0\, dy_0 \\ &= \frac{jkn}{2\pi z} A e^{-jknz}\int_{-\infty}^{\infty} \exp\left\{-\frac{x_0^2}{w_1^2} - j\frac{kn}{2n}(x-x_0)^2\right\} dx_0 \\ &\quad \times \int_{-\infty}^{\infty} \exp\left\{-\frac{y_0^2}{w_2^2} - j\frac{kn}{2z}(y-y_0)^2\right\} dy_0, \end{aligned} \tag{2.101}$$

where the Fresnel approximation to r has been used. Since the integral in Eq. (2.101) for x_0 and y_0 has the same form, detailed calculation only for x_0 will be described. When we define the parameter p as

$$p = \frac{1}{w_1^2} + j\frac{\pi n}{\lambda z}, \tag{2.102}$$

the integral with respect to x_0 in Eq. (2.101) becomes

$$\int_{-\infty}^{\infty} \exp\left\{-\frac{x_0^2}{w_1^2} - j\frac{kn}{2z}(x-x_0)^2\right\} dx_0$$

$$= \exp\left\{-j\frac{\pi n}{\lambda z}x^2 - \frac{\pi^2 n^2 x^2}{p\lambda^2 z^2}\right\} \int_{-\infty}^{\infty} \exp\left\{-p\left(x_0 - j\frac{\pi n x}{p\lambda z}\right)^2\right\} dx_0$$

$$= \sqrt{\frac{\pi}{p}} \exp\left\{-j\frac{\pi n}{\lambda z}x^2 - \frac{\pi^2 n^2 x^2}{p\lambda^2 z^2}\right\}$$

$$= \sqrt{\frac{\pi}{p}} \exp\left\{-j\frac{\pi n x^2}{\lambda}\frac{\left(z - j\dfrac{\pi n w_1^2}{\lambda}\right)}{\left(z^2 + \dfrac{\pi^2 n^2 w_1^4}{\lambda^2}\right)}\right\}. \tag{2.103}$$

We further introduce new variables, whose physical meanings are explained later, as

$$W_1(z) = w_1\sqrt{1 + \left(\frac{\lambda z}{\pi n w_1^2}\right)^2}, \tag{2.104a}$$

$$R_1(z) = z\left[1 + \left(\frac{\pi n w_1^2}{\lambda z}\right)^2\right], \tag{2.104b}$$

$$\Theta_1(z) = \tan^{-1}\left(\frac{\lambda z}{\pi n w_1^2}\right). \tag{2.104c}$$

Parameter p of Eq. (2.102) can be rewritten by using (2.104) as

$$p = j\frac{\pi n W_1(z)}{\lambda z w_1} e^{-j\Theta_1}. \tag{2.105}$$

Substituting Eq. (2.105) into (2.103), Eq. (2.103) is finally expressed as

$$\int_{\infty}^{\infty} \exp\left\{-\frac{x_0^2}{w_1^2} - j\frac{kn}{2z}(x-x_0)^2\right\} dx_0$$

$$= \sqrt{\frac{\lambda w_1 z}{jnW_1(z)}} \exp\left\{-\left[\frac{1}{W_1^2(z)} + \frac{jkn}{2R_1(z)}\right]x^2 + j\frac{\Theta_1(z)}{2}\right\}. \tag{2.106}$$

Similarly, the integral with respect y_0 in Eq. (2.101) is given by

$$\int_{-\infty}^{\infty} \exp\left\{-\frac{y_0^2}{w_2^2} - j\frac{kn}{2z}(y-y_0)^2\right\} dy_0$$

$$= \sqrt{\frac{\lambda w_2 z}{jnW_2(z)}} \exp\left\{-\left[\frac{1}{W_2^2(z)} + \frac{jkn}{2R_2(z)}\right]y^2 + j\frac{\Theta_2(z)}{2}\right\}, \tag{2.107}$$

where the parameters W_2, R_2 and Θ_2 are defined by

$$W_2(z) = w_2\sqrt{1+\left(\frac{\lambda z}{\pi n w_2^2}\right)^2}, \tag{2.108a}$$

$$R_2(z) = z\left[1+\left(\frac{\pi n w_2^2}{\lambda z}\right)^2\right], \tag{2.108b}$$

$$\Theta_2(z) = \tan^{-1}\left(\frac{\lambda z}{\pi n w_2^2}\right). \tag{2.108c}$$

Substituting Eqs. (2.106) and (2.107) into (2.101), the radiation pattern from the rectangular waveguide $f(x, y, z)$ is expressed by

$$f(x, y, z) = \sqrt{\frac{w_1 w_2}{W_1 W_2}}A\exp\left\{-\left[\frac{x^2}{W_1^2}+\frac{y^2}{W_2^2}\right]\right.$$
$$\left.-jkn\left[\frac{x^2}{2R_1}+\frac{y^2}{2R_2}+z\right]+j\frac{(\Theta_1+\Theta_2)}{2}\right\}. \tag{2.109}$$

It is known from the above equation that $W_1(z)$ and $W_2(z)$ represent the spot sizes of the radiation field, and $R_1(z)$ and $R_2(z)$ represent the radii of curvature of the wavefronts, respectively. If the observation point P is sufficiently far from the endface of the waveguide, and the following conditions $z \gg \pi n w_1^2/\lambda$ and $\pi n w_2^2/\lambda$ are satisfied in the Fraunhofer region, Eqs. (2.104) and (2.108) are approximated as

$$\begin{cases} W_1(z) \cong \dfrac{\lambda z}{\pi n w_1} \\ W_2(z) \cong \dfrac{\lambda z}{\pi n w_2} \\ R_1(z) \cong R_2(z) \cong z. \end{cases} \tag{2.110}$$

In this Fraunhofer region, the divergence angles θ_1 (Fig. 2.19) and θ_2 of the radiation field along the x- and y-axis directions are expressed by

$$\theta_1 = \tan^{-1}\left(\frac{W_1(z)}{z}\right) = \tan^{-1}\left(\frac{\lambda}{\pi n w_1}\right), \tag{2.111a}$$

$$\theta_2 = \tan^{-1}\left(\frac{W_2(z)}{z}\right) = \tan^{-1}\left(\frac{\lambda}{\pi n w_2}\right). \tag{2.111b}$$

Let us calculate the divergence angles of the radiation field from a semiconductor laser diode operating at $\lambda = 1.55\ \mu\text{m}$ and having the active-layer (core) refractive

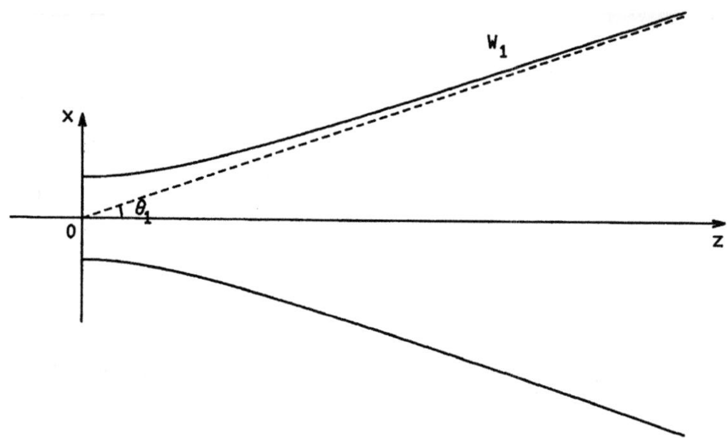

Figure 2.19 Variation of the spot size along x-axis direction, $W_1(z)$.

index $n_1 = 3.5$, cladding index $n_0 = 3.17$, and core width and thickness of $2a = 1.5\,\mu\text{m}$ and $2d = 0.15\,\mu\text{m}$, respectively. The electric field distribution of the waveguide is calculated by using the finite element method waveguide analysis, which will be described in Chapter 6, and is Gaussian fitted to obtain the spot sizes w_1 and w_2 along x- and y-axis directions. Gaussian-fitted spot sizes w_1 and w_2 are

$$\begin{cases} w_1 = 0.88\,\mu\text{m} \\ w_2 = 0.35\,\mu\text{m}. \end{cases} \tag{2.112}$$

The divergence angles θ_1 and θ_2 are then obtained, by Eqs. (2.111b) and (2.112) as

$$\begin{cases} \theta_1 = 0.51 \text{ (rad.)} = 29.4 \text{ (degree)} \\ \theta_2 = 0.95 \text{ (rad.)} = 54.4 \text{ (degree)}. \end{cases} \tag{2.113}$$

It is known from the above result that the radiation field from the semiconductor laser diode has an elliptic shape and the divergence angle along the thin active-layer (y-axis direction) is much larger than that along the wide active-layer direction (x-axis direction).

2.4. MULTIMODE INTERFERENCE (MMI) DEVICE

Multimode interference devices, based on self-imaging effect [11,12], are very important integrated optical components which can perform many different splitting and combining functions [13–16]. Figure 2.20 shows a schematic

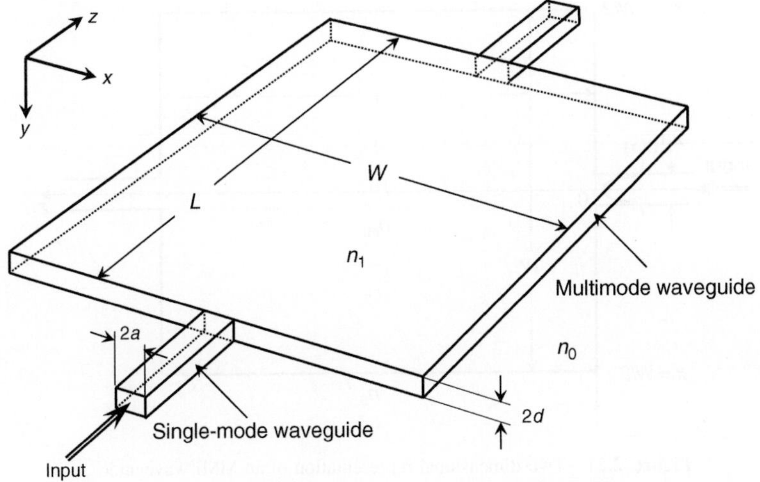

Figure 2.20 Schematic configuration of multimode interference (MMI) waveguide.

configuration of MMI waveguide. The key structure of an MMI device is a waveguide designed to support a large number of modes. The width, thickness and length of the multimode region are W, $2d$ and L, respectively. Single-mode waveguide with core width $2a$ and thickness $2d$ is connected to the multimode waveguide. Refractive indices of the core of single-mode and multimode waveguides are equal to n_1 and the refractive index of the cladding is n_0. Three-dimensional waveguide structure can be reduced to a two-dimensional problem by using an effective index method. The effective index n_{eff} of the core is calculated by solving the eigen-mode equation along y-axis. Figure 2.21 shows two-dimensional configuration of an MMI waveguide of core effective index n_{eff} and cladding refractive index n_0. Electric field in the multimode waveguide is calculated by using Eqs. (2.7)–(2.15). Here waveguide parameters n_1, a and n_s in Eqs. (2.7)–(2.15) are replaced by n_{eff}, $W/2$ and n_0, respectively. Then electric field profile for TE$_m$ mode in the multimode waveguide is expressed by

$$E_y^m(x, y) = \begin{cases} A_m \cos\left(u_m + \dfrac{m\pi}{2}\right) \exp\left[\dfrac{2w_m}{W}\left(x + \dfrac{W}{2}\right) - j\beta_m z\right] & \left(x < -\dfrac{W}{2}\right) \\ A_m \cos\left(\dfrac{2u_m}{W}x - \dfrac{m\pi}{2}\right) \exp(-j\beta_m z) & \left(|x| \leqslant \dfrac{W}{2}\right) \\ A_m \cos\left(u_m - \dfrac{m\pi}{2}\right) \exp\left[-\dfrac{2w_m}{W}\left(x - \dfrac{W}{2}\right) - j\beta_m z\right] & \left(x > \dfrac{W}{2}\right), \end{cases} \tag{2.114}$$

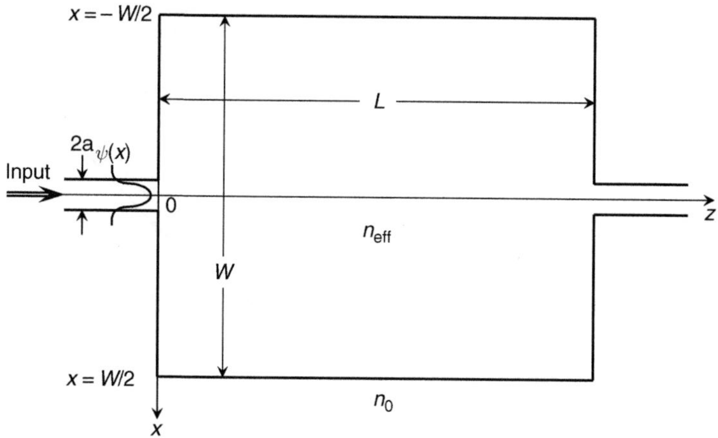

Figure 2.21 Two-dimensional representation of an MMI waveguide.

where u_m and w_m denote the transverse wavenumbers of the m-th mode in the core and cladding and A_m is constant. Transverse wavenumbers are obtained from the eigenvalue equation as

$$w_m = u_m \tan\left(u_m - \frac{m\pi}{2}\right) \tag{2.115}$$

and

$$u_m^2 + w_m^2 = k^2\left(\frac{W}{2}\right)^2 (n_{\text{eff}}^2 - n_0^2) \equiv v^2. \tag{2.116}$$

When the core width W of MMI region is large, the normalized frequency v also becomes large. It is known from Fig. 2.3 that when v becomes large, u_m approaches $u_m \cong (m+1)\,\pi/2$. Then the propagation constant β_m is approximately expressed as

$$\beta_m = \sqrt{k^2 n_{\text{eff}}^2 - (2u_m/W)^2} \cong k n_{\text{eff}} - \frac{(m+1)^2\lambda}{4 n_{\text{eff}} W^2}\pi. \tag{2.117}$$

The total electric field in the MMI region is obtained by

$$\Psi(x, z) = \sum_{m=0}^{M} E_y^m(x, z) = e^{-jkn_{\text{eff}} z} \sum_{m=0}^{M} A_m \cos\left[\frac{(m+1)\pi}{W}x - \frac{m\pi}{2}\right] \times \exp\left[j\frac{(m+1)^2\pi\lambda}{4 n_{\text{eff}} W^2} z\right], \tag{2.118}$$

where M denotes the maximum mode number. At $z=0$, $\Psi(x,0)$ coincides with the electric field of the input waveguide $\psi(x)$. Then the electric field amplitude A_m is obtained from Eq. (2.118) as

$$A_m = \frac{2}{W}\int_{-W/2}^{W/2} \psi(x)\cos\left[\frac{(m+1)\pi}{W}x - \frac{m\pi}{2}\right]dx. \tag{2.119}$$

For simplicity, we consider the case in which the input single-mode waveguide is connected to the center of the multimode waveguide. In this condition, modes in MMI region become only symmetrical modes; that is, m becomes an even number $m=2\ell$ (ℓ : integer). At the point $z=n_{\text{eff}}W^2/\lambda$, the phase term in Eq. (2.118) reduces to

$$\exp\left[j\frac{(m+1)^2\pi\lambda}{4n_{\text{eff}}W^2}z\right] = \exp\left[j\ell(\ell+1)\pi + j\frac{\pi}{4}\right] = \exp\left(j\frac{\pi}{4}\right). \tag{2.120}$$

We now define the characteristic length L_{MMI} as

$$L_{\text{MMI}} = \frac{n_{\text{eff}}W^2}{\lambda}. \tag{2.121}$$

The electric field profile at the MMI length L_{MMI} is then obtained from Eq. (2.118) as

$$\Psi(x, L_{\text{MMI}}) = e^{-jkn_{\text{eff}}\,L_{\text{MMI}}+j\pi/4}\sum_{m=0}^{M} A_m \cos\left[\frac{(m+1)\pi}{W}x - \frac{m\pi}{2}\right]. \tag{2.122}$$

Since $\Psi(x,0)$ in Eq. (2.118) is the electric field of the input waveguide $\psi(x)$, the above equation is rewritten as

$$\Psi(x, L_{\text{MMI}}) = \psi(x)e^{-jkn_{\text{eff}}\,L_{\text{MMI}+j\pi/4}}. \tag{2.123}$$

It is confirmed that the input electric field $\psi(x)$ is reproduced at the specific length L_{MMI} with slight phase retardation. Self-imaging characteristics in MMI waveguide are confirmed by the Beam Propagation Method (BPM) simulation. Figure 2.22 shows the image formation for light input at the center of MMI waveguide. Refractive-index difference of the waveguide is $\Delta = 0.75\%$ and the wavelength of light is $\lambda = 1.55\,\mu\text{m}$. Waveguide parameters of the single-mode input waveguide are $2a = 7\,\mu\text{m}$ and $2d = 6\,\mu\text{m}$ and those of MMI are $W = 150\,\mu\text{m}$ and $L = 25.99$ mm. Specific length L_{MMI} that is given by Eq. (2.121) is 25.89 mm. Since there is a Goos-Hanshen effect, light field slightly penetrates into cladding region. Therefore, slight correction is necessary for either width W or length L of the MMI region. In Fig. 2.22, correction length of $\delta_{\text{L}} = 100\,\mu\text{m}$ is

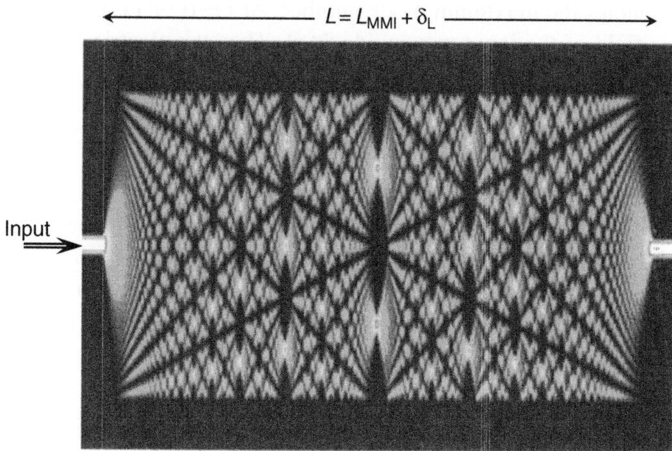

Figure 2.22 Image formation for light input at the center of MMI waveguide.

added to the analytical self-imaging length L_{MMI}. It is known from Fig. 2.22 that N images are formed at $z = L_{MMI}/N$, for any integer N. Figure 2.23 shows light-splitting characteristics of MMI waveguide with a length of $L_{MMI}/8 + \delta'_L$, where $\delta'_L = 105\,\mu$m. Output waveguides are located at $x_i = (4.5 - i)\,W/8$ for i-th ($i = 1, 2, \ldots, 8$) waveguide. Figure 2.24 shows theoretical and experimental splitting characteristics of 1×8 MMI splitter at $\lambda = 1.55\,\mu$m. MMI splitter is made of silica waveguide with $2a = 7\,\mu$m, $2d = 6\,\mu$m and $\Delta = 0.75\%$. Splitting

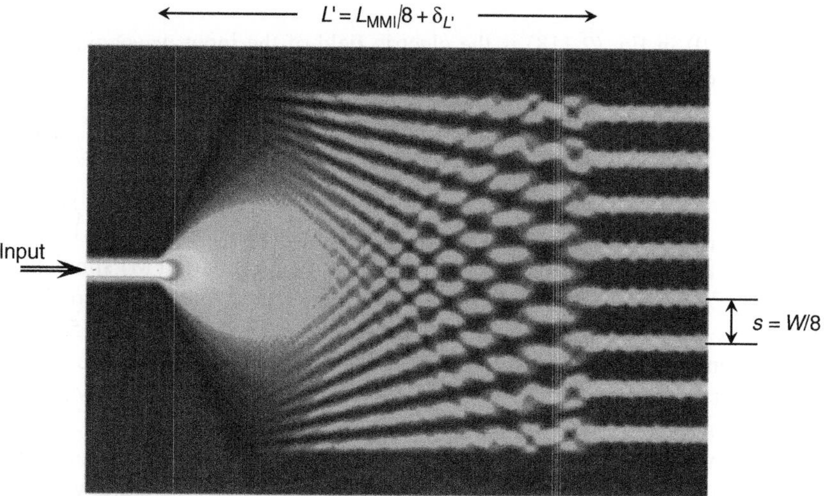

Figure 2.23 Light-splitting characteristics of MMI waveguide with a length of LMMI/8.

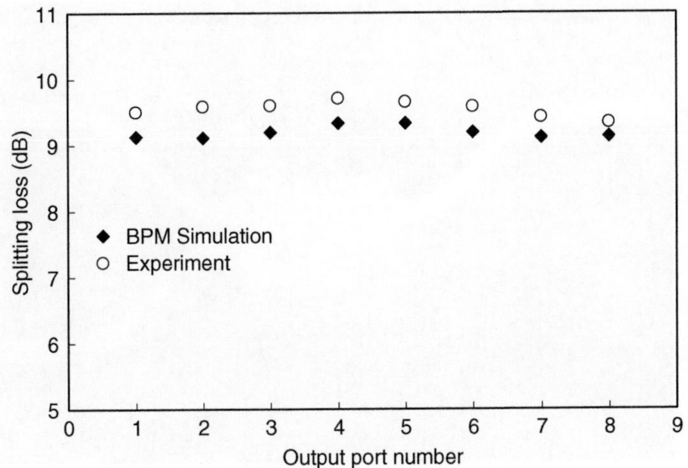

Figure 2.24 Theoretical and experimental splitting characteristics of 1×8 MMI splitter.

loss of 1/8 corresponds to 9 dB. Therefore, it is known that the excess loss of each output port is less than 1 dB.

When an input waveguide is placed at the proper position from the center of MMI waveguide, two-fold images are formed with equal amplitude at the distance of [17]

$$L_{3\,\mathrm{dB}} = \frac{2}{3} \cdot \frac{n_{\mathrm{eff}} W^2}{\lambda}, \tag{2.124a}$$

$$W = (N+1)s \qquad (N=2), \tag{2.124b}$$

where s denotes the separation of output waveguides. Figure 2.25 shows a 3-dB coupler based on the 2×2 MMI splitter. BPM simulation is required in order to accurately determine the 3-dB coupler configuration. Light propagation characteristics in the MMI 3-dB coupler are shown in Fig. 2.26. The length of 3-dB coupler is determined to be $L = L_{3\,\mathrm{dB}} + \delta_{3\,\mathrm{dB}} (\delta_{3\,\mathrm{dB}} = 200\,\mu\mathrm{m})$ by the BPM

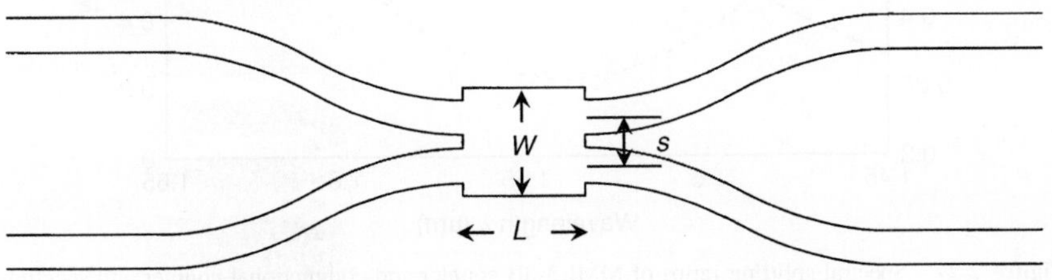

Figure 2.25 3-dB coupler based on the 2×2 MMI splitter.

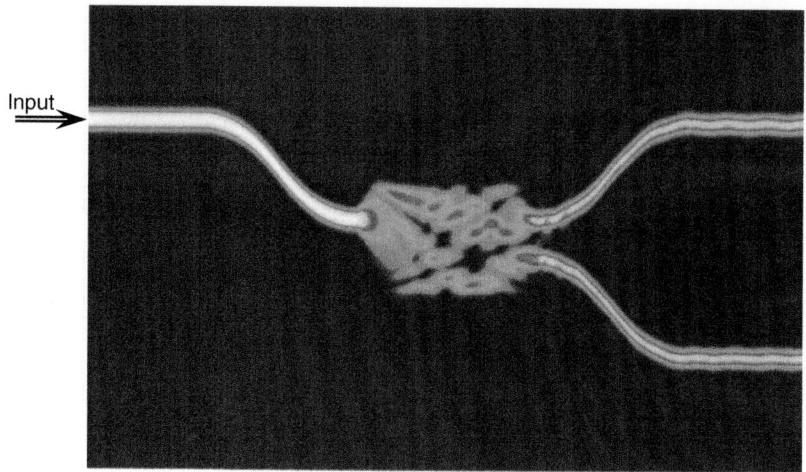

Figure 2.26 Light propagation characteristics of MMI 3-dB coupler.

calculation. Figure 2.27 shows spectral splitting ratios of MMI 3-dB coupler and codirectional coupler (see Section 4.2) and spectral insertion loss of MMI 3-dB coupler. It is known from the figure that coupling ratio of MMI 3-dB coupler is almost insensitive to wavelength as compared to codirectional coupler. This is a great advantage of MMI 3-dB coupler over a codirectional coupler. However,

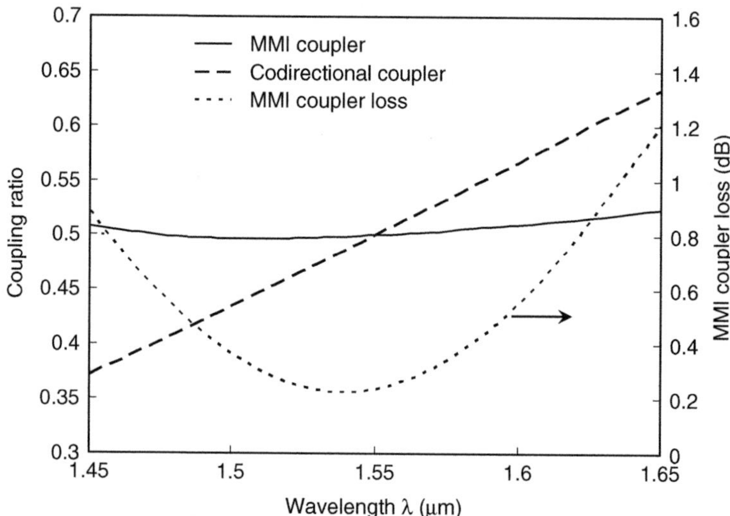

Figure 2.27 Spectral splitting ratios of MMI 3-dB coupler and codirectional coupler and spectral insertion loss of MMI 3-dB coupler.

we should take notice of two facts. First, insertion loss of MMI is not zero even in theoretical simulation. Theoretical insertion loss of the MMI 3-dB coupler is about 0.22 dB at the minimum. Second, the insertion loss of MMI coupler rapidly increases as wavelength departs from the optimal wavelength.

When phase of the input light is properly adjusted $1 \times N$ MMI splitter functions as $N \times 1$ combiner. Figure 2.28 shows light propagation characteristics in MMI 16×1 combiner. Complex electric field g_i in the i-th input waveguide is

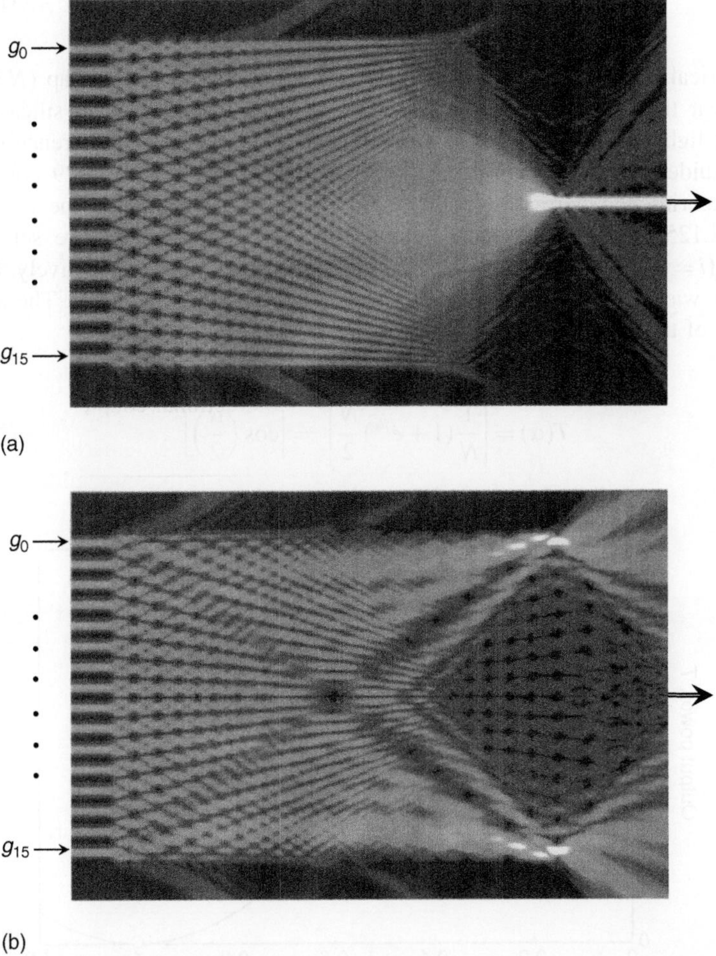

Figure 2.28 Light propagation characteristics in MMI 16×1 combiner: (a) Amplitudes of g_i's are equal and their phases are properly adjusted; and (b) amplitudes of g_i's are equal and their phases are completely out of phase.

given by $g_i = a_i \exp(j\theta_i)$, where a_i and θ_i denote amplitude and phase of g_i. In the BPM simulation shown in Fig. 2.28a, amplitudes of g_i's are set to be equal and their phases are properly adjusted. Every light beam from 16 input ports constructively interfere to form a single output image at the distance of $L = L_{\mathrm{MMI}}/16 + \delta_{\mathrm{L}}$, where $\delta_{\mathrm{L}} = 140\,\mu\mathrm{m}$. It is shown by a number of numerical simulations that MMI $N \times 1$ combiner has a unique property in which we can obtain coherent summation of the input electric field as

$$T = \left| \frac{1}{N} \sum_{i=0}^{N-1} g_i \right|^2 = \left| \frac{1}{N} \sum_{i=0}^{N-1} a_i e^{j\theta_i} \right|^2. \tag{2.125}$$

Numerical simulation was confirmed by the experiment using 16-tap ($N = 16$) coherent transversal filter [18]. The device was fabricated using silica-based planar lightwave circuits. The core size and refractive-index difference of the waveguides are $7\,\mu\mathrm{m} \times 7\,\mu\mathrm{m}$ and 0.75%, respectively. Figure 2.29 compares the experimental normalized output power with the theoretical one given by Eq. (2.125). Complex electric fields of even and odd ports were set to be $g_i = 1\ (i = 0, 2, \ldots, 14)$ and $g_i = \exp(j\alpha)\ (i = 1, 3, \ldots, 15)$, respectively. Phase shift α was introduced to the waveguide by the thermo-optic effect. The output power of the MMI $N \times 1$ combiner is given from Eq. (2.125) by

$$T(\alpha) = \left| \frac{1}{N}(1 + e^{j\alpha})\frac{N}{2} \right|^2 = \left| \cos\left(\frac{\alpha}{2}\right) \right|^2. \tag{2.126}$$

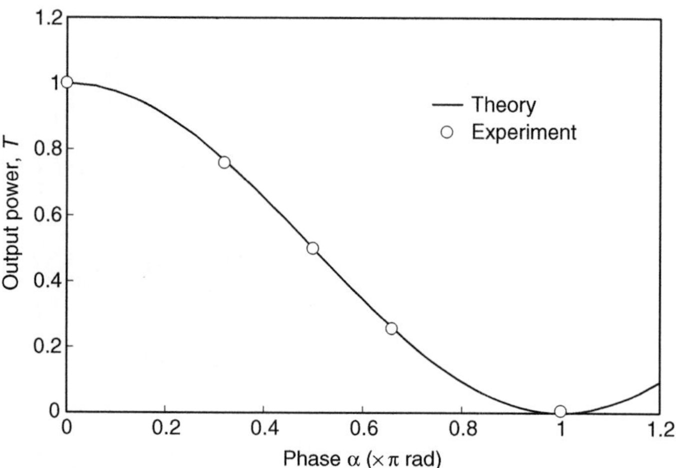

Figure 2.29 Normalized output power T of the 16×1 MMI combiner.

Solid line in Fig. 2.29 shows theoretical curve $|\cos(\alpha/2)|^2$ and circles are experimental values for $\alpha = 0, \pi/3, \pi/2, 2\pi/3$ and π, respectively. It is confirmed that the collective summation of complex electric fields is obtained by using MMI combiner.

REFERENCES

[1] Marcuse, D. 1982. *Light Transmission Optics*. New York: Van Nostrand Reinhold.

[2] Marcuse, D. 1974. *Theory of Optical Waveguides*. New York: Academic Press.

[3] Unger, H. G. 1977. *Planar Optical Waveguides and Fibers*. Oxford: Clarendon Press.

[4] Kressel, H. and J. K. Butler. 1977. *Semiconductor Lasers and Heterojunction LEDs*. New York: Academic Press.

[5] Marcatili, E. A. J. 1969. Dielectric rectangular waveguide and directional coupler for integrated optics. *Bell Syst. Tech. J.* 48:2071–2102.

[6] Kumar, A., K. Thyagarajan and A. K. Ghatak. 1983. Analysis of rectangular-core dielectric waveguides—An accurate perturbation approach. *Opt. Lett.* 8:63–65.

[7] Goell, J. E. 1969. A circular harmonic computer analysis of rectangular dielectric waveguides. *Bell Syst. Tech. J.* 48:2133–2160.

[8] Knox, R. M. and P. P. Toulios. 1970. Integrated circuits for the millimeter through optical frequency range. *Symposium on Submillimeter Waves*, Polytechnic Institute of Brooklyn, pp. 497–516.

[9] Tamir, T. 1975. *Integrated Optics*. Chap. 2, Berlin: Springer-Verlag.

[10] Born, M. and E. Wolf. 1970. *Principles of Optics*. Oxford: Pergamon Press.

[11] Bryngdahl, O. 1973. Image formation using self-imaging techniques. *J. Opt. Soc. Amer.* 63:416–419.

[12] Ulrich, R. 1975. Image formation by phase coincidences in optical waveguides. *Opt. Commun.* 13:259–264.

[13] Niemeier, T. and R. Ulrich. 1986. Quadrature outputs from fiber interferometer with 4 × 4 coupler. *Opt. Lett.* 11:677–679.

[14] Veerman, F. B., P. J. Schalkwijk, E. C. M. Pennings, M. K. Smit and B. H. Verbeek. 1992. An optical passive 3-dB TMI-coupler with reduced fabrication tolerance sensitivity. *IEEE J. Lightwave Tech.* 10:306–311.

[15] Bachmann, M., P. A. Besse and H. Melchior. 1994. General self-imaging properties in N × N multimode interference couplers including phase relations. *Appl. Opt.* 33:3905–3911.

[16] Heaton, J. M. and R. M. Jenkins. 1999. General matrix theory of self-imaging in multimode interference (MMI) couplers. *IEEE Photon. Tech. Lett.* 11:212–214.

[17] Soldano, L. B. and E. C. M. Pennings. 1995. Optical multi-mode interference devices based on self-imaging: Principles and applications. *IEEE J. Lightwave Tech.* 13:615–627.

[18] Okamoto, K., H. Yamada and T. Goh. 1999. Fabrication of coherent optical transversal filter consisting of MMI splitter/combiner and thermo-optic amplitude and phase controllers. *Electron. Lett.* 35:1331–1332.

Chapter 3

Optical Fibers

Silica-based optical fibers are the most important transmission medium for long-distance and large-capacity optical communication systems. The most distinguished feature of optical fiber is its low loss characteristics. The lowest transmission loss ever achieved is 0.154 dB/km at $\lambda = 1.55$-μm wavelength [1]. This means that the signal intensity of light becomes half of the original strength after propagating 20 km along the optical fiber. Together with such low loss properties, low dispersion is also required for signal transmission. Signal distortion due to dispersion of the fiber is closely related to the guiding structure of optical fibers. In order to realize low-dispersion fibers, it is necessary to understand the transmission characteristics of fibers and to design and analyze the arbitrarily shaped guiding structures. In this chapter, first a rigorous analysis of step-index fiber is presented, to understand the basic properties of optical fibers. Then linearly polarized (LP) modes, which are quite important mode designations for the practical weakly guiding fibers, will be described. The derivation of dispersion equations is explained in detail in order to understand the dispersion characteristics of fibers. Signal transmission bandwidths of graded-index multimode fibers and single-mode fibers are discussed and compared in connection with their dispersion values. Finally, the principle of polarization-maintaining properties in birefringent fibers and their polarization characteristics are described.

3.1. BASIC EQUATIONS

The electromagnetic fields in optical fibers are expressed in cylindrical coordinates as

$$\tilde{\mathbf{E}} = \mathbf{E}(r, \theta)\ e^{j(\omega t - \beta z)}, \tag{3.1a}$$

$$\tilde{\mathbf{H}} = \mathbf{H}(r, \theta)\ e^{j(\omega t - \beta z)}. \tag{3.1b}$$

Substituting Eq. (3.1) into Maxwell's Eq. (1.31), we obtain two sets of wave equations [2, 3] as

$$\begin{cases} \dfrac{\partial^2 E_z}{\partial r^2} + \dfrac{1}{r}\dfrac{\partial E_z}{\partial r} + \dfrac{1}{r^2}\dfrac{\partial^2 E_z}{\partial \theta^2} + [k^2 n(r,\theta)^2 - \beta^2]E_z = 0 & \text{(3.2a)} \\ \dfrac{\partial^2 H_z}{\partial r^2} + \dfrac{1}{r}\dfrac{\partial H_z}{\partial r} + \dfrac{1}{r^2}\dfrac{\partial^2 H_z}{\partial \theta^2} + [k^2 n(r,\theta)^2 - \beta^2]H_z = 0. & \text{(3.2b)} \end{cases}$$

In axially symmetric optical fibers, the refractive-index distribution is not dependent on θ and is expressed by $n(r)$. Then the transverse electromagnetic fields are related to E_z and H_z as follows:

$$\begin{cases} E_r = -\dfrac{j}{[k^2 n(r)^2 - \beta^2]}\left(\beta\dfrac{\partial E_z}{\partial r} + \dfrac{\omega\mu_0}{r}\dfrac{\partial H_z}{\partial \theta}\right) & \text{(3.3a)} \\ E_\theta = -\dfrac{j}{[k^2 n(r)^2 - \beta^2]}\left(\dfrac{\beta}{r}\dfrac{\partial E_z}{\partial \theta} - \omega\mu_0\dfrac{\partial H_z}{\partial r}\right) & \text{(3.3b)} \\ H_r = -\dfrac{j}{[k^2 n(r)^2 - \beta^2]}\left(\beta\dfrac{\partial H_z}{\partial r} - \dfrac{\omega\varepsilon_0 n(r)^2}{r}\dfrac{\partial E_z}{\partial \theta}\right) & \text{(3.3c)} \\ H_\theta = -\dfrac{j}{[k^2 n(r)^2 - \beta^2]}\left(\dfrac{\beta}{r}\dfrac{\partial H_z}{\partial \theta} + \omega\varepsilon_0 n(r)^2\dfrac{\partial E_z}{\partial r}\right). & \text{(3.3d)} \end{cases}$$

The azimuthal dependency of the electromagnetic fields in axially symmetric fibers is expressed by $\cos(n\theta + \psi)$ or $\sin(n\theta + \psi)$, where n is an integer and ψ denotes the phase. The modes in an optical fiber consists of TE modes ($E_z = 0$), TM modes ($H_z = 0$) and hybrid modes ($E_z \neq 0,\ H_z \neq 0$), respectively. In the following, electromagnetic fields, dispersion equations, and propagation characteristics of optical fibers are described in detail for step-index fibers as shown in Fig. 3.1, which has a uniform refractive index in the core.

3.2. WAVE THEORY OF STEP-INDEX FIBERS

3.2.1. TE Modes

When we have $E_z = 0$ in Eqs. (3.2) and (3.3), we have following set of equations for the TE mode:

$$\frac{\partial^2 H_z}{\partial r^2} + \frac{1}{r}\frac{\partial H_z}{\partial r} + \left[k^2 n(r)^2 - \beta^2 - \frac{n^2}{r^2}\right]H_z = 0, \tag{3.4}$$

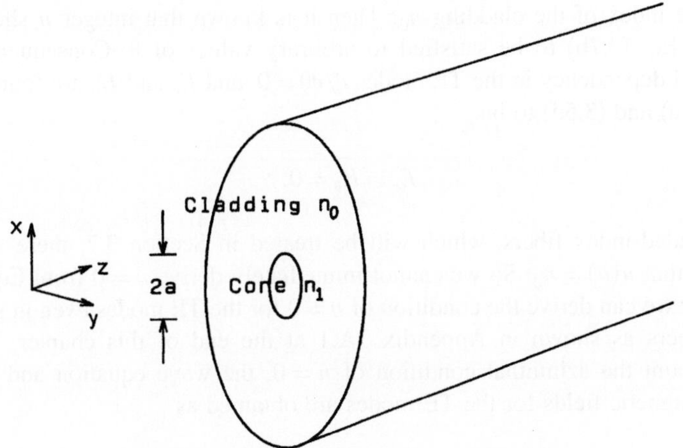

Figure 3.1 Waveguide structure of optical fiber.

$$\begin{cases} E_r = -\dfrac{j\omega\mu_0}{[k^2n(r)^2-\beta^2]}\dfrac{1}{r}\dfrac{\partial H_z}{\partial\theta} & (3.5a) \\ E_\theta = \dfrac{j\omega\mu_0}{[k^2n(r)^2-\beta^2]}\dfrac{\partial H_z}{\partial r} & (3.5b) \\ H_r = -\dfrac{j\beta}{[k^2n(r)^2-\beta^2]}\dfrac{\partial H_z}{\partial r} & (3.5c) \\ H_\theta = -\dfrac{j\beta}{[k^2n(r)^2-\beta^2]}\dfrac{1}{r}\dfrac{\partial H_z}{\partial\theta}. & (3.5d) \end{cases}$$

The magnetic field in the core and cladding are expressed as

$$H_z = \begin{Bmatrix} g(r) \\ h(r) \end{Bmatrix} \cos(n\theta+\psi) \qquad \begin{matrix} (0 \leqslant r \leqslant a) \\ (r > a). \end{matrix} \tag{3.6}$$

From the boundary condition that the tangential field components H_z and H_θ should be continuous at the core–cladding interface $r=a$, we obtain the following two conditions:

$$g(a) = h(a), \tag{3.7a}$$

$$\frac{j\beta}{[k^2n(a)^2-\beta^2]}\frac{n}{a}g(a)\sin(n\theta+\psi) = \frac{j\beta}{[k^2n_0^2-\beta^2]}\frac{n}{a}h(a)\sin(n\theta+\psi). \tag{3.7b}$$

Since in the step-index fiber, the refractive index at the boundary of the core $n(a)=n_1$ (n_1 is the refractive index of the core), $n(a)$ is not equal to the refractive index of the cladding n_0. Then it is known that integer n should be zero for Eq. (3.7b) to be satisfied to arbitrary values of θ. Consequently the azimuthal dependency in the TE modes $\partial/\partial\theta = 0$, and E_r and H_θ are found from Eqs. (3.5a) and (3.5d) to be

$$E_r = H_\theta = 0. \tag{3.8}$$

In graded-index fibers, which will be treated in Section 3.7, there may be the case that $n(a) = n_0$. So we cannot immediately derive $n = 0$ from Eq. (3.7). However we can derive the condition of $n = 0$ for the TE modes even in graded-index fibers as shown in Appendix 3A.1 at the end of this chapter. Taking into account the azimuthal condition of $n = 0$, the wave equation and related electromagnetic fields for the TE modes are obtained as

$$\frac{d^2 H_z}{dr^2} + \frac{1}{r}\frac{dH_z}{dr} + [k^2 n(r)^2 - \beta^2]\, H_z = 0, \tag{3.9}$$

$$\begin{cases} E_\theta = \dfrac{j\omega\mu_0}{[k^2 n(r)^2 - \beta^2]} \dfrac{dH_z}{dr}, & (3.10a) \\ H_r = -\dfrac{j\beta}{[k^2 n(r)^2 - \beta^2]} \dfrac{dH_z}{dr}, & (3.10b) \\ E_r = H_\theta = 0. & (3.10c) \end{cases}$$

Here, we define the wave number in the core and cladding along the transversal direction as

$$\kappa = \sqrt{k^2\, n_1^2 - \beta^2}, \tag{3.11a}$$

$$\sigma = \sqrt{\beta^2 - k^2\, n_0^2}. \tag{3.11b}$$

The wave Eq. (3.9) for the field in the core $H_z = g(r)$ is obtained as

$$\frac{d^2 g}{dr^2} + \frac{1}{r}\frac{dg}{dr} + \kappa^2 g = 0 \qquad (0 \leqslant r \leqslant a) \tag{3.12}$$

and the wave equation for the field in the cladding $H_z = h(r)$ is given by

$$\frac{d^2 h}{dr^2} + \frac{1}{r}\frac{dh}{dr} - \sigma^2 h = 0 \qquad (r > a). \tag{3.13}$$

The solutions for Eq. (3.12) are the 0th-order Bessel function $J_0(\kappa r)$ and the 0th-order Neumann function $N_0(\kappa r)$ [4, 5], respectively. However, $N_0(\kappa r)$

diverges infinitely at $r = 0$. Therefore $J_0(\kappa r)$ is the proper solution in the core. The solutions for Eq. (3.13) are modified Bessel function of the first kind $I_0(\sigma r)$ and modified Bessel functions of the second kind $K_0(\sigma r)$, respectively. However, $I_0(\sigma r)$ diverges infinitely at $r = \infty$. Therefore $K_0(\sigma r)$ is the proper solution in the cladding. Then the magnetic fields for the TE mode are given by

$$H_z = \begin{cases} AJ_0(\kappa r) & (0 \leqslant r \leqslant a) \\ BK_0(\sigma r) & (r > a), \end{cases} \tag{3.14}$$

where A and B are constants. The boundary conditions are given by the conditions that H_z and E_θ should be continuous at $r = a$:

$$AJ_0(\kappa a) = B\,K_0(\sigma a), \tag{3.15a}$$

$$\frac{A}{\kappa} J'_0(\kappa a) = -\frac{B}{\sigma} K'_0(\sigma a). \tag{3.15b}$$

By using the normalized transverse wave numbers

$$u = \kappa a = a\sqrt{k^2\,n_1^2 - \beta^2}, \tag{3.16a}$$

$$w = \sigma a = a\sqrt{\beta^2 - k^2\,n_0^2}, \tag{3.16b}$$

Eqs. (3.15a) and (3.15b) can be reduced to the following dispersion equation:

$$\frac{J'_0(u)}{u\,J_0(u)} = -\frac{K'_0(w)}{w\,K_0(w)}. \tag{3.17}$$

Based on the following Bessel function formulas:

$$J'_0(u) = -J_1(u) \tag{3.18a}$$

$$K'_0(w) = -K_1(w). \tag{3.18b}$$

Eq. (3.17) is rewritten as

$$\frac{J_1(u)}{u\,J_0(u)} = -\frac{K_1(w)}{w\,K_0(w)}. \tag{3.19}$$

Transverse wave numbers u and w are related, from Eq. (3.16), as

$$u^2 + w^2 = k^2(n_1^2 - n_0^2)\,a^2 = v^2. \tag{3.20}$$

Therefore when the normalized frequency v is given, the transverse wave numbers u and w are determined from Eqs. (3.19) and (3.20). Substituting Eqs. (3.14) and (3.15a) into (3.10), the electromagnetic fields for TE mode are obtained;

$$E_r = E_z = H_\theta = 0, \tag{3.21}$$

a. *Fields in the core* $(0 \leqslant r \leqslant a)$:

$$E_\theta = -j\omega\mu_0 \frac{a}{u} A J_1\left(\frac{u}{a} r\right), \tag{3.22a}$$

$$H_r = j\beta \frac{a}{u} A J_1\left(\frac{u}{a} r\right), \tag{3.22b}$$

$$H_z = A J_0\left(\frac{u}{a} r\right), \tag{3.22c}$$

b. *Fields in the cladding* $(r > a)$:

$$E_\theta = j\omega\mu_0 \frac{a}{w} \frac{J_0(u)}{K_0(w)} A K_1\left(\frac{w}{a} r\right), \tag{3.23a}$$

$$H_r = -j\beta \frac{a}{w} \frac{J_0(u)}{K_0(w)} A K_1\left(\frac{w}{a} r\right), \tag{3.23b}$$

$$H_z = \frac{J_0(u)}{K_0(w)} A K_0\left(\frac{w}{a} r\right). \tag{3.23c}$$

The constant A is determined in the relationship from the power P carried by the mode, as shown in Section 3.3.

3.2.2. TM Modes

When we set $H_z = 0$ in Eqs. (3.2) and (3.3) for TM modes and follow the same procedure as in the TE mode, we know that $n = 0$ holds also for the TM mode. Then the wave equation and other electromagnetic field components are expressed as

$$\frac{d^2 E_z}{dr^2} + \frac{1}{r} \frac{dE_z}{dr} + [k^2\ n(r)^2 - \beta^2]\ E_z = 0, \tag{3.24}$$

$$\begin{cases} E_r = \dfrac{-j\beta}{[k^2 n(r)^2 - \beta^2]} \dfrac{dE_z}{dr}, & (3.25\text{a}) \\[2ex] H_\theta = \dfrac{-j\omega\varepsilon_0 n^2}{[k^2 n(r)^2 - \beta^2]} \dfrac{dE_z}{dr}, & (3.25\text{b}) \\[2ex] E_\theta = H_r = 0. & (3.25\text{c}) \end{cases}$$

Solutions for Eq. (3.24) are given by the 0th-order Bessel functions as

$$E_z = \begin{cases} A J_0(\kappa r) & (0 \leqslant r \leqslant a) & (3.26\text{a}) \\ B K_0(\sigma r) & (r > a). & (3.26\text{b}) \end{cases}$$

where A and B are constants. Applying the boundary conditions that E_z and H_θ should be continuous at the core–cladding interface $r = a$, we obtain

$$\frac{J'_0(u)}{u\,J_0(u)} = -\left(\frac{n_0}{n_1}\right)^2 \frac{K'_0(w)}{w\,K_0(w)}. \tag{3.27}$$

Using the recurrence relation of Bessel functions (3.18), Eq. (3.27) can be rewritten into the dispersion equation for the TM modes:

$$\frac{J_1(u)}{u\,J_0(u)} = -\left(\frac{n_0}{n_1}\right)^2 \frac{K_1(w)}{w\,K_0(w)}. \tag{3.28}$$

The electromagnetic fields for TM mode are summarized as

$$E_\theta = H_r = H_z = 0, \tag{3.29}$$

a. *Fields in the core* $(0 \leqslant r \leqslant a)$:

$$E_r = j\beta \frac{a}{u} A J_1\left(\frac{u}{a} r\right), \tag{3.30a}$$

$$E_z = A J_0\left(\frac{u}{a} r\right), \tag{3.30b}$$

$$H_\theta = j\omega\varepsilon_0 n_1^2 \frac{a}{u} A J_1\left(\frac{u}{a} r\right), \tag{3.30c}$$

b. *Fields in the cladding* $(r > a)$:

$$E_r = -j\beta \frac{a}{w} \frac{J_0(u)}{K_0(w)} A K_1\left(\frac{w}{a} r\right), \tag{3.31a}$$

$$E_z = \frac{J_0(u)}{K_0(w)} A K_0\left(\frac{w}{a} r\right), \tag{3.31b}$$

$$H_\theta = -j\omega\varepsilon_0 n_0^2 \frac{a}{w} \frac{J_0(u)}{K_0(w)} A K_1\left(\frac{w}{a} r\right). \tag{3.31c}$$

3.2.3. Hybrid Modes

In hybrid modes the axial electromagnetic field components E_z and H_z are not zero. Therefore solutions for Eq. (3.2) are given by the product of nth-order Bessel functions and $\cos(n\theta + \psi)$ or $\sin(n\theta + \psi)$. E_z and H_z should be continuous at $r = a$. Also it is known from Eq. (3.3) that $\partial E_z/\partial r$ and $\partial H_z/\partial\theta$ (or $\partial E_z/\partial\theta$

and $\partial H_z/\partial r$) have the same θ dependencies. Taking these into consideration, the z-components of the electromagnetic field are expressed by

$$E_z = \begin{cases} AJ_n\left(\frac{u}{a}r\right)\cos(n\theta+\psi) & (0 \leqslant r \leqslant a) \quad (3.32a) \\ A\frac{J_n(u)}{K_n(w)}K_n\left(\frac{w}{a}r\right)\cos(n\theta+\psi) & (r > a) \quad (3.32b) \end{cases}$$

$$H_z = \begin{cases} CJ_n\left(\frac{u}{a}r\right)\sin(n\theta+\psi) & (0 \leqslant r \leqslant a) \quad (3.33a) \\ C\frac{J_n(u)}{K_n(w)}K_n\left(\frac{w}{a}r\right)\sin(n\theta+\psi) & (r > a). \quad (3.33b) \end{cases}$$

The transverse components are obtained, by substituting Eqs. (3.32) and (3.33) into (3.3), as follows.

a. *Core region* $(0 \leqslant r \leqslant a)$:

$$E_r = -\frac{ja^2}{u^2}\left[A\beta\frac{u}{a}J_n'\left(\frac{u}{a}r\right) + C\omega\mu_0\frac{n}{r}J_n\left(\frac{u}{a}r\right)\right]\cos(n\theta+\psi) \tag{3.34a}$$

$$E_\theta = -\frac{ja^2}{u^2}\left[-A\beta\frac{n}{r}J_n\left(\frac{u}{a}r\right) - C\omega\mu_0\frac{u}{a}J_n'\left(\frac{u}{a}r\right)\right]\sin(n\theta+\psi) \tag{3.34b}$$

$$H_r = -\frac{ja^2}{u^2}\left[A\omega\varepsilon_0 n_1^2\frac{n}{r}J_n\left(\frac{u}{a}r\right) + C\beta\frac{u}{a}J_n'\left(\frac{u}{a}r\right)\right]\sin(n\theta+\psi) \tag{3.34c}$$

$$H_\theta = -\frac{ja^2}{u^2}\left[A\omega\varepsilon_0 n_1^2\frac{u}{a}J_n'\left(\frac{u}{a}r\right) + C\beta\frac{n}{r}J_n\left(\frac{u}{a}r\right)\right]\cos(n\theta+\psi) \tag{3.34d}$$

b. *Cladding region* $(r > a)$:

$$E_r = \frac{ja^2}{w^2}\left[A\beta\frac{w}{a}K_n'\left(\frac{w}{a}r\right) + C\omega\mu_0\frac{n}{r}K_n\left(\frac{w}{a}r\right)\right]\frac{J_n(u)}{K_n(w)}\cos(n\theta+\psi) \tag{3.35a}$$

$$E_\theta = \frac{ja^2}{w^2}\left[-A\beta\frac{n}{r}K_n\left(\frac{w}{a}r\right) - C\omega\mu_0\frac{w}{a}K_n'\left(\frac{w}{a}r\right)\right]\frac{J_n(u)}{K_n(w)}\sin(n\theta+\psi) \tag{3.35b}$$

$$H_r = \frac{ja^2}{w^2}\left[A\omega\varepsilon_0 n_0^2\frac{n}{r}K_n\left(\frac{w}{a}r\right) + C\beta\frac{w}{a}K_n'\left(\frac{w}{a}r\right)\right]\frac{J_n(u)}{K_n(w)}\sin(n\theta+\psi) \tag{3.35c}$$

$$H_\theta = \frac{ja^2}{w^2}\left[A\omega\varepsilon_0 n_0^2\frac{w}{a}K_n'\left(\frac{w}{a}r\right) + C\beta\frac{n}{r}K_n\left(\frac{w}{a}r\right)\right]\frac{J_n(u)}{K_n(w)}\cos(n\theta+\psi) \tag{3.35d}$$

The boundary condition at $r=a$ that E_θ and H_θ should be continuous brings two relations, one is from Eqs. (3.34b) and (3.35b) as

$$A\beta\left(\frac{1}{u^2}+\frac{1}{w^2}\right)n=-C\omega\mu_0\left[\frac{J_n'(u)}{uJ_n(u)}+\frac{K_n'(w)}{wK_n(w)}\right] \tag{3.36}$$

and the other is from Eqs. (3.34d) and (3.35d):

$$A\omega\varepsilon_0\left[n_1^2\frac{J_n'(u)}{uJ_n(u)}+n_0^2\frac{K_n'(w)}{wK_n(w)}\right]=-C\beta\left(\frac{1}{u^2}+\frac{1}{w^2}\right)n. \tag{3.37}$$

We obtain the dispersion equation from Eqs. (3.36) and (3.37) in the form

$$\left[\frac{J_n'(u)}{uJ_n(u)}+\frac{K_n'(w)}{wK_n(w)}\right]\left[n_1^2\frac{J_n'(u)}{uJ_n(u)}+n_0^2\frac{K_n'(w)}{wK_n(w)}\right]=\frac{\beta^2}{k^2}\left(\frac{1}{u^2}+\frac{1}{w^2}\right)^2 n^2. \tag{3.38}$$

Substituting the following relation, which is derived from Eq. (3.16):

$$\frac{\beta^2}{k^2}\left(\frac{1}{u^2}+\frac{1}{w^2}\right)=\frac{n_1^2}{u^2}+\frac{n_0^2}{w^2}, \tag{3.39}$$

Eq. (3.38) may be rewritten

$$\left[\frac{J_n'(u)}{uJ_n(u)}+\frac{K_n'(w)}{wK_n(w)}\right]\left[\frac{J_n'(u)}{uJ_n(u)}+\left(\frac{n_0}{n_1}\right)^2\frac{K_n'(w)}{wK_n(w)}\right]$$
$$=n^2\left(\frac{1}{u^2}+\frac{1}{w^2}\right)\left[\frac{1}{u^2}+\left(\frac{n_0}{n_1}\right)^2\frac{1}{w^2}\right]. \tag{3.40}$$

The propagation constant of the hybrid modes is calculated by solving Eq. (3.40) using the u–w relation of Eq. (3.20). Although Eq. (3.40) is the strict solution of the hybrid modes in step-index fibers, it is rather difficult to investigate the propagation properties of optical fibers with Eq. (3.40). In practical fibers, the refractive-index difference Δ is of the order of 1%, so we can approximate $n_1 \cong n_0$ in some cases. In these cases Eq. (3.40) can be simplified as shown in Section 3.4 and much practical and useful information is obtained.

The constant C in the electromagnetic field expressions (3.34) and (3.35) can be written from Eq. (3.36) as

$$C=-A\frac{\beta}{\omega\mu_0}s \tag{3.41a}$$

where

$$s = \frac{n\left(\frac{1}{u^2} + \frac{1}{w^2}\right)}{\left[\frac{J_n'(u)}{uJ_n(u)} + \frac{K_n'(w)}{wK_n(w)}\right]}, \quad (3.41b)$$

when we apply the following recurrence relations for the Bessel functions

$$J_n'(z) = \frac{1}{2}[J_{n-1}(z) - J_{n+1}(z)], \quad (3.42a)$$

$$\frac{n}{z}J_n(z) = \frac{1}{2}[J_{n-1}(z) + J_{n+1}(z)], \quad (3.42b)$$

$$K_n'(z) = -\frac{1}{2}[K_{n-1}(z) + K_{n+1}(z)], \quad (3.43a)$$

$$\frac{n}{z}K_n(z) = -\frac{1}{2}[K_{n-1}(z) - K_{n+1}(z)], \quad (3.43b)$$

Eqs. (3.34) and (3.35) become the following.

a. *Core region* $(0 \leqslant r \leqslant a)$:

$$E_r = -jA\beta\frac{a}{u}\left[\frac{(1-s)}{2}J_{n-1}\left(\frac{u}{a}r\right) - \frac{(1+s)}{2}J_{n+1}\left(\frac{u}{a}r\right)\right]\cos(n\theta + \psi) \quad (3.44a)$$

$$E_\theta = jA\beta\frac{a}{u}\left[\frac{(1-s)}{2}J_{n-1}\left(\frac{u}{a}r\right) + \frac{(1+s)}{2}J_{n+1}\left(\frac{u}{a}r\right)\right]\sin(n\theta + \psi) \quad (3.44b)$$

$$E_z = AJ_n\left(\frac{u}{a}r\right)\cos(n\theta + \psi) \quad (3.44c)$$

$$H_r = -jA\omega\varepsilon_0 n_1^2\frac{a}{u}\left[\frac{(1-s_1)}{2}J_{n-1}\left(\frac{u}{a}r\right) + \frac{(1+s_1)}{2}J_{n+1}\left(\frac{u}{a}r\right)\right]\sin(n\theta + \psi) \quad (3.44d)$$

$$H_\theta = -jA\omega\varepsilon_0 n_1^2\frac{a}{u}\left[\frac{(1-s_1)}{2}J_{n-1}\left(\frac{u}{a}r\right) - \frac{(1+s_1)}{2}J_{n+1}\left(\frac{u}{a}r\right)\right]\cos(n\theta + \psi) \quad (3.44e)$$

$$H_z = -A\frac{\beta}{\omega\mu_0}s\, J_n\left(\frac{u}{a}r\right)\sin(n\theta + \psi) \quad (3.44f)$$

b. *Cladding region* $(r > a)$:

$$E_r = -jA\beta\frac{aJ_n(u)}{wK_n(w)}\left[\frac{(1-s)}{2}K_{n-1}\left(\frac{w}{a}r\right) + \frac{(1+s)}{2}K_{n+1}\left(\frac{w}{a}r\right)\right] \times \cos(n\theta+\psi) \tag{3.45a}$$

$$E_\theta = jA\beta\frac{aJ_n(u)}{wK_n(w)}\left[\frac{(1-s)}{2}K_{n-1}\left(\frac{w}{a}r\right) - \frac{(1+s)}{2}K_{n+1}\left(\frac{w}{a}r\right)\right] \times \sin(n\theta+\psi) \tag{3.45b}$$

$$E_z = A\frac{J_n(u)}{K_n(w)}K_n\left(\frac{w}{a}r\right)\cos(n\theta+\psi) \tag{3.45c}$$

$$H_r = -jA\omega\varepsilon_0 n_0^2\frac{aJ_n(u)}{wK_n(w)}\left[\frac{(1-s_0)}{2}K_{n-1}\left(\frac{w}{a}r\right) - \frac{(1+s_0)}{2}K_{n+1}\left(\frac{w}{a}r\right)\right]\sin(n\theta+\psi) \tag{3.45d}$$

$$H_\theta = -jA\omega\varepsilon_0 n_0^2\frac{aJ_n(u)}{wK_n(w)}\left[\frac{(1-s_0)}{2}K_{n-1}\left(\frac{w}{a}r\right) + \frac{(1+s_0)}{2}K_{n+1}\left(\frac{w}{a}r\right)\right]\cos(n\theta+\psi) \tag{3.45e}$$

$$H_z = -A\frac{\beta}{\omega\mu_0}s\frac{J_n(u)}{K_n(w)}K_n\left(\frac{w}{a}r\right)\sin(n\theta+\psi), \tag{3.45f}$$

where

$$s_1 = \frac{\beta^2}{k^2n_1^2}s \tag{3.46a}$$

$$s_0 = \frac{\beta^2}{k^2n_0^2}s. \tag{3.46b}$$

3.3. OPTICAL POWER CARRIED BY EACH MODE

The time averaged Poynting vector component along the z-axis per unit area is expressed, by Eq. (1.45), as

$$S_z = \frac{1}{2}(\mathbf{E}\times\mathbf{H}^*)\cdot\mathbf{u}_z = \frac{1}{2}(E_rH_\theta^* - E_\theta H_r^*), \tag{3.47}$$

where $\mathbf{u}_z$ is a unit vector in the z-direction. The power carried by the optical fiber is then given by

$$P = \int_0^{2\pi}\int_0^{\infty} S_z r\,dr\,d\theta = \frac{1}{2}\int_0^{2\pi}\int_0^{\infty}(E_r H_\theta^* - E_\theta H_r^*) r\,dr\,d\theta. \tag{3.48}$$

The analytical expressions for the transmission power in each mode are described in the following.

3.3.1. TE Modes

The transmission power in the core and cladding are calculated from Eqs. (3.21)–(3.23) and (3.48) as follows:

$$\begin{aligned} P_{\text{core}} &= \pi\omega\mu_0\beta|A|^2\frac{a^2}{u^2}\int_0^a J_1^2\left(\frac{u}{a}r\right) r\,dr \\ &= \frac{\pi}{2}\omega\mu_0\beta|A|^2\frac{a^4}{u^2}\left[J_1^2(u) - J_0(u)J_2(u)\right], \end{aligned} \tag{3.49}$$

$$\begin{aligned} P_{\text{clad}} &= \pi\omega\mu_0\beta|A|^2\frac{a^2 J_0^2(u)}{w^2 K_0^2(w)}\int_a^{\infty} K_1^2\left(\frac{w}{a}r\right) r\,dr \\ &= \frac{\pi}{2}\omega\mu_0\beta|A|^2\frac{a^4 J_0^2(u)}{w^2 K_0^2(w)}\left[K_0(w)K_2(w) - K_1^2(w)\right], \end{aligned} \tag{3.50}$$

where we used the integral formula of the Bessel functions

$$\int_0^a J_m^2\left(\frac{u}{a}r\right) r\,dr = \begin{cases} \dfrac{a^2}{2}\left[J_0^2(u) + J_1^2(u)\right] & (m=0) \\ \dfrac{a^2}{2}\left[J_m^2(u) - J_{m-1}(u)J_{m+1}(u)\right] & (m \geqslant 1) \end{cases} \tag{3.51}$$

$$\int_0^{\infty} K_m^2\left(\frac{w}{a}r\right) r\,dr = \begin{cases} \dfrac{a^2}{2}\left[K_1^2(w) - K_0^2(w)\right] & (m=0) \\ \dfrac{a^2}{2}\left[K_{m-1}(w)K_{m+1}(w) - K_m^2(w)\right] & (m \geqslant 1). \end{cases} \tag{3.52}$$

For the calculation of Eq. (3.49), we first rewrite it in the following form:

$$\left[J_1^2(u) - J_0(u)J_2(u)\right] = J_1^2\left[1 - \frac{J_0 J_2}{J_1^2}\right]. \tag{3.53}$$

Then we substitute the dispersion equation for the TE mode (3.19) into the recurrence relation of Bessel function $J_2(u)$ [$n=1$ in Eq. (3.42b)]:

$$J_2(u) = \frac{2J_1(u)}{u} - J_0(u), \tag{3.54}$$

and we also use the recurrence relation for the modified Bessel function of the second kind to obtain the expression for $J_2(u)$:

$$J_2(u) = -\frac{2K_1(w)J_0(u)}{w\,K_0(w)} - J_0(u) = -\frac{K_2(w)}{K_0(w)}J_0(u). \tag{3.55}$$

Putting Eq. (3.55) into (3.53) and using the dispersion Eq. (3.19) again, Eq. (3.53) is reduced to

$$[J_1^2(u) - J_0(u)J_2(u)] = J_1^2(u)\left[1 + \frac{w^2}{u^2}\frac{K_0(w)K_2(w)}{K_1^2(w)}\right]. \tag{3.56}$$

Then the optical power carried in the core and cladding regions is

$$P_{\text{core}} = \frac{\pi}{2}\omega\mu_0\beta|A|^2\frac{a^4}{u^2}J_1^2(u)\left[1 + \frac{w^2}{u^2}\frac{K_0(w)K_2(w)}{K_1^2(w)}\right], \tag{3.57}$$

$$P_{\text{clad}} = \frac{\pi}{2}\omega\mu_0\beta|A|^2\frac{a^4}{u^2}J_1^2(u)\left[\frac{K_0(w)K_2(w)}{K_1^2(w)} - 1\right]. \tag{3.58}$$

The total power carried by the TE mode is given by

$$P = P_{\text{core}} + P_{\text{clad}} = \frac{\pi}{2}\omega\mu_0\beta|A|^2\frac{a^4v^2}{u^4}J_1^2(u)\frac{K_0(w)K_2(w)}{K_1^2(w)}. \tag{3.59}$$

The unknown constant A can be determined from Eq. (3.59) when we specify the total power flow P in optical fiber. Ratios of the power confinement ratios to the total power in each core and cladding region are expressed as

$$\frac{P_{\text{core}}}{P} = 1 - \frac{u^2}{v^2}\left[1 - \frac{K_1^2(w)}{K_0(w)K_2(w)}\right], \tag{3.60a}$$

$$\frac{P_{\text{clad}}}{P} = \frac{u^2}{v^2}\left[1 - \frac{K_1^2(w)}{K_0(w)K_2(w)}\right]. \tag{3.60b}$$

3.3.2. TM Modes

Substituting Eqs. (3.29)–(3.31) into (3.48) and applying similar procedures to those for the TE mode, the power in the core and cladding for the TM mode is given by

$$P_{\text{core}} = \frac{\pi}{2}\omega\varepsilon_0 n_1^2\beta|A|^2\frac{a^4}{u^2}[J_1^2(u) - J_0(u)J_2(u)], \tag{3.61}$$

$$P_{\text{clad}} = \frac{\pi}{2}\omega\varepsilon_0 n_0^2\beta|A|^2\frac{a^4J_0^2(u)}{w^2K_0^2(w)}[K_0(w)K_2(w) - K_1^2(w)]. \tag{3.62}$$

Equations (3.61) and (3.62) are rewritten using the recurrence relations of Bessel function and the dispersion Eq. (3.28) into

$$P_{\text{core}} = \frac{\pi}{2}\omega\varepsilon_0 n_1^2\beta|A|^2\frac{a^4}{u^2}J_1^2(u) \times\left[1+\frac{n_1^2}{n_0^2}\frac{w^2}{u^2}\frac{K_0(w)K_2(w)}{K_1^2(w)}+\left(1-\frac{n_0^2}{n_1^2}\right)\frac{J_0^2(u)}{J_1^2(u)}\right], \tag{3.63}$$

$$P_{\text{clad}} = \frac{\pi}{2}\omega\varepsilon_0 n_1^2\beta|A|^2\frac{a^4}{u^2}J_1^2(u)\frac{n_1^2}{n_0^2}\left[\frac{K_0(w)K_2(w)}{K_1^2(w)}-1\right], \tag{3.64}$$

$$\begin{aligned} P &= P_{\text{core}} + P_{\text{clad}} \\ &= \frac{\pi}{2}\omega\varepsilon_0 n_1^2\beta|A|^2\frac{a^4}{u^2}J_1^2(u) \\ &\quad\times\left[\frac{n_1^2}{n_0^2}\frac{v^2}{u^2}\frac{K_0(w)K_2(w)}{K_1^2(w)}+\left(1-\frac{n_1^2}{n_0^2}\right)\left(1-\frac{n_0^2}{n_1^2}\frac{J_0^2(u)}{J_1^2(u)}\right)\right]. \end{aligned} \tag{3.65}$$

When the weakly guiding approximation $n_1/n_0 \cong 1$ is satisfied, Eqs. (3.63)–(3.65) are simplified into equations similar to Eqs. (3.57)–(3.59) for the TE mode.

3.3.3. Hybrid Modes

The analytical expressions of the power flow for the hybrid modes are rather complicated. Here we show only the derivation equations of P_{core} and P_{clad}:

$$\begin{aligned} P_{\text{core}} = \frac{\pi}{4}\omega\varepsilon_0 n_1^2\beta|A|^2\frac{a^2}{u^2}\bigg[&(1-s)(1-s_1)\int_0^a J_{n-1}^2\left(\frac{u}{a}r\right)r\,dr \\ &+(1+s)(1+s_1)\int_0^a J_{n+1}^2\left(\frac{u}{a}r\right)r\,dr\bigg], \end{aligned} \tag{3.66}$$

$$\begin{aligned} P_{\text{clad}} = \frac{\pi}{4}\omega\varepsilon_0 n_0^2\beta|A|^2\frac{a^2J_n^2(u)}{w^2K_n^2(w)}\bigg[&(1-s)(1-s_0)\int_a^\infty K_{n-1}^2\left(\frac{w}{a}r\right)r\,dr \\ &+(1+s)(1+s_0)\int_a^\infty K_{n+1}^2\left(\frac{w}{a}r\right)r\,dr\bigg]. \end{aligned} \tag{3.67}$$

P_{core} and P_{clad} can be calculated by applying the integral formulas Eqs. (3.51) and (3.52) to Eqs. (3.66) and (3.67). If the approximation of $n_1/n_0 \cong 1$ holds as shown in upcoming Section 3.4.3, P_{core} and P_{clad} are expressed in more simple forms.

3.4. LINEARLY POLARIZED (LP) MODES

In the preceding sections, rigorous analyses for the TE, TM and hybrid modes in a step-index fibers have been described. The refractive-index difference Δ of practical fiber is of the order of 1%. Moreover index differences of the most important single-mode fibers for optical communication are about $\Delta \cong 0.3$–0.8%. Then we can approximate as $n_1/n_0 \cong 1$. This approximation allows us to simplify the analysis of optical fibers drastically and enables us to obtain quite clear results. The analysis of fibers based on the approximation with $n_1/n_0 \cong 1$ was first presented by Snyder [6]. Afterwards such mode groups with the approximation $n_1/n_0 \cong 1$ were designated LP (linearly polarized) modes by Gloge [7]. Since an LP mode is derived by the approximation of $n_1/n_0 \cong 1$, it means that the light confinement in the core is not so tight. Therefore this approximation is called weakly guiding approximation. We will study LP modes in detail in the following sections.

3.4.1. Unified Dispersion Equation for LP Modes

The strict solution [Eq. (3.19)] for the TE modes is adopted as it is. For the TM modes the weakly guiding approximation $n_1/n_0 \cong 1$ is applied to the rigorous dispersion Eq. (3.28) to obtain the approximate form

$$\frac{J_1(u)}{uJ_0(u)} = -\frac{K_1(w)}{wK_0(w)}. \tag{3.68}$$

This equation is known to be the same as the dispersion equation for TE modes (3.19). For the hybrid modes, we apply the weakly guiding approximation $n_1/n_0 \cong 1$ into the strict dispersion equation (3.40) and obtain a pair of equations:

$$\frac{J_n'(u)}{uJ_n(u)} + \frac{K_n'(w)}{wK_n(w)} = \pm n\left(\frac{1}{u^2} + \frac{1}{w^2}\right), \tag{3.69}$$

where $n \geqslant 1$. This equation is rewritten by using the recurrence relation of Bessel functions (3.42a) and (3.43a) into

$$\frac{J_{n+1}(u)}{uJ_n(u)} = -\frac{K_{n+1}(w)}{wK_n(w)} \tag{3.70}$$

and

$$\frac{J_{n-1}(u)}{uJ_n(u)} = \frac{K_{n-1}(w)}{wK_n(w)}, \tag{3.71}$$

where Eq. (3.70) is obtained from the plus sign of Eq. (3.69), and Eq. (3.71) is obtained from the negative sign of Eq. (3.69), respectively. The modes corresponding to the plus sign of Eq. (3.69) are called EH modes; those corresponding to the negative sign of Eq. (3.69) are called HE modes. The mode designations of EH and HE have no particular rationale and are merely conventional. Historically, microwave engineers first referred to the lowest-order mode (mode without cutoff) in a dielectric rod waveguide as the HE_{11} mode [3, 8]. Later, designations of HE and EH modes were derived in accordance with this custom. It is worth stating, however, that in EH modes the axial magnetic field H_z is relatively strong, whereas in HE modes the axial electric filed E_z is relatively strong.

The approximation $n_1 \cong n_0$ allows us to rewrite the expressions (3.46) into $s_1 \cong s$ and $s_0 \cong s$. Therefore equations representing the electromagnetic fields (3.44) and (3.45) are also simplified. Since $s = 1$ for the EH modes, from Eqs. (3.41b) and (3.69), we obtain the approximation $s_1 \cong 1$ and $s_0 \cong 1$. Then the electromagnetic field of the EH modes is given by putting $s_1 \cong 1$ and $s_0 \cong 1$ into Eqs. (3.44) and (3.45). It is known that the terms with $J_{n+1}(ur/a)$ and $K_{n+1}(wr/a)$ are predominant in the EH modes. On the other hand, since $s = -1$ for the HE modes from Eqs. (3.41b) and (3.69), we obtain the approximations $s_1 \cong -1$ and $s_0 \cong -1$. Then the electromagnetic field of the HE modes is found by putting $s_1 \cong -1$ and $s_0 \cong -1$ into Eqs. (3.44) and (3.45). It is known that the terms with $J_{n-1}(ur/a)$ and $K_{n-1}(wr/a)$ are predominant in the HE modes.

The dispersion equation for the HE modes having the azimuthal mode number $n \geqslant 2$ can be rewritten as follows. First, Eq. (3.71) is reversed. Then the recurrence relations for Bessel functions (3.42b) and (3.43b) are applied to $J_n(u)$ and $K_n(w)$ to derive the following relation:

$$\frac{J_{n-1}(u)}{uJ_{n-2}(u)} = -\frac{K_{n-1}(w)}{wK_{n-2}(w)}. \tag{3.72}$$

This dispersion equation is used for the HE modes having the azimuthal mode number $n \geqslant 2$. The dispersion equations for TE, TM and hybrid EH and HE modes under the weakly guiding approximation are summarized in Table 3.1. Integer n is a mode order in the azimuthal θ direction and $\ell(\geqslant 1)$ is a mode order in the radial direction, respectively. More precisely, ℓ represents the ℓth solution of each dispersion equation. Considering the similarity between the LP modes in Table 3.1, we introduce a new parameter defined by

$$m = \begin{cases} 1 & \text{(TE andTM mode)} \\ n+1 & \text{(EH mode)} \\ n-1 & \text{(HE mode).} \end{cases} \tag{3.73}$$

Table 3.1
Dispersion equations under the weakly-guiding approximation

Mode designation ($\ell \geqslant 1$)	Dispersion equation
$TE_{0\ell}$ mode, $TM_{0\ell}$ mode	$\frac{J_1(u)}{uJ_0(u)} = -\frac{K_1(w)}{wK_0(w)}$
$EH_{n\ell}$ mode ($n \geqslant 1$)	$\frac{J_{n+1}(u)}{uJ_n(u)} = -\frac{K_{n+1}(w)}{wK_n(w)}$
$HE_{1\ell}$ mode	$\frac{J_0(u)}{uJ_1(u)} = \frac{K_0(w)}{wK_1(w)}$
$HE_{n\ell}$ mode ($n \geqslant 2$)	$\frac{J_{n-1}(u)}{uJ_{n-2}(u)} = -\frac{K_{n-1}(w)}{wK_{n-2}(w)}$

Then the dispersion equations of the LP modes can be expressed in the unified form

$$\frac{J_m(u)}{uJ_{m-1}(u)} = -\frac{K_m(w)}{wK_{m-1}(w)}. \tag{3.74}$$

For the $HE_{1\ell}$ mode with $m = 0$ ($n = 1$), the Bessel function formulas of $J_{-1}(u) = -J_1(u)$ and $K_{-1}(w) = K_1(w)$ should be used in Eq. (3.74).

It is known from Eq. (3.74) that the mode which has the same mode parameter m (and ℓ) has the identical eigenvalue under the weakly guiding approximation. Of course, since they are not the strict modes, the eigenvalues are slightly different in the rigorous dispersion equations. Therefore LP modes are approximate modes classified by the eigenvalues.

Table 3.2 compares the relation between LP modes and conventional modes. Three kinds of mode corresponding to $m = 1$, $TE_{0\ell}$, $TM_{0\ell}$ and $HE_{2\ell}$ satisfy approximately the same dispersion equation. Also, mode combination $EH_{m-1,\ell}$ and $HE_{m+1,\ell}$, which corresponds to $m \geqslant 2$, satisfies the same dispersion equation. This means that the propagation constants of these mode groups are nearly degenerate. Moreover the EH and HE modes have two independent azimuthal components $\cos(n\theta)$ and $\sin(n\theta)$ [$\psi = 0$ and $\pi/2$ in Eqs. (3.32)–(3.35)]. The TE and TM modes are not degenerate in terms of polarization, since they have axially symmetric ($n = 0$) field distributions. Then the solution of the dispersion equation corresponding to the combination of (m, ℓ) is two fold degenerate for $m = 0$ and four fold for $m \geqslant 1$, respectively.

Figure 3.2 shows the relation between the electric field vectors and intensity profiles of E_x for the LP modes and conventional modes in the three mode groups of $LP_{01}(HE_{11})$, $LP_{11}(TE_{01}, TM_{01}, HE_{21})$ and $LP_{21}(EH_{11}, HE_{31})$ [2, 3],

Table 3.2

Comparision of LP modes with conventional modes

LP mode ($\ell \geqslant 1$)	Conventional mode ($\ell \geqslant 1$)	Dispersion equation
$LP_{0\ell}$ mode (m = 0)	$HE_{1\ell}$ mode	$\frac{J_0(u)}{uJ_1(u)} = \frac{K_0(w)}{wK_1(w)}$
	$TE_{0\ell}$ mode	
$LP_{1\ell}$ mode ($m = 1$)	$TM_{0\ell}$ mode	$\frac{J_1(u)}{uJ_0(u)} = -\frac{K_1(w)}{wK_0(w)}$
	$HE_{2\ell}$ mode	
$LP_{m\ell}$ mode ($m \geqslant 2$)	$EH_{m-1,\ell}$ mode	$\frac{J_m(u)}{uJ_{m-1}(u)} = -\frac{K_m(w)}{wK_{m-1}(w)}$
	$HE_{m+1,\ell}$ mode	

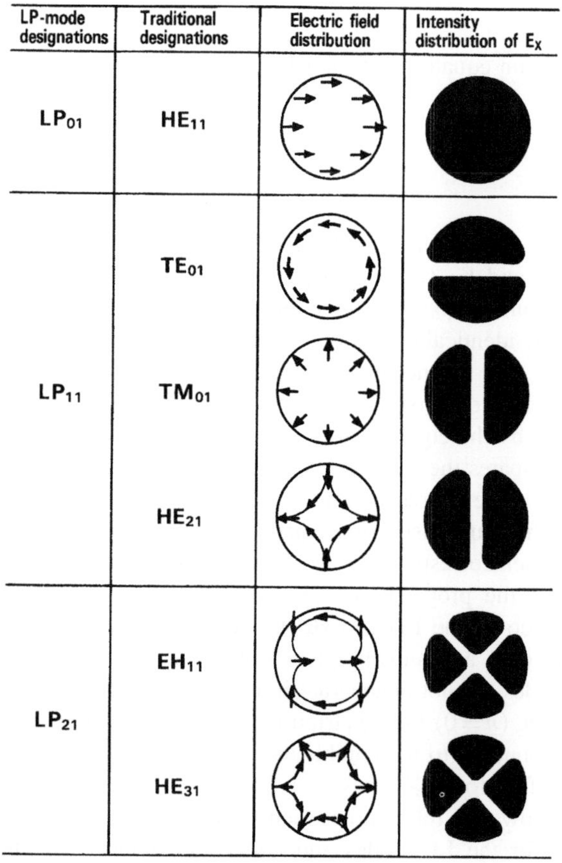

LP-mode designations	Traditional designations	Electric field distribution	Intensity distribution of E_x
LP_{01}	HE_{11}		
LP_{11}	TE_{01}		
	TM_{01}		
	HE_{21}		
LP_{21}	EH_{11}		
	HE_{31}		

Figure 3.2 Electric field vectors and intensity profiles of LP modes and conventional modes.

respectively. It is known that the intensity profiles of transverse electric fields (E_x or E_y) belonging to the same LP mode have the same distribution.

3.4.2. Dispersion Characteristics of LP Modes

The propagation constant of the step-index fiber is obtained by solving the dispersion equation in Table 3.2 under the condition of $u^2 + w^2 = v^2$. The relations between the transverse wavenumbers u and w, which are calculated via the dispersion equation itself and $u^2 + w^2 = v^2$ for $v = 5$, are shown as in Fig. 3.3.

The number attached to each curve indicates the mode number $m\ell$ of the LP mode. The crossing points of the vertical curves and the semicircle give the set of eigenvalues u and w. The cutoff v-values are obtained by the following

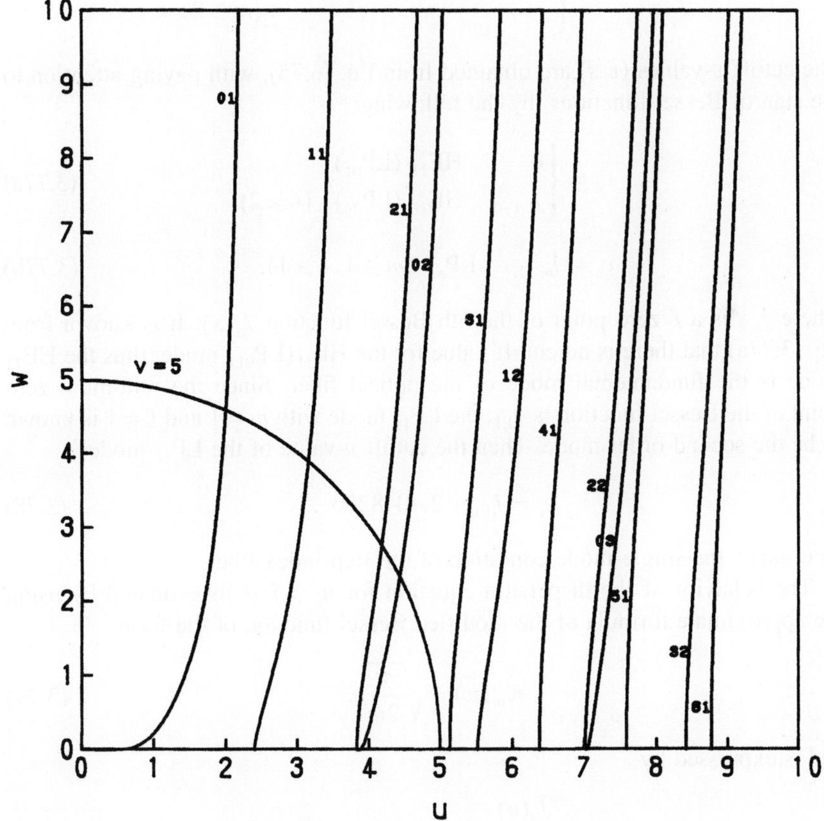

Figure 3.3 u–w relation in the step-index fiber.

equations when we set $w \to 0$ (and simultaneously $u \to v$) in the dispersion equation:

$$\frac{J_0(v)}{vJ_1(v)} \to \infty \qquad (m=0) \tag{3.75a}$$

$$\frac{J_m(v)}{vJ_{m-1}(v)} \to -\infty \qquad (m \geqslant 1). \tag{3.75b}$$

In the derivation of these two equations, we used the approximate formula for the modified Bessel functions for $w \ll 1$:

$$K_m(w) \cong \begin{cases} -\ell n(w) + 0.1159315\ldots & (m=0) \\ \dfrac{1}{w} & (m=1) \\ \dfrac{(m-1)!\, 2^{m-1}}{w^m} & (m \geqslant 2). \end{cases} \tag{3.76}$$

The cutoff v-values ($v_c s$) are obtained from Eq. (3.75), with paying attention to the sign of Bessel functions, by the following:

$$v_c = \begin{cases} 0 & \mathrm{HE}_{11}\ (\mathrm{LP}_{01}) \\ j_{1,\ell-1} & \mathrm{HE}_{1\ell}\ (\mathrm{LP}_{0\ell}),\ (\ell \geqslant 2) \end{cases} \tag{3.77a}$$

$$v_c = j_{m-1,\ell} \quad \mathrm{LP}_{m\ell}\ (m \geqslant 1, \ell \geqslant 1), \tag{3.77b}$$

where $j_{n,\ell}$ is a ℓ zero point of the nth Bessel function $J_n(x)$. It is known from Eq. (3.77a) that there is no cutoff value for the $\mathrm{HE}_{11}(\mathrm{LP}_{01})$ mode; thus the HE_{11} mode is the fundamental mode of the optical fiber. Since the minimum zero point of the Bessel function is $j_{0,1}$, the LP_{11} mode with $m=1$ and $\ell=1$ is known to be the second-order mode. Then the cutoff v-value of the LP_{11} mode

$$v_c = j_{0,1} = 2.4048256\ldots \tag{3.78}$$

determines the single-mode condition of the step-index fiber.

The behavior of the dispersion equation for $w \gg 1$ is investigated by using the approximate formula of the modified Bessel function of the form

$$K_m(w) \cong \sqrt{\frac{\pi}{2w}} e^{-w} \tag{3.79}$$

and is expressed by

$$\frac{J_0(u)}{uJ_1(u)} \to 0 \qquad (m=0) \tag{3.80a}$$

or

$$-\frac{J_m(u)}{uJ_{m-1}(u)} \to 0 \qquad (m \geqslant 1). \tag{3.80b}$$

It is known that $w \gg 1$, u approaches

$$u = j_{m,\ell} \qquad (m \geqslant 0). \tag{3.81}$$

The variation range of u for the LP modes is then given, from Eqs. (3.77) and (3.81) by

$$\begin{array}{ll} LP_{01}(HE_{11}) \text{ mode} & u = 0 - j_{0,1}, \\ LP_{0\ell}(HE_{1\ell} : \ell \geqslant 2) \text{ mode} & u = j_{1,\ell-1} - j_{0,\ell}, \\ LP_{m\ell}(m \geqslant 1,\ \ell \geqslant 1) \text{ mode} & u = j_{m-1,\ell} - j_{m,\ell}. \end{array}$$

Figure 3.4 shows dispersion curves of LP modes for the step-index fiber. They are calculated by numerically solving the dispersion equations (Table 3.1) under the constraints of $u^2 + w^2 = v^2$ [Eq. (3.20)]. The horizontal axis of Fig. 3.4 is

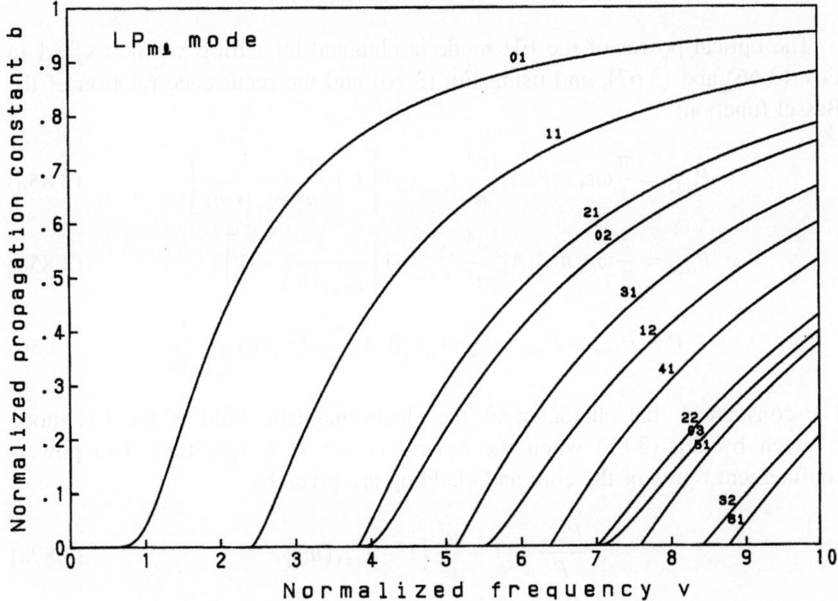

Figure 3.4 Dispersion curves of LP modes in step-index fibers.

the normalized frequency v and the vertical axis is the normalized propagation constant

$$b=\frac{(\beta/k)^2-n_0^2}{n_1^2-n_0^2}. \tag{3.82}$$

3.4.3. Propagating Power of LP Modes

The rigorous Eqs. (3.59) and (3.60) are applied to the TE mode. For the TM mode, if we apply the weakly guiding approximation $n_1 \cong n_0$ to Eqs. (3.63)–(3.65), we obtain the same expression as the TE mode. Then the power carried by TE and TM modes is given by

$$\frac{P_{\text{core}}}{P}=1-\frac{u^2}{v^2}[1-\xi_1(w)] \tag{3.83a}$$

$$\frac{P_{\text{clad}}}{P}=\frac{u^2}{v^2}[1-\xi_1(w)], \tag{3.83b}$$

where

$$\xi_m(w)=\frac{K_m^2(w)}{K_{m-1}(w)K_{m+1}(w)}. \tag{3.84}$$

The optical power of the EH mode is obtained by setting $s \cong s_1 \cong s_0 \cong 1$ in Eqs. (3.66) and (3.67), and using Eq. (3.70) and the recurrence relation of the Bessel function:

$$P_{\text{core}}=\frac{\pi}{2}\omega\varepsilon_0 n_1^2\beta|A|^2\frac{a^4}{u^2}J_{n+1}^2(u)\left[1+\frac{w^2}{u^2}\frac{1}{\xi_{n+1}(w)}\right], \tag{3.85a}$$

$$P_{\text{clad}}=\frac{\pi}{2}\omega\varepsilon_0 n_0^2\beta|A|^2\frac{a^4}{u^2}J_{n+1}^2(u)\left[\frac{1}{\xi_{n+1}(w)}-1\right], \tag{3.85b}$$

$$P=P_{\text{core}}+P_{\text{clad}}=\frac{\pi}{2}\omega\varepsilon_0 n_1^2\beta|A|^2\frac{a^4}{u^4}J_{n+1}^2(u)\frac{v^2}{\xi_{n+1}(w)}. \tag{3.86}$$

The constant A that characterizes the electromagnetic field of the EH mode is given by Eq. (3.86) when the optical power P is specified. The power-confinement ratios of the core and cladding are given by

$$\frac{P_{\text{core}}}{P}=1-\frac{u^2}{v^2}\left[1-\xi_{n+1}(w)\right], \tag{3.87a}$$

$$\frac{P_{\text{clad}}}{P}=\frac{u^2}{v^2}\left[1-\xi_{n+1}(w)\right]. \tag{3.87b}$$

The optical power of the HE mode is obtained by setting $s \cong s_1 \cong s_0 \cong -1$ in Eqs. (3.66) and (3.67), and using Eq. (3.71) and the recurrence relation of the Bessel function to give

$$P = P_{\text{core}} + P_{\text{clad}} = \frac{\pi}{2}\omega\varepsilon_0 n_1^2 \beta |A|^2 \frac{a^4}{u^4} J_{n-1}^2(u) \frac{v^2}{\xi_{n-1}(w)} \tag{3.88}$$

$$\frac{P_{\text{core}}}{P} = 1 - \frac{u^2}{v^2}[1 - \xi_{n-1}(w)], \tag{3.89a}$$

$$\frac{P_{\text{clad}}}{P} = \frac{u^2}{v^2}[1 - \xi_{n-1}(w)], \tag{3.89b}$$

where $\xi_0(w) = K_0^2(w)/K_1^2(w)$. When we use the mode parameter m defined by Eq. (3.73), the power carried by the LP mode is given in the unified expression by

$$\frac{P_{\text{core}}}{P} = 1 - \frac{u^2}{v^2}[1 - \xi_m(w)], \tag{3.90a}$$

$$\frac{P_{\text{clad}}}{P} = \frac{u^2}{v^2}[1 - \xi_m(w)]. \tag{3.90b}$$

Figure 3.5 shows the dependence of the power-confinement factor in the core P_{core}/P on the normalized frequency v. It is known from Fig. 3.5 that (1)

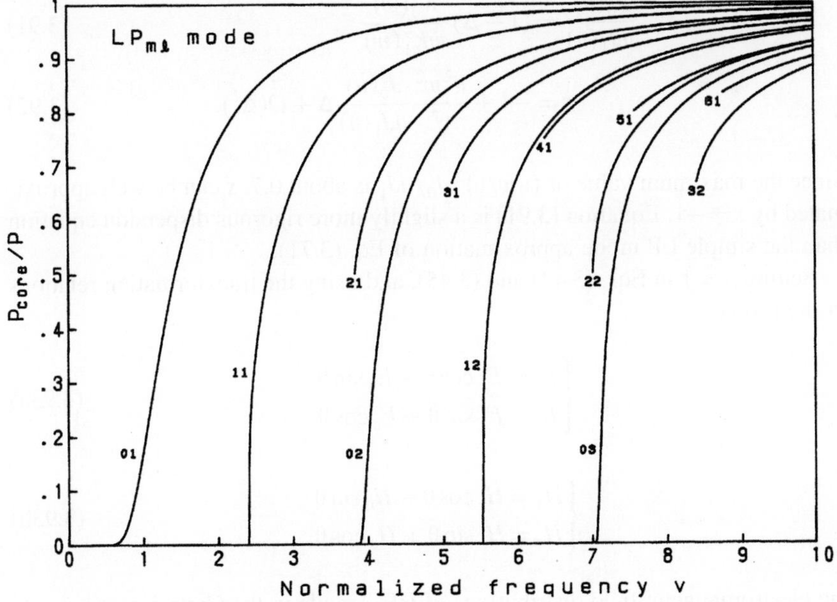

Figure 3.5 Power-confinement factor in the core P_{core}/P of the step-index fiber.

$P_{core}/P \cong 1$ for almost all modes in multimode fibers ($v \gg 1$), and (2) more than 10% of the optical power in single-mode fibers is carried in the cladding even at $v = 2.4$.

3.5. FUNDAMENTAL HE_{11} MODE

It has been clarified in the previous sections that the fundamental mode of the optical fiber is the HE_{11} mode. Therefore it is indispensible to understand the propagation characteristics of the HE_{11} mode in order to grasp the signal transmission properties of single-mode fibers. Here the dispersion characteristics and electromagnetic field distributions of the HE_{11} mode are investigated in detail. In order to rewrite Eqs. (3.40) and (3.41b) to easily understand expressions, we use the recurrence formulae of $J' = J_0 - J_1/u$ and $K' = -K_0 - K_1/w$. Noticing that $\Delta \ll 1$ in practical fibers and also that the dispersion equation in the form

$$\frac{J_1'(u)}{uJ_1(u)} + \frac{K_1'(w)}{wK_1(w)} \cong -\left(\frac{1}{u^2} + \frac{1}{w^2}\right)$$

can be adopted for the HE_{11} mode, Eqs. (3.40) and (3.41b) are reduced to

$$\frac{J_0(u)}{uJ_1(u)} = (1 - \Delta)\frac{K_0(w)}{wK_1(w)} \tag{3.91}$$

$$s = -1 + \frac{u^2 w^2}{v^2}\frac{J_0(u)}{uJ_1(u)}\Delta + O(\Delta^2). \tag{3.92}$$

Since the maximum value of $(uw/v)^2\, J_0/uJ_1$ is about 0.7, s can be well approximated by $s \cong -1$. Equation (3.91) is a slightly more rigorous dispersion equation than the simple LP mode approximation of Eq. (3.71).

Setting $n = 1$ in Eqs. (3.44) and (3.45), and using the transformation relations in the forms

$$\begin{cases} E_x = E_r \cos\theta - E_\theta \sin\theta \\ E_y = E_r \sin\theta + E_\theta \cos\theta, \end{cases} \tag{3.93a}$$

$$\begin{cases} H_x = H_r \cos\theta - H_\theta \sin\theta \\ H_y = H_r \sin\theta + H_\theta \cos\theta, \end{cases} \tag{3.93b}$$

the electromagnetic field distributions of HE_{11} mode in the Cartesian coordinate become the following.

a. *Core region* ($0 \leqslant r \leqslant a$):

$$E_x = -jA\beta\frac{a}{u}\left[\frac{(1-s)}{2}J_0\left(\frac{u}{a}r\right)\cos\psi - \frac{(1+s)}{2}J_2\left(\frac{u}{a}r\right)\cos(2\theta+\psi)\right], \quad (3.94a)$$

$$E_y = jA\beta\frac{a}{u}\left[\frac{(1-s)}{2}J_0\left(\frac{u}{a}r\right)\sin\psi + \frac{(1+s)}{2}J_2\left(\frac{u}{a}r\right)\sin(2\theta+\psi)\right], \quad (3.94b)$$

$$E_z = AJ_1\left(\frac{u}{a}r\right)\cos(\theta+\psi), \quad (3.94c)$$

$$H_x = -jA\omega\varepsilon_0 n_1^2\frac{a}{u}\left[\frac{(1-s_1)}{2}J_0\left(\frac{u}{a}r\right)\sin\psi + \frac{(1+s_1)}{2}J_2\left(\frac{u}{a}r\right)\sin(2\theta+\psi)\right], \quad (3.94d)$$

$$H_y = -jA\omega\varepsilon_0 n_1^2\frac{a}{u}\left[\frac{(1-s_1)}{2}J_0\left(\frac{u}{a}r\right)\cos\psi - \frac{(1+s_1)}{2}J_2\left(\frac{u}{a}r\right)\cos(2\theta+\psi)\right], \quad (3.94e)$$

$$H_z = -A\frac{\beta}{\omega\mu_0}s\,J_1\left(\frac{u}{a}r\right)\sin(\theta+\psi), \quad (3.94f)$$

b. *Cladding region* ($r \geqslant a$):

$$E_x = -jA\beta\frac{aJ_1(u)}{wK_1(w)}\left[\frac{(1-s)}{2}K_0\left(\frac{w}{a}r\right)\cos\psi + \frac{(1+s)}{2}K_2\left(\frac{w}{a}r\right)\cos(2\theta+\psi)\right], \quad (3.95a)$$

$$E_y = jA\beta\frac{aJ_1(u)}{wK_1(w)}\left[\frac{(1-s)}{2}K_0\left(\frac{w}{a}r\right)\sin\psi - \frac{(1+s)}{2}K_2\left(\frac{w}{a}r\right)\sin(2\theta+\psi)\right], \quad (3.95b)$$

$$E_z = A\frac{J_1(u)}{K_1(w)}K_1\left(\frac{w}{a}r\right)\cos(\theta+\psi), \quad (3.95c)$$

$$H_x = -jA\omega\varepsilon_0 n_0^2\frac{aJ_1(u)}{wK_1(w)}\left[\frac{(1-s_0)}{2}K_0\left(\frac{w}{a}r\right)\sin\psi - \frac{(1+s_0)}{2}K_2\left(\frac{w}{a}r\right)\sin(2\theta+\psi)\right], \quad (3.95d)$$

$$H_y = -jA\omega\varepsilon_0 n_0^2 \frac{aJ_1(u)}{wK_1(w)} \left[\frac{(1-s_0)}{2} K_0\left(\frac{w}{a}r\right)\cos\psi \right.$$
$$\left. + \frac{(1+s_0)}{2} K_2\left(\frac{w}{a}r\right)\cos(2\theta+\psi) \right], \quad (3.95e)$$
$$H_z = -A\frac{\beta}{\omega\mu_0} s \frac{J_1(u)}{K_1(w)} K_1\left(\frac{w}{a}r\right)\sin(\theta+\psi). \quad (3.95f)$$

There are two independent polarization modes in Eqs. (3.94) and (3.95), which correspond to $\psi = 0$ and $\psi = \pi/2$. The electric field components in the core with $\psi = 0$ are expressed as

$$E_x = -jA\beta\frac{a}{u}\left[\frac{(1-s)}{2}J_0\left(\frac{u}{a}r\right) - \frac{(1+s)}{2}J_2\left(\frac{u}{a}r\right)\cos(2\theta)\right] \quad (3.96a)$$
$$E_y = jA\beta\frac{a}{u}\frac{(1+s)}{2}J_2\left(\frac{u}{a}r\right)\sin(2\theta) \quad (3.96b)$$
$$E_z = AJ_1\left(\frac{u}{a}r\right)\cos(\theta) \quad (3.96c)$$

and those corresponding to $\psi = \pi/2$ are

$$E_x = -jA\beta\frac{a}{u}\frac{(1+s)}{2}J_2\left(\frac{u}{a}r\right)\sin(2\theta) \quad (3.97a)$$
$$E_y = jA\beta\frac{a}{u}\left[\frac{(1-s)}{2}J_0\left(\frac{u}{a}r\right) + \frac{(1+s)}{2}J_2\left(\frac{u}{a}r\right)\cos(2\theta)\right] \quad (3.97b)$$
$$E_z = -AJ_1\left(\frac{u}{a}r\right)\sin(\theta). \quad (3.97c)$$

Equations (3.94)–(3.97) are rigorous electromagnetic field distributions for the HE_{11} mode. It is known that E_x is the dominant mode in Eq. (3.96) while E_y is the dominant mode in Eq. (3.97), since we know the relation $(1-s)/2 \cong 1$ and $(1+s)/2 \cong \Delta \ll 1$ from Eq. (3.92). Therefore, the polarization mode in Eq. (3.96) with $\psi = 0$ is called HE_{11}^x mode and that in Eq. (3.97) with $\psi = \pi/2$ is called HE_{11}^y mode, respectively. It is shown that the two perpendicularly polarized HE_{11} modes are degenerate in the so–called "single-mode fiber". Although $E_x(E_y)$ mode is the dominant mode in the $HE_{11}^x(HE_{11}^y)$ mode, a quite small E_y (E_x) component having the perpendicular polarization exists in the strict sense. The amplitude ratio of such a minor component to the major one is of the order of Δ ($\ll 1$) and thus can be neglected in most cases. Actually, in the LP mode (weakly guiding approximation), those minor components are neglected. Under this LP mode approximation, the electric field of the HE_{11}^x (HE_{11}^y) mode becomes only the E_x (E_y) component in the cross-sectional plane and thus the electric field vector becomes linear. This is the reason that the mode with a weakly guiding approximation is called "linearly polarized mode."

Substituting Eqs. (3.94) and (3.95), having the approximation of $s \cong s_1 \cong s_0 \cong -1$, into the transmission power equation (3.48)

$$P = \frac{1}{2}\int_0^{2\pi}\int_0^{\infty}\left(E_x H_y^* - E_y H_x^*\right) r\,dr\,d\theta \tag{3.98}$$

and considering the transformation relation of Eq. (3.93), the amplitude coefficient A of the field is given by

$$A = \frac{uw}{\beta a^2 v J_1(u)}\sqrt{\frac{2P}{\pi\varepsilon_0 n_1 c}}, \tag{3.99}$$

where c is the velocity of light in vacuum. Though the eigenvalue of the HE_{11} mode is given by the numerical solution of Eq. (3.91), a useful approximation was derived by Marcuse [9]:

$$u = v\sqrt{1-b} = 2.4048\ e^{-0.8985/v}. \tag{3.100}$$

When we compare the eigenvalue u, which is obtained by numerically solving Eq. (3.91) by setting $\Delta = 0$, with that of Eq. (3.100), the eigenvalue u, by Eq. (3.100) gives a slightly smaller value than the rigorous one. The error of the eigenvalue u given by Eq. (3.100) is less than 0.75% in the range of $v = 0.9$–10 and is less than 0.5% in the range of $v = 0.9$–2.4048, respectively.

3.6. DISPERSION CHARACTERISTICS OF STEP-INDEX FIBERS

3.6.1. Signal Distortion Caused by Group Velocity Dispersion

Let us consider the response when an optical pulse having the Gaussian envelope of the form

$$f(t) = A\exp\left[-\left(\frac{t}{t_{\mathrm{in}}}\right)^2 + j\omega_0 t\right] \tag{3.101}$$

is injected into a fiber. Here ω_0 is a center angular frequency, t_{in} is the input pulse width (which is related with the full width at the half maximum (FWHM) pulse width τ_0 by $\tau_0 = t_{\mathrm{in}}\sqrt{2\ln 2} \cong 1.177 t_{\mathrm{in}}$), and A is a constant. The optical pulse waveform after propagating along the fiber over distance z is expressed by [10]

$$g(t) = \frac{1}{2\pi}\int_{-\infty}^{\infty} F(\omega)e^{-\alpha z + j(\omega t - \beta z)}\,d\omega, \tag{3.102}$$

where $\alpha(\omega)$ and $\beta(\omega)$ denote the amplitude attenuation coefficient and propagation constant of the fiber and $F(\omega)$ is the frequency spectrum of the optical pulse, respectively. The frequency spectrum $F(\omega)$ is given, from Eq. (3.101), as

$$\begin{aligned} F(\omega) &= \int_{-\infty}^{\infty} f(t)e^{-j\omega t}\,dt \\ &= \sqrt{\pi}At_{\text{in}}\exp\left\{-\left[\frac{(\omega-\omega_0)t_{\text{in}}}{2}\right]^2\right\}. \end{aligned} \tag{3.103}$$

Since the attenuation coefficient $\alpha(\omega)$ of the optical fiber is almost independent of ω over the spectral range of $\omega_0 - 2/t_{\text{in}} \leqslant \omega \leqslant \omega_0 + 2/t_{\text{in}}$, $\alpha(\omega)$ is treated as a constant in Eq. (3.102). The propagation constant $\beta(\omega)$ is approximated by the Taylor series around the center angular frequency ω_0 as

$$\beta(\omega) = \beta(\omega_0) + \beta'(\omega_0)(\omega-\omega_0) + \frac{1}{2}\beta''(\omega_0)(\omega-\omega_0)^2 + \cdots, \tag{3.104}$$

where $\beta' = d\beta/d\omega$ and $\beta'' = d^2\beta/d\omega^2$. The output pulse waveform $g(t, z)$ is calculated by substituting Eqs. (3.103) and (3.104) into Eq. (3.102):

$$g(t,z) = \frac{A}{\sqrt{t_{\text{out}}/t_{\text{in}}}}\exp\left\{-\alpha z - \left[\frac{(t-\beta' z)}{t_{\text{out}}}\right]^2 + j[\omega_0 t - \beta_0 z + \theta(t,z)]\right\}, \tag{3.105}$$

where

$$t_{\text{out}} = \left[t_{\text{in}}^2 + \left(\frac{2}{t_{\text{in}}}\beta'' z\right)^2\right]^{1/2}, \tag{3.106}$$

$$\theta(t,z) = \frac{2\beta'' z}{t_{\text{in}}^2}\left(\frac{t-\beta' z}{t_{\text{out}}}\right)^2 - \frac{1}{2}\tan^{-1}\left(\frac{2\beta'' z}{t_{\text{in}}^2}\right). \tag{3.107}$$

It is known from Eq. (3.105) that the relation $(t - \beta' z)$ represents the progression of the optical pulse. The velocity of the optical pulse (signal) is then given by

$$v_g = \frac{dz}{dt} = \frac{1}{\beta'} = \frac{1}{d\beta/d\omega}, \tag{3.108}$$

where v_g is called the group velocity. In Eq. (3.106) t_{out} is an output pulse width (FWHM pulse width is $\tau_{\text{out}} = t_{\text{out}}\sqrt{2\ln 2}$) after propagating the distance z. Since t_{in} is the input pulse width,

$$\delta t = \left| \frac{2}{t_{\text{in}}} \beta'' z \right| \tag{3.109}$$

is the pulse spreading (signal distortion) caused by the optical fiber. The second derivative of β is related with the group velocity by $\beta''/(\beta')^2 = -dv_g/d\omega$. Therefore if the group velocity varies with the signal frequency $dv_g/d\omega \neq 0$ (or varies with signal wavelength component $dv_g/d\lambda \neq 0$), the second derivative of β becomes $\beta'' \neq 0$ and it brings the signal distortion. The variation of group velocity with the signal frequency (wavelength) is called *group velocity dispersion* (GVD).

It is known from Eq. (3.103) that $\delta\omega = 2/t_{\text{in}}$ is approximately spectral width of the signal pulse. Thus the pulse spreading is known to become large for large $|\beta''|$ and large spectral width $\delta\omega$ (small input pulse width t_{in}).

The typical β'' value at 1.55-μm wavelength is about $\beta'' = -2 \times 10^{-2}\,\text{ps}^2/\text{m}$. Figure 3.6 shows the output pulse waveform of a $B = 10$-Gbit/s pulse train with the PCM (pulse code modulation) code of "110111", when it was coupled into the fiber having $\beta'' = -2 \times 10^{-2}\,\text{ps}^2/\text{m}$. The FWHM width of the input pulse is $\tau_0 = 20\,\text{ps}$ and bit rate $B = 1/T$, where T is the pulse repetition rate. It is shown that the pulse broadening becomes large as the propagation length increases and that the signal is almost completely lost at $z = 50\,\text{km}$ (propagation loss of the fiber is assumed to be $\alpha = 0$ in Fig. 3.6). It should be noted here that even though the optical power itself is not dissipated, the signal can be lost by the fiber dispersion as shown in Fig. 3.6(c). In practical fibers, signal energy is further lost by the attenuation of the fiber. Therefore there are two factors limiting the transmission distance (or repeater spacing) of the signal in the fiber: dispersion and attenuation. Two cases are considered, depending on the dominance of the effects. First is a case where attenuation is larger than dispersion. For example, for the case shown in Fig. 3.6(b), the signal cannot be received when the peak intensity of the signal pulse of bit "1" becomes lower than the detection level of the receiver, even though the signal distortion caused by dispersion is not so large. This situation is called the "*loss limit*". In contrast is the second case, where dispersion is larger than attenuation. As shown in Fig. 3.6(c), when the signal component is lost due to dispersion, the signal cannot be received even though the optical energy itself is larger than the detection level. Such a situation is called the "*dispersion limit*".

The reduction in the attenuation of optical fibers owes much to improvements in fabrication technologies, and the ultralow attenuation of 0.154 dB/km ($\alpha = 1.77 \times 10^{-6}\text{m}^{-1}$) has been achieved in the 1.55-μm region [1]. In contrast, the

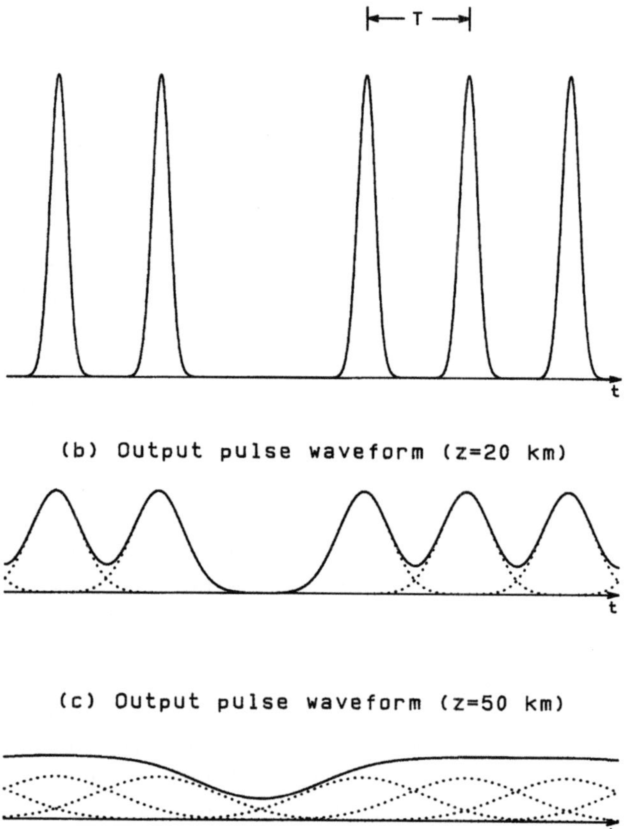

Figure 3.6 Several pulse waveforms with PCM code of "11011." (a) Input pulse waveform, (b) output pulse waveform after $z = 20\,\text{km}$ of the fiber with $\beta'' = -2 \times 10^{-2}\,\text{ps}^2/\text{m}$, and (c) output pulse after $z = 50$-km propagation.

dispersion characteristics of optical fiber are closely related with the refractive-index profile. Therefore, an analysis method that enables the calculation of the propagation constant β and its second derivative β'' for arbitrary index profiles is strongly required.

The spectral intensity distribution of the pulse repetition sequence [Fig. 3.6(a)] of the form

$$f(t) = \sum_{n=-\infty}^{\infty} A \exp\left\{-\left[\frac{(t - nT)}{t_{\text{in}}}\right]^2 + j\omega_0 t\right\} \tag{3.110}$$

is given by

$$S(\omega) = \left| \int_{-\infty}^{\infty} f(t) e^{-j\omega t} dt \right|^2. \tag{3.111}$$

When the peak intensity of $S(\omega)$ is normalized to unity, it is expressed as

$$S(\omega) = \lim_{N\to\infty} \left\{ \left[\frac{\sin(N\phi)}{2N\sin(\phi/2)} \right]^2 e^{-[(\omega-\omega_0)t_{\text{in}}]^2/2} \right\}, \tag{3.112}$$

where ϕ denotes

$$\phi = (\omega - \omega_0)T = 2\pi(f - f_0)T. \tag{3.113}$$

The value in the parenthesis of Eq. (3.112) is unity for $\phi = 2m\pi$ (m is an integer) and zero for all other value of ϕ. Therefore, the spectral intensity distribution $S(\omega)$ becomes a line spectrum, as shown in Fig. 3.7. The interval in the line spectrum is $f_m - f_{m-1} = 1/T$. The envelope of $S(\omega)$ is a Gaussian shape with spectral FWHM of

$$\delta f = \frac{0.44}{\tau_0}. \tag{3.114}$$

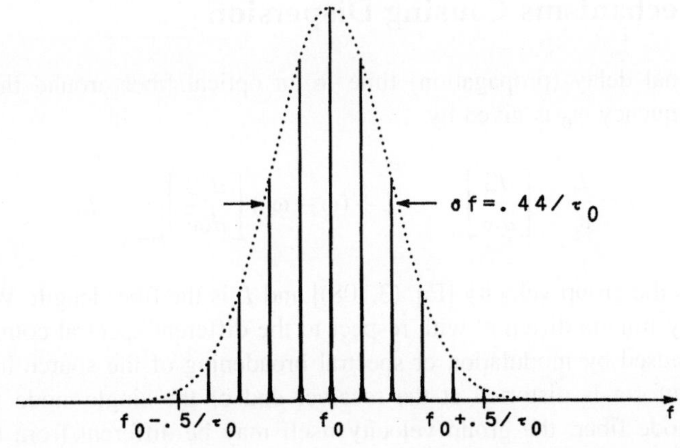

Figure 3.7 Spectral intensity distribution of the pulse repetition sequence having the FWHM pulse width of τ_0.

The spectrum occupies the frequency width of about $f_0 - 0.5/\tau_0 \leqslant f \leqslant f_0 + 0.5/\tau_0$. Taking into account the relation $\tau_0 = t_{\text{in}}\sqrt{2\ln 2}$, the FWHM width in terms of angular frequency is

$$\delta\omega = 2\pi\delta f = \frac{2.35}{t_{\text{in}}}. \tag{3.115}$$

Substituting Eq. (3.115) into Eq. (3.109) the pulse broadening due to the dispersion is expressed approximately by

$$\delta t \cong |\beta'' z \delta\omega| . \tag{3.116}$$

There are two basic modulation formats in PCM (pulse code modulation) as shown in Fig. 3.8. One is a RZ (return-to-zero) pulse waveform as shown in Fig. 3.8(a): the other is a NRZ (nonreturn-to-zero) pulse waveform, as shown in 3.8(b). The pulse width of the RZ pulse for 1 bit is roughly $\tau_{RZ} = 0.5/B$, where B is a bitrate. On the other hand, the minimum pulse width of the NRZ is about $\tau_{NRZ} = 1/B$. From the relation (3.114) between pulse width and spectral width for the Gaussian pulse, the spectral FWHM of the RZ pulse becomes $\delta f_{RZ} \cong 0.5/\tau_{RZ} = B$ and that of the NRZ pulse is $\delta f_{NRZ} \cong 0.5/\tau_{NRZ} = B/2$. It is known that the bandwidth occupation in the NRZ pulse is half that in the RZ pulse when transmitting the same bitrate B. The signal frequency range of an NRZ pulse is known to be about $f_0 - B/2 \leqslant f \leqslant f_0 + B/2$ when considering $\tau_0 = \tau_{NRZ} = 1/B$ in Fig. 3.7.

3.6.2. Mechanisms Causing Dispersion

The signal delay (propagation) time in an optical fiber around the center angular frequency ω_0 is given by

$$t = \frac{L}{v_g} = \left[\frac{d\beta}{d\omega}\right]_{\omega=\omega_0} \cdot L + (\omega - \omega_0)\left[\frac{d^2\beta}{d\omega^2}\right]_{\omega=\omega_0} \cdot L, \tag{3.117}$$

where v_g is the group velocity [Eq. (3.108)] and L is the fiber length. When the signal delay time is different with respect to the different spectral components, which is caused by modulation or spectral broadening of the source itself, the signal waveform is distorted at the receiver end of the single-mode fiber. In the multimode fiber, the group velocity itself may be different from mode to mode, and this causes the pulse broadening. There are four kinds of delay-time dispersion of fibers.

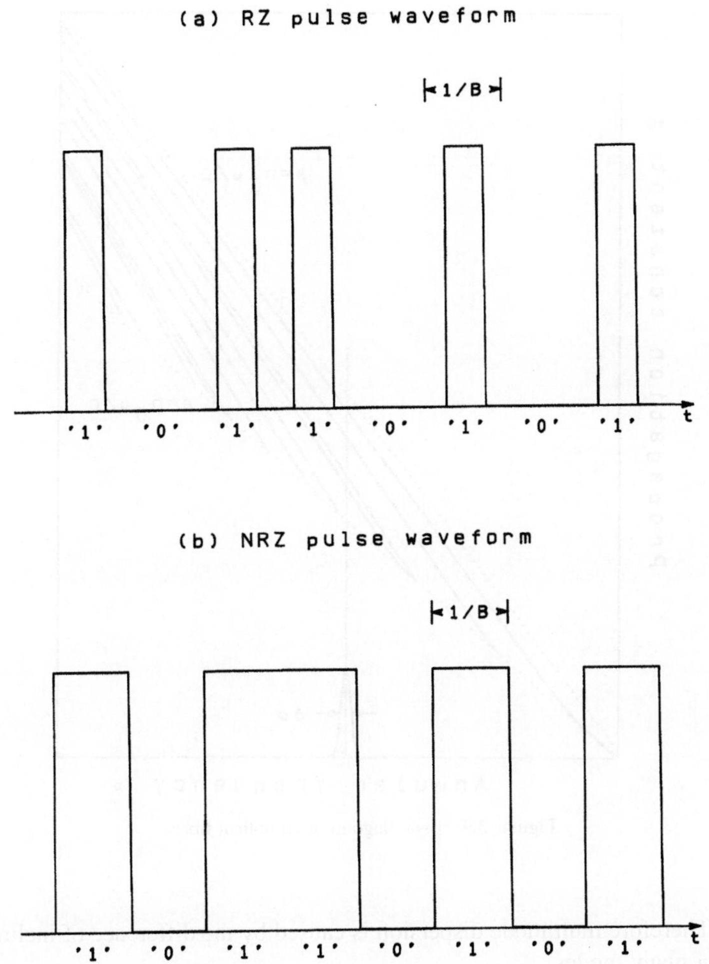

Figure 3.8 Two modulation formats in PCM: (a) RZ pulse and (b) NRZ pulse waveform.

3.6.2.1. Multimode Dispersion

Multimode dispersion is the delay-time dispersion caused by the difference of group velocity of the various modes [the first term in rightmost equation of Eq. (3.117)] in a multimode fiber. The $\beta-\omega$ diagram in Fig. 3.9 shows the transmission characteristics of an optical fiber. There are many dispersion curves corresponding to the modes between the two lines $\beta = n_1\omega/c$ and $\beta = n_0\omega/c$. The inclination of the curve $d\beta/d\omega$ at the intersection point of the curve with the constant-frequency line (dash-dotted line) gives the group velocity for each

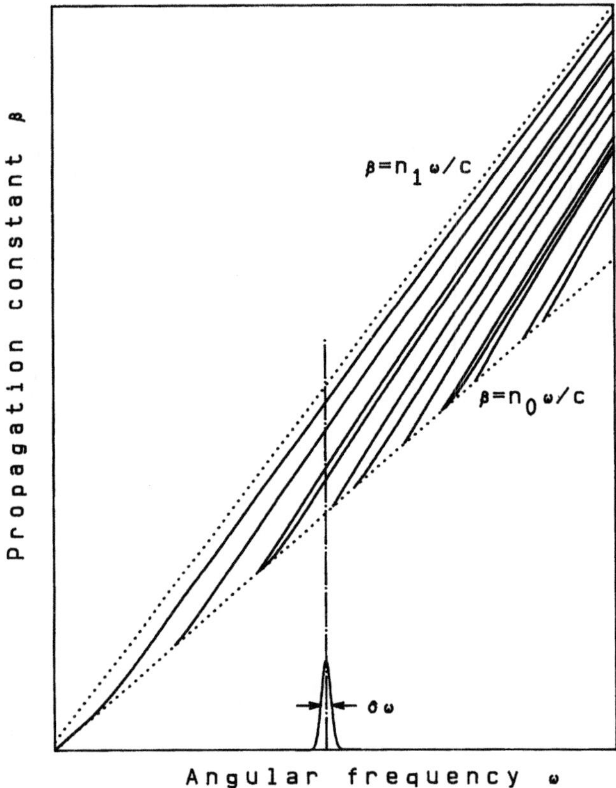

Figure 3.9 β–ω diagram of an optical fiber.

mode. Therefore multimode dispersion is caused by the difference of inclination between many modes.

3.6.2.2. Polarization Mode Dispersion

Polarization mode dispersion is a delay-time difference between the orthogonally polarized HE_{11}^x and HE_{11}^y modes in the "nominally" single-mode fibers or birefringent fibers (which will be described in Section 3.9). The slight birefringence in the single-mode fiber is caused by the non concentricity of the core and the elliptical deformation of the core.

The next two dispersions exist even when the fiber is truly single-moded. They are caused by the last term in Eq. (3.117) and are proportional to the signal spectral width $(\omega - \omega_0)$.

3.6.2.3. Material Dispersion

Material dispersion is a delay-time dispersion caused by the fact that the refractive index of the glass material changes in accordance with the change of the signal frequency (or wavelength). Figure 3.10 shows the dependence of refractive indices of the core and cladding on the frequency for an optical fiber with relative refractive-index difference $\Delta = 0.6\%$. It is known from Fig. 3.10 that the two dotted lines $\beta = n_1\omega/c$ and $\beta = n_0\omega/c$, depicted as straight lines in Fig. 3.9 are slightly, curved; that is, they are nonlinearly frequency dependent. This nonlinearity of the refractive index causes a non zero value for $d^2\beta/d\omega^2$.

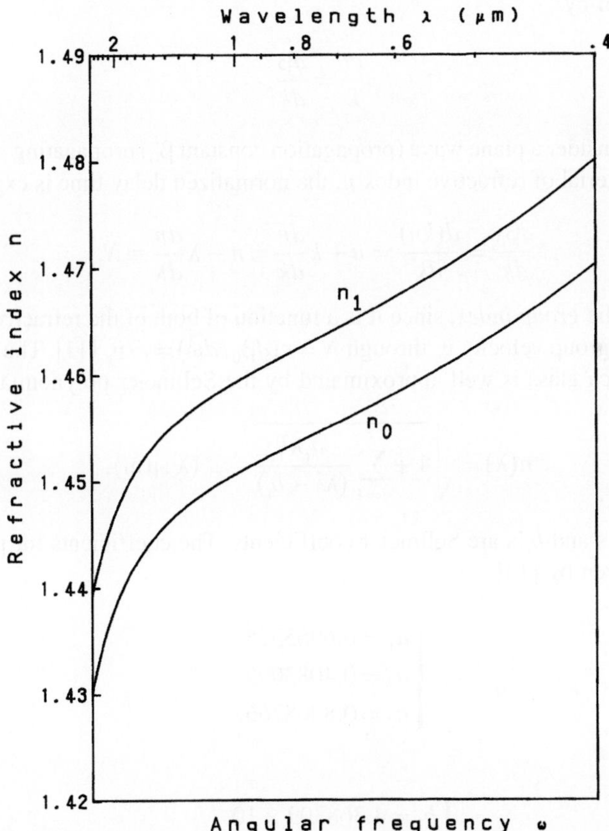

Figure 3.10 Refractive indices of silica glass as a function of the angular frequency ω (or wavelength λ).

3.6.2.4. Waveguide Dispersion

Waveguide dispersion is a delay-time dispersion caused by the confinement of light in the waveguide structure. As shown in Fig. 3.9 or 3.4, the dependence of the propagation constant β (or normalized propagation constant b) on the angular frequency ω (or normalized frequency v) is nonlinear for light propagating in the waveguide. Therefore waveguide dispersion is an essential dispersion that inevitably exists in waveguides.

3.6.3. Derivation of Delay-time Formula

Let us calculate the first term of Eq. (3.117) which is related to the multimode dispersion. The delay time t in the fiber relative to the delay time in a vacuum, L/c, is given by

$$\frac{ct}{L} = \frac{d\beta}{dk}. \tag{3.118}$$

When we consider a plane wave (propagation constant β_0) propagating in a homogeneous material of refractive index n, the normalized delay time is expressed as

$$\frac{d\beta_0}{dk} = \frac{d(kn)}{dk} = n + k\frac{dn}{dk} = n - \lambda\frac{dn}{d\lambda} \equiv N. \tag{3.119}$$

N is called the *group index*, since it is a function of both of the refractive index n and also the group velocity v_g through $N = c(d\beta_0/d\omega) = c/v_g$ [11]. The refractive index of silica glass is well approximated by the Sellmeier polynomial [12]

$$n(\lambda) = \sqrt{1 + \sum_{i=1}^{3} \frac{a_i\lambda^2}{(\lambda^2 - b_i)}} \qquad (\lambda : \mu\text{m}), \tag{3.120}$$

where the a_i's and b_i's are Sellmeier coefficients. The coefficients for pure silica glass are given by [13]

$$\begin{cases} a_1 = 0.6965325 \\ a_2 = 0.4083099 \\ a_3 = 0.8968766, \end{cases} \tag{3.121a}$$

$$\begin{cases} b_1 = 4.368309 \times 10^{-3} \\ b_2 = 1.394999 \times 10^{-2} \\ b_3 = 9.793399 \times 10^{1}. \end{cases} \tag{3.121b}$$

The Sellmeier coefficients in doped silica glasses depend on the dopant material and concentration. For example, the Sellmeier coefficients of G_eO_2-doped glass with 6.3 mol% concentration are given by

$$\begin{cases} a_1 = 0.7083952 \\ a_2 = 0.4203993 \\ a_3 = 0.8663412, \end{cases} \tag{3.122a}$$

$$\begin{cases} b_1 = 7.290464 \times 10^{-3} \\ b_2 = 1.050294 \times 10^{-2} \\ b_3 = 9.793428 \times 10^{1}. \end{cases} \tag{3.122b}$$

The relative refractive-index difference between G_eO_2-doped glass of 6.3 mol% concentration and pure silica glass is about $\Delta = 0.6\%$. Figure 3.10 shows the refractive-index dispersion of a fiber having 6.3 mol% G_eO_2-doped glass as the core (n_1) and pure silica glass as the cladding (n_0).

The propagation constant β is expressed in terms of the normalized propagation constant b as

$$\beta = k\sqrt{n_0^2 + (n_1^2 - n_0^2)b} \cong k[n_0 + (n_1 - n_0)b]. \tag{3.123}$$

Substituting the above equation into (3.118), we obtain

$$\frac{d\beta}{dk} = N_0 + (N_1 - N_0)b + k(n_1 - n_0)\frac{db}{dk}. \tag{3.124}$$

Noticing the relation of $k \propto v$ and that the difference between the core–cladding refractive indices are almost the same as that between the group indices, we can approximate as

$$(n_1 - n_0) \cong (N_1 - N_0), \tag{3.125}$$

Then Eq. (3.124) can be rewritten

$$\frac{d\beta}{dk} \cong N_0 + (N_1 - N_0)\frac{d(vb)}{dv}. \tag{3.126}$$

The normalized delay time $d\beta/dk$ can be calculated from the v–b dispersion curve and group indices N_1 and N_0 as follows.

Group indices N_1 and N_0 are calculated from Eqs. (3.119) and (3.120). Figure 3.11 shows the group indices of a fiber consisting of a core with 6.3 mol%

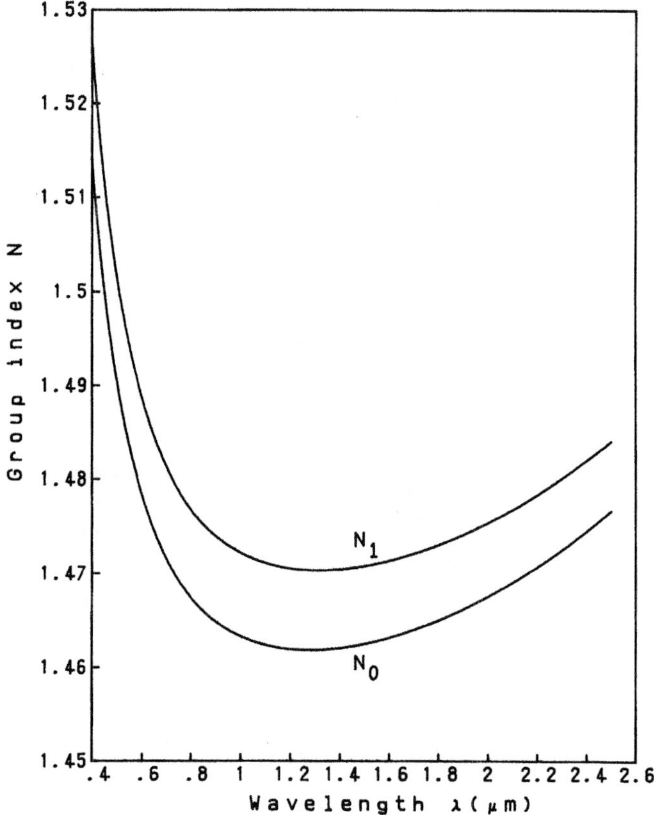

Figure 3.11 Group indices of a fiber consisting of a core with 6.3 mol% G_eO_2-doped glass and a pure silica cladding.

G_eO_2-doped glass and a pure silica cladding. Next we will consider the calculation of $d(vb)/dv$. First, the unified dispersion equation (3.74) for the $LP_{m\ell}$ mode is differentiated by v. Here it is expressed by reversing the denominator and numerator:

$$\frac{uJ_{m-1}(u)}{J_m(u)} = -\frac{wK_{m-1}(w)}{K_m(w)} \tag{3.127}$$

so that the differentiation becomes easy.

The differentiation of both terms in Eq. (3.127) with respect to v gives

$$\frac{d}{du}\left[\frac{uJ_{m-1}}{J_m}\right]\frac{du}{dv} = -\frac{d}{dw}\left[\frac{wK_{m-1}}{K_m}\right]\frac{dw}{dv}, \tag{3.128}$$

where

$$\frac{d}{du}\left[\frac{uJ_{m-1}}{J_m}\right]=u\left[\frac{J_{m-1}(u)J_{m+1}(u)}{J_m^2(u)}-1\right], \tag{3.129a}$$

and

$$\frac{d}{dw}\left[\frac{wK_{m-1}}{K_m}\right]=w\left[\frac{K_{m-1}(w)K_{m+1}(w)}{K_m^2(w)}-1\right]. \tag{3.129b}$$

Here we can be express (3.127) in a different form when we notice the recurrence relation of Bessel functions (3.42) and (3.43) and obtain

$$\frac{uJ_{m+1}(u)}{J_m(u)}=\frac{wK_{m+1}(w)}{K_m(w)}. \tag{3.130}$$

Combining Eqs. (3.127) and (3.130), we obtain the relation

$$\frac{J_{m-1}(u)J_{m+1}(u)}{J_m^2(u)}=-\frac{w^2}{u^2}\frac{K_{m-1}(w)K_{m+1}(w)}{K_m^2(w)}. \tag{3.131}$$

Moreover, when we put the relation $u^2+w^2=v^2$ and Eqs. (3.84), (3.129) and (3.131) into Eq. (3.128), it is reduced to

$$\frac{du}{dv}=\frac{u}{v}[1-\xi_m(w)]. \tag{3.132}$$

Considering the relation of $u=v\sqrt{1-b}$, we obtain the expression for $d(vb)/dv$ as

$$\frac{d(vb)}{dv}=b+2(1-b)\xi_m(w). \tag{3.133}$$

Figure 3.12 shows the dependence of $d(vb)/dv$ for the $\mathrm{LP}_{m\ell}$ mode on the normalized frequency v. When the electromagnetic energy is tightly confined in the core—in other words for large v—the normalized group delay $d(vb)/dv$ approaches unity. In such a condition, it is known from Eqs. (3.118) and (3.126) that $d\beta/dk=N_1$, and the delay time becomes

$$t=\frac{N_1L}{c}. \tag{3.134}$$

Multimode dispersion is defined as the dispersion of the group delay time of each mode at a certain frequency. Therefore, multimode dispersion of a step-index fiber can be obtained by calculating the variance of the value $d(vb)/dv$ of

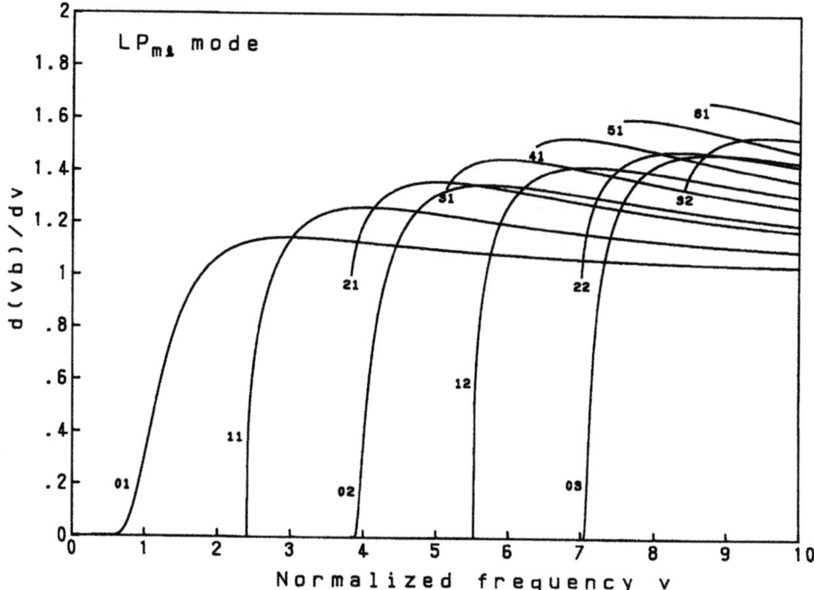

Figure 3.12 Normalized group delay for the step-index fiber.

each mode at the intersecting point of the normalized group delay curve with the straight line at a fixed v-value in Fig. 3.12. However, there are several hundreds of modes [refer to Eq. (3.186) in Section 3.7.2] in the multimode fiber with $\Delta = 1\%$ and $2a = 50\,\mu\text{m}$, and therefore it is quite tedious to calculate $d(vb)/dv$ for each mode. Moreover, the optimum refractive-index profile of a multimode fiber, in which multimode dispersion becomes a minimum, is a quadratic-index profile rather than a step-index profile. The WKB (Wentzel–Kramers–Brillouin) method is a suitable way to analyze the propagation characteristics and dispersion properties of graded-index fibers. Analysis of graded-index fibers using the WKB method will be described in Section 3.7.

3.6.4. Chromatic Dispersion

The sum of material dispersion and waveguide dispersion is called *chromatic dispersion.* Group delay-time dispersion is given, as shown in Eq. (3.116) or (3.117), by

$$\delta t = \left[\frac{d^2\beta}{d\omega^2}\right]_{\omega=\omega_0} \cdot L\ \delta\omega. \tag{3.135}$$

This equation can be rewritten using the relations $\omega = kc$ and $k = 2\pi/\lambda$ as

$$\delta t = -\frac{\delta\lambda}{\lambda}\frac{L}{c}k\frac{d^2\beta}{dk^2}, \tag{3.136}$$

where $\delta\lambda/\lambda$ represents the relative spectral width of the signal source. Differentiation of Equation (3.126) by k while keeping the relation $v \propto k$ in mind gives

$$k\frac{d^2\beta}{dk^2} = k\frac{dN_0}{dk} + k\frac{d(N_1 - N_0)}{dk}\frac{d(vb)}{dv} + (N_1 - N_0)v\frac{d^2(vb)}{dv^2}, \tag{3.137}$$

The derivative of the group index N given by Eq. (3.119) with respect to k is then reduced to

$$k\frac{dN}{dk} = -\lambda\frac{dN}{d\lambda} = \lambda^2\frac{d^2n}{d\lambda^2} \equiv s. \tag{3.138}$$

s is a normalized material dispersion and is readily obtained by differentiating the refractive index n expressed by the Sellmeier polynomial. Figure 3.13 shows the normalized material dispersions of a fiber consisting of a core with 6.3 mol% G_eO_2-doped glass and pure silica cladding. It is known that the material dispersion of silica-based optical fiber becomes zero in the 1.3-μm region.

In Eq. (3.137), $vd^2(vb)/dv^2$ is obtained by differentiating Eq. (3.133) by v and may be written

$$v\frac{d^2(vb)}{dv^2} = 2(1-b)\xi_m(w)\left[(1 - 2\,\xi_m) + \left(1 + \frac{(1-b)}{b}\xi_m\right)(2 - \zeta_m)\right], \tag{3.139}$$

where ζ_m is given by

$$\zeta_m(w) = w\left[\frac{K_{m-1}(w)}{K_m(w)} + \frac{K_{m+1}(w)}{K_m(w)} - \frac{K_m(w)}{K_{m+1}(w)} - \frac{K_m(w)}{K_{m-1}(w)}\right], \tag{3.140}$$

and

$$\frac{d\xi_m}{dw} = \frac{\xi_m}{w}(2 - \zeta_m). \tag{3.141}$$

Figure 3.14 shows the normalized waveguide dispersion $vd^2(vb)/dv^2$ of the $LP_{m\ell}$ modes for a step-index fiber. It is shown that $vd^2(vb)/dv^2 > 0$ in the

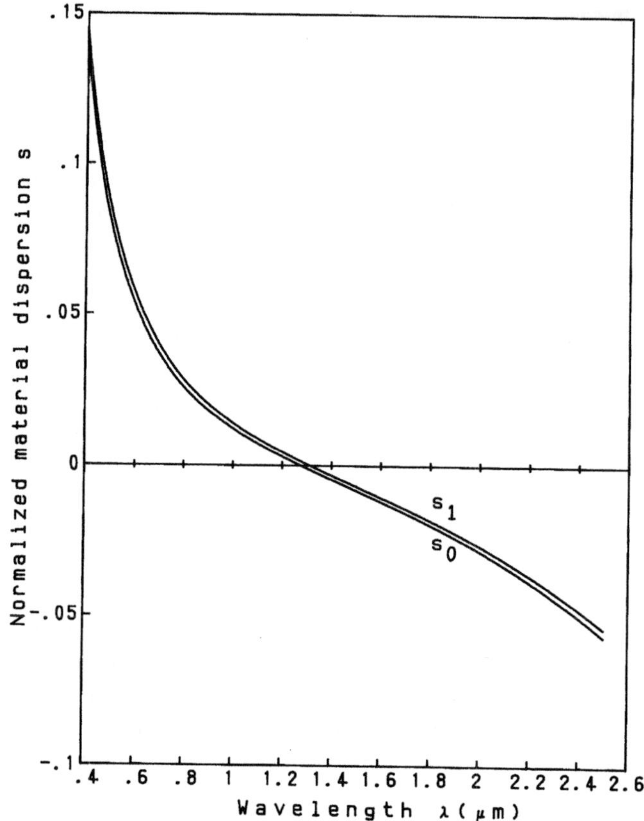

Figure 3.13 Normalized material dispersions of a fiber consisting of a core with 6.3 mol% G_eO_2-doped glass and pure silica cladding.

single-mode region ($v < 2.405$) of the step-index fiber. Equation (3.137) can then be simplified to

$$k\frac{d^2\beta}{dk^2} = s_0 + (s_1 - s_0)\frac{d(vb)}{dv} + (N_1 - N_0)v\frac{d^2(vb)}{dv^2}. \qquad (3.142)$$

Strictly speaking, material dispersion and waveguide dispersion are complicatedly mixed and cannot be separated into two independent dispersions. However, the third term in Eq. (3.142) clearly represents the influence of the waveguide structure. Therefore, here the third term is defined as the waveguide dispersion and the sum of the first and second terms is defined as the material dispersion, respectively. Although the pulse broadening due to chromatic dispersion is given

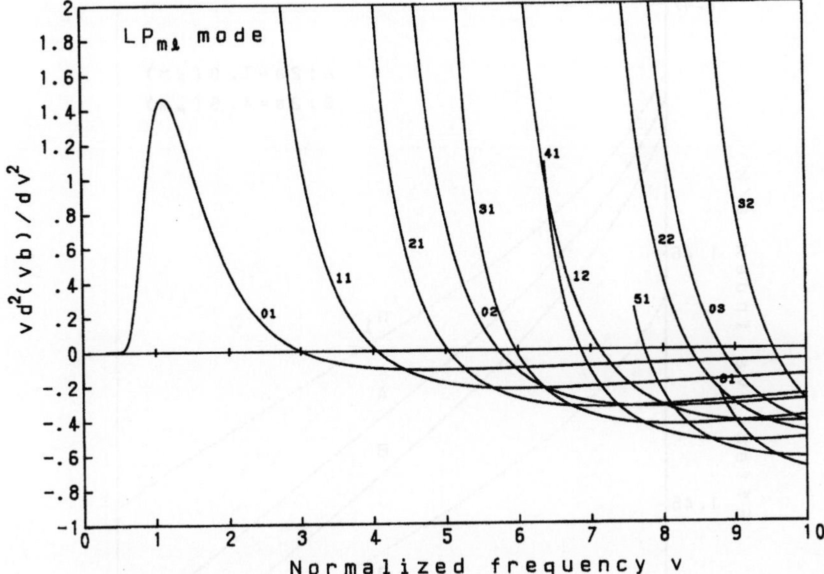

Figure 3.14 Normalized waveguide dispersion for the step-index fiber.

by (3.136), the dispersion is usually expressed in terms of unit fiber length and unit spectral broadening:

$$\sigma = \frac{\delta t}{L\,\delta\lambda} = -\frac{1}{c\lambda}k\frac{d^2\beta}{dk^2}. \tag{3.143}$$

The chromatic dispersion is then expressed as

$$\sigma = \sigma_m + \sigma_w, \tag{3.144}$$

where

$$\sigma_m = -\frac{1}{c\lambda}\left[s_0 + (s_1 - s_0)\frac{d(vb)}{dv}\right] \tag{3.145a}$$

and

$$\sigma_w = -\frac{(N_1 - N_0)}{c\lambda}v\frac{d^2(vb)}{dv^2}. \tag{3.145b}$$

Figures 3.15, 3.16, and 3.17 show the effective indices β/k [Eq. (3.123)], normalized delay times $d\beta/dk$ [Eq. (3.126)] and chromatic dispersions σ [Eq. (3.144)]

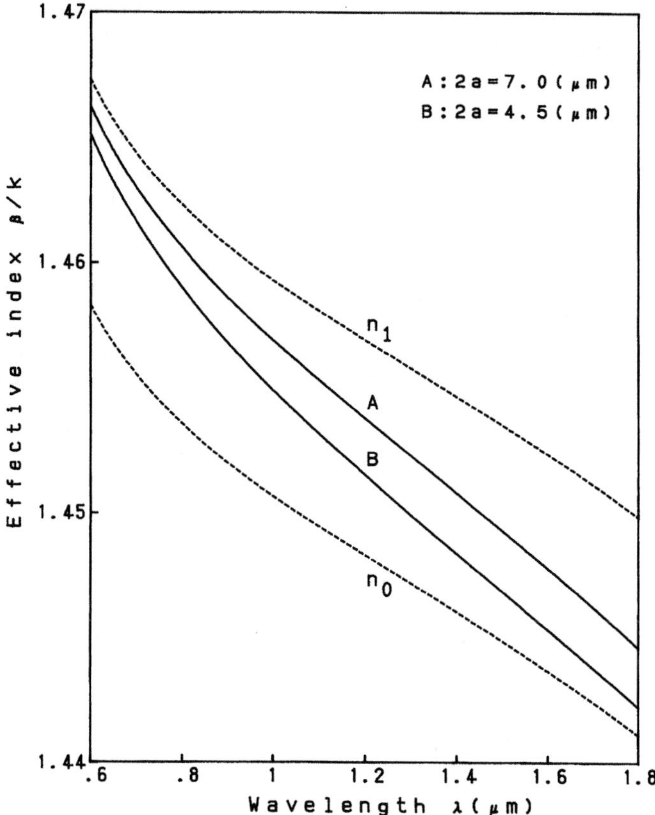

Figure 3.15 Effective indices β/k of a fiber consisting of a core with 6.3 mol% G_eO_2-doped glass and pure silica cladding. (Dotted lines indicate the refractive indices of core and cladding).

for the two core diameters $2a = 7.0\,\mu m$ and $2a = 4.5\,\mu m$ in a fiber consisting of a core with 6.3 mol% G_eO_2-doped glass and a pure silica cladding. As shown in Figs. 3.13 and 3.17, the material dispersion of G_eO_2-doped glass is almost the same as that of pure silica glass ($s_1 - s_0 \approx 0$). The dependence of the waveguide dispersion on the normalized frequency v, which is shown in Fig. 3.14, is plotted in Fig. 3.18 as a function of the normalized wavelength λ/λ_c, where λ_c is the cutoff wavelength of the LP_{11} mode. The normalized waveguide dispersion at the cutoff $v = v_c(\lambda/\lambda_c = 0)$ is

$$-\frac{c\lambda}{(N_1 - N_0)}\sigma_w = v\frac{d^2(vb)}{dv^2} = 0.193,$$

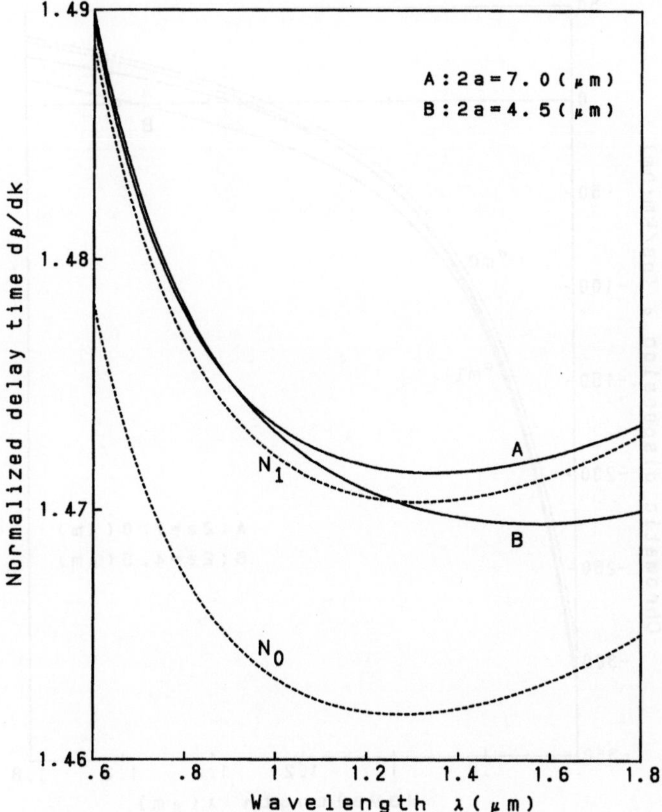

Figure 3.16 Normalized delay times $d\beta/dk$ of a fiber consisting of a core with 6.3 mol% G_eO_2-doped glass and pure silica cladding. (Dotted lines indicate the group indices of core and cladding).

and becomes a maximum at $v = 1.131(\lambda/\lambda_c = 2.126)$ given by

$$-\frac{c\lambda}{(N_1 - N_0)}\sigma_w = v\frac{d^2(vb)}{dv^2} = 1.464.$$

It is known that the value of the waveguide dispersion σ_w can be controlled by selecting appropriate values of the waveguide parameters N_1, N_0 and wavelength λ.

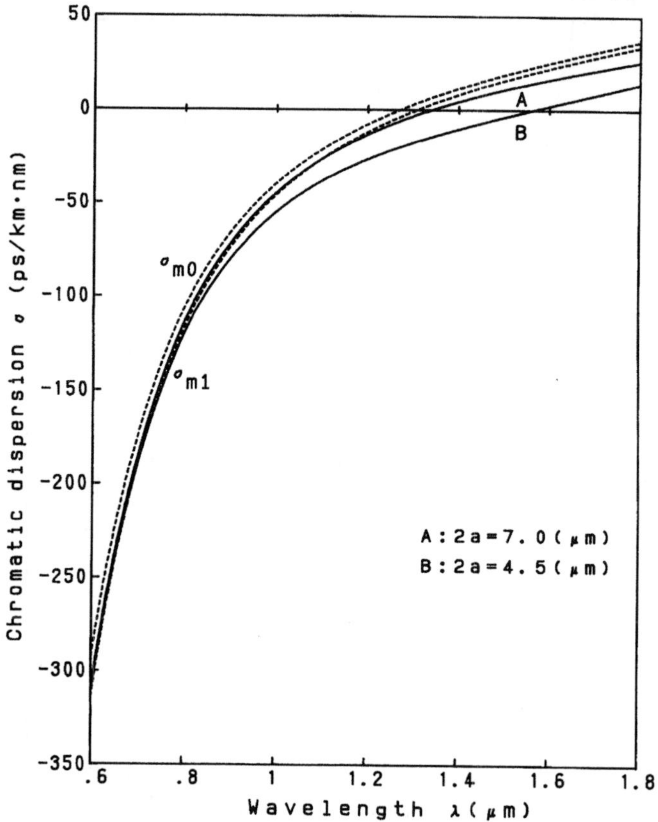

Figure 3.17 Chromatic dispersions σ of a fiber consisting of a core with 6.3 mol% G_eO_2-doped glass and pure silica cladding. (Dotted lines indicate the normalized dispersions of core and cladding).

3.6.5. Zero-dispersion Wavelength

Chromatic dispersion in a single-mode fiber is the sum of material dispersion and waveguide dispersion, as shown in Eqs. (3.144) and (3.145). As described in the previous section, the waveguide dispersion can be controlled by proper choice of the waveguide parameters, while the material dispersion is almost independent of these parameters. Therefore, the zero dispersion wavelength, at which the sum of material and waveguide dispersions becomes zero, can also be controlled by changing the core diameter $2a$ and relative refractive-index difference Δ (more generally the cutoff wavelength λ_c). Figures 3.19(a) and (b) show material, waveguide and total dispersions of fibers having (a) $\Delta = 0.3\%$ and $2a = 8.2\,\mu\text{m}$ and (b) $\Delta = 0.7\%$ and $2a = 4.6\,\mu\text{m}$, respectively. It is confirmed

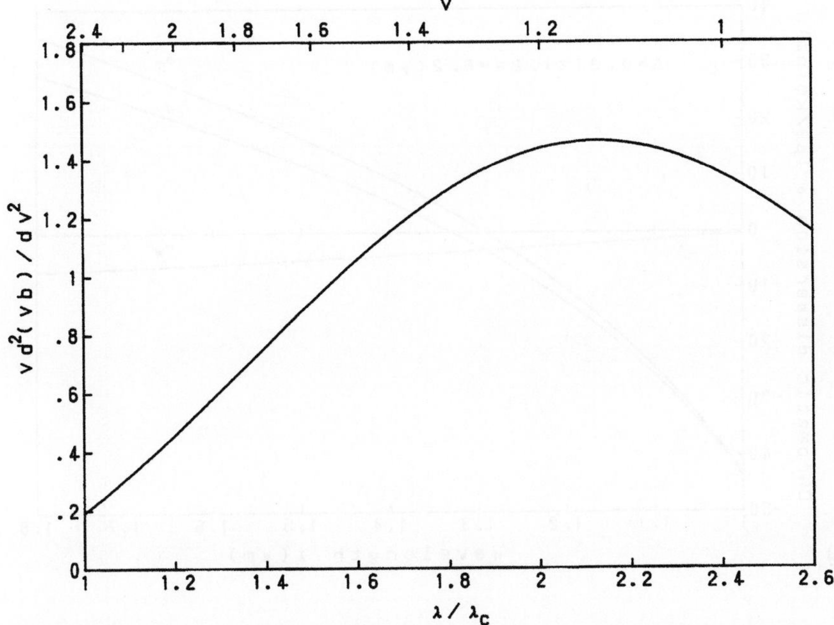

Figure 3.18 Normalized waveguide dispersion of the LP_{01} mode in a step-index fiber.

from the figure that the zero dispersion wavelength can be made coincident with the 1.55-μm minimum loss wavelength of optical fibers.

3.7. WAVE THEORY OF GRADED-INDEX FIBERS

3.7.1. Basic Equations and Mode Concepts in Graded-index Fibers

First, the basic equations for wave propagation in graded-index fibers are derived. The detailed treatment is described in Ref. 3. We express the refractive-index distribution and the propagation constant in the forms

$$n^2(r) = n_1^2[1 - f(r)], \tag{3.146}$$

$$\beta^2 = k^2 n_1^2(1 - \chi), \tag{3.147}$$

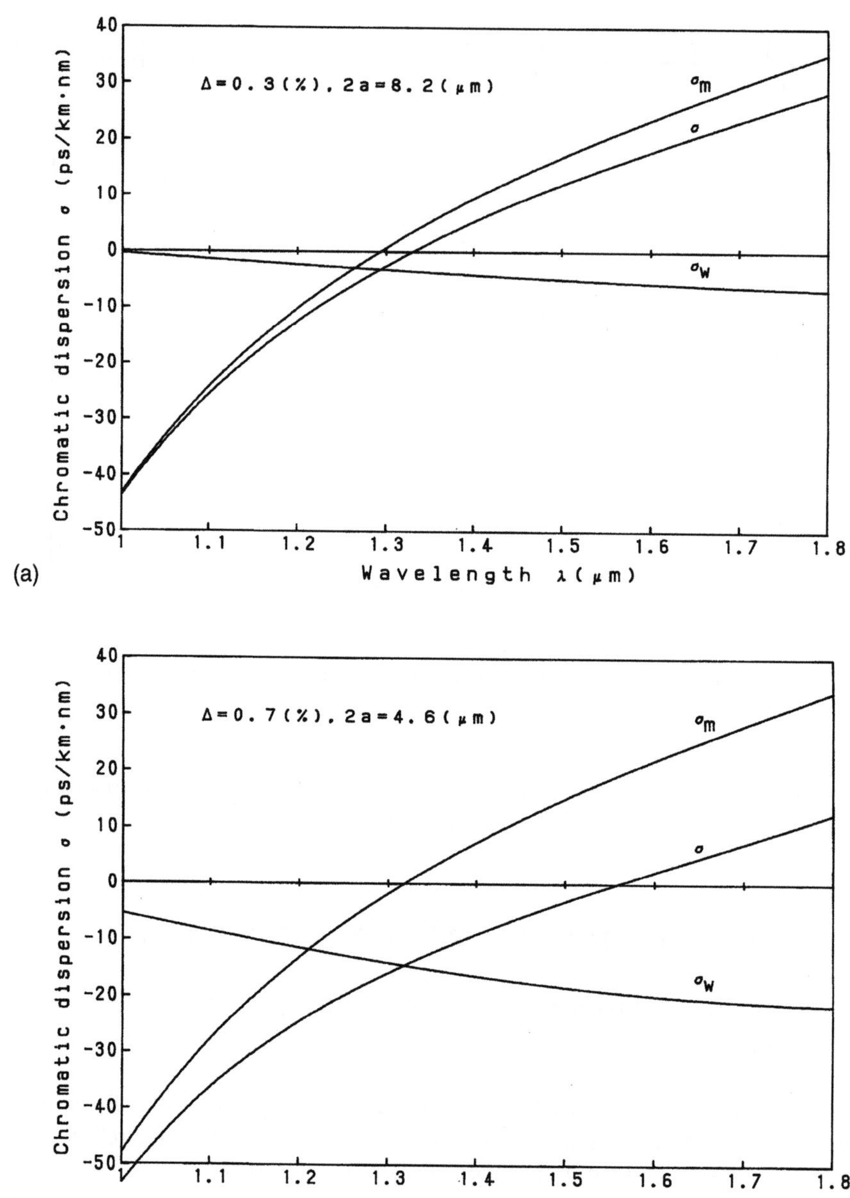

Figure 3.19 Material (σ_m), waveguide (σ_w) and total dispersions ($\sigma = \sigma_m + \sigma_w$) of fibers having (a) $\Delta = 0.3\%$ and $2a = 8.2\,\mu m$ and (b) $\Delta = 0.7\%$ and $2a = 4.6\,\mu m$, respectively.

where n_1 is the maximum refractive index in the core and therefore f is assumed to be $f(r) > 0$. Let us express E_z and H_z as products of functions of r and θ:

$$E_z = \frac{k^2 n_1^2}{\beta} \Phi(r) \cos(n\theta + \varphi_n), \tag{3.148a}$$

$$H_z = \omega\varepsilon_1 \Psi(r) \sin(n\theta + \varphi_n), \tag{3.148b}$$

where n denotes an integer and $\varphi_n = 0$ or $\pi/2$. Substituting Eqs. (3.146)–(3.148) into Maxwell's equation (refer to Eqs. (3.250) and (3.251) in Appendix 3A) and using the weakly guiding approximation

$$1 - f \cong 1 \qquad 1 - \chi = \frac{\beta^2}{k^2 n_1^2} \cong 1, \tag{3.149}$$

we obtain

$$\begin{aligned}(\chi - f)\frac{1}{r}\frac{d}{dr}\left[\frac{1}{(\chi - f)} r \frac{d\Phi}{dr}\right] + \left[k^2 n_1^2 (\chi - f) - \frac{n^2}{r^2}\right]\Phi \\ + \frac{n}{r}(\chi - f)\Psi \frac{d}{dr}\left(\frac{1}{\chi - f}\right) = 0,\end{aligned} \tag{3.150}$$

$$\begin{aligned}(\chi - f)\frac{1}{r}\frac{d}{dr}\left[\frac{1}{(\chi - f)} r \frac{d\Psi}{dr}\right] + \left[k^2 n_1^2 (\chi - f) - \frac{n^2}{r^2}\right]\Psi \\ + \frac{n}{r}(\chi - f)\Phi \frac{d}{dr}\left(\frac{1}{\chi - f}\right) = 0.\end{aligned} \tag{3.151}$$

The transverse electromagnetic field components are expressed in terms of Φ and Ψ:

$$E_r = -j\frac{1}{\chi - f}\left[\frac{d\Phi}{dr} + \frac{n}{r}\Psi\right]\cos(n\theta + \varphi_n), \tag{3.152}$$

$$E_\theta = j\frac{1}{\chi - f}\left[\frac{d\Psi}{dr} + \frac{n}{r}\Phi\right]\sin(n\theta + \varphi_n), \tag{3.153}$$

$$H_r = -j\frac{\beta}{\omega\mu_0}\frac{1}{(\chi - f)}\left[\frac{d\Psi}{dr} + \frac{n}{r}\Phi\right]\sin(n\theta + \varphi_n), \tag{3.154}$$

$$H_\theta = -j\frac{\beta}{\omega\mu_0}\frac{1}{\chi - f}\left[\frac{d\Phi}{dr} + \frac{n}{r}\Psi\right]\cos(n\theta + \varphi_n). \tag{3.155}$$

The case with $\Phi = 0$ and $n = 0$ in Eqs. (3.150)–(3.155) corresponds to the TE mode and the case with $\Psi = 0$ and $n = 0$ corresponds to the TM mode, respectively. If we write

$$R(r) = \begin{cases} j\dfrac{1}{\chi - f}\dfrac{d\Psi}{dr} & \text{TE mode} \quad (3.156a) \\[2ex] -j\dfrac{1}{\chi - f}\dfrac{d\Phi}{dr} & \text{TM mode} \quad (3.156b) \end{cases}$$

for each TE or TM mode and substitute them to Eqs. (3.150) and (3.151), we obtain

$$\Psi = \frac{j}{k^2 n_1^2}\left[\frac{dR}{dr} + \frac{1}{r}R\right] \qquad \text{TE mode,} \tag{3.157a}$$

$$\Phi = \frac{-j}{k^2 n_1^2}\left[\frac{dR}{dr} + \frac{1}{r}R\right] \qquad \text{TM mode.} \tag{3.157b}$$

Further, substituting each of the equations into Eqs. (3.156a) or (3.156b), we obtain the unified wave equation for TE and TM modes:

$$\frac{1}{r}\frac{d}{dr}\left(r\frac{dR}{dr}\right) + \left[k^2 n_1^2(\chi - f) - \frac{1}{r^2}\right]R = 0. \tag{3.158}$$

We next consider the hybrid modes. We introduce two new variables:

$$\phi = \frac{\Phi + \Psi}{2}, \tag{3.159}$$

$$\psi = \frac{\Phi - \Psi}{2}. \tag{3.160}$$

If we take the sum and difference of Eqs. (3.150) and (3.151) and rewrite these equations in terms of ϕ and ψ, we obtain

$$(\chi - f)\frac{1}{r}\frac{d}{dr}\left[\frac{1}{(\chi - f)}r\frac{d\psi}{dr}\right] + \left[k^2 n_1^2(\chi - f) - \frac{n^2}{r^2}\right]\psi - \frac{n}{r}(\chi - f)\psi\frac{d}{dr}\left(\frac{1}{\chi - f}\right) = 0, \tag{3.161}$$

$$(\chi - f)\frac{1}{r}\frac{d}{dr}\left[\frac{1}{(\chi - f)}r\frac{d\phi}{dr}\right] + \left[k^2 n_1^2(\chi - f) - \frac{n^2}{r^2}\right]\phi + \frac{n}{r}(\chi - f)\phi\frac{d}{dr}\left(\frac{1}{\chi - f}\right) = 0. \tag{3.162}$$

It is now understood that if we make appropriate approximations [Eq. (3.149)] and transformation of the variables [Eqs. (3.159) and (3.160)], the original simultaneous differential equations [Eqs. (3.150) and (3.151)] can be separated into two independent equations for two scalar quantities ϕ and ψ. Therefore, as in the cases for TE and TM modes, we have two independent cases; they are (1) $\phi=0, \psi\neq 0$ and (2) $\phi\neq 0, \psi=0$. Waves satisfying condition (1) correspond to EH modes, and those satisfying condition (2) correspond to HE modes, which are identified by comparing the electromagnetic fields of these modes with those of step-index fibers.

a. *EH Mode*:

From $\phi=0$ we obtain $\psi=\Phi=-\Psi$. Hence, if we write

$$R(r)=-j\frac{1}{\chi-f}\left[\frac{d\psi}{dr}-\frac{n}{r}\psi\right], \tag{3.163}$$

and substitute this into Eq. (3.161), we obtain

$$\psi=\frac{-j}{k^2n_1^2}\left[\frac{dR}{dr}+\frac{n+1}{r}R\right]. \tag{3.164}$$

Furthermore, by substituting Eq. (3.164) into Eq. (3.163), we obtain the differential equation

$$\frac{1}{r}\frac{d}{dr}\left(r\frac{dR}{dr}\right)+\left[k^2n_1^2(\chi-f)-\frac{(n+1)^2}{r^2}\right]R=0. \tag{3.165}$$

This equation is the wave equation for EH modes.

b. *HE Mode*:

From $\psi=0$ we obtain $\phi=\Phi=\Psi$. Therefore, if we write

$$R(r)=-j\frac{1}{\chi-f}\left[\frac{d\phi}{dr}+\frac{n}{r}\phi\right], \tag{3.166}$$

and substitute this into Eq. (3.162), we obtain

$$\phi=\frac{-j}{k^2n_1^2}\left[\frac{dR}{dr}-\frac{n-1}{r}R\right]. \tag{3.167}$$

By substituting Eq. (3.167) into Eqs. (3.166), we obtain the differential equation

$$\frac{1}{r}\frac{d}{dr}\left(r\frac{dR}{dr}\right)+\left[k^2n_1^2(\chi-f)-\frac{(n-1)^2}{r^2}\right]R=0. \tag{3.168}$$

This is the wave equation for HE modes.

Comparing Eqs. (3.158), (3.165) and (3.168), we now find that the basic wave equation for graded-index fibers is given by

$$\frac{1}{r}\frac{d}{dr}\left(r\frac{dR}{dr}\right)+\left[k^2n^2(r)-\beta^2-\frac{m^2}{r^2}\right]R=0, \tag{3.169}$$

where the integer m has already been defined in Eq. (3.73) as

$$m=\begin{cases}1 & \text{TE andTM modes} \quad (\mathrm{n}=0)\\ n+1 & \text{EH mode} \quad (\mathrm{n}\geqslant 1)\\ n-1 & \text{HE mode} \quad (\mathrm{n}\geqslant 1).\end{cases} \tag{3.170}$$

In most practical fibers, the refractive index varies in the core but is constant in the cladding; moreover, an index step is often present at the core–cladding boundary. Therefore, it is usually much more convenient to solve the wave equation in the core and cladding separately (an analytical solution is obtained in the cladding, since the refractive index is uniform) and to match those solutions at the core–cladding boundary in accordance with the physical boundary conditions. If the transverse field functions in the core and cladding are denoted by $R(r)$ and $R_{\text{clad}}(r)$, respectively, the boundary conditions under the weakly guiding approximation are given by

$$R(a)=R_{\text{clad}}(a), \tag{3.171}$$

$$\left[\frac{dR}{dr}\right]_{r=a}=\left[\frac{dR_{\text{clad}}}{dr}\right]_{r=a}. \tag{3.172}$$

Several methods are known for the analysis of graded-index fibers: the WKB (Wentzel–Kramers–Brillouin) method [14], finite element method (FEM) [15], among others. The WKB method is suitable for the analysis of multimode fibers of large v-value. On the other hand, the FEM is suitable for the analysis of single-mode graded-index fibers, since it requires a numerical calculation. The WKB method of analysis is described in the following section, and FEM is explained in detail in Chapter 6.

3.7.2. Analysis of Graded-index Fibers by the WKB Method

Here we describe the analysis of multimode graded-index fibers using the WKB method in accordance with the treatment in Ref. 16. When we apply the

WKB method to the wave equation of graded-index fibers (3.169), the dispersion equation that determines the propagation constant of the (m, ℓ) mode is given by

$$\int_{r_1}^{r_2} \left[k^2 n^2(r) - \beta^2 - \frac{m^2 - 1/4}{r^2} \right]^{1/2} dr = \left(\ell - \frac{1}{2} \right) \pi, \tag{3.173}$$

where r_1 and r_2 denote the turning points where the value in the brackets in Eq. (3.173) becomes zero. In practical multimode fibers with $\Delta = 1\%$ and $2a = 50\,\mu\text{m}$, the total number of propagation modes is several hundreds. Therefore, we can assume in Eq. (3.173) that $m \gg 1$ and $\ell \gg 1$. Then Eq. (3.173) is approximated

$$\int_{r_1(m)}^{r_2(m)} \left[k^2 n^2(r) - \beta^2 - \frac{m^2}{r^2} \right]^{1/2} dr \cong \ell \pi. \tag{3.174}$$

Although Eq. (3.174) has some errors for small m and ℓ, it can be applied to the majority of the modes in multimode fibers. Henceforth, we proceed as if Eq. (3.174) holds for any set of m and ℓ. If the maximum radial mode number of a propagation mode with an azimuthal mode number m is denoted by $\ell_{\max}(m)$, we may write, directly from Eq. (3.174),

$$\ell_{\max}(m) = \frac{1}{\pi} \int_{r_1(m)}^{r_2(m)} \left[k^2 n^2(r) - \beta_{\min}^2 - \frac{m^2}{r^2} \right]^{1/2} dr, \tag{3.175}$$

where $\beta_{\min}$ is the minimum β for the azimuthal mode number m under consideration. From Eq. (3.175) we see that $\ell_{\max}(m)$ radial modes ($\ell = 1, 2, \ldots, \ell_{\max}$) are included for each azimuthal mode $m (m = 0, 1, \ldots, m_{\max})$. The larger the azimuthal mode number m, the smaller the maximum radial mode number $\ell_{\max}(m)$. This relation is illustrated in Fig. 3.20. The maximum propagation constant $\beta_{\max}$ is when $m = 0$ and $\ell = 1$. The minimum propagation constant $\beta_{\min}$ is given, from the cutoff condition, by $\beta_{\min} = kn_0$. Therefore, if the number of modes having a propagation constant between β and $\beta_{\max}$ is denoted by $v(\beta)$, it can be found approximately by counting the number of circles plotted beneath the lower left of the dashed curve in Fig. 3.20:

$$\mathrm{v}(\beta) = 4 \int_0^{m_0(\beta)} \ell(m) dm = \frac{4}{\pi} \int_0^{m_0(\beta)} \int_{r_1(m)}^{r_2(m)} \left[k^2 n^2(r) - \beta^2 - \frac{m^2}{r^2} \right]^{1/2} dr\, dm, \tag{3.176}$$

where $m_0(\beta)$ is the maximum m for a given β. The factor 4 in the right-hand side of Eq. (3.176) expresses the fact that four conventional modes belong to each LP mode (refer to Table 3.2). Note also that the summation for m is replaced by

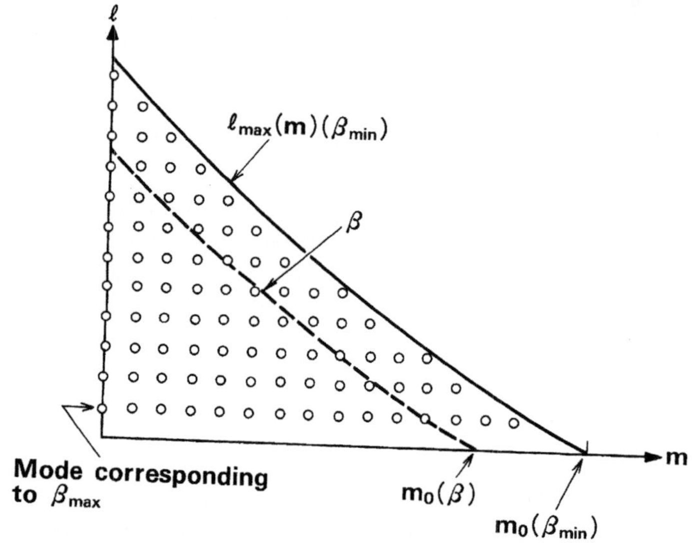

Figure 3.20 Relation between the propagation constant β and mode numbers m and ℓ.

the integration with respect to m because $m_0 \gg 1$ is assumed. From Eq. (3.176) we see that $[k^2n^2(r) - \beta^2 - m^2/r^2]^{1/2}$ should be integrated in the hatched region of Fig. 3.21. Exchanging the order of integration, we can rewrite Eq. (3.176) as

$$v(\beta) = \frac{4}{\pi}\int_0^{r_2(0)}\int_0^{r(k^2n^2-\beta^2)^{1/2}}\left[k^2n^2(r) - \beta^2 - \frac{m^2}{r^2}\right]^{1/2} dm\,dr. \tag{3.177}$$

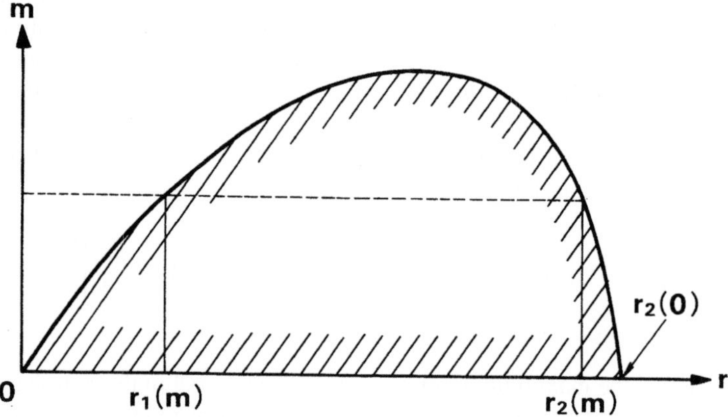

Figure 3.21 Region of integration in Eq. (3.176).

In this expression, the upper limit of the integral $m_0(\beta)$ is replaced by

$$m_0 = r\left[k^2 n^2(r) - \beta^2\right]^{1/2} \tag{3.178}$$

because m_0 is obtained by putting $\ell = 0$ into Eq. (3.174). The integration with respect to m can be performed without difficulty to obtain

$$\mathrm{v}(\beta) = \int_0^{r_2(0)} \left[k^2 n^2(r) - \beta^2\right] r\,dr. \tag{3.179}$$

We consider here the so-called α-power refractive-index profile

$$n(r) = n_1\left[1 - 2\Delta\left(\frac{r}{a}\right)^{\alpha}\right]^{1/2} \qquad (0 \leqslant r \leqslant a), \tag{3.180}$$

$$n_0 = n_1(1 - 2\Delta)^{1/2} \qquad (r > a), \tag{3.181}$$

where the power coefficient α is assumed to range between 1 and ∞. Profiles for various values of α are shown in Fig. 3.22. The usefulness of this profile lies in the fact that it approximates the actual profiles found in many fibers. For example, $\alpha = 2$ represents the quadratic-index profile and $\alpha = \infty$ corresponds to the step-index fiber.

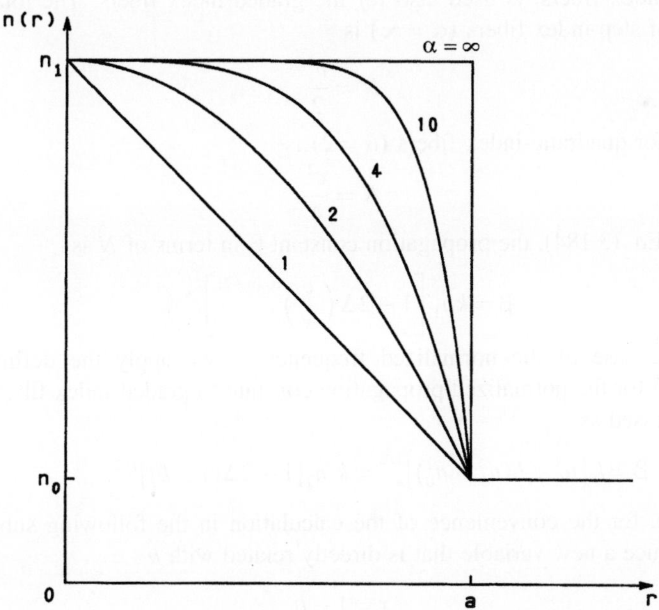

Figure 3.22 α-power refractive-index profile given by Eqs. (3.180) and (3.181).

Substituting Eqs. (3.180) and (3.181) into Eq. (3.179) and performing the integration, we obtain

$$\nu(\beta) = k^2 n_1^2 \Delta r_2(0)^2 \left[\frac{k^2 n_1^2 - \beta^2}{k^2 n_1^2 2\Delta} - \frac{2}{\alpha+2} \left(\frac{r_2(0)}{a} \right)^{\alpha} \right]. \tag{3.182}$$

In this equation, $r_2(0)$ denotes the outer turning point for $m=0$; that is, the solution of the equation $k^2 n^2(r_2) - \beta^2 = 0$. Then we have the relation for $r_2(0)/a$ in the form

$$\frac{r_2(0)}{a} = \left(\frac{k^2 n_1^2 - \beta^2}{k^2 n_1^2 2\Delta} \right)^{1/\alpha}. \tag{3.183}$$

Substitution of Eq. (3.183) into Eq. (3.182) gives

$$v(\beta) = \frac{\alpha}{\alpha+2} k^2 n_1^2 \Delta a^2 \left(\frac{k^2 n_1^2 - \beta^2}{k^2 n_1^2 2\Delta} \right)^{(\alpha+2)/\alpha}. \tag{3.184}$$

The total number of propagating modes N obtained by setting $\beta = \beta_{\min} = kn_0$ in Eq. (3.184) is

$$N = \frac{\alpha}{\alpha+2} k^2 n_1^2 \Delta a^2 = \frac{\alpha}{\alpha+2} \frac{v^2}{2}, \tag{3.185}$$

where the normalized frequency v, which is a quantity defined by Eq. (3.20) for step-index fibers, is used also for the graded-index fibers. The total mode number of step-index fibers ($\alpha = \infty$) is

$$N = \frac{v^2}{2}, \tag{3.186}$$

and that for quadratic-index fibers ($\alpha = 2$) is

$$N = \frac{v^2}{4}. \tag{3.187}$$

From Eq. (3.184), the propagation constant β in terms of N is

$$\beta = kn_1 \left[1 - 2\Delta \left(\frac{v}{N} \right)^{\alpha/(\alpha+2)} \right]^{1/2}. \tag{3.188}$$

As in the case of the normalized frequency v, we apply the definition of Eq. (3.82) for the normalized propagation constant to graded-index fibers. Then β is expressed as

$$\beta = k \left[n_0^2 + b(n_1^2 - n_0^2) \right]^{1/2} = k\, n_1 [1 - 2\Delta(1-b)]^{1/2}. \tag{3.189}$$

Moreover, for the convenience of the calculation in the following subsection, we introduce a new variable that is directly related with b

$$x = 1 - b. \tag{3.190}$$

Comparing each term of Eqs. (3.188) and (3.189) and using Eq. (3.190), we obtain

$$\frac{\mathrm{v}}{N} = x^{(\alpha+2)/\alpha}. \tag{3.191}$$

3.7.3. Dispersion Characteristics of Graded-index Fibers

The group delay time in optical fibers is given by Eq. (3.117). In multimode fibers, the first term in the right-hand side equation has a dominant effect over multimode dispersion. Then the delay time is expressed by

$$t = \frac{L}{v_g} = \left[\frac{d\beta}{d\omega}\right]_{\omega=\omega_0} \cdot L = \frac{L}{c}\frac{d\beta}{dk}. \tag{3.192}$$

Substituting this equation into Eq. (3.188) and noting that the refractive index n_1 and relative index difference Δ are all wavelength dependent, we obtain

$$t = \frac{L\,N_1}{c}\frac{1}{(1-2\Delta x)^{1/2}}\left[1-\left(2+\frac{y}{2}+\frac{n_1}{N_1}\frac{k}{x}\frac{dx}{dk}\right)\Delta x\right], \tag{3.193}$$

where N_1 is the group index and y is a quantity measuring the wavelength dependence of Δ, which is defined by [17]

$$y = \frac{2n_1}{N_1}\frac{k}{\Delta}\frac{d\Delta}{dk} = -\frac{2n_1}{N_1}\frac{\lambda}{\Delta}\frac{d\Delta}{d\lambda}. \tag{3.194}$$

Figure 3.23 shows the wavelength dependence of Δ and y in a G_eO_2-doped optical fiber. Here, when we consider the relation $dN/dk = (N/k)(2+y/2)$, which is derived from Eq. (3.185), we obtain

$$\frac{k}{x}\frac{dx}{dk} = -\frac{\alpha}{\alpha+2}\left(2+\frac{y}{2}\right). \tag{3.195}$$

Substituting Eq. (3.195) into Eq. (3.193) and using the Taylor series expansion $(1-2\Delta x)^{-1/2} \cong 1+\Delta x+(3/2)\Delta^2 x^2$, the delay time can be rewritten as

$$t = \frac{LN_1}{c}\left[1+\frac{(\alpha-2-y)}{(\alpha+2)}\Delta x+\frac{(3\alpha-2-2y)}{2(\alpha+2)}\Delta^2 x^2+O(\Delta^3)\right]. \tag{3.196}$$

The second and third terms this equation represent the dependence of the delay time on the mode order x. Since $\Delta \ll 1$, the delay-time difference is determined mainly by the second term. Therefore, multimode dispersion becomes quite small when the index profile

$$\alpha = \alpha_0 = 2 + y. \tag{3.197}$$

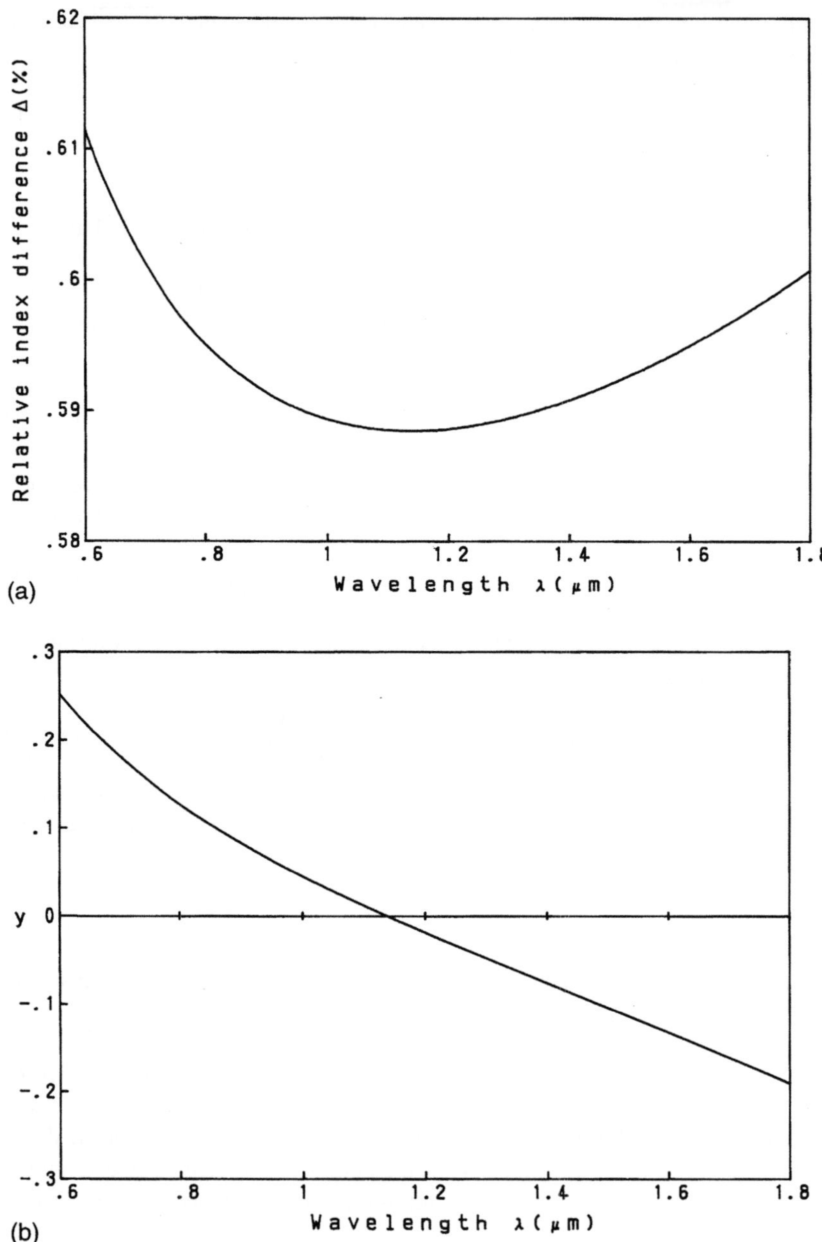

Figure 3.23 Wavelength dependence of (a) index difference Δ and (b) parameter y of a fiber consisting of a core with 6.3 mol% G_eO_2-doped glass and pure silica cladding.

More precisely, the multimode dispersion is a function of the delay time t. Then the multimode dispersion δt is obtained from the impulse response $h(t)$ as

$$\delta t = \left[\int_{-\infty}^{\infty} h(t) t^2 dt - \langle t \rangle^2 \right]^{1/2}, \tag{3.198a}$$

where the average delay time $\langle t \rangle$ is given by

$$\langle t \rangle = \int_{-\infty}^{\infty} h(t) t \, dt. \tag{3.198b}$$

The impulse response of the α-power fiber is given by Ref. 16 as

$$h(t) = \begin{cases} \dfrac{(\alpha+2)}{\alpha} \left| \dfrac{(\alpha+2)}{(\alpha-2-y)} \Delta \right|^{(\alpha+2)/\alpha} \tau^{2/\alpha} & (\alpha \neq 2+y), \quad (3.199a) \\ \dfrac{2}{\Delta^2} & (\alpha = 2+y), \quad (3.199b) \end{cases}$$

where τ denotes the normalized delay-time difference, which is defined by

$$\tau = \frac{ct}{N_1 L} - 1. \tag{3.200}$$

Figure 3.24 shows the impulse responses for several α-power graded-index fibers. Since $h(\tau) = 1/\Delta$ in step-index fibers, the multimode dispersion is obtained from Eq. (3.198) as

$$\delta t = 0.289 \frac{N_1 L}{c} \Delta. \tag{3.201}$$

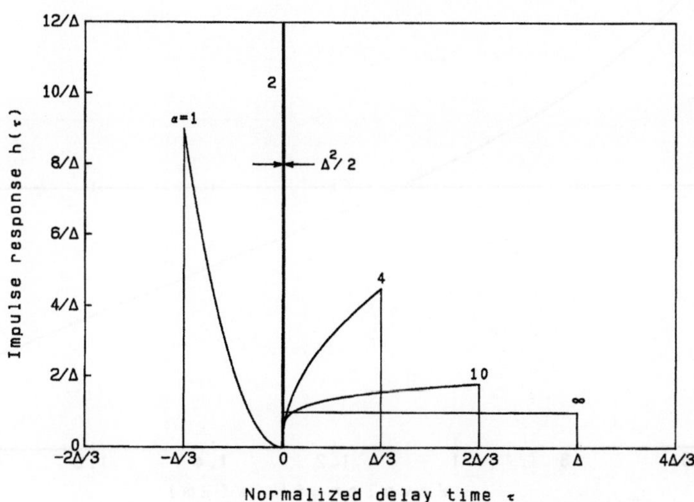

Figure 3.24 Impulse response of α-power graded-index fibers.

Substituting Eqs. (3.196) and (3.199) into Eqs. (3.198) and finding out the value which minimizes δt, the optimum α value for graded-index fibers is obtained by [17]

$$\alpha_{\text{opt}} = 2 + y - \Delta \frac{(4+y)(3+y)}{(5+2y)}. \tag{3.202}$$

The multimode dispersion in a fiber having an α_{opt}-power profile is

$$\delta t = 0.022 \frac{N_1 L}{c} \Delta^2. \tag{3.203}$$

When we compare Eq. (3.203) with Eq. (3.201), we find that the dispersion of an α_{opt}-power profile is about $\Delta/13(1/1300$ for $\Delta = 1\%)$ smaller than that of step-index fibers. However, it is quite difficult to fabricate graded-index fibers having the optimum α_{opt}-power profile, since multimode dispersion is very sensitive to slight changes in the profile parameter. When, for example, the profile parameter deviates slightly from the optimum value to $\alpha = \alpha_{\text{opt}}(1 \pm \Delta)$, the multimode dispersion becomes six times larger than the minimum value of Eq. (3.203).

The optimum profile parameter α_{opt} depends on the dopant material and the wavelength. Figure 3.25 shows the wavelength dependence of $\alpha_{\text{opt}}(\lambda)$ in

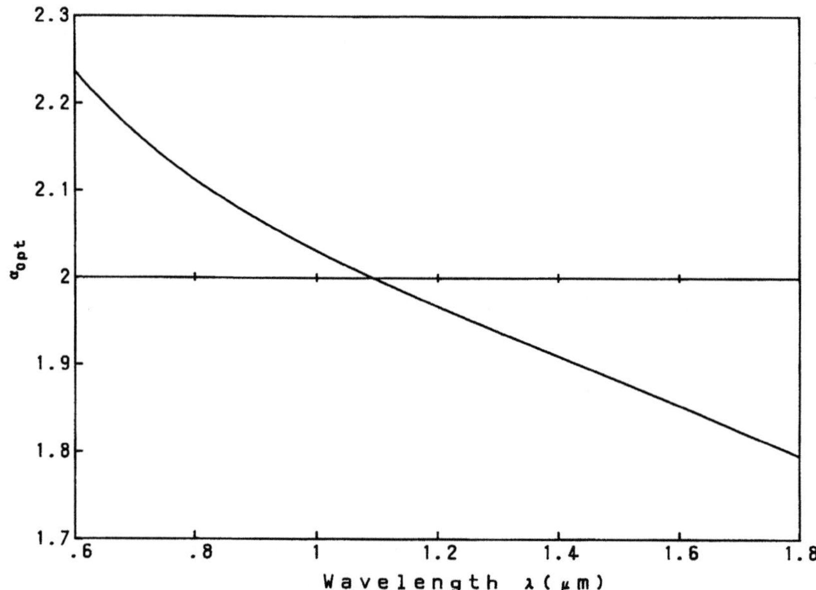

Figure 3.25 Wavelength dependence of α_{opt} (λ) in the G_eO_2-doped core fiber.

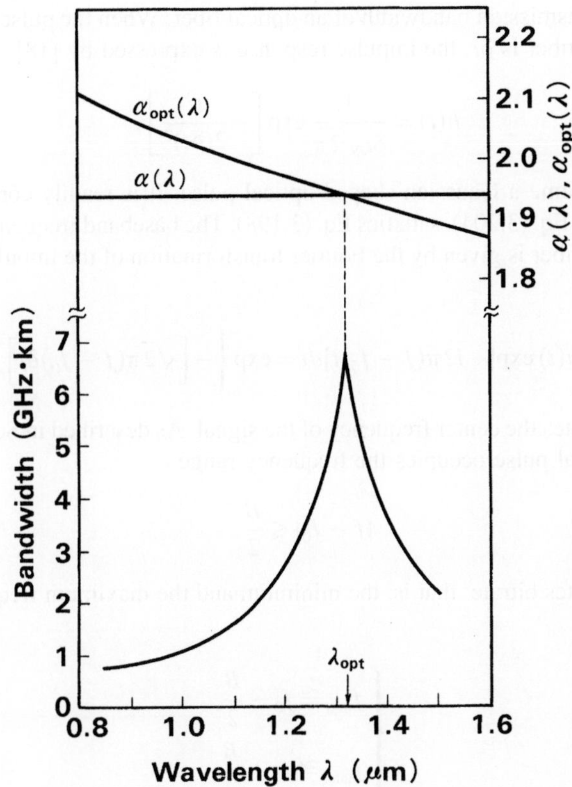

Figure 3.26 Wavelength dependence of the bandwidth of graded-index multimode fiber.

G_eO_2-doped core fiber. To the contrary, the profile parameter $\alpha(\lambda)$ of the fabricated fiber is known to be almost independent of the wavelength. Therefore, the transmission bandwidth of graded-index fiber (refer to the Section 3.8) becomes maximum at the wavelength λ_{opt} where $\alpha(\lambda) = \alpha_{opt}(\lambda)$ is satisfied and decreases rapidly on both sides of the optimum wavelength, as shown in Fig. 3.26.

3.8. RELATION BETWEEN DISPERSION AND TRANSMISSION CAPACITY

We have investigated the influence and the magnitude of several kinds of dispersion (multimode, material and waveguide) on the delay-time dispersion δt (pulse broadening). Here let us consider the relation between the pulse broadening

δt and the transmission bandwidth of an optical fiber. When the pulse broadening of an optical fiber is δt, the impulse response is expressed by [18]

$$h(t) = \frac{1}{\delta t \sqrt{2\pi}} \exp\left[-\frac{t^2}{2(\delta t)^2}\right], \tag{3.204}$$

where we assume a Gaussian-shaped optical pulse. It is readily confirmed that $h(t)$, given by Eq. (3.204), satisfies Eq. (3.198). The baseband frequency response of an optical fiber is given by the Fourier transformation of the impulse response $h(t)$ as

$$H(f) = \int_{-\infty}^{\infty} h(t) \exp[-j2\pi(f - f_0)t]dt = \exp\left\{-\left[\sqrt{2}\pi(f - f_0)\delta t\right]^2\right\}, \tag{3.205}$$

where f_0 denotes the center frequency of the signal. As described in Section 3.6.1, the NRZ signal pulse occupies the frequency range

$$|f - f_0| \leqslant \frac{B}{2},$$

where B denotes bitrate; that is, the minimum and the maximum frequencies are given by

$$\begin{cases} f_{\min} \cong f_0 - \dfrac{B}{2}, \\ f_{\max} \cong f_0 + \dfrac{B}{2}. \end{cases} \tag{3.206}$$

It is known from Eq. (3.205) that the baseband frequency response decreases as the modulation frequency f (or bitrate B) increases. We define here the maximum modulation frequency $f_{\max}$ as the frequency which satisfies the following relation [18]:

$$10 \log \frac{H(f_{\max})}{H(f_0)} \geqslant -1 \quad [\text{dB}]. \tag{3.207}$$

This equation means that the baseband frequency response $H(f)$ becomes 1 dB smaller than $H(f_0)(=1)$ at $f_{\max}$. Combining Eqs. (3.205)–(3.207), we obtain

$$B \cdot \delta t \leqslant \frac{1}{\pi}\sqrt{2 \ln 10^{0.1}} \cong 0.22. \tag{3.208}$$

Then the upper limit of the bitrate is given by

$$B \leqslant \frac{0.22}{\delta t} \qquad [\text{bit/s}], \tag{3.209}$$

when the pulse broadening due to the dispersion of the fiber is δt. We will investigate the signal transmission capacity for several typical cases in multimode and single-mode fibers.

3.8.1. Multimode Fiber

The transmission capacities of a step-index multimode fiber and a graded-index fiber having an α_{opt} profile are expressed from Eqs. (3.201) and (3.203) as

$$B \leqslant \begin{cases} \dfrac{15.4}{L} & [\text{Mbit/s}] \quad \text{step-index profile} \qquad (3.210a) \\ \dfrac{20.3}{L} & [\text{Gbit/s}] \quad \alpha_{opt} \text{ profile}, \qquad (3.210b) \end{cases}$$

where L denotes the fiber length, in kilometers, and an index difference of $\Delta = 1\%$ and group index of $N_1 = 1.48$ are assumed.

3.8.2. Single-mode Fiber

The pulse broadening of single-mode fiber is given by

$$\delta t = \sigma L \delta\lambda$$

as shown in Eq. (3.143). δt is proportional to the chromatic dispersion of the fiber σ and the spectral width of the signal source $\delta\lambda$. Let us consider the case that the signal center wavelength is $\lambda_0 = 1.55\,\mu\text{m}$ and the chromatic dispersion is $\sigma = 1\,\text{ps/km}\cdot\text{nm}$, respectively. There are two possible situations, depending on the magnitude of spectral broadening due to the laser itself and the signal modulation.

3.8.2.1. Case I-Spectral Broadening Due to the Signal Modulation is Larger than that of the Laser.

The signal frequency range of an NRZ pulse is given by Eq. (3.206). If we rewrite this in terms of the wavelength, we obtain

$$B = f_{max} - f_{min} = \frac{c}{(\lambda_0 - \delta\lambda)} - \frac{c}{(\lambda_0 + \delta\lambda)} \cong \frac{2c\delta\lambda}{\lambda_0^2}, \tag{3.211}$$

where $\delta\lambda$ is the spectral broadening caused by the signal modulation. It is then known that the spectral broadening due to the signal modulation at a bitrate of B is given by

$$\delta\lambda = \frac{\lambda_0^2}{2c} B. \tag{3.212}$$

For example, when the bitrate of the NRZ pulse is $B = 10$ Gbit/s the spectral broadening becomes $\delta\lambda = 0.04$ nm. Substituting Eqs. (3.212) and (3.143) into Eq. (3.209), we obtain the relation between the bitrate B and chromatic dispersion σ:

$$B \leqslant \sqrt{\frac{0.44c}{\lambda_0^2 \sigma L}} = \frac{234}{\sqrt{L}} \qquad [\text{Gbit/s}]. \tag{3.213}$$

3.8.2.2. Case II: Spectral Broadening of the Laser is Larger than that Due to the Signal Modulation.

Since the spectral broadening $\delta\lambda$ for the expression $\delta t = \sigma L \delta\lambda$ is determined by the spectral width $\delta\lambda$ of the laser, we readily obtain B from Eq. (3.209):

$$B \leqslant \frac{0.22}{\sigma \cdot \delta\lambda \cdot L} \qquad [\text{Gbit/s}]. \tag{3.214}$$

For example, when the spectral broadening of the laser is $\delta\lambda = 1$ nm, we obtain the maximum bitrate B as

$$B \leqslant \frac{220}{L} \qquad [\text{Gbit/s}].$$

When we compare Eqs. (3.213) and (3.214), we readily understand that the fiber length dependences are different for the two spectral broadening cases. The maximum bitrates for the fiber length $L = 100$ km are

$$B = \begin{cases} 23.4 & [\text{Gbit/s}] \quad \text{Case I,} \\ 2.2 & [\text{Gbit/s}] \quad \text{Case II.} \end{cases}$$

It is obvious that the maximum bitrate is high when the spectral width of the laser is narrower than that caused by the signal modulation. It is also known that the bandwidth of a single-mode fiber is higher than that of a multimode fiber, even with the optimum α_{opt} profile.

3.9. BIREFRINGENT OPTICAL FIBERS

3.9.1. Two Orthogonally-polarized Modes in Nominally Single-mode Fibers

In the axially symmetric single-mode fiber, there exist two orthogonally polarized modes, as shown in Section 3.5. They are known as HE_{11}^x and HE_{11}^y modes in accordance with their polarization directions. If the fiber waveguide structure is truly axially symmetric, these orthogonally polarized modes have the same propagation constants and thus they are degenerate. This is why such fiber is called "single-mode" fiber. In practical fibers, however, an axial nonsymmetry is generated by the core deformation and/or core eccentricity to the outer diameter, and it causes a slight difference in the propagation constants of the two polarization modes. In such fibers, the state of polarization (SOP) of the output light randomly varies, since the mode coupling take place between HE_{11}^x and HE_{11}^y modes, which is caused by fluctuations in core diameter along the z-direction, vibration and temperature variations. Therefore, such fibers cannot be used for applications in optical fiber sensors and in coherent optical communications in which SOP and interference effects are utilized.

Birefringent fibers have been proposed and fabricated to solve such polarization fluctuation problems [19]. The difference of the propagation constants between HE_{11}^x and HE_{11}^y modes are intentionally made large in birefringent fibers. Birefringent fibers are also called *polarization-maintaining fibers*.

Mode coupling (or mode conversion) between HE_{11}^x and HE_{11}^y modes occurs strongly (refer to Chapter 4) when there exists the same, or nearly equal, frequency components in the longitudinal fluctuations as the difference of the propagation constants $\delta\beta = \beta_x - \beta_y$ between the two modes. The strength of the mode coupling is proportional to the magnitude of the spatial frequency component of the fluctuation. Figure 3.27 shows the measured power density of the spatial frequency in the fluctuations in the outer diameter of a single-mode optical fiber [20]. The power spectrum of the core fluctuation is considered to be the same as that of Fig. 3.27. It is known that the power spectrum of fluctuation is high for the low-spatial-frequency components and decreases rapidly for the high-spatial-frequency components. Then, if we make a birefringent fiber having

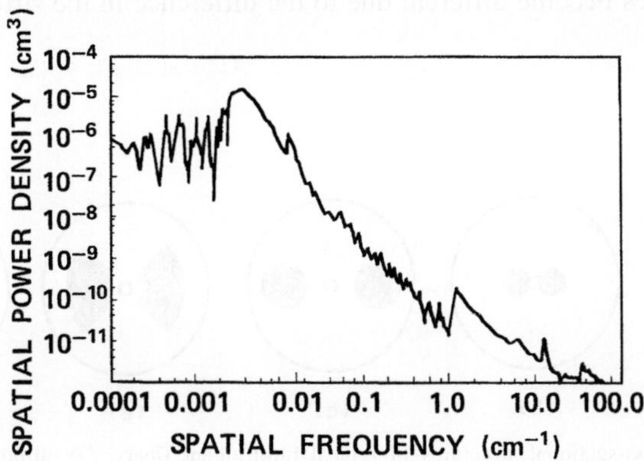

Figure 3.27 Measured power density of the spatial frequency in the fluctuations in the outer diameter of single-mode optical fiber. (After Ref. [20]).

a very large propagation constant difference $\delta\beta$ between the HE_{11}^x and HE_{11}^y modes, the mode coupling decreases, since the spatial frequency component of the fluctuation with the magnitude of $\delta\beta$ is quite small.

Birefringent fibers are classified into two categories: (1) geometrical birefringence type and (2) stress-induced birefringence type [21]. In the geometrical birefringence type, the birefringence is produced by the axially asymmetrical core or core vicinity structures. To the contrary, birefringence in the stress-induced birefringence type is generated by a nonsymmetric stress in the core. In the geometrical birefringence fiber, however, there generally exists nonsymmetrical stress distributions if there is an axial nonsymmetry in the waveguide structure. Therefore, practically it is quite difficult to realize the purely geometrical birefringence type fibers. On the contrary, it is possible to generate the difference $\delta\beta$ of the propagation constants purely by the stress effect.

Figure 3.28 shows the cross-sectional structures of typical birefringent fibers. Figures 3.28(a) and (b) belong to the geometrical birefringence type. The difference $\delta\beta$ of the propagation constants between HE_{11}^x and HE_{11}^y modes is produced by the elliptic-core deformation [22] in (a) and by the lower refractive-index regions than the core [23] or air holes [24] on both sides of the core in (b). On the other hand, Figs. 3.28(c)–(e) belong to the stress-induced type fibers [25–27]. The dark regions in these figures are stress-applying parts in which doped silica glasses having large thermal expansion coefficients are inserted. When stress-applying parts are cooled after the fiber drawing, they apply a large stress (or strain) to the core since they shrink tightly. Generally, a large tensile force is generated along the x-axis direction and a compressive force along the y-axis direction [21], respectively, since stress-applying parts are allocated in the x-axis direction. The refractive index of the glass under stress is changed by the photoelastic effect [28]. Therefore the refractive indices of the core for HE_{11}^x and HE_{11}^y modes become different due to the difference in the stress in the core region.

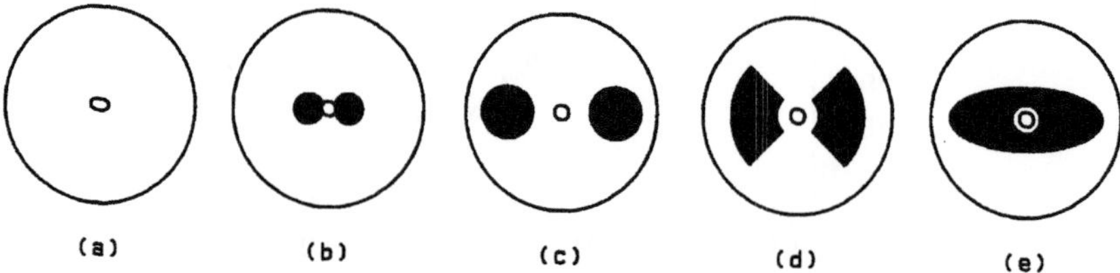

Figure 3.28 Cross-sectional structures of typical birefringent fibers: (a) elliptic-core fiber, (b) side-pit or side-tunnel fibers, (c) PANDA fiber, (d) Bow-tie fiber, and (e) elliptical-jacket fiber.

The modal birefringence B is defined as the normalized difference of the propagation constants between the HE_{11}^x and HE_{11}^y modes to the wavenumber k:

$$B = \frac{(\beta_x - \beta_y)}{k} = \frac{\delta\beta}{k}. \tag{3.215}$$

As described later, the modal birefringence of a typical birefringent fiber is $B = 1 \times 10^{-4} - 6 \times 10^{-4}$. The corresponding spatial frequency at $\lambda = 1\,\mu\text{m}$ is $\delta B = 6.3–7.7\ \text{cm}^{-1}$. The power densities of the core fluctuations for such high-spatial-frequency components are confirmed to be quite small in Fig. 3.27. Therefore, mode coupling is well suppressed in birefringent fibers.

3.9.2. Derivation of Basic Equations

In order to calculate the electromagnetic fields $\tilde{\mathbf{E}}$ and $\tilde{\mathbf{H}}$ in birefringent fibers, we should consider both the nonsymmetrical waveguide structure and the nonsymmetrical stress distribution. For the strict analysis of such waveguides, we should rely on the numerical analysis using, for example, the finite element method [15]. The combined analyses of FEM stress and FEM waveguide analysis will be described in Chapter 6. Although FEM analysis gives rigorous results, it does not always give a clear insight since it requires numerical calculations. Therefore, here the analytical method based on the perturbation method will be described. The refractive-index change due to the nonsymmetrical stress is of the order of 10^{-4} in practical birefringent fibers, which is sufficiently smaller than the refractive-index difference Δ. Therefore, the electromagnetic fields $\tilde{\mathbf{E}}$ and $\tilde{\mathbf{H}}$ in birefringent fibers under stress are considered to be the perturbation from the fields $\tilde{\mathbf{E}}_p$ and $\tilde{\mathbf{H}}_p$ ($p = 1$ corresponds to $\mathbf{HE}_{11}^x$ mode and $p = 2$ to $\mathbf{HE}_{11}^y$ mode, respectively) without stress. The perturbed electromagnetic fields $\tilde{\mathbf{E}}$ and $\tilde{\mathbf{H}}$ are expressed by using the nonperturbed fields $\tilde{\mathbf{E}}_p$ and $\tilde{\mathbf{H}}_p$ [29]:

$$\begin{cases} \tilde{\mathbf{E}} = A(z)\tilde{\mathbf{E}}_1 + B(z)\tilde{\mathbf{E}}_2, \\ \tilde{\mathbf{H}} = A(z)\tilde{\mathbf{H}}_1 + B(z)\tilde{\mathbf{H}}_2. \end{cases} \tag{3.216}$$

Each pair of the nonperturbed fields satisfies Maxwell's equations

$$\begin{cases} \nabla \times \tilde{\mathbf{E}}_p = -j\omega\mu_0\tilde{\mathbf{H}}_p, \\ \nabla \times \tilde{\mathbf{H}}_p = j\omega\varepsilon_0 K\tilde{\mathbf{E}}_p, \end{cases} \quad (p = 1, 2) \tag{3.217}$$

where $\mathbf{K}$ denotes the relative permittivity tensor of the fiber without nonsymmetrical stress. Here, the geometrical effect of nonsymmetrical core structure is considered in **K**. Substituting Eq. (3.216) into Maxwell's equations having the perturbed relative permitivity tensor $\tilde{\mathbf{K}}$

$$\begin{cases} \nabla \times \tilde{\mathbf{E}} = -j\omega\mu_0 \tilde{\mathbf{H}}, \\ \nabla \times \tilde{\mathbf{H}} = j\omega\varepsilon_0 \tilde{\mathbf{K}}\tilde{\mathbf{E}}, \end{cases} \tag{3.218}$$

and rewriting the equations by using Eq. (3.217), we have (refer to Appendix 3B)

$$\begin{cases} \dfrac{dA}{dz} = -j\Gamma_1 A, \\ \dfrac{dB}{dz} = -j\Gamma_2 B. \end{cases} \tag{3.219}$$

In this equation, Γ_p is given by

$$\Gamma_p = \frac{\omega\varepsilon_0 \int_0^{2\pi} \int_0^{\infty} \mathbf{E}_p^* \cdot (\tilde{\mathbf{K}} - \mathbf{K})\mathbf{E}_p r\, dr\, d\theta}{\int_0^{2\pi} \int_0^{\infty} \mathbf{u}_z \cdot (\mathbf{E}_p^* \times \mathbf{H}_p + \mathbf{E}_p \times \mathbf{H}_p^*)\, r\, dr\, d\theta}, \tag{3.220}$$

where $\mathbf{E}_p$ and $\mathbf{H}_p$ are cross-sectional electromagnetic fields of the nonperturbed fields $\tilde{\mathbf{E}}_p$ and $\tilde{\mathbf{H}}_p$, which are expressed by separating the z dependence as

$$\begin{cases} \tilde{\mathbf{E}}_p(r, \theta, z) = \mathbf{E}_p(r, \theta) \exp(-j\beta_p z), \\ \tilde{\mathbf{H}}_p(r, \theta, z) = \mathbf{H}_p(r, \theta) \exp(-j\beta_p z). \end{cases} \quad (p = 1, 2) \tag{3.221}$$

β_p is the propagation constant of the HE_{11}^x $(p = 1)$ and HE_{11}^y mode $(p = 2)$, respectively. The solutions of Eq. (3.219) are given by

$$\begin{cases} A(z) \propto \exp(-j\Gamma_1 z), \\ B(z) \propto \exp(-j\Gamma_2 z). \end{cases} \tag{3.222}$$

Then, the propagation constants of the HE_{11}^x and HE_{11}^y modes of the birefringent fiber under nonsymmetrical stress are

$$\begin{cases} \beta_x = \beta_1 + \Gamma_1, \\ \beta_y = \beta_2 + \Gamma_2. \end{cases} \tag{3.223}$$

Substituting this into Eq. (3.215), we obtain the expression for the modal birefringence:

$$B = \frac{\beta_1 - \beta_2}{k} + \frac{\Gamma_1 - \Gamma_2}{k}. \tag{3.224}$$

The first term of Eq. (3.224) represents the birefringence due to the nonsymmetrical waveguide structure and is called *geometrical birefringence*. The second term represents the birefringence caused by the nonsymmetrical stress distribution and is called *stress-induced birefringence*. Geometrical and stress-induced birefringences are expressed separately as

$$B_g = \frac{\beta_1 - \beta_2}{k}, \tag{3.225a}$$

$$B_s = \frac{\Gamma_1 - \Gamma_2}{k}. \tag{3.225b}$$

Geometrical birefringence B_g can be calculated by the collocation method [30] or the finite element waveguide analysis. On the other hand, stress-induced birefringence B_s is calculated by the finite element stress analysis.

The relative permitivity tensor $\tilde{\mathbf{K}}$ under stress effect is expressed by [31]

$$\tilde{\mathbf{K}} = \begin{pmatrix} (n - C_1\sigma_x - C_2(\sigma_y + \sigma_z))^2 & 2n(C_2 - C_1)\tau_{xy} & 0 \\ 2n(C_2 - C_1)\tau_{xy} & (n - C_1\sigma_y - C_2(\sigma_z + \sigma_x))^2 & 0 \\ 0 & 0 & (n - C_1\sigma_z - C_2(\sigma_x + \sigma_y))^2 \end{pmatrix}, \tag{3.226}$$

where n denotes the unstressed refractive index, σ_x, σ_y and σ_z are principal stresses along the x-, y-and z-directions, τ_{xy} is a shear stress, and C_1 and C_2 denote the photoelastic constants. The photoelastic constants of silica glass are given by [32]

$$\begin{cases} C_1 = 7.42 \times 10^{-6} & (\text{mm}^2/\text{kg}) \\ C_2 = 4.102 \times 10^{-5} & (\text{mm}^2/\text{kg}). \end{cases} \tag{3.227}$$

The relative permitivity tensor under the unstressed condition $\mathbf{K}$ is given by

$$\mathbf{K} = \begin{pmatrix} n^2 & 0 & 0 \\ 0 & n^2 & 0 \\ 0 & 0 & n^2 \end{pmatrix}. \tag{3.228}$$

Therefore the term $(\tilde{\mathbf{K}} - \mathbf{K})$ in Eq. (3.220) may be written

$$\tilde{\mathbf{K}} - \mathbf{K} = \begin{pmatrix} -2n(C_1\sigma_x - C_2(\sigma_y + \sigma_z)) & 2n(C_2 - C_1)\tau_{xy} & 0 \\ 2n(C_2 - C_1)\tau_{xy} & -2n(C_1\sigma_y + C_2(\sigma_z + \sigma_x)) & 0 \\ 0 & 0 & -2n(C_1\sigma_z + C_2(\sigma_x + \sigma_y)) \end{pmatrix}. \tag{3.229}$$

where we ignored the small terms C_1^2, C_1C_2, and C_2^2. Substituting this into Eq. (3.220) and taking into account that E_x and $H_y \cong (\omega\varepsilon_0 n^2/\beta)E_x$ are the dominant components in the $(\mathbf{E}_1, \mathbf{H}_1)$ of the HE_{11}^x mode and E_y and $H_x \cong -(\omega\varepsilon_0 n^2/\beta)E_y$ are the dominant components in the $(\mathbf{E}_2, \mathbf{H}_2)$ of the HE_{11}^y mode, we obtain

$$\frac{\Gamma_1}{k} = -\frac{\int_0^{2\pi}\int_0^{\infty}[C_1\sigma_x + C_2(\sigma_y + \sigma_z)]|\mathbf{E}_1|^2\, r\, dr\, d\theta}{\int_0^{2\pi}\int_0^{\infty}|\mathbf{E}_1|^2\, r\, dr\, d\theta}, \tag{3.230}$$

$$\frac{\Gamma_2}{k} = -\frac{\int_0^{2\pi}\int_0^{\infty}[C_1\sigma_y + C_2(\sigma_z + \sigma_x)]|\mathbf{E}_2|^2\, r\, dr\, d\theta}{\int_0^{2\pi}\int_0^{\infty}|\mathbf{E}_2|^2\, r\, dr\, d\theta}, \tag{3.231}$$

It is known from Eqs. (3.230) and (3.231) that the stress contributions to the propagation constants are obtained by the overlap integral of stress distribution and the optical intensity distribution.

3.9.3. Elliptical-core Fibers

We first define the geometry of an elliptical-core fiber, as shown in Fig. 3.29. The core radii along the x- and y-axis directions are a_x and a_y, where a_x is assumed to be larger than a_y. The refractive indices of core and cladding are denoted by n_1 and n_0. The core ellipticity ε is defined by

$$\varepsilon = \frac{a_x - a_y}{a_x}. \tag{3.232}$$

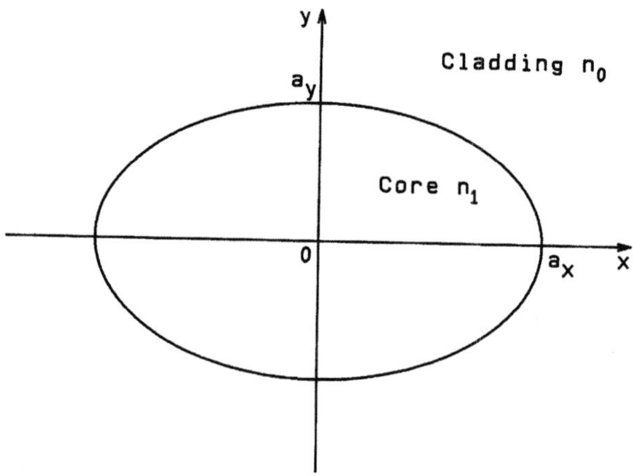

Figure 3.29 Geometry of an elliptical-core fiber.

In order to calculate the geometrical birefringence of elliptical-core fibers and other nonsymmetrical-core fibers, the rigorous analysis without using the LP mode approximation (scalar approximation) is necessary to calculate the propagation constants of HE_{11}^x and HE_{11}^y modes. The rigorous analysis is called the *vector analysis*, since it rigorously considers the orientation of electric field vector. The collocation method [30] and vectorial finite element method are known as *vectorial analyses*. The perturbation method analysis [33] is also applicable to calculate the geometrical birefringence, under the restriction that the ellipticity of the core is sufficiently small.

Geometrical birefringence B_g is analytically obtained by the perturbation method:

$$B_g = n_1 \Delta^2 \varepsilon G(v), \tag{3.233}$$

where v denotes the normalized frequency defined by

$$v = k n_1 a_x \sqrt{2\Delta}, \tag{3.234}$$

and the normalized geometrical birefringence $G(v)$ is given by

$$G(v) = \frac{w^2}{u^4}\left\{u^2 + (u^2 - w^2)\left[\frac{J_0(u)}{J_1(u)}\right]^2 + uw^2\left[\frac{J_0(u)}{J_1(u)}\right]^3\right\}. \tag{3.235}$$

Equation (3.233) is applicable to small ellipticities of about $\varepsilon \approx 0.1$. Even for a relatively large ellipticity, the Eq. (3.233) still holds approximately. However, the normalized geometrical birefringence $G(v)$ has different v dependencies with respect to ε, as shown in Fig. 3.30. Normalized geometrical birefringences in Fig. 3.30 are calculated numerically by using the collocation method [30].

3.9.4. Modal Birefringence

The effective indices of the HE_{11}^x and HE_{11}^y modes in a birefringent fiber are obtained from Eqs. (3.223), (3.230), and (3.231) as

$$n_x = \frac{\beta_x}{k} = n_{x0} - C_1\hat{\sigma}_x - C_2(\hat{\sigma}_y + \hat{\sigma}_z), \tag{3.236}$$

$$n_y = \frac{\beta_y}{k} = n_{y0} - C_1\hat{\sigma}_y - C_2(\hat{\sigma}_z + \hat{\sigma}_x), \tag{3.237}$$

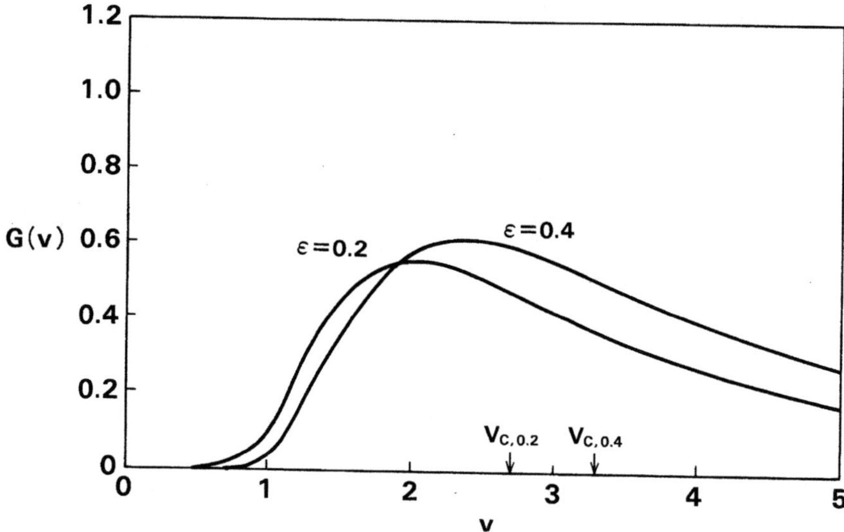

Figure 3.30 Normalized geometrical birefringence $G(v)$ for an elliptical-core fiber.

where $n_{x0}(=\beta_1/k)$ and $n_{y0}(=\beta_2/k)$ denote the effective indices neglecting the nonsymmetrical stress effect. In other words, $n_{x0} - n_{y0}$ represents the geometrical birefringence B_g. The effective principal stress $\hat{\sigma}_s$ $(s = x, y, z)$ is calculated by the overlap integral of stress distribution and optical intensity:

$$\hat{\sigma}_s = \frac{\int_0^{2\pi}\int_0^{\infty} \sigma_s(r,\theta)|\mathbf{E}|^2\, r\, dr\, d\theta}{\int_0^{2\pi}\int_0^{\infty} |\mathbf{E}|^2\, r\, dr\, d\theta} \qquad (s = x, y, z). \tag{3.238}$$

The electric field $\mathbf{E}(r,\theta)$ for the circular symmetric core is analytically given by Eqs. (3.94) and (3.95). On the other hand, the electric field $\mathbf{E}(r,\theta)$ for the nonsymmetricl core fiber should be calculated by using the collocation method or the finite element method. The stress-induced birefringence B_s is obtained from Eqs. (3.225b), (3.236), and (3.237) as

$$B_s = (C_2 - C_1)(\hat{\sigma}_x - \hat{\sigma}_y). \tag{3.239}$$

The stress-induced birefringence is usually approximated by using the principal stress difference at the core center $\sigma_{x0} - \sigma_{y0}$:

$$B_{s0} = (C_2 - C_1)(\sigma_{x0} - \sigma_{y0}). \tag{3.240}$$

Generally B_{s0} represents the maximum stress-induced birefringence. The normalized stress-induced birefringence is then defined by

$$H(v) = \frac{B_s}{B_s 0}. \tag{3.241}$$

Figures 3.31 and 3.32 show the normalized stress-induced birefringences of the elliptical-core and the PANDA fiber, respectively [34]. It is shown from the figures that $H(v) \leqslant 0.5$ in the elliptical-core fiber and $H(v) \cong 1.0$ in the PANDA fiber at the normal operating conditions. Figures 3.33 and 3.34 compare geometrical and stress-induced birefringences of the elliptical-core fiber calculated by using the combination of the collocation method for B_g and the finite element method for B_s [35]. In the FEM stress analyses, Young's modulus $E = 7830$ kg/mm^2, Poisson's ratio $v = 0.186$ and the temperature differences ΔT from the fictive temperature to the room temperature, as listed in Table 3.3, have been used [3]. Also, the normalized frequency v is chosen at $v = 0.9v_c$ for each elliptical-core fiber. B_g and B_s in the elliptical-core fiber have the same sign and then contribute to the total birefringence additively. It is seen from Figs. 3.33 and 3.34 that (1) B_g and B_s are proportional to Δ^2 and Δ, (2) B_s is larger than B_g by more than one order of magnitude for the small refractive-index fibers ($\Delta = 0.2$–0.4%), and (3) B_g becomes larger than B_s for large refractive-index

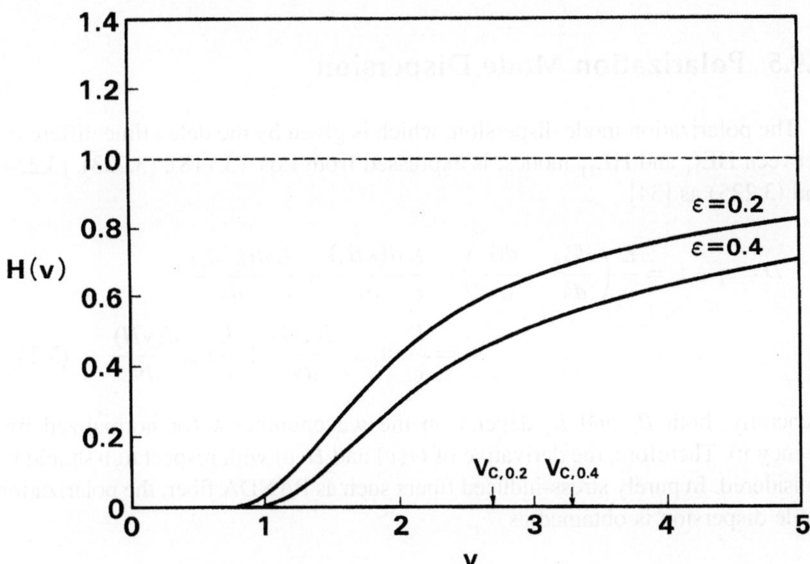

Figure 3.31 Normalized stress-induced birefringence $H(v)$ for an elliptical-core fiber.

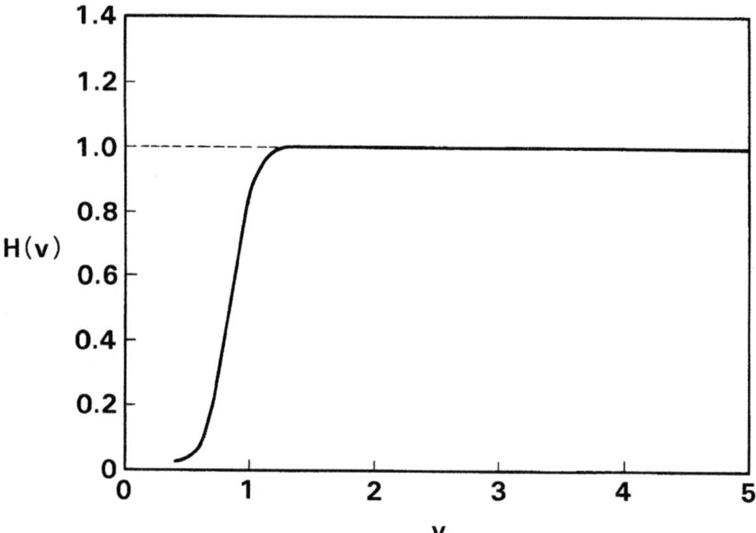

Figure 3.32 Normalized stress-induced birefringence $H(v)$ for a PANDA fiber.

fibers ($\Delta > 1.5\%$). Therefore, the elliptical-core fiber is not always the geometrical birefringence type of fiber.

3.9.5. Polarization Mode Dispersion

The polarization mode dispersion, which is given by the delay time difference between HE_{11}^{x} and HE_{11}^{y} modes, is expressed from Eqs. (3.118), (3.223), (3.224) and (3.225) as [34]

$$D = t_x - t_y = \frac{L}{c}\left(\frac{d\beta_x}{dk} - \frac{d\beta_y}{dk}\right) = \frac{L}{c}\frac{d(kB_g)}{dk} + \frac{L}{c}\frac{d(k\,B_s)}{dk}$$
$$= \frac{L}{c}\varepsilon n_1 \Delta^2 \frac{d(vG)}{dv} + \frac{L}{c}B_{s0}\frac{d(vH)}{dv}. \qquad (3.242)$$

Generally, both B_g and B_s depend on the wavenumber k (or normalized frequency v). Therefore, the derivative of $G(v)$ and $H(v)$ with respect to v should be considered. In purely stress-induced fibers such as PANDA fiber, the polarization mode dispersion is obtained as

$$D = \frac{L}{c}B_{s0} = \frac{L}{c}(C_2 - C_1)(\sigma_{x0} - \sigma_{y0}), \qquad (3.243)$$

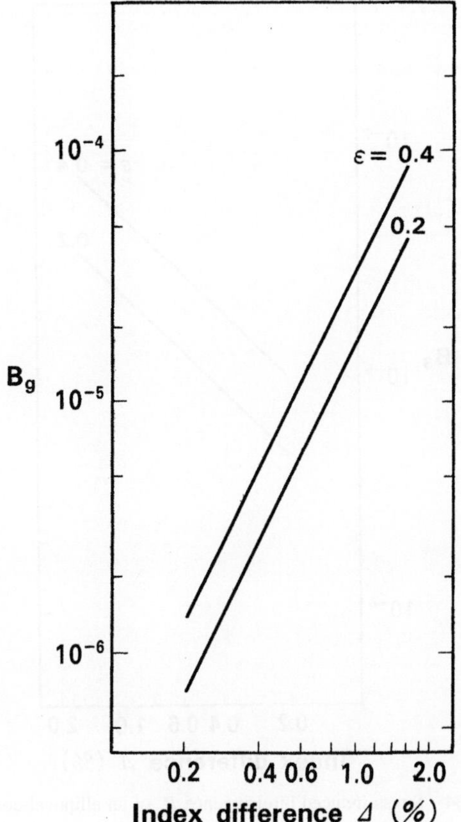

Figure 3.33 Geometrical birefringence B_g of an elliptical-core fiber.

since the geometrical birefringence $B_g = 0$ and the stress-induced birefringence are almost constant as shown in Fig. 3.32 ($v > 1.5$).

Behavior of pulse waveform in the two-mode optical fibers, in which two modes exchange their energy through mode coupling, was investigated in Ref. [36] and [37]. Delay time difference at the center of two modes is expressed by

$$T_{DGD} = \frac{1 - e^{-2hL}}{2h} \cdot \frac{1}{c} \frac{d(\delta\beta)}{dk}, \tag{3.244}$$

where $\delta\beta = \beta_x - \beta_y$ and $h(\mathrm{m}^{-1})$ denotes the mode coupling (or conversion) coefficient. T_{DGD} is called differential group delay (DGD). For the two limiting

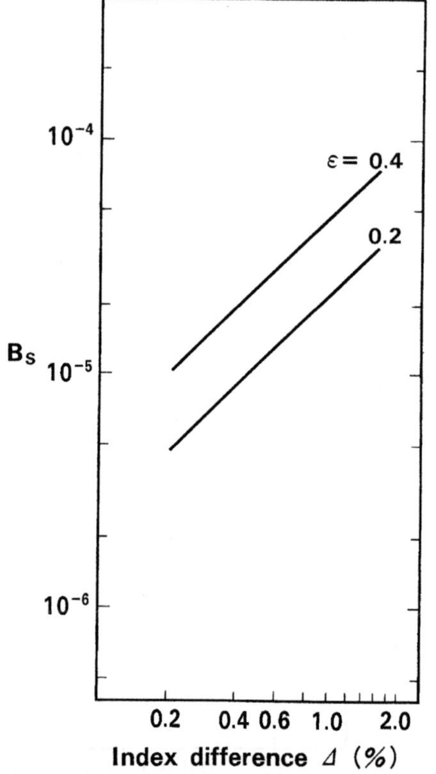

Figure 3.34 Stress-induced birefringence B_s of an elliptical-core fiber.

Table 3.3

Thermal expansion coefficients and temperature differences

$\Delta(\%)$	$\alpha[\times 10^{-7}{}^{\circ}\mathrm{C}^{-1}]$	$\Delta T[{}^{\circ}\mathrm{C}]$
0.2	6.6	−980
0.4	8.0	−950
0.8	10.6	−850
1.6	17.6	−700

cases with $hL \ll 1$ and $hL \gg 1$, T_{DGD} reduces to

$$T_{DGD} = \begin{cases} \dfrac{L}{c}\dfrac{d(\delta\beta)}{dk} & (h\,L \ll 1) \\[2ex] \dfrac{1}{2hc}\dfrac{d(\delta\beta)}{dk} & (h\,L \gg 1). \end{cases} \tag{3.245}$$

The root-mean-square (rms) pulse width $\delta\tau_{PMD}$ is obtained by solving the mode coupling equation [36] and is given by

$$\delta\tau_{PMD} = \sqrt{\langle(\delta\tau)^2\rangle} = \frac{\sqrt{(e^{-2hL}-1)/2+hL}}{h}\cdot\frac{1}{c}\frac{d(\delta\beta)}{dk}, \tag{3.246}$$

$\delta\tau_{PMD}$ represents polarization mode dispersion in the nominal single-mode fibers. The rms pulse width $\delta\tau_{PMD}$ reduces to

$$\delta\tau_{PMD} \simeq \begin{cases} \dfrac{L}{c}\dfrac{d(\delta\beta)}{dk} & (h\,L \ll 1) \\[2ex] \dfrac{\sqrt{L/h}}{c}\dfrac{d(\delta\beta)}{dk} & (h\,L \gg 1) \end{cases} \tag{3.247}$$

for the two limiting cases with $hL \ll 1$ and $hL \gg 1$. In the limit of negligible mode coupling the principal states of polarization become the polarization modes of the fiber, and the differential delay time between the principal states is determined simply by the difference in group velocity for the two polarization modes. Consequently, $\delta\tau_{PMD}$ takes on the values of $\delta\tau_{PMD} \propto L$. In the limit of extensive mode coupling, the principal states and differential delay time in a fiber are no longer correlated with local fiber properties since they depend on the collective effects of the random mode coupling over the entire propagation path. The mode coupling thus has an equalizing effect in that it reduces the variance of $\delta\tau$ by a factor of $1/\sqrt{hL}$ relative to the no-mode-coupling case.

Mode coupling coefficient h is expressed by [38]

$$h = \frac{h_0}{1+(\beta_x-\beta_y)^2 L_0^2}, \tag{3.248}$$

where typical values of h_0 and L_0 are known to be $h_0 = 5.3\times10^{-3}(\mathrm{m}^{-1})$ and $L_0 = 2.7\times10^{-2}(\mathrm{m})$. $(L/c)[d(\delta\beta)/dk]$ for the elliptical-core fiber is given from Eq. (3.242) as

$$\frac{L}{c}\frac{d(\delta\beta)}{dk} = \frac{L}{c}\varepsilon n_1\Delta^2\frac{d(vG)}{dv} + \frac{L}{c}B_{s0}\frac{d(vH)}{dv}. \tag{3.249}$$

The values of $d(vG)/dv$ and $d(vH)/dv$ are numerically calculated using $G(v)$ and $H(v)$ in Figs. 3.30 and 3.31, respectively. Figure 3.35 shows length dependence of rms pulse width (PMD) in elliptical-core fibers with $\Delta = 0.8\%$ and $v = 2.2$. From Figures 3.30 and 3.31, $G(v) = 0.4353$, $d(vG)/dv = 0.132$, $H(v) = 0.477$ and $d(vH)/dv = 1.10$. It is known from Fig. 3.35 that the rms pulse width

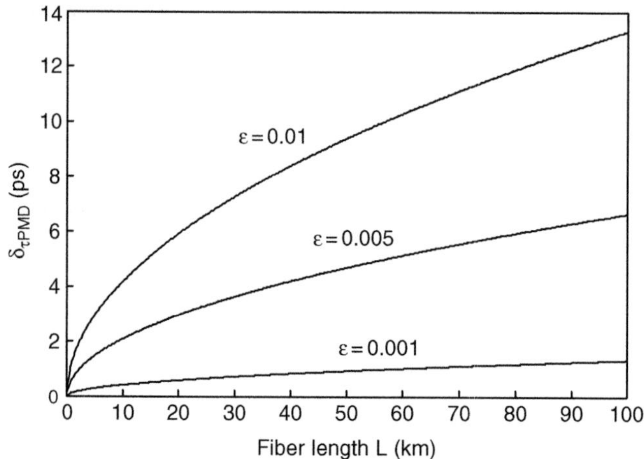

Figure 3.35 Length dependence of rms pulse width in elliptical-core fibers.

is expressed by $\delta\tau_{PMD} \propto 1.33\,\text{ps/km}^{1/2}$ for $\varepsilon = 0.01$, $\delta\tau_{PMD} \propto 0.66\,\text{ps/km}^{1/2}$ for $\varepsilon = 0.005$ and $\delta\tau_{PMD} \propto 0.13\,\text{ps/km}^{1/2}$ for $\varepsilon = 0.001$, respectively.

3.10. DISPERSION CONTROL IN SINGLE-MODE OPTICAL FIBERS

3.10.1. Dispersion Compensating Fibers

Single-mode optical fibers in which zero-dispersion wavelengths are shifted to 1.55-μm regions (Fig. 3.19(b)) are called dispersion-shifted fibers (DSFs). In order to distinguish standard single-mode fibers having zero-dispersion wavelengths around 1.3 μm regions (Fig. 3.19(a)) from DSFs, standard single-mode fibers are simply called single-mode fibers (SMFs). As described in Section 3.8, the maximum bit-rate B of fiber is given by $B = 234/\sqrt{\sigma L}$ (Gbit/s) where σ is chromatic dispersion in ps/km/nm and L is fiber length in km. Since chromatic dispersion σ of SMF is about 17 ps/km/nm at 1.55 μm region, the maximum bit-rate of SMF is about $B = 5.7\,\text{Gbit/s}$ for $L = 100\,\text{km}$. Then we cannot transmit 10 Gbit/s signal in such SMF fibers. Dispersion compensating fibers (DCFs) are quite attractive fiber-based components for upgrading the existing SMFs. Figure 3.36 shows chromatic dispersions of SMF and DCF, respectively. Refractive-index difference Δ of DCF is 2.8% and core diameter $2a = 1.6\,\mu\text{m}$ ($\lambda c = 0.74\,\mu\text{m}$). Chromatic dispersion of DCF at 1.55 μm is $-105\,\text{ps/km/nm}$. It is known that when we connect 16.2-km length of DCF to

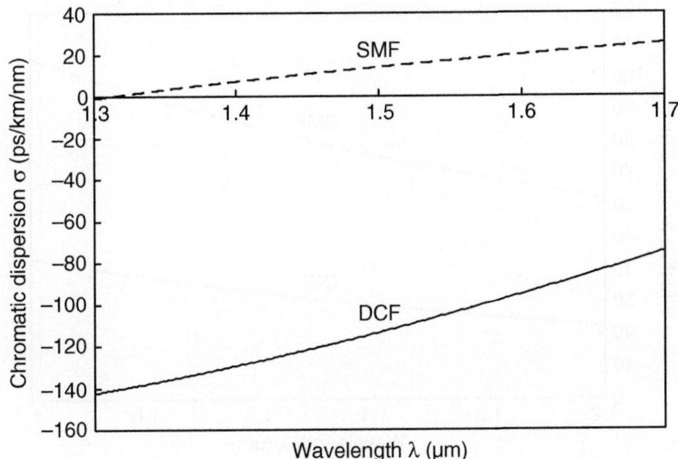

Figure 3.36 Chromatic dispersions of SMF with $\Delta = 0.3\%$, $2a = 9.2\,\mu m$ (dotted line) and DCF with $\Delta = 2.8\%$, $2a = 1.6\,\mu m$ (solid line).

100-km length of SMF the total chromatic dispersion of the transmission fiber becomes zero at $1.55\,\mu m$.

3.10.2. Dispersion-shifted Fibers

Dispersion-shifted fibers based on step-index profile are already described in Section 3.6.5. Cutoff wavelength of the step-index DSF is typically $\lambda c = 1.0\,\mu m$ so as to make the waveguide dispersion σ_W large at $1.55\,\mu m$ region. Under the waveguide parameters of $\Delta = 0.7\%$ and $2a = 4.6\,\mu m$, the cutoff wavelength $\lambda c = 1.03\,\mu m$. Therefore it is susceptible to large bending loss because light confinement to the core becomes weak. Moreover, since step-index DSF has small core diameter, spot size of the light field becomes small. Nonlinear optical effect in optical fibers depends on intensity of the light field as described in Chapter 5. Optical intensity I is expressed by

$$I = \frac{P}{A_{\text{eff}}}, \tag{3.250}$$

where P is a power carried by the mode and A_{eff} denotes the effective core area defined by Eq. (5.42). Figure 3.37 shows effective core area of SMF with $\Delta = 0.3\%$, $2a = 8.2\,\mu m$ (dotted line) and DSF with $\Delta = 0.75\%$, $2a = 4.6\,\mu m$ (solid line), respectively. The effective area of DSF ($A_{\text{eff}} = 35.3\,\mu m^2$) is about

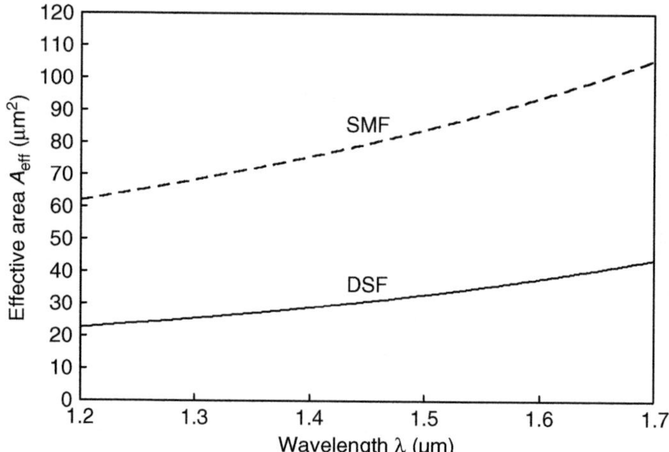

Figure 3.37 Effective core area of SMF with $\Delta = 0.3\%$, $2a = 8.2\,\mu m$ (dotted line) and DSF with $\Delta = 0.75\%$, $2a = 4.6\,\mu m$ (solid line).

1/2.5 of that of SMF. Nonlinear optical effects normally cause signal waveform distortion through self-phase modulation and four-wave mixing effect, which will be described in Chapter 5.

In order to enlarge the effective core area of DSFs, various kinds of refractive-index configurations have been proposed. Among them (a) dual-shape core DSF [39] and (b) segmented core DSF [40] will be described. Figures 3.38(a) and

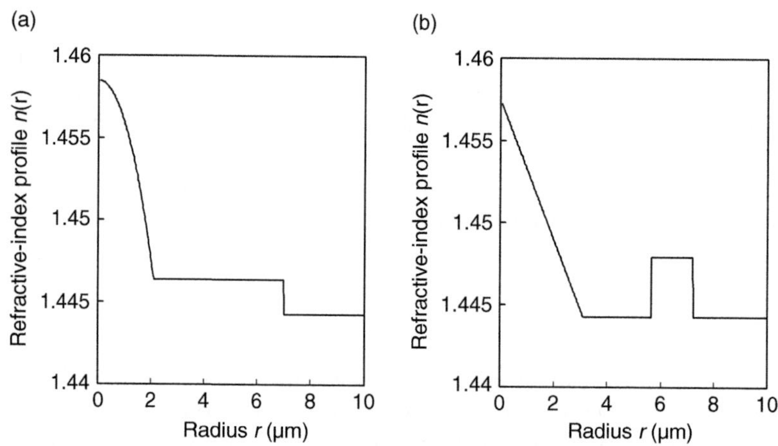

Figure 3.38 Refractive-index profiles of (a) dual-shape core DSF and (b) segmented core DSF.

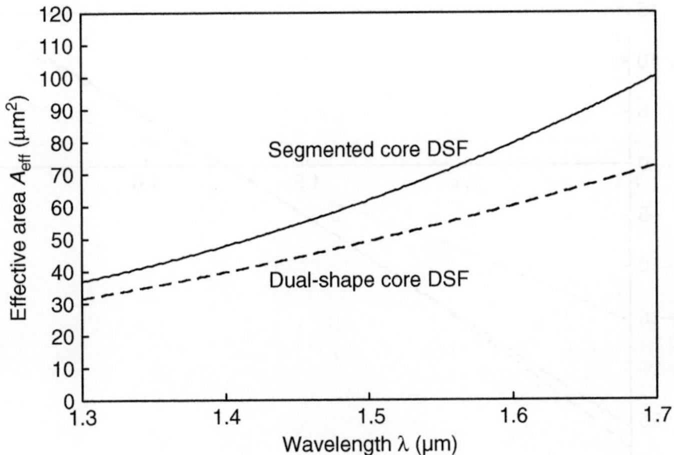

Figure 3.39 Effective core area of dual-shape core DSF (dotted line) and segmented core DSF (solid line).

(b) show refractive-index profiles of (a) dual-shape core DSF and (b) segmented core DSF. Dual-shape core fiber has pedestal region and segmented core fiber has outer ring region so as to tightly confine the light field. The role of these regions is twofold: one is to reduce the bending loss and the other is to enlarge the effective core area. Figure 3.39 shows effective core area of dual-shape core DSF and segmented core DSF. The effective area of dual-shape core DSF and segmented core DSF at 1.55 μm are enlarged to $A_{\text{eff}} = 54.4\,\mu\text{m}^2$ and $A_{\text{eff}} = 70.2\,\mu\text{m}^2$.

Figure 3.40 shows chromatic dispersions of dual-shape core DSF (dotted line), segmented core DSF (thick solid line) and step-index DSF (thin solid line). It is known that the inclination of chromatic dispersion in dual-shape core DSF and segmented core DSF becomes two times larger than that of step-index DSF. The inclination of chromatic dispersion is called dispersion slope, which is given by

$$\rho = \frac{d\sigma}{d\lambda}. \tag{3.251}$$

Figure 3.41 shows dispersion slopes of dual-shape core DSF (dotted line), segmented core DSF (thick solid line) and step-index DSF (thin solid line). In large dispersion-slope fibers, chromatic dispersion quickly becomes large when signal wavelength goes apart from the zero-dispersion wavelength. Then high bit-rate signals, which have broad frequency spectra, tend to suffer signal distortions.

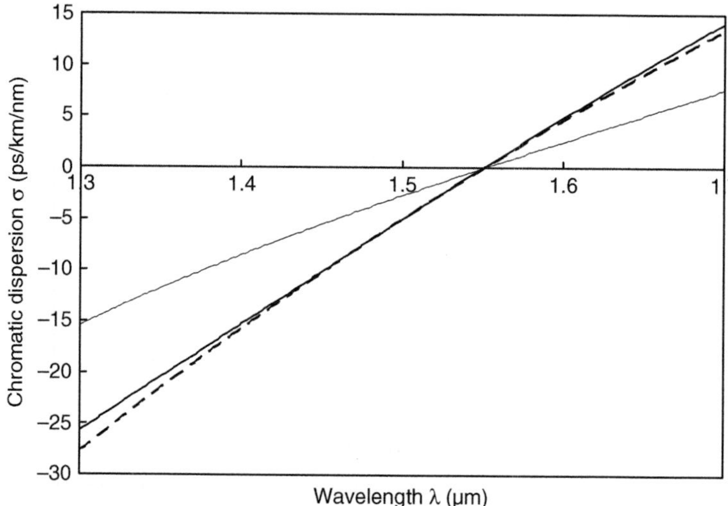

Figure 3.40 Chromatic dispersions of dual-shape core DSF (dotted line), segmented core DSF (thick solid line) and step-index DSF (thin solid line).

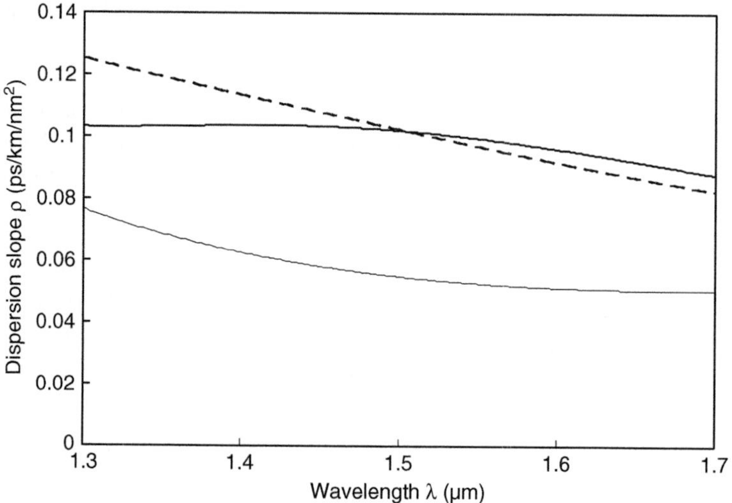

Figure 3.41 Dispersion slopes of dual-shape core DSF (dotted line), segmented core DSF (thick solid line) and step-index DSF (thin solid line).

Large dispersion slope fibers also cause problem in wavelength division multiplexing (WDM) systems. Signal channels that are separated from the zero-dispersion wavelength suffer higher signal distortion due to large chromatic dispersions.

3.10.3. Dispersion Flattened Fibers

As discussed in the previous section, minimizing the dispersion slope is important for high bit-rate transmissions and WDM systems. Optical fibers that have very small dispersion over a wide wavelength range are called dispersion flattened fibers (DFFs). The first proposal of DFF was made by Okamoto [41, 42] using single-mode fibers with W-type refractive-index profiles [43]. Refractive-index profile of W-type DFF is shown in Fig. 3.42. Core radius a, inner cladding thickness b, refractive-index difference of core and inner cladding $\Delta 1$ and $\Delta 2$, respectively, are optimized such that the waveguide dispersion cancels material dispersion almost completely. Figure 3.43 shows chromatic dispersion characteristics of W-type DFF. It is known that chromatic dispersion σ is reduced to less than ± 1 ps/km/nm over 1.47–1.6 μm wavelength (λ) range. The effective area of W-type DFF is about $A_{\text{eff}} = 30\,\mu\text{m}^2$ at 1.55 μm wavelength (Fig. 3.44), which is not large enough to suppress the signal waveform distortion due to nonlinear optical effect. In order to enlarge the effective core area while maintaining low dispersion over a wide spectral range, a quadruple-clad (QC) DFF was proposed [44]. Figure 3.45 shows the refractive-index profile of QC-type DFF. Ring-shaped region of $r = 7$–14 μm and outer ring of the depressed cladding

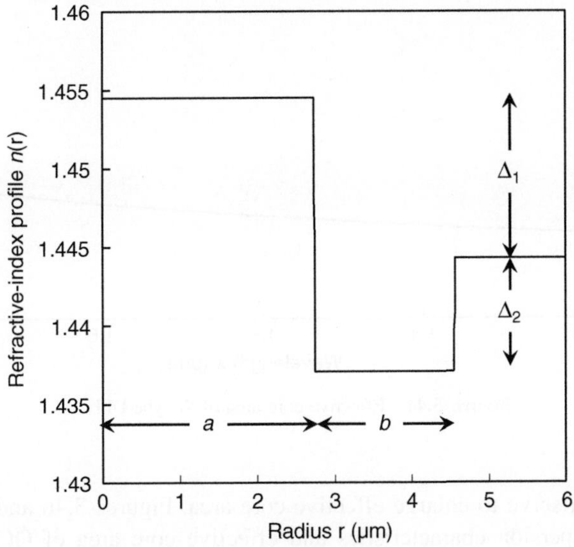

Figure 3.42 Refractive-index profile of W-type DFF. $\boldsymbol{a} = 2.73\,\mu\text{m}$, $\boldsymbol{b} = 1.77\,\mu\text{m}$, $\Delta_1 = 0.7\%$ and $\Delta_2 = -0.5\%$.

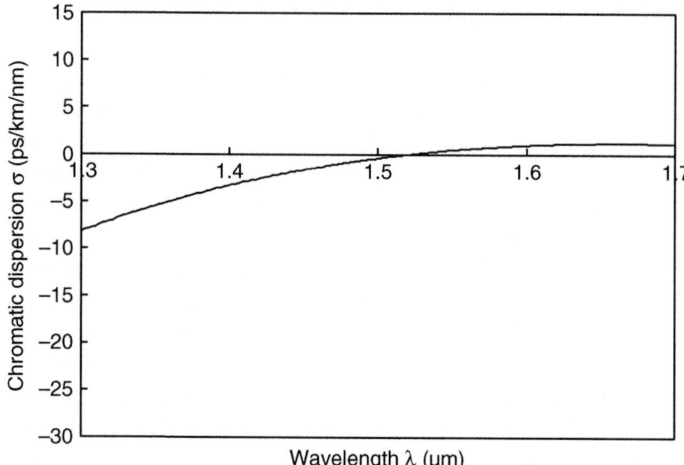

Figure 3.43 Chromatic dispersion characteristics of W-type DFF.

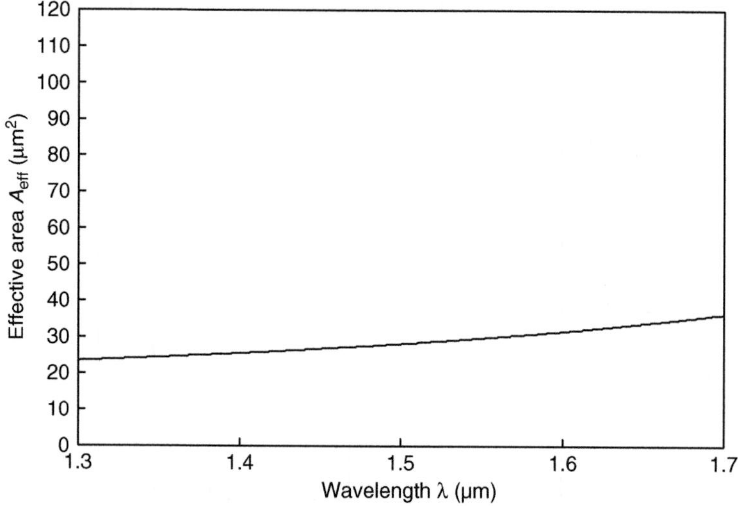

Figure 3.44 Effective core area of W-type DFF.

$r = 14$–$22\,\mu$m serve to enlarge effective core area. Figures 3.46 and 3.47 show chromatic dispersion characteristics and effective core area of QC-type DFF. Chromatic dispersion σ is reduced to less than ± 1 ps/km/nm over 1.43–1.6 μm wavelength (λ) range. The effective area of QC-type DFF is about $A_{eff} = 55\,\mu\text{m}^2$

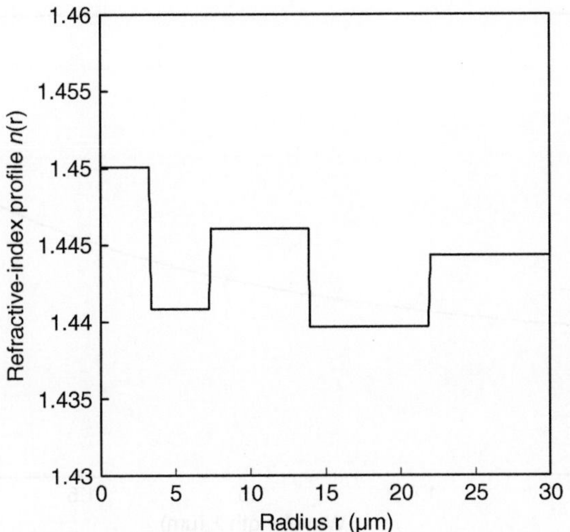

Figure 3.45 Refractive-index profile of QC-type DFF.

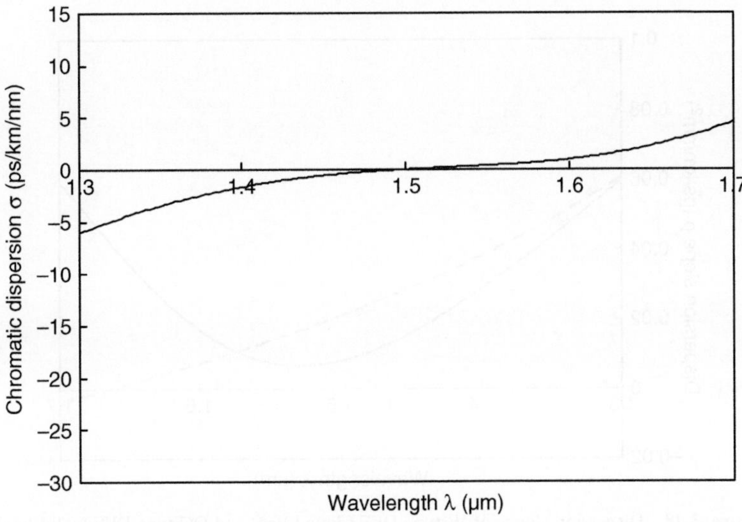

Figure 3.46 Chromatic dispersion characteristics of QC-type DFF.

at 1.55 μm wavelength, which is almost two times larger than that of W-type DFF. Figure 3.48 shows dispersion slopes of W-type DFF (dotted line) and QC-type DFF (solid line). It is confirmed that dispersion slopes in 1.4–1.6 μm wavelength (λ) range are very small because dispersions are flattened in these spectral regions.

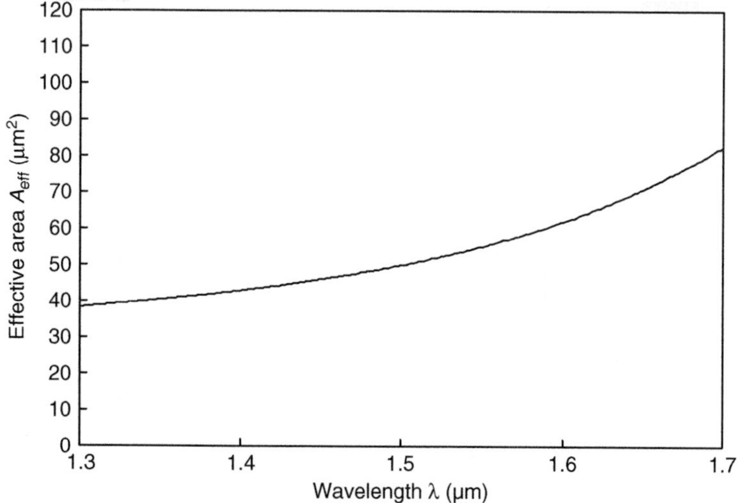

Figure 3.47 Effective core area of QC-type DFF.

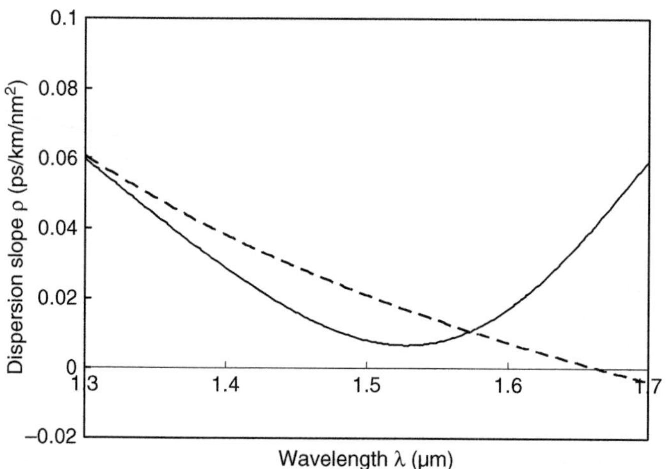

Figure 3.48 Dispersion slopes of W-type DFF (dotted line) and QC-type DFF (solid line).

3.10.4. Broadly Dispersion Compensating Fibers

The DFF is an ideal transmission medium for single-channel ultra-high bit-rate systems. In WDM systems, however, inter-channel nonlinear optical effects such as four-wave mixing (refer to Section 5.10) and cross-phase modulation

(XPM) [45] cause severe signal waveform degradations since optical signals having different wavelengths travel with almost the same group velocities. Cross-phase modulation is always accompanied by self-phase modulation (SPM) and occurs because the effective refractive index of a wave depends not only on the intensity of that wave but also on the intensity of other co-propagating waves in WDM. Broadly dispersion compensating fibers (BDCFs) [46, 47] were proposed to reduce the nonlinear signal impairment while maintaining the flatness of dispersion. Figure 3.49 shows a refractive-index profile of typical BDCF. Basically, BDCF has W-type [46] or segmented core [47] refractive-index profiles. Chromatic dispersion of BDCF is designed such that it almost completely cancels the dispersion of SMF when two fibers are connected with a certain ratio of lengths. Figure 3.50 shows chromatic dispersions of 1-km SMF (dotted line), 197-m BDCF (dot-broken line) and total dispersion of SMF + BDCF (solid line), respectively. Chromatic dispersion of the total SMF + BDCF is reduced to less than ± 0.5 ps/km/nm over $\lambda = 1.524$–$1.624\ \mu$m range. The advantage of the transmission line consisting of SMF and BDCF is that the local dispersion of each fiber is substantially large. It means that optical signals having different wavelengths in WDM systems travel with different group velocities in SMF and BDCF. Then, nonlinear interactions between WDM channels are minimized. Though local dispersions are large, the total dispersions for all WDM channels are made almost zero as shown in Fig. 3.50. Therefore, ultra-high bit-rate signals can be transmitted over long distances without suffering inter-channel nonlinear signal impairments.

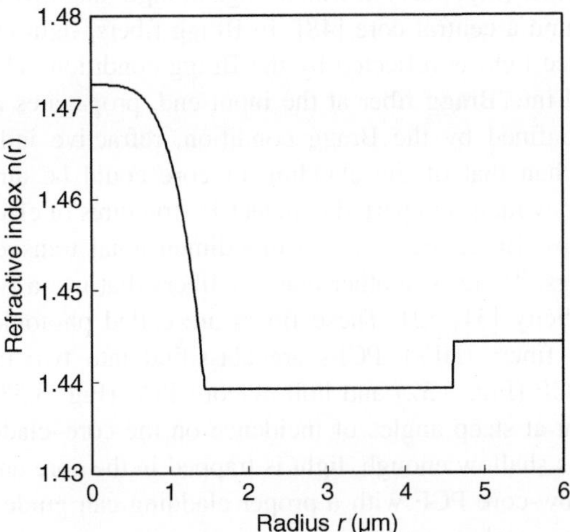

Figure 3.49 Refractive-index profile of BDCF.

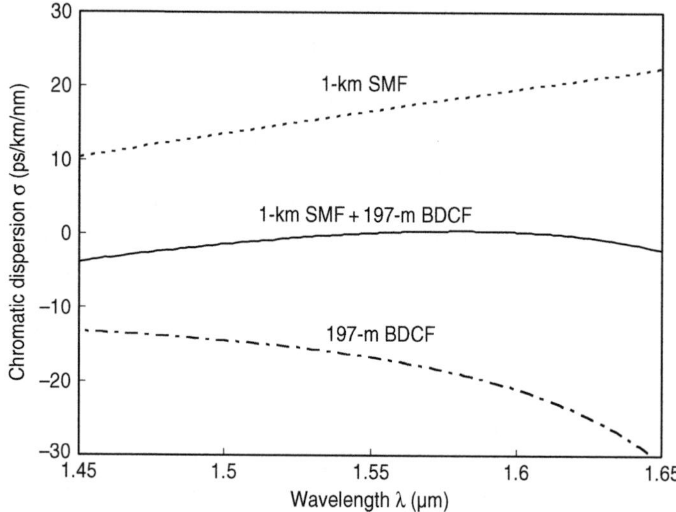

Figure 3.50 Chromatic dispersions of 1-km SMF (dotted line), 197-m BDCF (dot-broken line) and total dispersion of SMF + BDCF (solid line).

3.11. PHOTONIC CRYSTAL FIBERS

Traditional optical fibers, whose refractive index of core is higher than that of the cladding, confine light field by the total internal reflection. Yeh et al. proposed Bragg fiber (Fig. 3.51) in which rings of high- and low-refractive index are arranged around a central core [48]. In Bragg fibers, light cannot penetrate into cladding since light is reflected by the Bragg condition. Then, light beam, which is coupled into Bragg fiber at the input end, propagates along the fiber. Since light is confined by the Bragg condition, refractive index of the core could be lower than that of the cladding or core could be air [49, 50]. The forbidden frequency ranges in periodic dielectric structures of cladding are called photonic bandgaps. Bragg fibers use a one-dimensional transverse periodicity of concentric rings. There is another class of fibers that use a two-dimensional transverse periodicity [51, 52]. These fibers are called photonic crystal fibers (PCFs) or holey fibers (HFs). PCFs are classified into two categories: they are, solid-core PCF (Fig. 3.52) and hollow-core PCF (Fig. 3.53). A solid-core PCF refracts light at steep angles of incidence on the core–cladding boundary. When the angle is shallow enough, light is trapped in the core and guided along the fiber. A hollow-core PCF with a proper cladding can guide light at angles of incidence where a photonic band gap operates. Therefore, hollow-core PCF requires strict control of the periodic cladding structures.

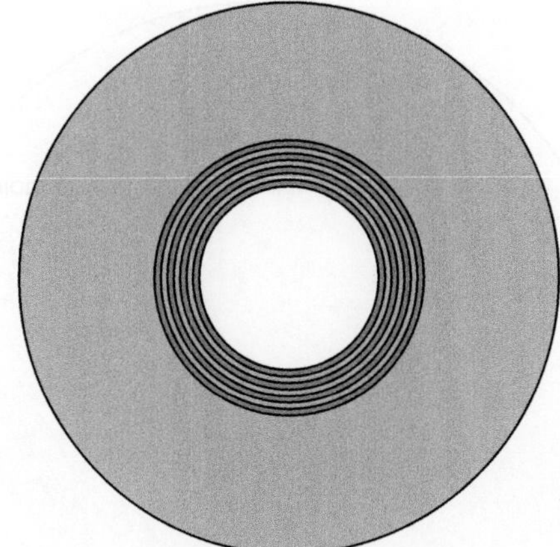

Figure 3.51 Bragg fiber.

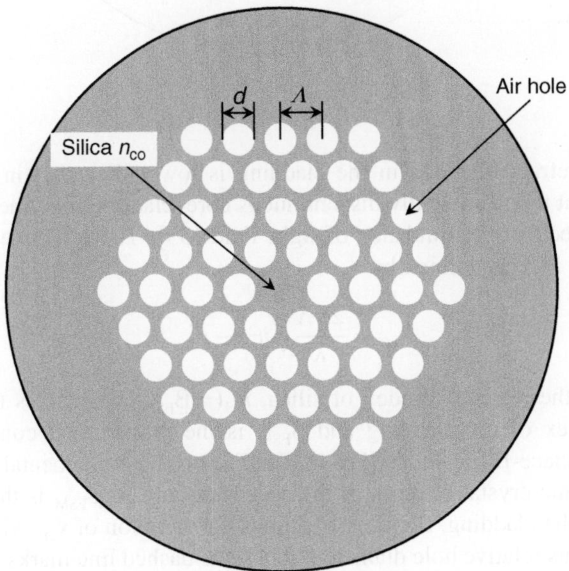

Figure 3.52 Solid-core PCF.

Fiber structure of PCF is determined by (a) pitch of the air hole Λ, (b) diameter of the air hole d and (c) number of air holes N_{AH}. Light guiding principle of the solid-core PCF is basically similar to that of the traditional optical fibers. However, there is no definite boundary between solid-core region and air-hole cladding region. On the other hand, there is a refractive-index difference because

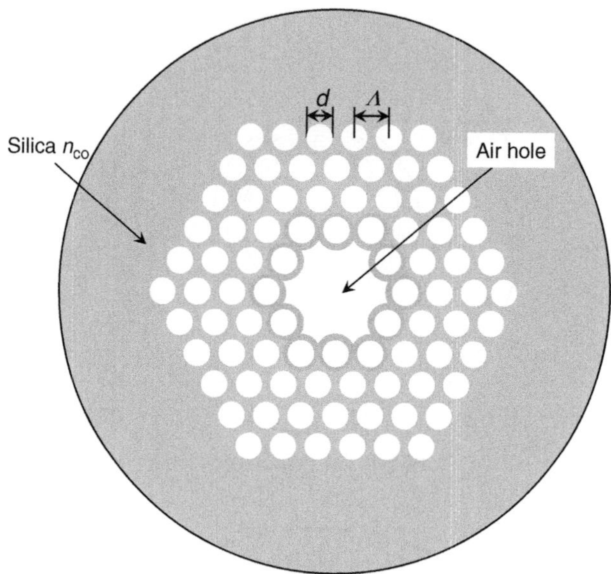

Figure 3.53 Hollow-core PCF.

the average refractive index in the cladding is lower than that in the core. It was found that the azimuthally discontinuous core–cladding interface has a very important effect on the guidance of light field [53]. The effective normalized frequency for PCF is defined by

$$\mathbf{v}_{\mathrm{eff}} = \frac{2\pi\Lambda}{\lambda}\sqrt{n_{\mathrm{co}}^2 - n_{\mathrm{cl}}^2}, \tag{3.252}$$

where n_{co} is the refractive index of silica, $n_{\mathrm{cl}}(=\beta_{\mathrm{FSM}}/k)$ denotes the effective refractive index of the cladding and β_{FSM} is the propagation constant of the fundamental space-filling mode (FSM). The FSM is the fundamental mode of the infinite photonic crystal cladding if the core is absent, so β_{FSM} is the maximum β allowed in the cladding. Figure 3.54 shows the variation of $\mathbf{v}_{\mathrm{eff}}$ with respect to Λ/λ for various relative hole diameters d/Λ. The dashed line marks $\mathbf{v}_{\mathrm{c}} = 4.1$, the cutoff $\mathbf{v}$ value for PCF [54]. For the relative hole diameters d/Λ less than about 0.4, the second-order mode is never guided even at infinite frequency; that is, $\mathbf{v}$ is always less than $\mathbf{v}_{\mathrm{c}}$ and the PCF is endlessly single-mode. Figures 3.55(a) and (b) show the intensity contour plots of the fundamental mode in solid-core PCF with relative hole diameter $d/\Lambda = 0.4$ ($d = 0.84\,\mu\mathrm{m}$ and $\Lambda = 2.1\,\mu\mathrm{m}$) at $\lambda = 0.4\,\mu\mathrm{m}$ and $\lambda = 1.55\,\mu\mathrm{m}$. Mode field distribution was calculated by using FEM (refer to Chapter 6.6). The second-order mode does not appear even at wavelength shorter than $\lambda = 0.4\,\mu\mathrm{m}$. Endlessly single-mode phenomenon is explained by noting that

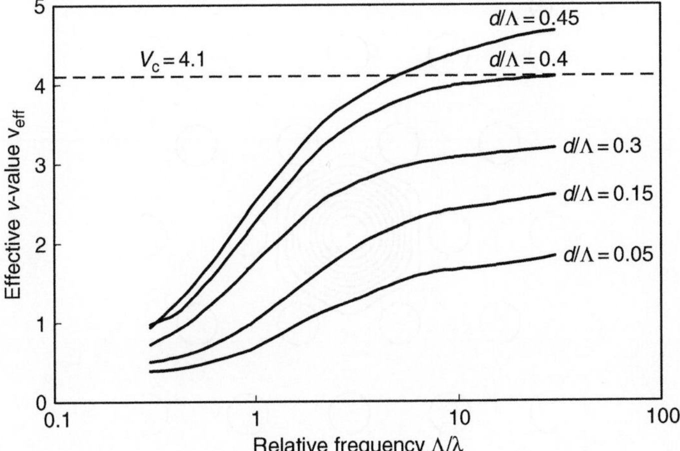

Figure 3.54 Variation of $\mathbf{v}_{\mathrm{eff}}$ with Λ/λ for various relative hole diameters d/Λ. The dashed line marks $\mathbf{v}_c = 4.1$, the cutoff v value for PCF.

the fundamental mode has a transverse effective wavelength that is roughly equal to twice the hole period Λ. The light is thus unable to escape because it cannot "image" the gaps between the air-holes, i.e., it cannot "squeeze between" them. The fundamental mode is then effectively trapped inside a "sieve", whereas the higher order modes, with smaller transverse effective wavelengths, can leak away rapidly through the gaps between the air holes [55].

The chromatic dispersion characteristics of PCF are distinctively different from that of the traditional optical fibers. This is mainly due to the fact that the waveguide dispersion in PCF becomes very large. In the derivation of waveguide dispersion of traditional optical fibers, we have neglected the wavelength (or frequency) dispersion of the term $n_{\mathrm{co}}^2 - n_{\mathrm{cl}}^2$ in Eq. (3.123). However, the effective refractive-index difference $\Delta_{\mathrm{eff}} = (n_{\mathrm{co}}^2 - n_{\mathrm{cl}}^2)/2n_{\mathrm{co}}^2$ strongly depends on the wavelength (or frequency). Figure 3.56 shows the effective refractive-index difference Δ_{eff} of solid-core PCF with relative hole diameter $d/\Lambda = 0.4$ ($d = 0.84\,\mu\mathrm{m}$ and $\Lambda = 2.1\,\mu\mathrm{m}$). The large wavelength dependence of Δ_{eff} enhances the waveguide dispersion in PCF. In Figure 3.57 the chromatic dispersions (waveguide dispersion σ_{w}, material dispersion σ_{m} and the total dispersion σ) are plotted against wavelength in the range from $0.5\,\mu\mathrm{m}$ to $1.3\,\mu\mathrm{m}$. Inset of Fig. 3.57 shows the contour plot of optical intensity at $\lambda = 1.05\,\mu\mathrm{m}$. Bulk silica glass has normal (negative) dispersion in this range. In the conventional single-mode fiber, the zero-dispersion wavelength is normally larger than $1.3\,\mu\mathrm{m}$ because the waveguide dispersion is negative in single-mode region. However, the zero-dispersion wavelength of PCF is shifted down to $1.05\,\mu\mathrm{m}$ since the waveguide dispersion

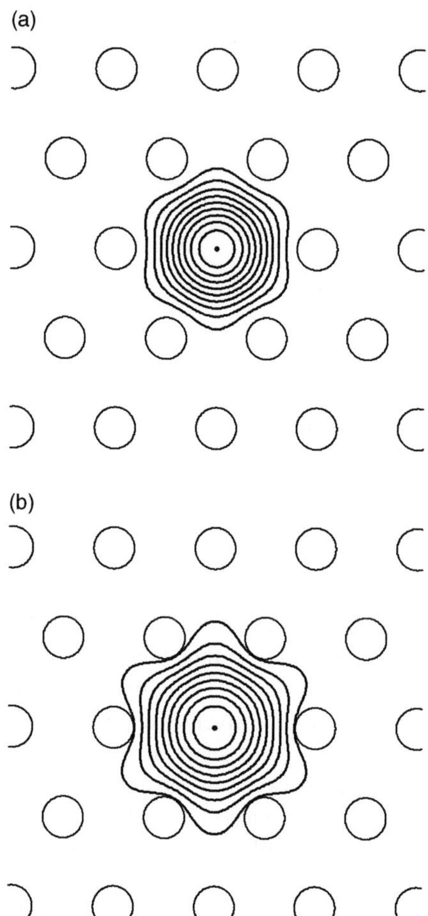

Figure 3.55 (a) Intensity contour plot of the fundamental mode at $\lambda = 0.4\,\mu m$ in solid-core PCF with relative hole diameter $d/\Lambda = 0.4$ ($d = 0.84\,\mu m$ and $\Lambda = 2.1\,\mu m$). (b) Intensity contour plot of the fundamental mode at $\lambda = 1.55\,\mu m$ in solid-core PCF with relative hole diameter $d/\Lambda = 0.4$ ($d = 0.84\,\mu m$ and $\Lambda = 2.1\,\mu m$).

has large positive value even in the single-mode region. As the air-holes become bigger the core becomes increasingly isolated and begins to look like a strand of silica glass sitting in the air. The waveguide dispersion of such a strand is very strong compared with the material dispersion. Figure 3.58 shows the chromatic dispersion characteristics of solid-core PCF with relative hole diameter $d/\Lambda = 0.8$ ($d = 1.68\,\mu m$ and $\Lambda = 2.1\,\mu m$). Inset of Fig. 3.58 shows the contour plot of optical intensity at $\lambda = 0.86\,\mu m$. The zero-dispersion wavelength

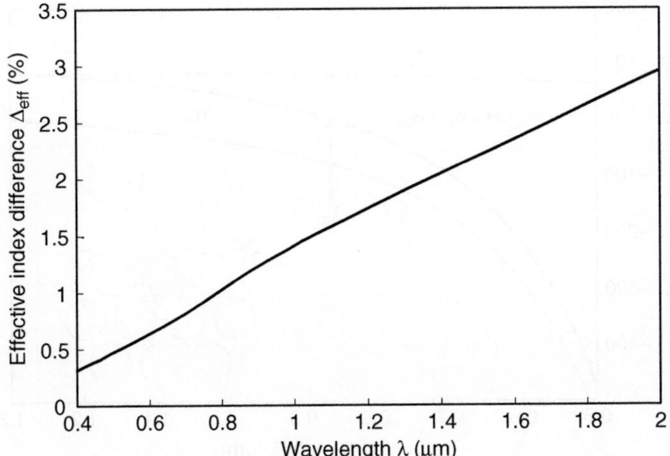

Figure 3.56 Effective refractive-index difference Δ_{eff} of solid-core PCF with relative hole diameter $d/\Lambda = 0.4$ ($d = 0.84\,\mu m$ and $\Lambda = 2.1\,\mu m$).

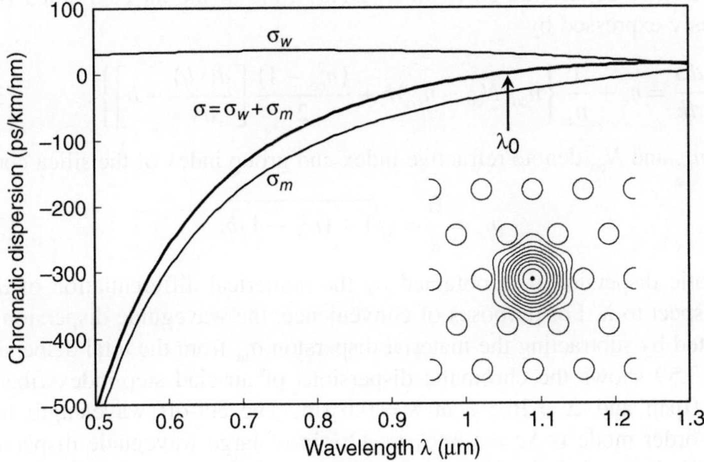

Figure 3.57 Chromatic dispersion characteristics of solid-core PCF with relative hole diameter $d/\Lambda = 0.4$ ($d = 0.84\,\mu m$ and $\Lambda = 2.1\,\mu m$).

is further shifted down to $0.86\,\mu m$ compared to the PCF with relative air-hole diameter $d/\Lambda = 0.4$. Different from the case of $d/\Lambda = 0.4$, PCF with $d/\Lambda = 0.8$ becomes multi-moded at $0.86\,\mu m$.

Since PCF with large air-hole diameter tends toward the step-index fiber with air cladding, it is worthwhile to investigate the chromatic dispersion

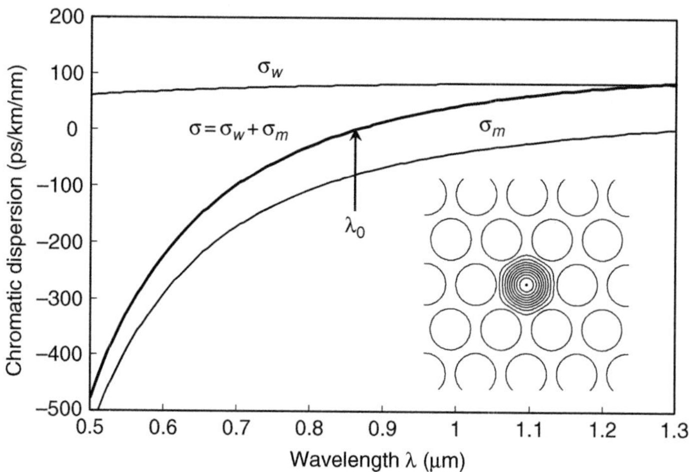

Figure 3.58 Chromatic dispersion characteristics of solid-core PCF with relative hole diameter $d/\Lambda = 0.8$ ($d = 1.68\,\mu\text{m}$ and $\Lambda = 2.1\,\mu\text{m}$).

characteristics of air-clad silica fiber. Delay time of the air-clad silica fiber is rigorously expressed by

$$\frac{d\beta}{dk} = n_e + \frac{1}{n_e}\left\{n_{co}(N_{co} - n_{co})b + \frac{(n_{co}^2 - 1)}{2}\left[\frac{d(vb)}{dv} - b\right]\right\}, \qquad (3.253)$$

where n_{co} and N_{co} denote refractive index and group index of the silica core and

$$n_e = \frac{\beta}{k} = \sqrt{1 + (n_{co}^2 - 1)b}. \qquad (3.254)$$

Chromatic dispersion σ is obtained by the numerical differentiation of $d\beta/dk$ with respect to λ. For purposes of convenience, the waveguide dispersion σ_w is calculated by subtracting the material dispersion σ_m from the total dispersion σ. Figure 3.59 shows the chromatic dispersions of air-clad step-index fiber with $2a = 1.0\,\mu\text{m}$ and $\Delta = 26.5\%$ at $\lambda = 0.6\,\mu\text{m}$. The cut-off wavelength for the second-order mode is $\lambda c = 1.386\,\mu\text{m}$. Origin of large waveguide dispersion in PCF with large air-hole diameter and the step-index air-clad silica fiber can be explained to be large refractive-index difference between silica core and air cladding [56].

One of the most interesting and useful applications of PCF is to the generation of broad-band supercontinuum light from short-pulse laser systems [57]. This is made possible by a combination of ultra-small cores and dispersion zeros that can be shifted to coincide with the pump laser wavelength. Broad-band supercontinuum light is very important not only in telecommunications but also in applications such as optical coherence tomography [58] and frequency metrology [59].

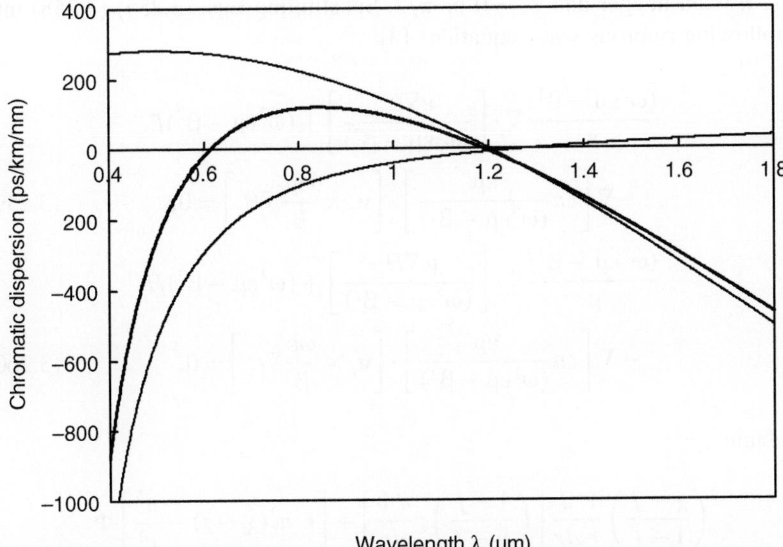

Figure 3.59 Chromatic dispersions of air-clad step-index fiber with $2a = 1.0\,\mu$m and $\Delta = 26.5\%$ at $\lambda = 0.6\,\mu$m. The cut-off wavelength for the second-order mode is $\lambda c = 1.386\,\mu$m.

Appendix 3A Vector wave equations in graded-index fibers

We express the refractive-index distribution and the propagation constant in the forms

$$n^2(r) = n_1^2[1 - f(r)], \tag{3.255}$$

$$\beta^2 = k^2 n_1^2 (1 - \chi), \tag{3.256}$$

where n_1 is the maximum refractive index in the core and therefore f is assumed to be $f(r) \geqslant 0$. The axial electromagnetic field components E_z and H_z are expressed as

$$E_z = \frac{k^2 n_1^2}{\beta} \Phi(r) \cos(n\theta + \varphi_n), \tag{3.257}$$

$$H_z = \omega\varepsilon_1 \Psi(r) \sin(n\theta + \varphi_n), \tag{3.258}$$

where n is an integer and $\varphi_n = 0$ or $\pi/2$. Substituting Eqs. (3.255)-(3.258) into the following rigorous wave equations [3]:

$$\frac{(\omega^2\varepsilon\mu - \beta^2)}{\varepsilon}\nabla\cdot\left[\frac{\varepsilon\nabla E_z}{(\omega^2\varepsilon\mu - \beta^2)}\right] + (\omega^2\varepsilon\mu - \beta^2)E_z - \nabla\left[\ell n\frac{\varepsilon\mu}{(\omega^2\varepsilon\mu - \beta^2)}\right]\cdot\left[\mathbf{u}_z \times \frac{\omega\mu}{\beta}\nabla H_z\right] = 0, \tag{3.259}$$

$$\frac{(\omega^2\varepsilon\mu - \beta^2)}{\mu}\nabla\cdot\left[\frac{\mu\nabla H_z}{(\omega^2\varepsilon\mu - \beta^2)}\right] + (\omega^2\varepsilon\mu - \beta^2)H_z + \nabla\left[\ell n\frac{\varepsilon\mu}{(\omega^2\varepsilon\mu - \beta^2)}\right]\cdot\left[\mathbf{u}_z \times \frac{\omega\varepsilon}{\beta}\nabla E_z\right] = 0, \tag{3.260}$$

we obtain

$$\left(\frac{\chi - f}{1 - f}\right)\frac{1}{r}\frac{d}{dr}\left[\left(\frac{1 - f}{\chi - f}\right)r\frac{d\Phi}{dr}\right] + \left[k^2 n_1^2(\chi - f) - \frac{n^2}{r^2}\right]\Phi + \frac{n}{r}\left(\frac{\chi - f}{1 - f}\right)\Psi\frac{d}{dr}\left(\frac{1 - f}{\chi - f}\right) = 0, \tag{3.261}$$

$$(\chi - f)\frac{1}{r}\frac{d}{dr}\left[\frac{1}{(\chi - f)}r\frac{d\Psi}{dr}\right] + \left[k^2 n_1^2(\chi - f) - \frac{n^2}{r^2}\right]\Psi + \frac{n}{r}(\chi - f)\Phi\frac{d}{dr}\left(\frac{1}{\chi - f}\right) = 0. \tag{3.262}$$

When we set $E_z = \Phi = 0$ for TE modes, we obtain from Eqs. (3.261) and (3.262),

$$\frac{n}{r}\left(\frac{\chi - f}{1 - f}\right)\Psi\frac{d}{dr}\left(\frac{1 - f}{\chi - f}\right) = 0, \tag{3.263}$$

$$(\chi - f)\frac{1}{r}\frac{d}{dr}\left[\frac{1}{(\chi - f)}r\frac{d\Psi}{dr}\right] + \left[k^2 n_1^2(\chi - f) - \frac{n^2}{r^2}\right]\Psi = 0. \tag{3.264}$$

The derivative of the term containing $f(r)$ is not zero in Eq. (3.263) since we are dealing with graded-index fibers. Therefore, the azimuthal mode number should be

$$n = 0, \tag{3.265}$$

in order that Eq. (3.263) holds for the arbitrary functional shape of $f(r)$.

Appendix 3B Derivation of equation (3.219)

Substituting Eq. (3.216) into Eq. (3.218) and using Eq. (3.217), we obtain

$$(\mathbf{u}_z \times \tilde{\mathbf{E}}_1)\frac{dA}{dz} + (\mathbf{u}_z \times \tilde{\mathbf{E}}_2)\frac{dB}{dz} = 0, \tag{3.266}$$

$$(\mathbf{u}_z \times \tilde{\mathbf{H}}_1)\frac{dA}{dz} - j\omega\varepsilon_0\, A(\tilde{\mathbf{K}} - \mathbf{K})\tilde{\mathbf{E}}_1 + (\mathbf{u}_z \times \tilde{\mathbf{H}}_2)\frac{dB}{dz} - j\omega\varepsilon_0\, B(\tilde{\mathbf{K}} - \mathbf{K})\tilde{\mathbf{E}}_2 = 0, \tag{3.267}$$

where $\mathbf{u}_z$ denotes the unit vector along z-axis direction. In the derivation of Eqs. (3.266) and (3.267), the following vector formula has been used:

$$\nabla \times (A\mathbf{E}) = A\nabla \times \mathbf{E} + \nabla A \times \mathbf{E} = A\nabla \times \mathbf{E} + \frac{dA}{dz}\mathbf{u}_z \times \mathbf{E}. \tag{3.268}$$

Noting that Eqs. (3.266) and (3.267) are zero, we consider here the following integration:

$$\int_0^{2\pi}\int_0^{\infty} [\tilde{\mathbf{E}}_1^* \cdot (3.256) - \tilde{\mathbf{H}}_1^* \cdot (3.255)]rd\,rd\theta = 0, \tag{3.269}$$

$$\int_0^{2\pi}\int_0^{\infty} [\tilde{\mathbf{E}}_2^* \cdot (3.256) - \tilde{\mathbf{H}}_2^* \cdot (3.255)]rd\,rd\theta = 0. \tag{3.270}$$

Equations (3.269) and (3.270) are rewritten as

$$\begin{aligned}
&\frac{dA}{dz}\int_0^{2\pi}\int_0^{\infty} \mathbf{u}_z \cdot (\tilde{\mathbf{E}}_1^* \times \tilde{\mathbf{H}}_1 + \tilde{\mathbf{E}}_1 \times \tilde{\mathbf{H}}_1^*)rd\,rd\theta \\
&+\frac{dB}{dz}\int_0^{2\pi}\int_0^{\infty} \mathbf{u}_z \cdot (\tilde{\mathbf{E}}_1^* \times \tilde{\mathbf{H}}_2 + \tilde{\mathbf{E}}_2 \times \tilde{\mathbf{H}}_1^*)rd\,rd\theta \\
&+j\omega\varepsilon_0 A\int_0^{2\pi}\int_0^{\infty} \tilde{\mathbf{E}}_1^* \cdot (\tilde{\mathbf{K}} - \mathbf{K})\tilde{\mathbf{E}}_1 rd\,rd\theta \\
&+j\omega\varepsilon_0 B\int_0^{2\pi}\int_0^{\infty} \tilde{\mathbf{E}}_1^* \cdot (\tilde{\mathbf{K}} - \mathbf{K})\tilde{\mathbf{E}}_2 rd\,rd\theta = 0,
\end{aligned} \tag{3.271}$$

$$\begin{aligned}
&\frac{dA}{dz}\int_0^{2\pi}\int_0^{\infty} \mathbf{u}_z \cdot (\tilde{\mathbf{E}}_2^* \times \tilde{\mathbf{H}}_1 + \tilde{\mathbf{E}}_1 \times \tilde{\mathbf{H}}_2^*)rd\,rd\theta \\
&+\frac{dB}{dz}\int_0^{2\pi}\int_0^{\infty} \mathbf{u}_z \cdot (\tilde{\mathbf{E}}_2^* \times \tilde{\mathbf{H}}_2 + \tilde{\mathbf{E}}_2 \times \tilde{\mathbf{H}}_2^*)rd\,rd\theta \\
&+j\omega\varepsilon_0 A\int_0^{2\pi}\int_0^{\infty} \tilde{\mathbf{E}}_2^* \cdot (\tilde{\mathbf{K}} - \mathbf{K})\tilde{\mathbf{E}}_1 rd\,rd\theta \\
&+j\omega\varepsilon_0 B\int_0^{2\pi}\int_0^{\infty} \tilde{\mathbf{E}}_2^* \cdot (\tilde{\mathbf{K}} - \mathbf{K})\tilde{\mathbf{E}}_2 rd\,rd\theta = 0,
\end{aligned} \tag{3.272}$$

Since E_x and H_y are dominant electromagnetic field components in HE_{11}^x mode $(\tilde{\mathbf{E}}_1, \tilde{\mathbf{H}}_1)$ and E_y and H_x are dominant electromagnetic field components in HE_{11}^y mode $(\tilde{\mathbf{E}}_2, \tilde{\mathbf{H}}_2)$ as described in Section 3.5, the fourth term in Eq. (3.271) and the third term in Eq. (3.272) can be neglected.

In order to further simplify Eqs. (3.271) and (3.272), we should derive the orthogonality relationship for the eigen modes $\tilde{\mathbf{E}}_p$ and $\tilde{\mathbf{H}}_p$ in the nonperturbed waveguides. We first consider integration of vector products over entire fiber cross-sectional area as

$$\iint \nabla \cdot (\tilde{\mathbf{E}}_p^* \times \tilde{\mathbf{H}}_q + \tilde{\mathbf{E}}_q \times \tilde{\mathbf{H}}_p^*)dS \quad (p, q = 1, 2). \tag{3.273}$$

Rewriting Eq. (3.273) by using Eq. (3.217) and vector formula

$$\nabla \cdot (\mathbf{A} \times \mathbf{B}) = \mathbf{B} \cdot \nabla \times \mathbf{A} - \mathbf{A} \cdot \nabla \times \mathbf{B}, \tag{3.274}$$

we obtain

$$\iint \nabla \cdot (\tilde{\mathbf{E}}_p^* \times \tilde{\mathbf{H}}_q + \tilde{\mathbf{E}}_q \times \tilde{\mathbf{H}}_p^*)dS = j\omega\varepsilon_0 \iint \tilde{\mathbf{E}}_p^* \cdot (\mathbf{K}^* - \mathbf{K})\tilde{\mathbf{E}}_q dS = 0. \tag{3.275}$$

Since relative permittivity tensor is real $(\mathbf{K}^* = \mathbf{K})$ in the lossless dielectric waveguides, Eq. (3.275) is zero. We separate here the eigen modes $\tilde{\mathbf{E}}_p$ and $\tilde{\mathbf{H}}_p$ into transversal and longitudinal components:

$$\begin{cases} \tilde{\mathbf{E}}_p(r, \theta, z) = \mathbf{E}_p(r, \theta)\exp(-j\beta_p z), \\ \tilde{\mathbf{H}}_p(r, \theta, z) = \mathbf{H}_p(r, \theta)\exp(-j\beta_p z), \end{cases} \quad (p = 1, 2) \tag{3.276}$$

Substituting Eq. (3.276) into Eq. (3.275) we obtain

$$\iint \nabla \cdot \{(\mathbf{E}_p^* \times \mathbf{H}_q + \mathbf{E}_q \times \mathbf{H}_p^*)\exp[j(\beta_p - \beta_q)z]\}dS = 0. \tag{3.277}$$

By using a vector formula of the form

$$\nabla \cdot (\mathbf{A}\phi) = \phi\nabla \cdot \mathbf{A} + \mathbf{A} \cdot \nabla\phi = \phi\nabla_t \cdot \mathbf{A} + \frac{d\phi}{dz}\mathbf{u}_z \cdot \mathbf{A}, \tag{3.278}$$

Eq. (3.277) can be rewritten into

$$\iint \nabla_t \cdot (\mathbf{E}_p^* \times \mathbf{H}_q + \mathbf{E}_q \times \mathbf{H}_p^*)dS + j(\beta_p - \beta_q) \iint \mathbf{u}_z \cdot (\mathbf{E}_p^* \times \mathbf{H}_q + \mathbf{E}_q \times \mathbf{H}_p^*)dS = 0, \tag{3.279}$$

where ∇_t denotes a differential operator in the cross-sectional area. The first term in Eq. (3.279) can be modified into line integral by using Gauss' theorem as

$$\iint \nabla_t \cdot (\mathbf{E}_p^* \times \mathbf{H}_q + \mathbf{E}_q \times \mathbf{H}_p^*) dS + \oint (\mathbf{E}_p^* \times \mathbf{H}_q + \mathbf{E}_q \times \mathbf{H}_p^*) \cdot \mathbf{n} d\ell, \tag{3.280}$$

where $\oint d\ell$ represents line integral along the peripheral of the cross-sectional area S and $\mathbf{n}$ denotes outward directed unit normal vector, respectively. Since electromagnetic field $\mathbf{E}_p$ and $\mathbf{H}_p$ become zero when line integral is carried out on the peripheral sufficiently far from the core center, Eq. (3.280) also becomes zero. Then Eq. (3.279) reduces to

$$j(\beta_p - \beta_q) \iint \mathbf{u}_z \cdot (\mathbf{E}_p^* \times \mathbf{H}_q + \mathbf{E}_q \times \mathbf{H}_p^*) dS = 0. \tag{3.281}$$

It is known from Eq. (3.281) that orthogonality relation

$$\iint \mathbf{u}_z \cdot (\mathbf{E}_p^* \times \mathbf{H}_q \times \mathbf{E}_q \times \mathbf{H}_p^*) dS = 0 \qquad (p \neq q) \tag{3.282}$$

holds between modes having different propagation constants $(\beta_p \neq \beta_q)$.

In case of the circular symmetric fiber, HE_{11}^x and HE_{11}^y are degenerated and have the same propagation constants. Therefore, we can not prove the orthogonality relation from Eq. (3.281). In such a case, however, we can derive the orthogonality relation by directly putting the electromagnetic fields for HE_{11}^x and HE_{11}^y modes [Eqs. (3.94) and (3.95)] into Eq. (3.282). Substituting Eq. (3.282) into Eqs. (3.271) and (3.272), we obtain

$$\frac{dA}{dz} = -jA \frac{\omega\varepsilon_0 \int_0^{2\pi} \int_0^{\infty} \mathbf{E}_1^* \cdot (\tilde{\mathbf{K}} - \mathbf{K}) \mathbf{E}_1 r\, dr\, d\theta}{\int_0^{2\pi} \int_0^{\infty} \mathbf{u}_z \cdot (\mathbf{E}_1^* \times \mathbf{H}_1 + \mathbf{E}_1 \times \mathbf{H}_1^*) r\, dr\, d\theta}, \tag{3.283}$$

$$\frac{dB}{dz} = -jB \frac{\omega\varepsilon_0 \int_0^{2\pi} \int_0^{\infty} \mathbf{E}_2^* \cdot (\tilde{\mathbf{K}} - \mathbf{K}) \mathbf{E}_2 r\, dr\, d\theta}{\int_0^{2\pi} \int_0^{\infty} \mathbf{u}_z \cdot (\mathbf{E}_2^* \times \mathbf{H}_2 + \mathbf{E}_2 \times \mathbf{H}_2^*) r\, dr\, d\theta}. \tag{3.284}$$

REFERENCES

[1] Yokota, H., H. Kanamori, Y. Ishiguro, G. Tanaka, S. Tanaka, H. Takada, M. Watanabe, S. Suzuki, K. Yano, M. Hoshikawa, and H. Shinba. 1986. Ultra low-loss pure silica core single-mode fiber and transmission experiment. *Tech. Digest of Opt. Fiber Commun.*, Atlanta, Postdeadline Paper, PD3.

[2] Snitzer, E. 1961. Cylindrical dielectric waveguide modes. *J. Opt. Soc. Amer.* 51:491–498.

[3] Okoshi, T. 1982. *Optical Fibers*. New York: Academic Press.

[4] Abramowitz, M., and J. A. Stegun. 1965. *Handbook of Mathematical Functions*. New York: Dover Publications.

[5] Watson, G. N. 1962. *Theory of Bessel Functions*. New York: Cambridge University Press.

[6] Snyder, A. W. 1969. Asymptotic expression for eigenfunctions and eigenvalues of dielectric optical waveguides. *IEEE Trans. on Microwave Theory and Tech.* MTT-17:1130–1138.

[7] Gloge, D. 1971. Weakly guiding fibers. *Appl. Opt.* 10:2252–2258.

[8] Carson, J. R., S. P. Mead, and S. A. Schelkunoff. 1936. Hyper frequency waveguides—Mathematical theory. *Bell. Syst. Tech. J.* 15:310–333.

[9] Marcuse, D. 1976. Microbending losses of single-mode step-index and multimode, parabolic-index fibers. *Bell. Syst. Tech. J.* 55:937–955.

[10] Collin, R. E. 1960. *Field Theory of Guided Waves*. New York: McGraw-Hill.

[11] Gloge, D. 1971. Dispersion in weakly guiding fibers. *Appl. Opt.* 10:2442–2445.

[12] Malitson, I. H. 1965. Interspecimen comparison of the refractive index of fused silica. *J. Opt. Soc. Amer.* 55:1205–1209.

[13] Shibata, N. and T. Edahiro. 1980. Refractive index dispersion properties of glasses for optical fibers (in Japanese). Paper of Technical Group, IEICE Japan, no.OQE80, pp.114–118.

[14] Morse, P. M. and H. Feshbach. 1953. *Methods of Theoretical Physics*. New York: McGraw-Hill.

[15] Koshiba, M. 1973. *Optical waveguide analysis*. New York: McGraw-Hill.

[16] Gloge, D., and E. A. J. Marcatili. 1973. Multimode theory of graded-core fibers *Bell. Syst. Tech. J.* 52:1563–1578.

[17] Olshansky, R., and D. B. Keck. 1976. Pulse broadening in graded-index optical fibers. *Appl. Opt.* 15:483–491.

[18] Henry, P. S. 1985. Lightwave primer. *IEEE J. of Quantum Electron.* QE-21:1862–1879.

[19] Kaminow, I. P. 1981. Polarization in optical fibers. *IEEE J. of Quantum Electron.* QE-17:15–22.

[20] Krawarik, P. H., and L. S. Watkins. 1978. Fiber geometry specifications and its relation to measured fiber statistics. *Appl. Opt.* 17:3984–3989.

[21] Noda, J., K. Okamoto, and Y. Sasaki. 1986. Polarization-maintaining fibers and their applications. *J. Lightwave Tech.* LT-4:1071–1089.

[22] Dyott, R. B., J. R. Cozens, and D. G. Morris. 1979. Preservation of polarization in optical-fiber waveguides with elliptical cores. *Electron. Lett.* 15:380–382.

[23] Hosaka, T., K. Okamoto, Y. Sasaki, and T. Edahiro. 1981. Single-mode fibers with asymmetrical refractive-index pits on both sides of the core. *Electron. Lett.* 17:191–193.

[24] Okoshi, T., K. Oyamada, M. Nishimura, and H. Yokota. 1982. Side-tunnel fiber–An approach to polarization-maintaining optical waveguiding scheme. *Electron. Lett.* 18:824–826.

[25] Hosaka, T., K. Okamoto, T. Miya, Y. Sasaki, and T. Edahiro. 1981. Low-loss single-polarization fibers with asymmetrical strain birefringence. *Electron. Lett.* 17:530–531.

[26] Birch, R. D., M. P. Varnham, D. N. Payne, and E. J. Tarbox. 1982. Fabrication of polarization-maintaining fibers using gas-phase etching. *Electron. Lett.* 18:1036–1038.

[27] Katsuyama, T., H. Matsumura, and T. Suganuma. 1981. Low-loss single-polarization fibers. *Electron. Lett.* 17:473–474.

[28] Nye, J. F. 1957. *Physical Properties of Crystals*. Oxford: Oxford University Press.

[29] Marcuse, D. 1972. *Light Transmission Optics*. New York: Van Nostrand Reinhold.

[30] Goell, J. E. 1969. A circular-harmonic computer analysis of rectangular dielectric waveguides. *Bell. Syst. Tech. J.* 48:2133–2160.

[31] Scherer, G. W. 1980. Stress-induced index profile distribution in optical waveguides. *Appl. Opt.* 19:2000–2006.

[32] Sinha, N. K. 1978. Normalized dispersion of birefringence of quartz and stress optical coefficient of fused and plate glass. *Phys. and Chem. of Glass.* 19:69–77.

[33] Sakai, J., and T. Kimura. 1981. Birefringence and polarization characteristics of single-mode optical fibers under elastic deformations. *IEEE J. of Quantum Electron.* QE-17:1041–1051.

[34] Okamoto, K., T. Edahiro, and N. Shibata. 1982. Polarization properties of single-polarization fibers. *Opt. Lett.* 7:569–571.

[35] Okamoto, K., T. Hosaka, and T. Edahiro. 1981. Stress analysis of optical fibers by a finite element method. *IEEE J. of Quantum Electron.* QE-17:2123–2129.

[36] Kawakami, S. and M. Ikeda. Transmission characteristics of a two-mode optical waveguide. *IEEE J. Quantum Electron.* QE-14:608–614.

[37] Poole, C. D. Statistical treatment of polarization dispersion in single-mode fiber. *Opt. Lett.* 8:687–689.

[38] Tsubokawa, M. N. Shibata and S. Seikai. Evaluation of polarization mode coupling coefficient from measurement of polarization mode dispersion. *IEEE J. Lightwave Tech.* LT-3:850–854.

[39] Kuwaki, N. M. Ohashi, C. Tanaka, N. Uesugi, S. Seikai and Y. Negishi. 1987. Characteristics of dispersion-shifted dual shape core single-mode fibers. *IEEE J. Lightwave Tech.* LT-5(6):792–797.

[40] Croft, T. D. J. E. Ritter and V. A. Bhagavatula. 1985. Low-loss dispersion-shifted single-mode fiber manufactured by the OVD process. *IEEE J. Lightwave Tech.* LT-3(5):931–934.

[41] Okamoto, K., T. Edahiro, A. Kawana and T. Miya. 1979. Dispersion minimization in single mode fibers over a wide spectral range. *Electron. Lett.* 15(22):729–731.

[42] Miya, T. K. Okamoto, Y. Ohmori and Y. Sasaki. 1981. Fabrication of low dispersion single mode fibers over a wide spectral range. *IEEE J. Quantum Electron.* QE-17(6):858–861.

[43] Kawakami S. and S. Nishida. 1974. Characteristics of a doubly clad optical fiber with a low-index inner cladding. *IEEE J. Quantum Electron.* 10(12):879–887.

[44] Cohen, L. G. W. L. Mammel and S. J. Jang. 1982. Low-loss quadruple-clad single-mode lightguide with dispersion below 2 ps/km/nm over the 1.28 μm–1.65 μm wavelength range. *Electron. Lett.* 18:1023–1024.

[45] Agrawal G. P. 1989. *Nonlinear Fiber Optics.* San Diego, Academic Press.

[46] Mukasa, K. Y. Akasaka, Y. Suzuki and T. Kamiya. 1997. Novel network fiber to manage dispersion at 1.55 μm with combination of 1.3 μm zero dispersion single mode fiber. *ECOC'97, Mo3C*, pp. 127–130, Sept. 22–25, Edinburgh, UK.

[47] Hirano, M. A. Tada, T. Kato, M. Onishi, Y. Makio and M. Nishimura. 2001. Dispersion compensating fiber over 140 nm-bandwidth, *ECOC '01*, Th.M.1.4, pp. 494–495, Sept. 30–Oct. 4, Amsterdam, The Netherlands.

[48] Yeh, P. A. Yariv and E. Marom. 1978. Theory of Bragg fiber. *J. Opt. Soc. Am.* 68:1196–1201.

[49] Miyagi M. and S. Kawakami. 1984. Design theory of dielectric-coated circular metallic waveguides for infrared transmission. *J. Lightwave Tech.* LT-2(2):116–126.

[50] Johnson, S. G. M. Ibanescu, M. Skorobogatiy, O. Weisberg, T. D. Engeness, M. Soljacic, S. A. Jacobs, J. D. Joannopoulos and Y. Fink. 2001. Low-loss asymptotically single-mode propagation in large-core omniguide fibers. *Optics Express* 9(13):748–779.

[51] Birks, T. A. P. J. Roberts, P. St. J. Russell, D. M. Atkin and T. J. Shepherd. 1995. Full 2-D photonic band gaps in silica/air structures. *Electron. Lett.* 31:1941–1942.

[52] Monro, T. M. D. J. Richardson, N. G. R. Broderick and P. J. Bennett. 1999. Holey optical fibers: An efficient modal model. *J. Lightwave Tech.* LT-17:1093–1102.

[53] Birks, T. A. J. C. Knight and P. St. J. Russell. 1997. Endlessly single-mode photonic crystal fiber. *Opt. Lett.* 22:961–963.

[54] Birks, T. A. D. Mogilevtsev, J. C. Knight, P. St. J. Russell, J. Broeng and P. J. Roberts. 1999. The analogy between photonic crystal fibers and step index fibers. *OFC/IOOC '99*, San Diego, CA Feb. 21–26, FG4, pp. 114–116.

[55] Russell, P. St. J. 2000. Photonic crystal fibers. *Science* 299:358–362.

[56] Birks, T. A. W. J. Wadsworth and P. St. J. Russell. 2000. Supercontinuum generation in tapered fibers. *Opt. Lett.* 25:1415–1417.

[57] Ranka, J. K. R. S. Windeler and A. J. Stentz. 2000. Visible continuum generation in air-silica microstructure optical fibers with anormalous dispersion at 800 nm. *Opt. Lett.* 25:25–27.

[58] Holzwarth, R. A. Y. Nevsky, M. Zimmermann, T. Udem, T. W. Hänsch, J. Von Zanthier, H. Walther, J. C. Knight, W. J. Wadsworth, P. St. J. Russell, M. N. Skvortsov and S. N. Bagayev. 2001. Absolute frequency measurement of iodine lines with a femtosecond optical synthesizer. *Appl. Phys. B* 73:269–271.

[59] Hundertmark, H. D. Kracht, D. Wandt, C. Fallnich, V. V. Ravi Kanth Kumar, A. K. George, J. C. Knight and P. St. J. Russell. 2003. Supercontinuum generation with 200 pJ laser pulses in an extruded SF6 fiber at 1560 nm. *Opt. Exp.* 11:3196–3201.

Chapter 4

Coupled Mode Theory

In the preceding two chapters, the transmission characteristics of independent planar optical waveguides and optical fibers have been investigated. For the construction of practical optical devices, it is very important to utilize the mutual lightwave interaction between the two copropagating light beams in the adjacent waveguides or interaction between the contrapropagating two beams in the corrugated optical waveguides. Coupled mode theory deals with the mutual lightwave interactions between the two propagation modes. In this chapter derivation of coupled mode equations based on perturbation theory is first presented and then concrete methods calculating the coupling coefficients for several practically important devices are explained in detail. Finally, several waveguide devices using directional couplers such as Mach–Zehnder interferometers, ring resonators, and bistable devices are described.

4.1. DERIVATION OF COUPLED MODE EQUATIONS BASED ON PERTURBATION THEORY

In axially uniform optical waveguides, a number of propagation modes exist, as has been described in the previous chapters. These propagation modes are specific to each waveguide and satisfy the orthogonality conditions between the modes.

If two waveguides are brought close together as shown in Fig. 4.1, optical modes of each waveguide either couple or interfere with each other. When the electromagnetic field distributions after mode coupling do not differ substantially from those before coupling, the propagation characteristics of the coupled waveguides can be analyzed by the perturbation method [1].

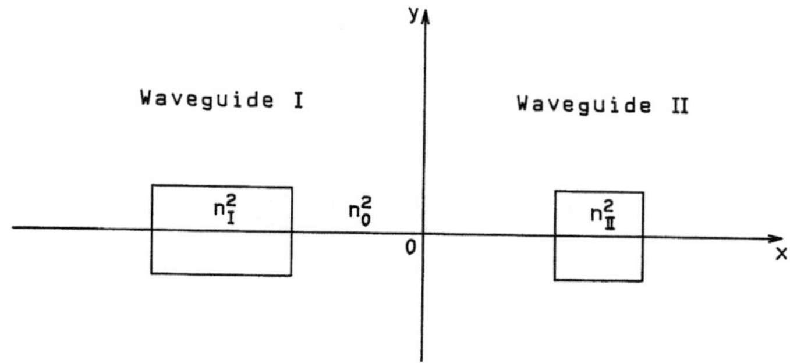

Figure 4.1 Directionally coupled optical waveguides.

When we denote the eigen modes in each optical waveguide before mode coupling as $\tilde{\mathbf{E}}_p, \tilde{\mathbf{H}}_p (p = 1, 2)$, they satisfy the following Maxwell's equations:

$$\begin{cases} \nabla \times \tilde{\mathbf{E}}_p = -j\omega\mu_0\tilde{\mathbf{H}}_p \\ \nabla \times \tilde{\mathbf{H}}_p = j\omega\varepsilon_0 N_p^2 \tilde{\mathbf{E}}_p, \end{cases} \qquad (p = 1, 2) \tag{4.1}$$

where $N_p^2(x, y)$ represents the refractive-index distribution of each waveguide. We assume that the electromagnetic fields of the coupled waveguide can be expressed as the sum of the eigen modes in each waveguide:

$$\begin{cases} \tilde{\mathbf{E}} = A(z)\tilde{\mathbf{E}}_1 + B(z)\tilde{\mathbf{E}}_2 \\ \tilde{\mathbf{H}} = A(z)\tilde{\mathbf{H}}_1 + B(z)\tilde{\mathbf{H}}_2. \end{cases} \tag{4.2}$$

The electromagnetic fields in the coupled waveguide $\tilde{\mathbf{E}}$ and $\tilde{\mathbf{H}}$ also should satisfy Maxwell's equations. Then substituting Eq. (4.2) into

$$\begin{cases} \nabla \times \tilde{\mathbf{E}} = -j\omega\mu_0\tilde{\mathbf{H}} \\ \nabla \times \tilde{\mathbf{H}} = j\omega\varepsilon_0 N^2 \tilde{\mathbf{E}}, \end{cases} \tag{4.3}$$

and using Eq. (4.1) and the vector formula

$$\nabla \times (A\mathbf{E}) = A\nabla \times \mathbf{E} + \nabla A \times \mathbf{E} = A\nabla \times \mathbf{E} + \frac{dA}{dz}\mathbf{u}_z \times \mathbf{E},$$

we obtain the following relations:

$$(\mathbf{u}_z \times \tilde{\mathbf{E}}_1)\frac{dA}{dz} + (\mathbf{u}_z \times \tilde{\mathbf{E}}_2)\frac{dB}{dz} = 0, \tag{4.4}$$

$$(\mathbf{u}_z \times \tilde{\mathbf{H}}_1)\frac{dA}{dz} - j\omega\varepsilon_0(N^2 - N_1^2)A\tilde{\mathbf{E}}_1$$
$$+ (\mathbf{u}_z \times \tilde{\mathbf{H}}_2)\frac{dB}{dz} - j\omega\varepsilon_0(N^2 - N_2^2)B\tilde{\mathbf{E}}_2 = 0. \tag{4.5}$$

Here, $N^2(x, y)$ denotes the refractive-index distribution in the entire coupled waveguide. Substituting Eqs. (4.4) and (4.5) into the following integral equations:

$$\int_{-\infty}^{\infty}\int_{-\infty}^{\infty} [\tilde{\mathbf{E}}_1^* \cdot (4.5) - \tilde{\mathbf{H}}_1^* \cdot (4.4)]\, dx\, dy = 0, \tag{4.6}$$

$$\int_{-\infty}^{\infty}\int_{-\infty}^{\infty} [\tilde{\mathbf{E}}_2^* \cdot (4.5) - \tilde{\mathbf{H}}_2^* \cdot (4.4)]\, dx\, dy = 0, \tag{4.7}$$

we obtain (see Appendix 4A at the end of this chapter)

$$\begin{aligned} &\frac{dA}{dz} + \frac{dB}{dz}\frac{\int_{-\infty}^{\infty}\int_{-\infty}^{\infty} \mathbf{u}_z \cdot (\tilde{\mathbf{E}}_1^* \times \tilde{\mathbf{H}}_2 + \tilde{\mathbf{E}}_2 \times \tilde{\mathbf{H}}_1^*) dx\, dy}{\int_{-\infty}^{\infty}\int_{-\infty}^{\infty} \mathbf{u}_z \cdot (\tilde{\mathbf{E}}_1^* \times \tilde{\mathbf{H}}_1 + \tilde{\mathbf{E}}_1 \times \tilde{\mathbf{H}}_1^*)\, dx\, dy} \\ &+ jA\frac{\omega\varepsilon_0 \int_{-\infty}^{\infty}\int_{-\infty}^{\infty} (N^2 - N_1^2)\tilde{\mathbf{E}}_1^* \cdot \tilde{\mathbf{E}}_1\, dx\, dy}{\int_{-\infty}^{\infty}\int_{-\infty}^{\infty} \mathbf{u}_z \cdot (\tilde{\mathbf{E}}_1^* \times \tilde{\mathbf{H}}_1 + \tilde{\mathbf{E}}_1 + \tilde{\mathbf{H}}_1^*)\, dx\, dy} \\ &+ jB\frac{\omega\varepsilon_0 \int_{-\infty}^{\infty}\int_{-\infty}^{\infty} (N^2 - N_2^2)\tilde{\mathbf{E}}_1^* \cdot \tilde{\mathbf{E}}_2\, dx\, dy}{\int_{-\infty}^{\infty}\int_{-\infty}^{\infty} \mathbf{u}_z \cdot (\tilde{\mathbf{E}}_1^* \times \tilde{\mathbf{H}}_1 + \tilde{\mathbf{E}}_1 \times \tilde{\mathbf{H}}_1^*)\, dx\, dy} = 0 \end{aligned} \tag{4.8}$$

$$\begin{aligned} &\frac{dB}{dz} + \frac{dA}{dz}\frac{\int_{-\infty}^{\infty}\int_{-\infty}^{\infty} \mathbf{u}_z \cdot (\tilde{\mathbf{E}}_2^* \times \tilde{\mathbf{H}}_1 + \tilde{\mathbf{E}}_1 \times \tilde{\mathbf{H}}_2^*)\, dx\, dy}{\int_{-\infty}^{\infty}\int_{-\infty}^{\infty} \mathbf{u}_z \cdot (\tilde{\mathbf{E}}_2^* \times \tilde{\mathbf{H}}_2 + \tilde{\mathbf{E}}_2 \times \tilde{\mathbf{H}}_2^*)\, dx\, dy} \\ &+ jA\frac{\omega\varepsilon_0 \int_{-\infty}^{\infty}\int_{-\infty}^{\infty} (N^2 - N_1^2)\tilde{\mathbf{E}}_2^* \cdot \tilde{\mathbf{E}}_1\, dx\, dy}{\int_{-\infty}^{\infty}\int_{-\infty}^{\infty} \mathbf{u}_z \cdot (\tilde{\mathbf{E}}_2^* \times \tilde{\mathbf{H}}_2 + \tilde{\mathbf{E}}_2 + \tilde{\mathbf{H}}_2^*)\, dx\, dy} \\ &+ jB\frac{\omega\varepsilon_0 \int_{-\infty}^{\infty}\int_{-\infty}^{\infty} (N^2 - N_2^2)\tilde{\mathbf{E}}_2^* \cdot \tilde{\mathbf{E}}_2\, dx\, dy}{\int_{-\infty}^{\infty}\int_{-\infty}^{\infty} \mathbf{u}_z \cdot (\tilde{\mathbf{E}}_2^* \times \tilde{\mathbf{H}}_2 + \tilde{\mathbf{E}}_2 \times \tilde{\mathbf{H}}_2^*)\, dx\, dy} = 0. \end{aligned} \tag{4.9}$$

Here we separate the transverse and axial dependencies of the electromagnetic fields:

$$\begin{cases} \tilde{\mathbf{E}}_p = \mathbf{E}_p \exp(-j\beta_p z) \\ \tilde{\mathbf{H}}_p = \mathbf{H}_p \exp(-j\beta_p z). \end{cases} \qquad (p = 1, 2) \tag{4.10}$$

Substituting Eq. (4.10) into Eqs. (4.8) and (4.9), we obtain

$$\frac{dA}{dz} + c_{12}\frac{dB}{dz}\exp[-j(\beta_2 - \beta_1)z] + j\chi_1 A + j\kappa_{12} B \exp[-j(\beta_2 - \beta_1)z] = 0 \tag{4.11}$$

$$\frac{dB}{dz} + c_{21}\frac{dA}{dz}\exp[+j(\beta_2 - \beta_1)z] + j\chi_2 B + j\kappa_{21} A \exp[+j(\beta_2 - \beta_1)z] = 0. \tag{4.12}$$

where

$$\kappa_{pq} = \frac{\omega\varepsilon_0 \int_{-\infty}^{\infty}\int_{-\infty}^{\infty}(N^2 - N_q^2)\mathbf{E}_p^* \cdot \mathbf{E}_q \, dx\, dy}{\int_{-\infty}^{\infty}\int_{-\infty}^{\infty}\mathbf{u}_z \cdot (\mathbf{E}_p^* \times \mathbf{H}_p + \mathbf{E}_p \times \mathbf{H}_p^*)\, dx\, dy} \tag{4.13}$$

$$c_{pq} = \frac{\int_{-\infty}^{\infty}\int_{-\infty}^{\infty}\mathbf{u}_z \cdot (\mathbf{E}_p^* \times \mathbf{H}_q + \mathbf{E}_q \times \mathbf{H}_p^*)\, dx\, dy}{\int_{-\infty}^{\infty}\int_{-\infty}^{\infty}\mathbf{u}_z \cdot (\mathbf{E}_p^* \times \mathbf{H}_p + \mathbf{E}_p \times \mathbf{H}_p^*)\, dx\, dy} \tag{4.14}$$

$$\chi_p = \frac{\omega\varepsilon_0 \int_{-\infty}^{\infty}\int_{-\infty}^{\infty}(N^2 - N_p^2)\mathbf{E}_p^* \cdot \mathbf{E}_p \, dx\, dy}{\int_{-\infty}^{\infty}\int_{-\infty}^{\infty}\mathbf{u}_z \cdot (\mathbf{E}_p^* \times \mathbf{H}_p + \mathbf{E}_p \times \mathbf{H}_p^*)\, dx\, dy} \tag{4.15}$$

and the pair of p and q are either $(p, q) = (1, 2)$ or (2, 1), respectively. κ_{pq} is a mode coupling coefficient of the directional coupler. The meaning of c_{pq} is described as follows. Let us consider the waveguide configurations shown in Fig. 4.2, where waveguide I exists only in the region $z < 0$ and waveguide II in $z \geqslant 0$. When the eigen mode $(\mathbf{E}_1, \mathbf{H}_1)$ of waveguide I propagates from the negative z-direction to $z = 0$, the electromagnetic field in the cladding excites the eigen mode $(\mathbf{E}_2, \mathbf{H}_2)$ at the point $z = 0$. This excitation efficiency is considered to be c_{12}. Therefore, c_{pq} represents the butt coupling coefficient between the two waveguides [2, 3].

Next we compare the magnitude of κ_{pq} and χ_p for the case of $p = 1$ and $q = 2$. As shown in Fig. 4.3(c), the actual value of $(N^2 - N_2^2)$ in waveguide I equals $(n_1^2 - n_0^2)$ and takes zero in all other regions. Then the integral of κ_{12} is carried out only inside the core region of waveguide I. The electric field $\mathbf{E}_2$

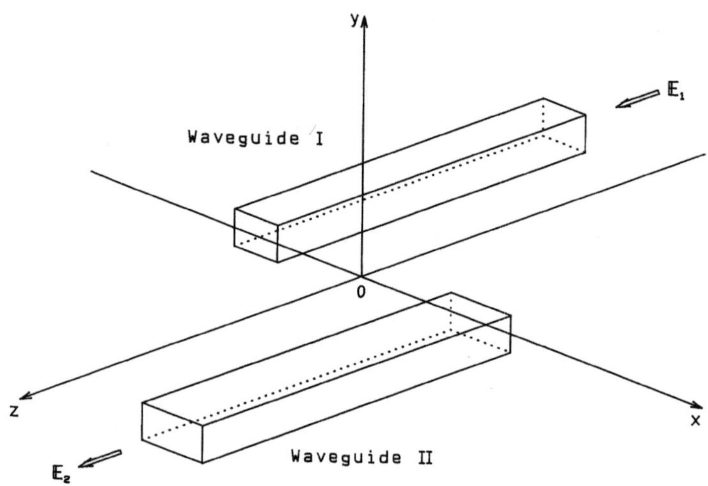

Figure 4.2 Explanation of butt coupling coefficient c_{12}.

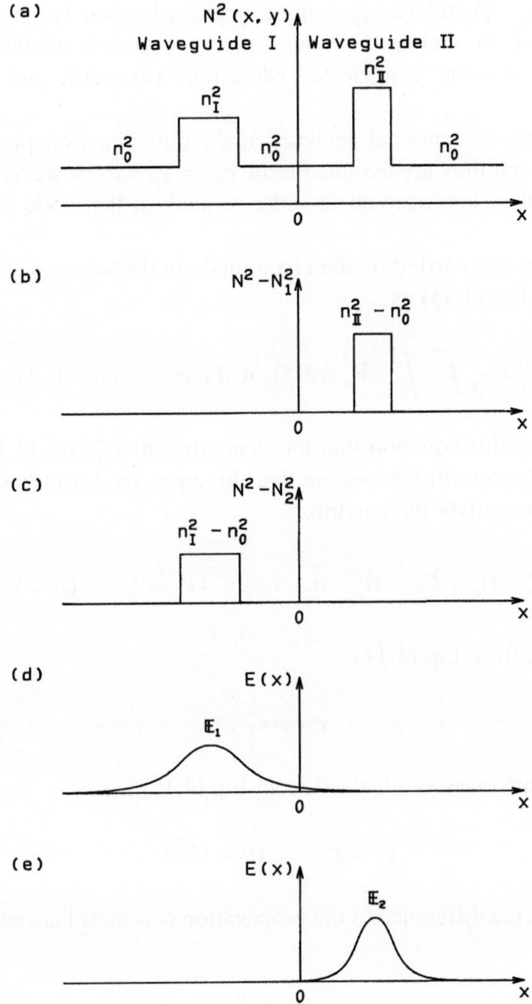

Figure 4.3 Refractive-index distribution $N^2(x, y)$ of the coupled waveguides, difference of the refractive-index distributions $(N^2 - N_p^2)$ and electric field $\mathbf{E}_p$ appearing in Eqs. (4.13) and (4.15).

inside waveguide I (we denote this $|\mathbf{E}_2| = \eta|\mathbf{E}_1|$) is quite small when compared to $\mathbf{E}_1$. Then the magnitude of the integral term of κ_{12} in the numerator is about $(n_1^2 - n_0^2)\eta$. The integral of χ_1 in Eq. (4.15) is carried out in waveguide II, where $(N^2 - N_1^2)$ is not zero. The magnitude of the integral term of χ_1 in the numerator is about $(n_1^2 - n_0^2)\eta^2$, since the electric field strength of $\mathbf{E}_1$ in waveguide II is about η. Based on the foregoing comparisons, it is known that χ_p is η times smaller than κ_{pq}. Therefore, χ_p can be neglected when two waveguides are sufficiently separated and $\eta \ll 1$ holds, since χ_p is much smaller than κ_{pq}. To the contrary, χ_p cannot be neglected when two waveguides are close to each other.

In most of the conventional analyses of the directional couplers, c_{pq} and χ_p were neglected and they are assumed to be $c_{pq} = \chi_p = 0$. However, both c_{pq} and χ_p should be taken into account in order to analyze the mode coupling effect strictly.

The optical power carried by the eigen mode in the waveguide $p(p = 1, 2)$ is expressed from Eq. (1.45) as

$$P_p = \frac{1}{2}\int_{-\infty}^{\infty}\int_{-\infty}^{\infty}(\mathbf{E}_p \times \mathbf{H}_p^*)\cdot \mathbf{u}_z\,dx\,dy \qquad (p = 1, 2). \tag{4.16}$$

It is known from this equation that the denominators of Eqs. (4.13)–(4.15) are equal to $4P_p$. Henceforth we assume that the eigen modes in both waveguides are normalized to satisfy the condition.

$$\int_{-\infty}^{\infty}\int_{-\infty}^{\infty}(\mathbf{E}_p^* \times \mathbf{H}_p + \mathbf{E}_p \times \mathbf{H}_p^*)\cdot \mathbf{u}_z\,dx\,dy = 4P_p = 1 \qquad (p = 1, 2). \tag{4.17}$$

Then we obtain, from Eq. (4.14),

$$c_{21} = c_{12}^*, \tag{4.18}$$

Next it is straightforwardly obtained from Eq. (4.15) as

$$\chi_p = \chi_p^* \qquad (p = 1, 2). \tag{4.19}$$

Here we express the difference of the propagation constants between waveguides I and II as

$$\delta = \frac{(\beta_2 - \beta_1)}{2}. \tag{4.20}$$

The optical power in the entire coupled waveguides is expressed by

$$P = \frac{1}{2}\int_{-\infty}^{\infty}\int_{-\infty}^{\infty}(\tilde{\mathbf{E}} \times \tilde{\mathbf{H}}^*)\cdot \mathbf{u}_z\,dx\,dy. \tag{4.21}$$

Substitution of Eqs. (4.2) and (4.10) in Eq. (4.21) gives

$$P = \frac{1}{2}[|A|^2 + |B|^2 + A^*Bc_{12}\exp(-j2\delta z) + AB^*c_{12}^*\exp(j2\delta z)]. \tag{4.22}$$

In the derivation of this last equation we used Eqs. (4.14), (4.17), and (4.18). In the loss-less waveguides, the optical power remains constant because we have

$$\frac{dP}{dz} = 0. \tag{4.23}$$

Substituting Eqs. (4.11), (4.12), and (4.22) in Eq. (4.23) we obtain

$$\begin{aligned} &jA^*B(\kappa_{21}^* - \kappa_{12} - 2\delta c_{12})\exp(-j2\delta z) \\ &-jAB^*(\kappa_{21} - \kappa_{12}^* - 2\delta c_{12}^*)\exp(j2\delta z) = 0. \end{aligned} \tag{4.24}$$

In order that Eq. (4.24) is satisfied independent of z, we should have

$$\kappa_{21} = \kappa_{12}^* + 2\delta c_{12}^*. \tag{4.25}$$

In most of the conventional analyses, reciprocity of the coupling coefficients was expressed by $\kappa_{21} = \kappa_{12}^*$, since c_{12} was assumed to be zero. However, $\kappa_{21} = \kappa_{12}^*$ holds only when (1) the propagation constants of the two waveguides are equal ($\delta = 0$) or (2) two waveguides are sufficiently separated ($c_{12} \cong 0$). Especially when two waveguides with different core geometries are placed close together, care should be taken, since the second term of the right-hand side of Eq. (4.25) cannot be neglected.

Next we derive the coupling mode equations using Eqs. (4.11) and (4.12). From the equality of Eqs. (4.11)–(4.12) $\times c_{12}\exp(-j2\delta z) = 0$, we obtain

$$\frac{dA}{dz} = -j\kappa_a B\exp(-j2\delta z) + j\alpha_a A. \tag{4.26}$$

Similarly, from the equality of Eqs. (4.12)–(4.11) $\times\, c_{21}\exp(j2\delta z) = 0$, we obtain

$$\frac{dB}{dz} = -j\kappa_b A\exp(2\delta z) + j\alpha_b B. \tag{4.27}$$

In the last two equations, parameters κ_a, κ_b, α_a, and α_b are defined by

$$\kappa_a = \frac{\kappa_{12} - c_{12}\chi_2}{1 - |c_{12}|^2}, \tag{4.28a}$$

$$\kappa_b = \frac{\kappa_{12} - c_{12}^*\chi_1}{1 - |c_{12}|^2}, \tag{4.28b}$$

$$\alpha_a = \frac{\kappa_{21}c_{12} - \chi_1}{1 - |c_{12}|^2}, \tag{4.29a}$$

$$\alpha_b = \frac{\kappa_{12}c_{12}^* - \chi_2}{1 - |c_{12}|^2}. \tag{4.29b}$$

In the following, the solution method of the coupled mode Eqs. (4.26) and (4.27) for the codirectional coupler ($\beta_1 > 0, \beta_2 > 0$) and contradirectional coupler ($\beta_1 > 0, \beta_2 < 0$) will be described. However, we assume $c_{pq} = \chi_p = 0\ (p, q = 1, 2)$ and rewrite Eqs. (4.26) and (4.27) into more simplified form, since the rigorous analysis becomes very complicated. Of course, the strict analysis based on the Eqs. (4.26) and (4.27) is possible and their solutions of the codirectional coupler are described in Appendix 4A at the chapter's end.

With the assumption of $c_{pq} = \chi_p = 0 (p, q = 1, 2)$, we can rewrite Eqs. (4.26) and (4.27) as

$$\frac{dA}{dz} = -j\kappa_{12} B \exp[-j(\beta_2 - \beta_1)z], \tag{4.30}$$

$$\frac{dB}{dz} = -j\kappa_{21} A \exp[+j(\beta_2 - \beta_1)z], \tag{4.31}$$

where κ_{pq} is given by Eq. (4.13). The reciprocity relation of the coupling coefficients are

$$\kappa_{21} = \kappa_{12}. \tag{4.32}$$

In most of the directional couplers, κ_{pq} is real. Therefore, we express $\kappa = \kappa_{21} = \kappa_{12}$. The reciprocity relation for the contradirectional coupler is expressed by

$$\kappa_{21} = -\kappa_{12}^*. \tag{4.33}$$

4.2. CODIRECTIONAL COUPLERS

The solutions of codirectional couplers ($\beta_1 > 0, \beta_2 > 0$) are assumed in the forms

$$A(z) = [a_1 e^{jqz} + a_2 e^{-jqz}] \exp(-j\delta z), \tag{4.34a}$$

$$B(z) = [b_1 e^{jqz} + b_2 e^{-jqz}] \exp(j\delta z), \tag{4.34b}$$

where q is an unknown parameter to be determined. Constants a_1, a_2, b_1, and b_2 should satisfy the initial conditions

$$a_1 + a_2 = A(0), \tag{4.35a}$$

$$b_1 + b_2 = B(0). \tag{4.35b}$$

Substituting Eqs. (4.34) into coupled mode Eqs. (4.30) and (4.31) and applying the initial conditions of Eqs. (4.35), we obtain

$$A(z) = \left\{ \left[\cos(qz) + j\frac{\delta}{q}\sin(qz) \right] A(0) - j\frac{\kappa}{q}\sin(qz)B(0) \right\} \exp(-j\delta z), \quad (4.36)$$

$$B(z) = \left\{ -j\frac{\kappa}{q}\sin(qz)A(0) + \left[\cos(qz) - j\frac{\delta}{q}\sin(qz) \right] B(0) \right\} \exp(j\delta z), \quad (4.37)$$

where q is given by

$$q = \sqrt{\kappa^2 + \delta^2}. \quad (4.38)$$

For the most practical case, in which light is coupled into waveguide I only at $z = 0$, we have the conditions of $A(0) = A_0$ and $B(0) = 0$. Then the optical power flow along the z-direction is given by

$$P_a(z) = \frac{|A(z)|^2}{|A_0|^2} = 1 - F\sin^2(qz), \quad (4.39)$$

$$P_b(z) = \frac{|B(z)|^2}{|A_0|^2} = F\sin^2(qz), \quad (4.40)$$

where F denotes the maximum power-coupling efficiency, defined by

$$F = \left(\frac{\kappa}{q} \right)^2 = \frac{1}{1 + (\delta/\kappa)^2}. \quad (4.41)$$

Figure 4.4 shows the dependence of P_a and P_b on the normalized length qz for the two directional coupler configurations $F = 1.0$ and $F = 0.2$, respectively. The power-coupling efficiency from excited waveguide I to waveguide II reaches maximum at

$$z = \frac{\pi}{2q}(2m + 1) \qquad (m = 0, 1, 2, \ldots). \quad (4.42)$$

The length z at $m = 0$ is called the *coupling length* and is given by

$$L_c = \frac{\pi}{2q} = \frac{\pi}{2\sqrt{\kappa^2 + \delta^2}}. \quad (4.43)$$

When the propagation constants of the two waveguides are equal ($\beta_1 = \beta_2$ and then $\delta = 0$), 100% power coupling occurs at the coupling length of

$$L_c = \frac{\pi}{2\kappa}. \quad (4.44)$$

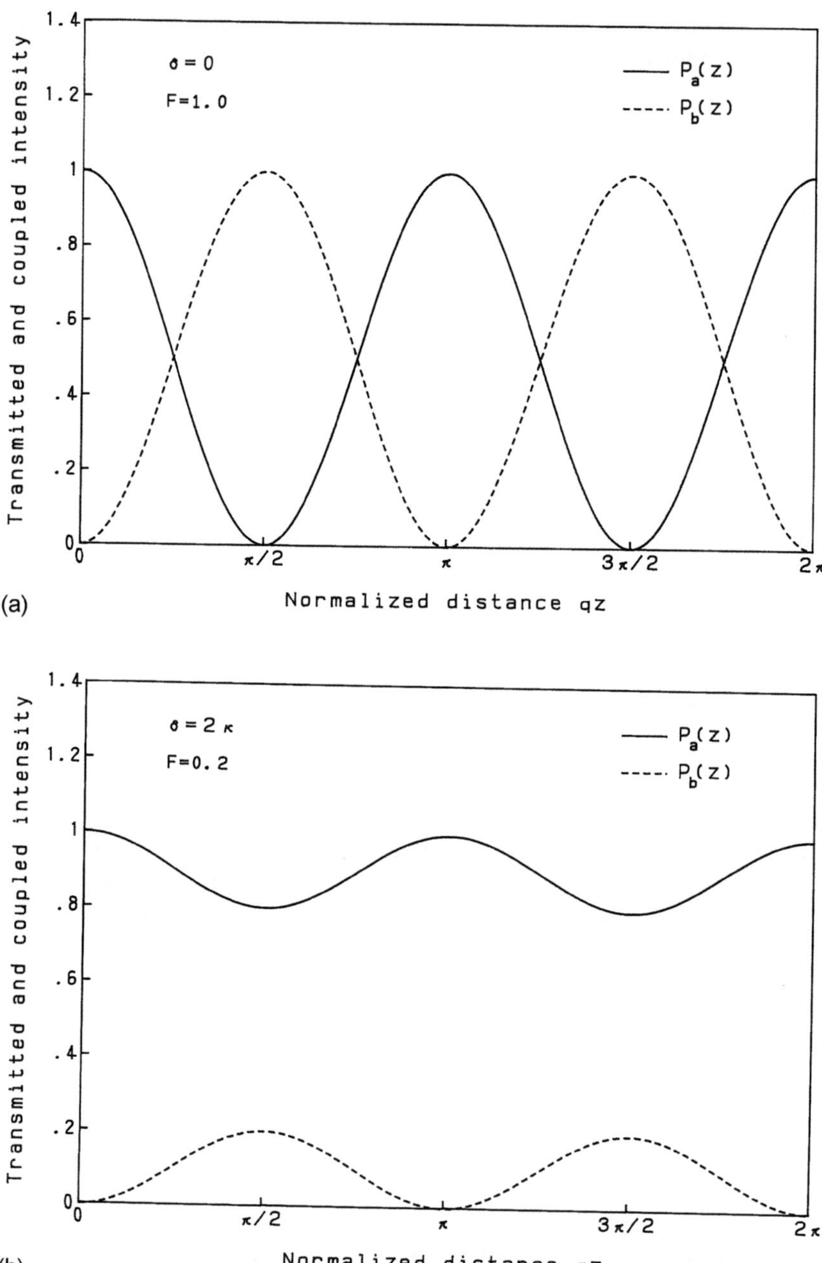

Figure 4.4 Variation of optical power in the codirectional coupler with (a) $F = 1.0$ and (b) $F = 0.2$.

4.3. CONTRADIRECTIONAL COUPLING IN CORRUGATED WAVEGUIDES

4.3.1. Transmission and Reflection Characteristics in Uniform Gratings

When the light propagation direction is opposite ($\beta_1 > 0, \beta_2 < 0$), light coupling does not occur by simply making waveguides I and II close to each other. Let us consider the coupler configuration where the medium (refractive index or effective index) between waveguides I and II are periodically perturbed, as shown in Fig. 4.5. We assume that the coupling coefficient is expressed by $\kappa_{12}(z) = \kappa_G \exp[-j(2\pi/\Lambda)z]$ (Λ is a period of the perturbation). The mode-coupling equations are reduced from Eqs. (4.30) and (4.31):

$$\frac{dA}{dz} = -j\kappa_G B \exp\left[j\left(\beta_1 - \beta_2 - \frac{2\pi}{\Lambda}\right)z\right], \tag{4.45}$$

$$\frac{dB}{dz} = j\kappa_G A \exp\left[-j\left(\beta_1 - \beta_2 - \frac{2\pi}{\Lambda}\right)z\right]. \tag{4.46}$$

In the derivation of Eqs. (4.45) and (4.46), we used the reciprocity relation

$$\kappa_{21} = -\kappa_{12}^* = -\kappa_G \exp\left(j\frac{2\pi}{\Lambda}z\right), \tag{4.47}$$

which is obtained from the power conservation theorem for $P \propto |A|^2 - |B|^2$ propagating along the positive z-direction:

$$\frac{d}{dz}(|A|^2 - |B|^2) = 0. \tag{4.48}$$

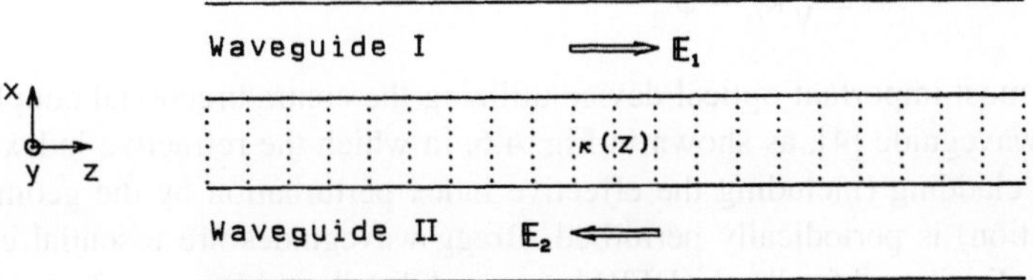

Figure 4.5 Contradirectional coupling waveguides.

We introduce here a new parameter that expresses the phase-matching condition as

$$\varphi = \frac{(\beta_1 - \beta_2 - 2\pi/\Lambda)}{2}. \tag{4.49}$$

The periodic perturbation exists over the region of $z = 0 - L$. The initial and boundary conditions for the light input to waveguide I are given by $A(0) = A_0$ and $B(L) = 0$ (light reflection at $z = L$ is zero since there is no perturbation in $z > L$). Under these boundary conditions, the solution of the coupled mode Eqs. (4.45) and (4.46) are given as follows for each phase-matching condition.

a. $|\varphi| > \kappa_G$:

$$A(z) = A_0 \frac{\rho \cos[\rho(z-L)] - j\varphi \sin[\rho(z-L)]}{\rho \cos(\rho L) + j\varphi \sin(\rho L)} \exp(j\varphi z), \tag{4.50}$$

$$B(z) = A_0 \frac{j\kappa_G \sin[\rho(z-L)]}{\rho \cos(\rho L) + j\varphi \sin(\rho L)} \exp(-j\varphi z), \tag{4.51}$$

$$\rho = \sqrt{\varphi^2 - \kappa_G^2}. \tag{4.52}$$

b. $|\varphi| = \kappa_G$:

$$A(z) = A_0 \frac{1 - j\varphi(z-L)}{1 + j\varphi L} \exp(j\varphi Z), \tag{4.53}$$

$$B(z) = A_0 \frac{j\kappa_G(z-L)}{1 + j\varphi L} \exp(-j\varphi Z), \tag{4.54}$$

c. $|\varphi| < \kappa_G$:

$$A(z) = A_0 \frac{\alpha \cosh[\alpha(z-L)] - j\varphi \sinh[\alpha(z-L)]}{\alpha \cosh(\alpha L) + j\varphi \sinh(\alpha L)} \exp(j\varphi z), \tag{4.55}$$

$$B(z) = A_0 \frac{j\kappa_G \sinh[\alpha(z-L)]}{\alpha \cosh(\alpha L) + j\varphi \sinh(\alpha L)} \exp(-j\varphi z), \tag{4.56}$$

$$\alpha = \sqrt{\kappa_G^2 - \varphi^2}. \tag{4.57}$$

The most important optical device utilizing the contradirectional coupler is a Bragg waveguide [4], as shown in Fig. 4.6, in which the refractive index of the core or cladding (including the effective index perturbation by the geometrical corrugation) is periodically perturbed. Bragg waveguides are essential components in distributed feedback (DFB) lasers and distributed Bragg reflector (DBR) lasers [5].

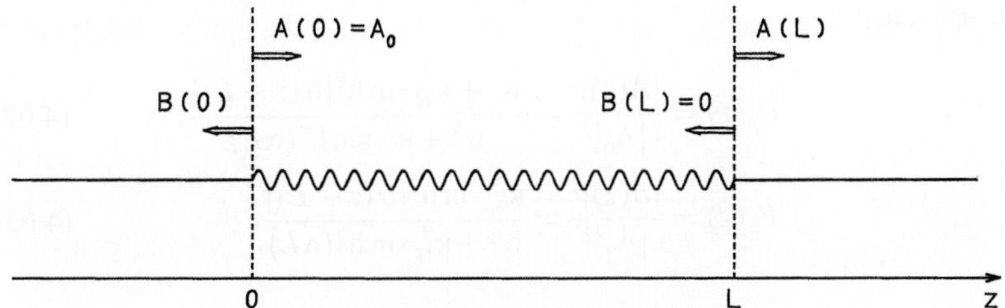

Figure 4.6 Bragg optical waveguide.

In the Bragg waveguide, the magnitude of the propagation constants are the same and have opposite signs, since waveguides I and II are the same. Then we can write

$$\beta_1 = -\beta_2 = kn_{\text{eff}}, \tag{4.58}$$

where n_{eff} denotes effective index. The phase-matching parameter φ is expressed from Eqs. (4.49) and (4.58) as

$$\varphi = kn_{\text{eff}} - \frac{\pi}{\Lambda}. \tag{4.59}$$

The normalized transmitted (forward) and reflected (backward) optical power in the Bragg grating waveguide are expressed, by using Eqs. (4.50) to (4.56), as follows.

a. $|\varphi| > \kappa_G$:

$$P_f(z) = \frac{|A(z)|^2}{|A_0|^2} = \frac{\rho^2 + \kappa_G^2 \sin^2[\rho(z-L)]}{\rho^2 + \kappa_G^2 \sin^2(\rho L)}, \tag{4.60a}$$

$$P_b(z) = \frac{|B(z)|^2}{|A_0|^2} = \frac{\kappa_G^2 \sin^2[\rho(z-L)]}{\rho^2 + \kappa_G^2 \sin^2(\rho L)}. \tag{4.60b}$$

b. $|\varphi| = \kappa_G$:

$$P_f(z) = \frac{|A(z)|^2}{|A_0|^2} = \frac{1 + \kappa_G^2 (z-L)^2}{1 + \kappa_G^2 L^2}, \tag{4.61a}$$

$$P_b(z) = \frac{|B(z)|^2}{|A_0|^2} = \frac{\kappa_G^2 (z-L)^2}{1 + \kappa_G^2 L}. \tag{4.61b}$$

c. $|\varphi| < \kappa_G$:

$$P_f(z) = \frac{|A(z)|^2}{|A_0|^2} = \frac{\alpha^2 + \kappa_G^2 \sinh^2[\alpha(z-L)]}{\alpha^2 + \kappa_G^2 \sinh^2(\alpha L)}, \tag{4.62a}$$

$$P_b(z) = \frac{|B(z)|^2}{|A_0|^2} = \frac{\kappa_G^2 \sinh^2[\alpha(z-L)]}{\alpha^2 + \kappa_G^2 \sinh^2(\alpha L)}. \tag{4.62b}$$

Figures 4.7(a) and (b) show the normalized forward and backward optical power in Bragg waveguides at the two different phase-matching conditions (a) $\rho = \pi/L, \kappa_G = 2/L(|\varphi| > \kappa_G)$ and (b) $\alpha = \kappa_G = 2/L(|\varphi| = 0)$, respectively. When $|\varphi| > \kappa_G$, the incident wave transmits from the opposite side of the Bragg waveguide, as shown in Fig. 4.7(a). The angular frequencies of the optical wave satisfying this condition are given by

$$\frac{\omega}{c} n_{\text{eff}} < \frac{\pi}{\Lambda} - \kappa_G, \tag{4.63a}$$

$$\frac{\omega}{c} n_{\text{eff}} > \frac{\pi}{\Lambda} - \kappa_G. \tag{4.63b}$$

This frequency span is called the *pass band*. In contrast, the light wave with the phase-matching condition of $|\varphi| < \kappa_G$ decays exponentially and is mostly reflected back, as shown in Fig. 4.7(b). This frequency span is called the *stop band* and is expressed by

$$\frac{\pi}{\Lambda} - \kappa_G < \frac{\omega}{c} n_{\text{eff}} > \frac{\pi}{\Lambda} + \kappa_G. \tag{4.64}$$

Especially, the optical wavelength satisfying $(\omega/c)n_{\text{eff}} = \pi/\Lambda$ [$\varphi = 0$ from Eq. (4.59)] is called the *Bragg wavelength* and is expressed by

$$\lambda_B = 2n_{\text{eff}}\Lambda. \tag{4.65}$$

The Bragg waveguide acts as the band elimination filter that reflects the light wave near the Bragg wavelength and transmits light outside of the Bragg wavelength. The transmittance and reflection characteristics of the Bragg waveguide with $\kappa_G L = 2$ are shown in Fig. 4.8. The horizontal axis is a detuning $\varphi L = (\omega - \omega_B) n_{\text{eff}} L/c$ from the Bragg angular frequency $\omega_B = (2\pi/\lambda_B)c$. The transmittance T and reflectance R are given by

$$T = \frac{|A(L)|^2}{|A_0|^2}. \tag{4.66a}$$

$$R = \frac{|B(0)|^2}{|A_0|^2}. \tag{4.66b}$$

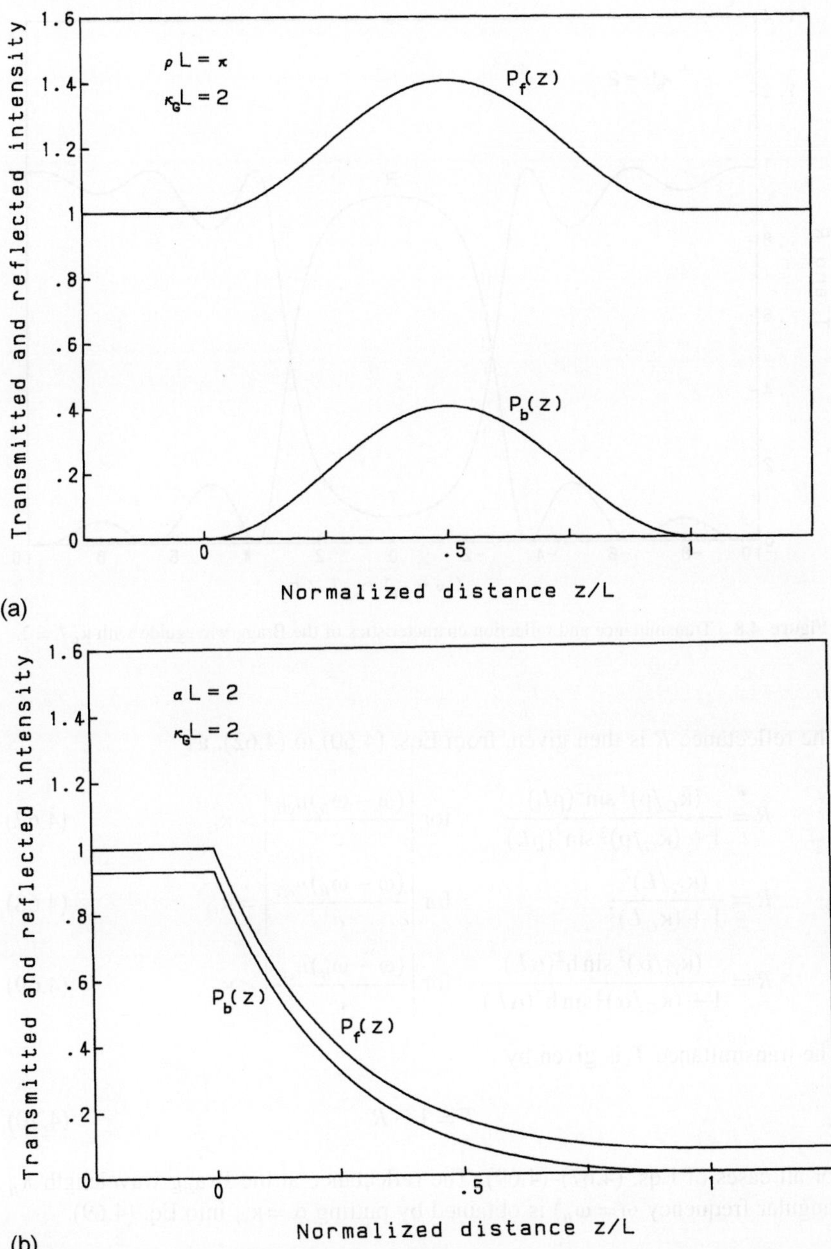

Figure 4.7 Normalized forward and backward optical power in Bragg waveguides for (a) $\rho = \pi/L$, $\kappa_G = 2/L(|\varphi| > \kappa_G)$ and (b) $\alpha = \kappa_G = 2/L(|\varphi| = 0)$.

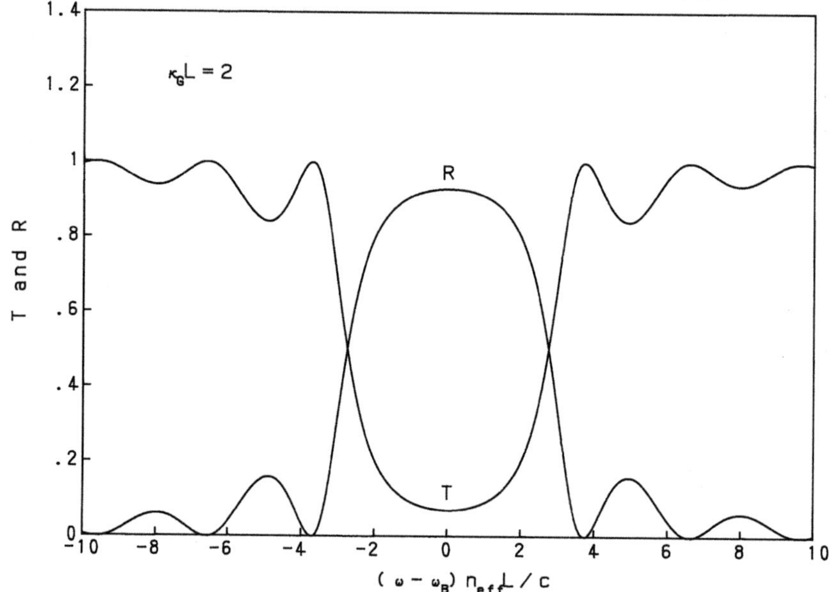

Figure 4.8 Transmittance and reflection characteristics of the Bragg waveguide with $\kappa_G L = 2$.

The reflectance R is then given, from Eqs. (4.60) to (4.62), as

$$R = \frac{(\kappa_G/\rho)^2 \sin^2(\rho L)}{1 + (\kappa_G/\rho)^2 \sin^2(\rho L)} \quad \text{for} \left| \frac{(\omega - \omega_B) n_{\text{eff}}}{c} \right| > \kappa_G \tag{4.67}$$

$$R = \frac{(\kappa_G/L)^2}{1 + (\kappa_G L)^2} \quad \text{for} \left| \frac{(\omega - \omega_B) n_{\text{eff}}}{c} \right| = \kappa_G \tag{4.68}$$

$$R = \frac{(\kappa_G/\alpha)^2 \sin\text{h}^2(\alpha L)}{1 + (\kappa_G/\alpha)^2 \sin\text{h}^2(\alpha L)} \quad \text{for} \left| \frac{(\omega - \omega_B) n_{\text{eff}}}{c} \right| < \kappa_G. \tag{4.69}$$

The transmittance T is given by

$$T = 1 - R \tag{4.70}$$

for all cases of Eqs. (4.67)–(4.69). The reflectance at the Bragg wavelength λ_B (angular frequency $\omega = \omega_B$) is obtained by putting $\alpha = \kappa_G$ into Eq. (4.69):

$$R = \tan\text{h}^2(\kappa_G L). \tag{4.71}$$

For example, $R = 0.93$ for the coupling strength of $\kappa_G L = 2$.

4.3.2. Phase-shift Grating

The phase of the reflected wave by the Bragg waveguide is very important for the applications to DFB and DBR lasers. Let us express the amplitude reflectance of the Bragg waveguide in Fig. 4.6 measured at $z=0$ as

$$r=\frac{B(0)}{A_0}=\sqrt{R}\,e^{-j\theta}. \tag{4.72}$$

The optical phase θ at the wavelength close to the Bragg wavelength is given from Eqs. (4.56), (4.69), and (4.72) as

$$\theta=\frac{\pi}{2}+\tan^{-1}\left[\frac{\varphi}{\alpha}\tan\mathrm{h}(\alpha L)\right]. \tag{4.73}$$

At the center of the Bragg wavelength ($\varphi=0$), we have $\theta=\pi/2$. The configuration of the DFB laser is considered to consist of two Bragg waveguides, as shown in Fig. 4.9. The total phase shift of one round trip at the Bragg wavelength is then given by $\varphi=2\times\pi/2=\pi$. Therefore, the phase-matching condition (phase shift of one round trip is an integer multiple of 2π) is not satisfied in the normal DFB configuration. To the contrary, the phase-matching condition is satisfied for two slightly separated wavelengths [6]. This generates two spectral oscillation peaks and causes the degradation of the signal transmission characteristics when used as the light source of optical fiber communications.

Let us next consider Bragg waveguides having 2Θ phase shift at $z=0$, as shown in Fig. 4.9. The coupled mode equations for the two Bragg waveguides are given, from Eqs. (4.45) and (4.46), as

$$\frac{dA_\ell}{dz}=-j\kappa_G B_\ell \exp(j2\varphi z\pm j\Theta) \tag{4.74a}$$

$$\frac{dB_\ell}{dz}=-j\kappa_G A_\ell \exp(-j2\varphi z\mp j\Theta) \qquad \ell=(1,2). \tag{4.74b}$$

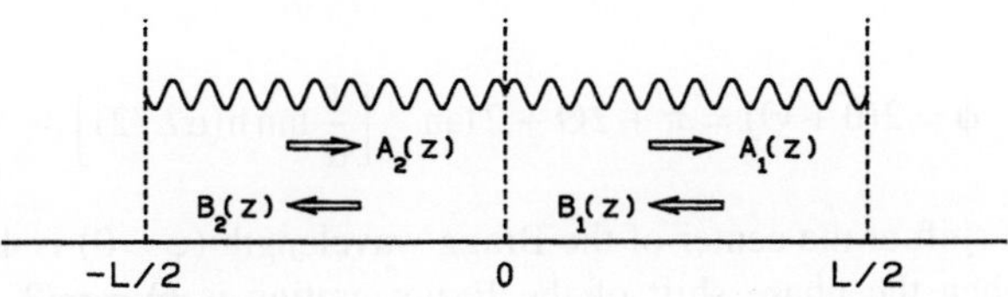

Figure 4.9 Phase-shifted Bragg waveguide.

In these equations, $\ell=1$ and $\ell=2$ correspond to the upper and the lower case of the plus or minus sign. Here we rewrite Eq. (4.74) as

$$\frac{d}{dz}\left[A_\ell \exp\left(\mp\frac{j\Theta}{2}\right)\right]=-j\kappa_G\left[B_\ell \exp\left(\pm\frac{j\Theta}{2}\right)\right]\exp(j2\varphi z), \quad (4.75a)$$

$$\frac{d}{dz}\left[B_\ell \exp\left(\pm\frac{j\Theta}{2}\right)\right]=j\kappa_G\left[A_\ell \exp\left(\mp\frac{j\Theta}{2}\right)\right]\exp(-j2\varphi z). \quad (4.75b)$$

When we compare Eqs. (4.75) with Eqs. (4.45) and (4.46), it is seen that the phase-shifted Bragg waveguide can be analyzed with Eqs. (4.45) and (4.46) by simply replacing the parameters as follows:

$$\begin{cases} A \to A_\ell \left(\mp\frac{j\Theta}{2}\right) \\ B \to B_\ell \exp\left(\pm\frac{j\Theta}{2}\right). \end{cases} \quad (4.76)$$

The amplitude reflectivity r_1 of the right-hand Bragg waveguide is given from Eq. (4.72) by noting the relation

$$\sqrt{R}\,e^{-j\theta}=\frac{B_1(0)\exp(j\Theta/2)}{A_1(0)\exp(-j\Theta/2)}=\frac{B_1(0)}{A_1(0)}\exp(j\Theta)$$

as

$$r_1=\frac{B_1(0)}{A_1(0)}=\sqrt{R}\,e^{-j(\theta+\Theta)}. \quad (4.77)$$

In a similar manner, the amplitude reflectivity r_2 of the lefthand Bragg waveguide is obtained as

$$r_2=\frac{A_2(0)}{B_2(0)}=\sqrt{R}\,e^{-j(\theta+\Theta)}. \quad (4.78)$$

Then the total phase shift of one round trip in the phase-shifted Bragg waveguide is given by

$$\psi=2(\theta+\Theta)=\pi+2\Theta+2\tan^{-1}\left[\frac{\varphi}{\alpha}\tan\mathrm{h}(\alpha L/2)\right]. \quad (4.79)$$

The phase shift at the center of the Bragg wavelength ($\varphi=0$) is $\psi=\pi+2\Theta$. Especially when the phase shift of the Bragg grating is $\Theta=\pi/2$, the optical phase shift at the center of the Bragg wavelength becomes $\psi=2\pi$ and therefore the phase-matching condition is satisfied. The grating phase shift of $2\Theta=\pi$ corresponds to the $\Lambda/2$ of the grating period and also corresponds to one-quarter of the wavelength $\lambda_B/n_{\rm eff}$ inside the waveguide. Therefore, the grating phase shift of $2\Theta=\pi$ is called the "$\lambda/4$ (quarter λ shift)" [7].

4.4. DERIVATION OF COUPLING COEFFICIENTS

The mode-coupling coefficient κ is very important for the calculation of the coupling length in the codirectional coupler [Eq. (4.44)], the reflectivity in the contradirectional coupler [Eq. (4.71)], and so on. In this subsection, the derivation of the coupling coefficient κ for several typical optical waveguide couplers will be described.

4.4.1. Coupling Coefficients for Slab Waveguides

Here we derive the coupling coefficient of the TE mode in the directional coupler consisting of symmetrical slab waveguides. The coupling coefficient $\kappa(=\kappa_{12}=\kappa_{12})$ is expressed from Eq. (4.13) as

$$\kappa=\frac{\omega\varepsilon_0\int_{-\infty}^{\infty}(N^2-N_2^2)\mathbf{E}_1^*\cdot\mathbf{E}_2dx}{\int_{-\infty}^{\infty}\mathbf{u}_z\cdot(\mathbf{E}_1^*\times\mathbf{H}_1+\mathbf{E}_1\times\mathbf{H}_1^*)dx}. \tag{4.80}$$

The electromagnetic field components of the TE mode is expressed from Eq. (2.5) as $E_x=H_y=0$ and $H_x=-(\beta/\omega\mu_0)E_y$. Therefore, we have the following equalities:

$$\mathbf{u}_z\cdot(\mathbf{E}_1^*\times\mathbf{H}_1+\mathbf{E}_1\times\mathbf{H}_1^*)=\frac{2\beta}{\omega\mu_0}|E_{1y}|^2, \tag{4.81a}$$

$$\mathbf{E}_1^*\cdot\mathbf{E}_2=E_{1y}^*\cdot E_{2y}. \tag{4.81b}$$

Since $(N^2-N_2^2)$ is zero outside of waveguide I, the integration of Eq. (4.80) needs to be done only inside of waveguide I. The origin of the x-axis is taken at the center of waveguide I, as shown in Fig. 4.10, and the core center separation is denoted by D. Substituting Eqs. (4.81) into Eq. (4.80), we obtain

$$\kappa=\frac{\omega\varepsilon_0(n_1^2-n_0^2)\int_{-a}^{a}E_{1y}^*\cdot E_{2y}dx}{\frac{2\beta}{\omega\mu_0}\int_{-\infty}^{\infty}|E_{1y}|^2dx} \tag{4.82}$$

The electric field components in the slab waveguides are given, from Eq. (2.7), as

$$E_{1y}=\begin{cases}A\cos\left(\dfrac{u}{a}x\right) & (|x|\leqslant a)\\ A\cos(u)\exp\left[-\dfrac{w}{a}(|x|-a)\right] & (|x|>a)\end{cases} \tag{4.83}$$

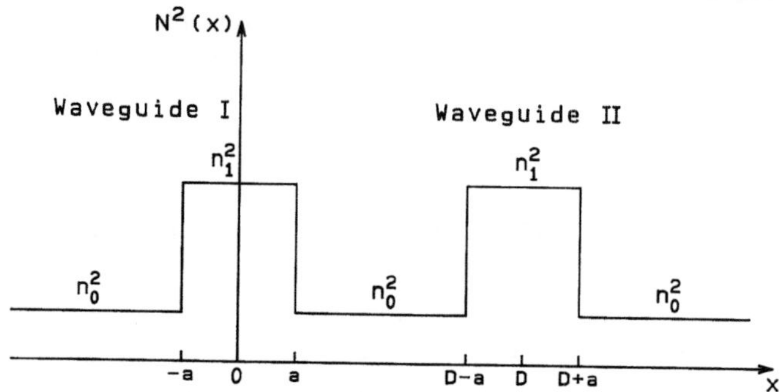

Figure 4.10 Directional coupler consisting of slab optical waveguides.

and

$$E_{2y} = A\cos(u)\exp\left[\frac{w}{a}(x - D + a)\right]$$
$$\text{(inside of core of waveguide } I;\ |x| \leqslant a). \tag{4.84}$$

Substituting Eqs. (4.83) and (4.84) into Eq. (4.82) and utilizing the eigenvalue equation for the TE mode [Eq. (2.24)] of the form

$$w = u\tan(u), \tag{4.85}$$

Eq. (4.82) reduces to

$$\kappa = \frac{k^2}{\beta}(n_1^2 - n_0^2)\frac{u^2w^2}{(1+w)v^4}\exp\left[-\frac{w}{a}(D - 2a)\right]. \tag{4.86}$$

Here Eq. (4.86) can be rewritten further by using $\beta \cong kn_1$ and $(n_1^2 - n_0^2) = 2n_1^2\Delta$:

$$\kappa = \frac{\sqrt{2\Delta}}{a}\frac{u^2w^2}{(1+w)v^3}\exp\left[-\frac{w}{a}(D - 2a)\right]. \tag{4.87}$$

For example, the mode-coupling coefficient of the directional coupler consisting of slab waveguides with $2a = 6\,\mu\text{m}$, $\Delta = 0.3\%$, $v = 1.5$, and core center separation of $D = 4a$ is calculated to be $\kappa = 0.39\,\text{mm}^{-1}$. The coupling length of this coupler is obtained from Eq. (4.44) as $L_c = 4\,\text{mm}$.

4.4.2. Coupling Coefficients for Rectangular Waveguides

Here we consider the directional coupler consisting of three-dimensional rectangular waveguides, as shown in Fig. 4.11. When we deal with the E_{11}^x mode,

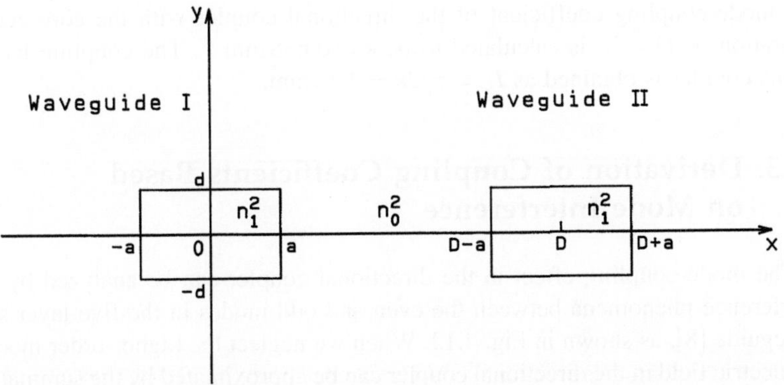

Figure 4.11 Directional coupler consisting of three-dimensional rectangular waveguides.

we have $H_x = 0$ from Eq. (2.41). Since we can assume $|E_x| \gg |E_y|$ for the E_{11}^x mode in Eq. (4.13), the mode-coupling coefficient is expressed by

$$\kappa = \frac{\omega\varepsilon_0(n_1^2 - n_0^2)\int_{-a}^{a}\int_{-d}^{d} E_{1x}^* \cdot E_{2x}\,dx\,dy}{2\int_{-\infty}^{\infty}\int_{-\infty}^{\infty} E_{1x}^* \cdot H_{1y}\,dx\,dy}. \tag{4.88}$$

Substituting Eq. (2.44) in Eq. (4.88) and using the relation $E_x \cong (\omega\mu_0/\beta)H_y$, the denominator and numerator of (4.88) are calculated as

$$2\int_{-\infty}^{\infty}\int_{-\infty}^{\infty} E_{1x}^* \cdot H_{1y}\,dx\,dy \cong \frac{2\omega\mu_0}{\beta}|A|^2\left(a + \frac{1}{\gamma_x}\right)\left(d + \frac{1}{\gamma_y}\right), \tag{4.89}$$

and

$$\omega\varepsilon_0(n_1^2 - n_0^2)\int_{-a}^{a}\int_{-d}^{d} E_{1x}^* \cdot E_{2x}\,dx\,dy$$
$$\cong \frac{2\omega\mu_0}{\beta^2}|A|^2\left(d + \frac{1}{\gamma_y}\right)\frac{k_x^2\gamma_x a^2}{v^2} \times \exp[-\gamma_x(D - 2a)]. \tag{4.90}$$

Here normalized frequency is defined as $v = kn_1 a\sqrt{2\Delta}$. The mode coupling coefficient is then given by

$$\kappa = \frac{\sqrt{2\Delta}}{a}\frac{(k_x a)^2(\gamma_x a)^2}{(1 + \gamma_x a)v^3}\exp[-\gamma_x(D - 2a)]. \tag{4.91}$$

Parameters k_x and γ_x are obtained by solving the eigenvalue equation (2.47). For example, we obtain $k_x a = 0.995$ and $\gamma_x a = 1.523$ for the rectangular waveguide with $2a = 8\,\mu\text{m}$, $2d = 8\,\mu\text{m}$, $\Delta = 0.3\%$, and $v = 1.819$ at $\lambda = 1.55\,\mu\text{m}$.

The mode-coupling coefficient of the directional coupler with the core center separation of $D = 3a$ is calculated to be $\kappa = 0.638\,\text{mm}^{-1}$. The coupling length of this coupler is obtained as $L_c = \pi/2\kappa = 2.46\,\text{mm}$.

4.4.3. Derivation of Coupling Coefficients Based on Mode Interference

The mode-coupling effect in the directional coupler can be analyzed by the interference phenomena between the even and odd modes in the five-layer slab waveguide [8], as shown in Fig. 4.12. When we neglect the higher-order modes, the electric field in the directional coupler can be approximated by the summation of the even mode (first-order mode in the five-layer waveguide) and the odd mode (second-order mode in the five-layer waveguide):

$$E(x, z) = E_e(x)\exp(-j\beta_e z) + E_o(x)\exp(-j\beta_o z), \tag{4.92}$$

where $E_e(x)$ and β_e denote electric field and propagation constant of the even mode and $E_o(x)$ and β_o denote those of the odd mode, respectively. The incident electric field, which is coupled to waveguide I at $z = 0$, is expressed by

$$|E(x, 0)| = |E_e(x) + E_o(x)| = E_1(x). \tag{4.93}$$

Here $E_1(x)$ denotes the eigen mode of waveguide I. When the cores of waveguides I and II are not so close, this expression holds with good accuracy. The electric field amplitude at z is given, from Eq. (4.92), as

$$|E(x, z)| = |E_e(x) + E_o(x)\exp[j(\beta_e - \beta_o)z]|. \tag{4.94}$$

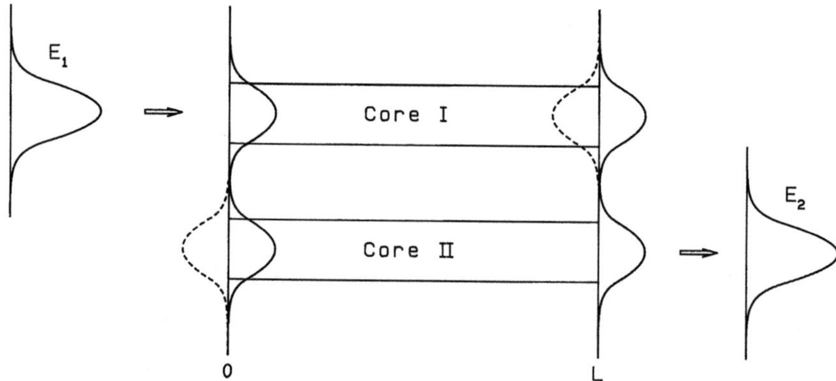

Figure 4.12 Even (solid line) and odd (dotted line) modes in the five-layer slab waveguide.

Electric field distribution at $z = \pi/(\beta_e - \beta_o)$ is then given by

$$|E(x, z)| = |E_e(x) - E_o(x)| = E_2(x), \tag{4.95}$$

where $E_2(x)$ denotes the eigen mode of waveguide II. Equation (4.95) means that the incident field coupled to waveguide I shifted to waveguide II at the distance

$$L_c = \frac{\pi}{\beta_e - \beta_o}. \tag{4.96}$$

L_c is a coupling length. The mode-coupling coefficient is obtained from Eqs. (4.44) and (4.96):

$$\kappa = \frac{\pi}{2L_c} = \frac{\beta_e - \beta_o}{2}. \tag{4.97}$$

Let us calculate the mode-coupling coefficient κ for the TE mode in the five-layer slab waveguide. The eigenvalue equations of the five-layer slab waveguide in the coordinate system shown in Fig. 4.13 are given by

$$2u = \tan^{-1}\left(\frac{w}{u}\right) + \tan^{-1}\left\{\frac{w}{u}\tanh\left[\left(\frac{D}{2a} - 1\right)w\right]\right\} \quad \text{(even mode)} \tag{4.98}$$

$$2u = \tan^{-1}\left(\frac{w}{u}\right) + \tan^{-1}\left\{\frac{w}{u}\coth\left[\left(\frac{D}{2a} - 1\right)w\right]\right\} \quad \text{(odd mode)}, \tag{4.99}$$

where

$$u = a\sqrt{k^2 n_1^2 - \beta^2}, \tag{4.100a}$$

$$w = a\sqrt{\beta^2 - k^2 n_0^2}. \tag{4.100b}$$

When the core center separation D approaches infinity ($D \to \infty$), Eqs. (4.98) and (4.99) both reduce to the eigen mode equation of the single-slab waveguide:

$$u_0 = \tan^{-1}\left(\frac{w_0}{u_0}\right). \tag{4.101}$$

We denote the propagation constant derived by Eq. (4.101) as $\beta^{(0)}$. When the mode coupling between the two waveguides is weak, eigen mode equations (4.98) and (4.99) are considered to be a perturbation from Eq. (4.101). Then the propagation constant for the even mode is expressed by

$$\beta_e = \beta^{(0)} + \delta\beta_e. \tag{4.102}$$

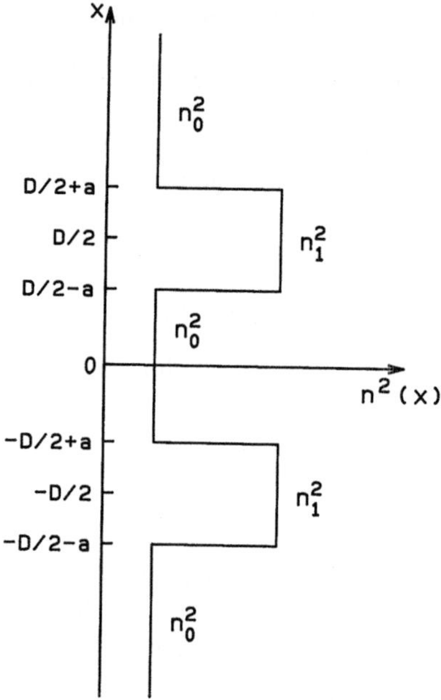

Figure 4.13 Refractive-index distribution of the five-layer slab waveguide.

Substituting Eq. (4.102) into Eq. (4.100a), we obtain

$$2u = 2a\sqrt{k^2 n_1^2 - (\beta^{(0)} + \delta\beta_e)^2} \cong 2u_0 - \frac{2\beta^{(0)} a^2}{u_0}\delta\beta_e. \tag{4.103}$$

In a similar manner, each term of the right-hand side of Eq. (4.98) can be approximated as

$$\tan^{-1}\left(\frac{w}{u}\right) \cong u_0 + \frac{\beta^{(0)} a^2}{u_0 w_0}\delta\beta_e, \tag{4.104a}$$

$$\tan^{-1}\left\{\frac{w}{u}\tanh\left[\left(\frac{D}{2a} - 1\right)w\right]\right\}$$
$$\cong -u_0 + \frac{\beta^{(0)} a^2}{u_0 w_0}\delta\beta_e - \frac{2u_0 w_0}{v_0^2}\exp\left[-2w_0\left(\frac{D}{2a} - 1\right)\right], \tag{4.104b}$$

where the approximation of $\tanh(z) \cong 1 - 2e^{-2z}$ has been used. Substituting Eqs. (4.103) and (4.104) into Eq. (4.98), we obtain

$$\frac{(1 + w_0)}{v_0 w_0}\beta^{(0)} a^2 \delta\beta_e = u_0 + \frac{u_0 w_0}{v_0^2}\exp\left[-\frac{w_0}{a}(D - 2a)\right]. \tag{4.105}$$

In a similar manner, the expression for $\delta\beta_o = \beta_o - \beta^{(0)}$ is obtained as

$$\frac{(1+w_0)}{v_0 w_0}\beta^{(0)} a^2 \delta\beta_o = u_0 - \frac{u_0 w_0}{v_0^2} \exp\left[-\frac{w_0}{a}(D-2a)\right]. \tag{4.106}$$

Substituting Eqs. (4.105) and (4.106) into Eq. (4.97), the mode-coupling coefficient κ is obtained as

$$\kappa = \frac{(\delta\beta_e - \delta\beta_o)}{2} = \frac{u_0^2 w_0^2}{\beta^{(0)} a^2 (1+w_0) v_0^2} \exp\left[-\frac{w_0}{a}(D-2a)\right]. \tag{4.107}$$

This equation reduces to Eq. (4.86) when we substitute $\beta^{(0)} \cong kn_1$ and $v_0^2 = k^2 a^2 (n_1^2 - n_0^2)$ into it.

4.4.4. Coupling Coefficients for Optical Fibers

We rewrite the mode-coupling coefficient in Eq. (4.13) as

$$\kappa = \frac{\omega\varepsilon_0 \int_{-\infty}^{\infty}\int_{-\infty}^{\infty}(N^2 - N_2^2)\mathbf{E}_1^* \cdot \mathbf{E}_2 \, dx\, dy}{\int_{-\infty}^{\infty}\int_{-\infty}^{\infty}\mathbf{u}_z \cdot (\mathbf{E}_1^* \times \mathbf{H}_1 + \mathbf{E}_1 \times \mathbf{H}_1^*)\, dx\, dy}. \tag{4.108}$$

Putting the relation of $s = s_1 = s_2 = -1$ and replacing A by $C = -j(\beta a/u)A$ in Eqs. (3.94) and (3.95), electromagnetic fields of the fundamental HE_{11} mode are expressed by the following.

a. *Core region* $(0 \leqslant r \leqslant a)$:

$$E_x = CJ_0\left(\frac{u}{a}r\right)\cos\psi, \tag{4.109a}$$

$$E_y = -CJ_0\left(\frac{u}{a}r\right)\sin\psi, \tag{4.109b}$$

$$E_z = j\frac{u}{\beta a}CJ_1\left(\frac{u}{a}r\right)\cos(\theta+\psi), \tag{4.109c}$$

$$H_x = \frac{\omega\varepsilon_0 n_1^2}{\beta}CJ_0\left(\frac{u}{a}r\right)\sin\psi, \tag{4.109d}$$

$$H_y = \frac{\omega\varepsilon_o n_1^2}{\beta}CJ_0\left(\frac{u}{a}r\right)\cos\psi, \tag{4.109e}$$

$$H_z = j\frac{u}{\omega\varepsilon_0 a}CJ_1\left(\frac{u}{a}r\right)\sin(\theta+\psi), \tag{4.109f}$$

b. *Cladding region* $(r > a)$:

$$E_x = C\frac{J_0(u)}{K_0(w)}K_0\left(\frac{w}{a}r\right)\cos\psi, \tag{4.110a}$$

$$E_y = -C\frac{J_0(u)}{K_0(w)}K_0\left(\frac{w}{a}r\right)\sin\psi, \tag{4.110b}$$

$$E_z = j\frac{u}{\beta a}C\frac{J_1(u)}{K_1(w)}K_1\left(\frac{w}{a}r\right)\cos(\theta+\psi), \tag{4.110c}$$

$$H_x = \frac{\omega\varepsilon_0 n_0^2}{\beta}C\frac{J_0(u)}{K_0(w)}K_0\left(\frac{w}{a}r\right)\sin\psi, \tag{4.110d}$$

$$H_y = \frac{\omega\varepsilon_0 n_0^2}{\beta}C\frac{J_0(u)}{K_0(w)}K_0\left(\frac{w}{a}r\right)\cos\psi \tag{4.110e}$$

$$H_z = j\frac{u}{\omega\varepsilon_0 a}C\frac{J_1(u)}{K_1(w)}K_1\left(\frac{w}{a}r\right)\sin(\theta+\psi). \tag{4.110f}$$

Constant C is related to optical power P by Eq. (3.99):

$$|C| = \frac{w}{avJ_1(u)}\sqrt{\frac{2P\sqrt{\mu_0/\varepsilon_0}}{\pi n_1}}, \tag{4.111}$$

where light velocity c was replaced by $1/\sqrt{\varepsilon_0\mu_0}$. The denominator of Eq. (4.108) is normalized, from Eq. (4.17), as

$$\int_{-\infty}^{\infty}\int_{-\infty}^{\infty}\mathbf{u}_z\cdot(\mathbf{E}_1^*\times\mathbf{H}_1+\mathbf{E}_1\times\mathbf{H}_1^*)\,dx\,dy = 4P. \tag{4.112}$$

Next we consider the integral of the numerator of Eq. (4.108). As shown in Fig. 4.14, $N^2(r,\theta) - N_2^2(r,\theta)$ is zero outside of core 1. Noting that the electric field of the core is used for $\mathbf{E}_1$ [Eq. (4.109)] and that the field of the cladding is used for $\mathbf{E}_2$ [Eq. (4.110)] for the integral inside the core 1, $\mathbf{E}_1^*\cdot\mathbf{E}_2$ is expressed by

$$\begin{aligned}\mathbf{E}_1^*\cdot\mathbf{E}_2 &= E_{x1}^*E_{x2}+E_{y1}^*E_{y2}+E_{z1}^*E_{z2}\\ &= |C|^2\frac{J_0(u)}{K_0(w)}J_0\left(\frac{u}{a}r\right)K_0\left(\frac{w}{a}R\right)+\left(\frac{u}{\beta a}\right)^2|C|^2\frac{J_1(u)}{K_1(w)}J_1\left(\frac{u}{a}r\right)K_1\left(\frac{w}{a}R\right)\\ &\quad\times\cos(\theta+\psi)\cos(\Theta+\psi),\end{aligned} \tag{4.113}$$

where (R, Θ) is a coordinate system having the origin at the center of core 2 as shown in Fig. 4.15. The separation of the two core centers is denoted by D. When $D \gg r$ holds, radius R can be approximated as

$$R = (D^2+r^2-2Dr\cos\theta)^{1/2} \cong D - r\cos\theta. \tag{4.114}$$

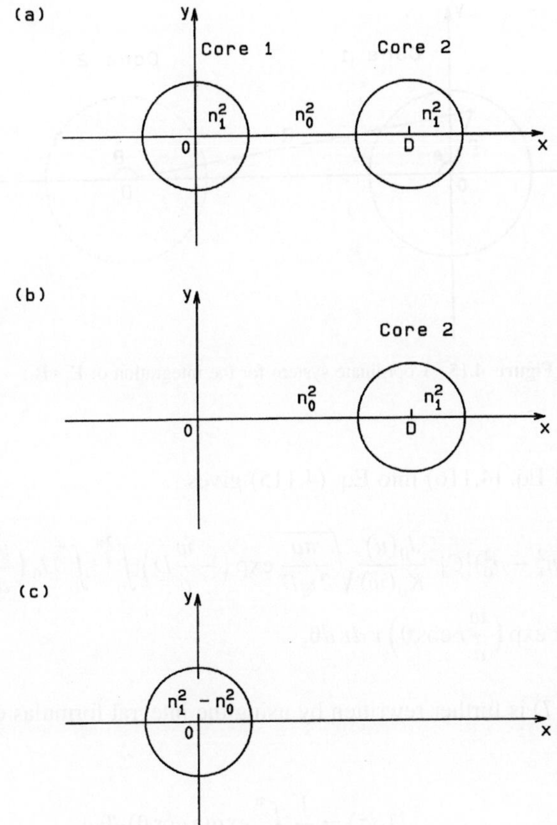

Figure 4.14 Geometries for the calculation of the mode-coupling coefficient. (a), (b), and (c) represent $N^2(r, \theta)$, $N_2^2(r, \theta)$, and $N^2(r, \theta) - N_2^2(r, \theta)$, respectively.

Since the second term of the right-hand side of Eq. (4.113) is sufficiently smaller than the first term, the integration of the numerator in Eq. (4.108) becomes [9, 10]:

$$S = \int_{-\infty}^{\infty}\int_{-\infty}^{\infty}(N^2 - N_2^2)\mathbf{E}_1^* \cdot \mathbf{E}_2\, dx\, dy = \int_0^{2\pi}\int_0^{a}(n_1^2 - n_0^2)|C|^2 \frac{J_0(u)}{K_0(w)} J_0\left(\frac{u}{a}r\right)$$
$$\times K_0\left(\frac{w}{a}R\right) r\, dr\, d\theta. \tag{4.115}$$

When the argument of the modified Bessel function $K_0(z)$ in Eq. (4.115) is large, it can be approximated as

$$K_0(z) \cong \sqrt{\frac{\pi}{2z}} \exp(-z). \tag{4.116}$$

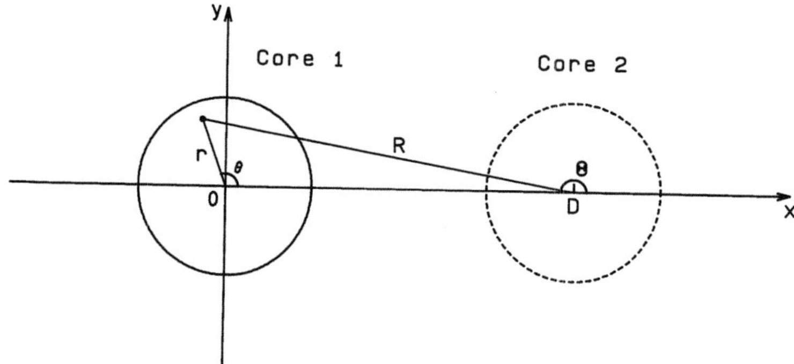

Figure 4.15 Coordinate system for the integration of $\mathbf{E}_1^* \cdot \mathbf{E}_2$.

Substitution of Eq. (4.116) into Eq. (4.115) gives

$$S = (n_1^2 - n_0^2)|C|^2 \frac{J_0(u)}{K_0(w)} \sqrt{\frac{\pi a}{2wD}} \exp\left(-\frac{w}{a}D\right) \int_0^{2\pi} \int_0^a J_0\left(\frac{u}{a}r\right) \times \exp\left(\frac{w}{a} r \cos\theta\right) r\, dr\, d\theta. \tag{4.117}$$

Equation (4.117) is further rewritten by using the integral formulas of the Bessel functions [11]:

$$I_0(z) = \frac{1}{\pi} \int_0^{\pi} \exp(z \cos\theta) d\theta, \tag{4.118a}$$

$$\int_0^1 J_0(uz) I_0(wz) z dz = \frac{J_0(u) w I_1(w) + I_0(w) u J_1(u)}{u^2 + w^2} \tag{4.118b}$$

into

$$S = 2\pi a^2 (n_1^2 - n_0^2)|C|^2 \frac{J_0(u)}{K_0(w)} \sqrt{\frac{\pi a}{2wD}} \exp\left(-\frac{w}{a}D\right) \times \frac{u J_1(u)}{v^2 K_1(w)} \times \left[\frac{J_0(u)}{u J_1(u)} w K_1(w) I_1(w) + K_1(w) I_0(w)\right]. \tag{4.119}$$

If we use the eigenvalue equation of the HE_{11} mode [Eq. (3.71) with $n = 1$] and the formula of the modified Bessel function

$$K_0(w) I_1(w) + K_1(w) I_0(w) = \frac{1}{w}, \tag{4.120}$$

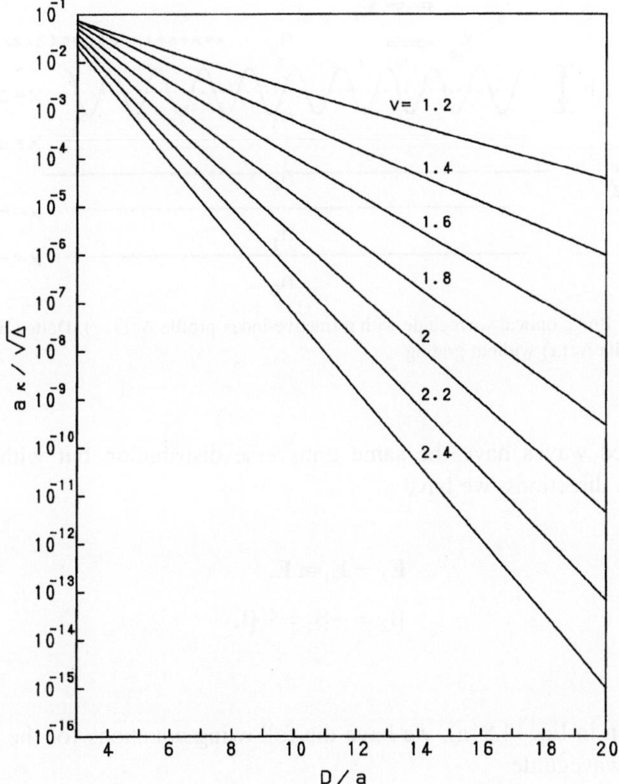

Figure 4.16 Dependencies of the normalized coupling coefficient $\kappa a/\sqrt{\Delta}$ on the relative core center separation D/a for various v-values.

then the mode-coupling coefficient of the optical fiber directional coupler is given by

$$\kappa = \frac{\sqrt{\Delta}}{a} \frac{u^2}{v^3 K_1^2(w)} \sqrt{\frac{\pi a}{wD}} \exp\left(-\frac{w}{a} D\right). \tag{4.121}$$

Figure 4.16 shows the dependencies of the normalized coupling coefficient $\kappa a/\sqrt{\Delta}$ on the relative core center separation D/a for various v-values.

4.4.5. Coupling Coefficients for Corrugated Waveguides

Here we describe the derivation method for the mode-coupling coefficient κ_G in the Bragg waveguide [12], as shown in Fig. 4.17. Since the incident

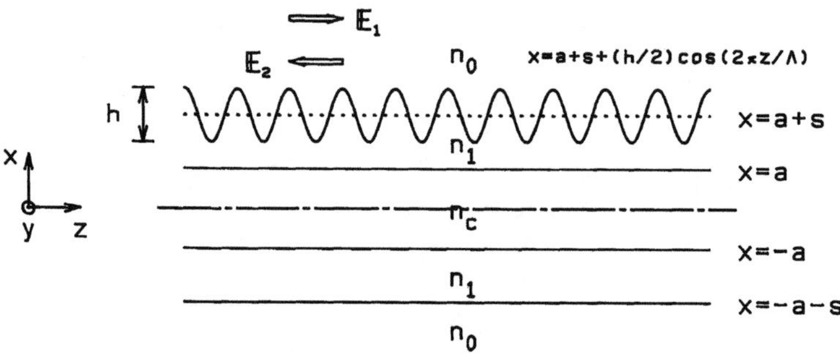

Figure 4.17 Bragg optical waveguide with refractive-index profile $N^2(x, z)$. Dotted line indicates the index profile $N_2^2(x)$ without grating.

and reflected waves have the same transverse distribution but with opposite propagation directions, we have

$$\mathbf{E}_2 = \mathbf{E}_1 \equiv \mathbf{E}, \tag{4.122a}$$

$$\beta_2 = -\beta_1 = -\beta. \tag{4.122b}$$

As shown in Eq. (4.81a), we have the following equations for the TE mode in the slab waveguide:

$$\mathbf{u}_z \cdot (\mathbf{E}_1^* \times \mathbf{H}_1 + \mathbf{E}_1 \times \mathbf{H}_1^*) = \frac{2\beta}{\omega\mu_0}|E_y|^2. \tag{4.123a}$$

$$\mathbf{u}_z \cdot (\mathbf{E}_2^* \times \mathbf{H}_2 + \mathbf{E}_2 \times \mathbf{H}_2^*) = -\frac{2\beta}{\omega\mu_0}|E_y|^2, \tag{4.123b}$$

$$\mathbf{E}_1^* \cdot \mathbf{E}_2 = \mathbf{E}_2^* \cdot \mathbf{E}_1 = |E_y|^2. \tag{4.123c}$$

Substituting Eqs. (4.13) and (4.123) into Eqs. (4.30) and (4.31), the mode-coupling equations for the Bragg optical waveguide are given by

$$\frac{dA}{dz} = -jB\exp(j2\beta z)\frac{k^2}{2\beta}\frac{\int_{-\infty}^{\infty}(N^2 - N_2^2)|E_y|^2 dx}{\int_{-\infty}^{\infty}|E_y|^2 dx}, \tag{4.124a}$$

$$\frac{dB}{dz} = jA\exp(-j2\beta z)\frac{k^2}{2\beta}\frac{\int_{-\infty}^{\infty}(N^2 - N_1^2)|E_y|^2 dx}{\int_{-\infty}^{\infty}|E_y|^2 dx}, \tag{4.124b}$$

where $N_1^2 = N_2^2$. As shown in Fig. 4.17, the perturbation term $[N^2(x, z) - N_2^2(x)]$ becomes zero outside of the grating region. Then it is expressed as

$$N^2 - N_2^2 = \begin{cases} 0 & \left(x > a + s + \dfrac{h}{2}\right) \\ \sum\limits_{m=-\infty}^{\infty} A_m(x) \exp\left(-j\dfrac{2\pi m}{\Lambda} z\right) & \left(a + s - \dfrac{h}{2} \leqslant x \leqslant a + s + \dfrac{h}{2}\right) \\ 0 & \left(x < a + s - \dfrac{h}{2}\right), \end{cases} \tag{4.125}$$

where s denotes the average thickness of the grating layer and h is a grating height. Fourier expansion coefficient A_m is obtained by

$$A_m(x) = \frac{1}{\Lambda} \int_{w_0}^{w_0+\Lambda} [N^2(x, z) - N_2^2(x)] \exp\left(j\frac{2\pi m}{\Lambda} z\right) dz, \tag{4.126}$$

where w_0 is given by

$$w_0 = -\frac{\Lambda}{2\pi} \cos^{-1}\left[\frac{2}{h}(x - a - s)\right]. \tag{4.127}$$

The integration of Eq. (4.126) is separated into two cases, corresponding to the sign of $(x - a - s)$, as shown in Fig. 4.18.

a. $x \geqslant a + s$ [Fig. 4.18(a)]:

$$A_m(x) = \begin{cases} \dfrac{2w_2}{\Lambda}(n_1^2 - n_0^2) & (m = 0) \\ \dfrac{n_1^2 - n_0^2}{\pi m} \sin\left(\dfrac{2\pi m}{\Lambda} w_2\right) & (m \neq 0) \end{cases} \tag{4.128}$$

$$w_2 = \frac{\Lambda}{2\pi} \cos^{-1}\left[\frac{2}{h}(x - a - s)\right] \tag{4.129}$$

b. $x < a < s$ [Fig. 4.18(b)]:

$$A_m(x) = \begin{cases} -\left(\dfrac{2w_4}{\Lambda} - 1\right)(n_1^2 - n_0^2) & (m = 0) \\ -\dfrac{n_1^2 - n_0^2}{\pi m} \sin\left(\dfrac{2\pi m}{\Lambda} w_4\right) & (m \neq 0) \end{cases} \tag{4.130}$$

$$w_4 = \frac{\Lambda}{2} + \frac{\Lambda}{2\pi} \cos^{-1}\left[\frac{2}{h}(a + s - x)\right]. \tag{4.131}$$

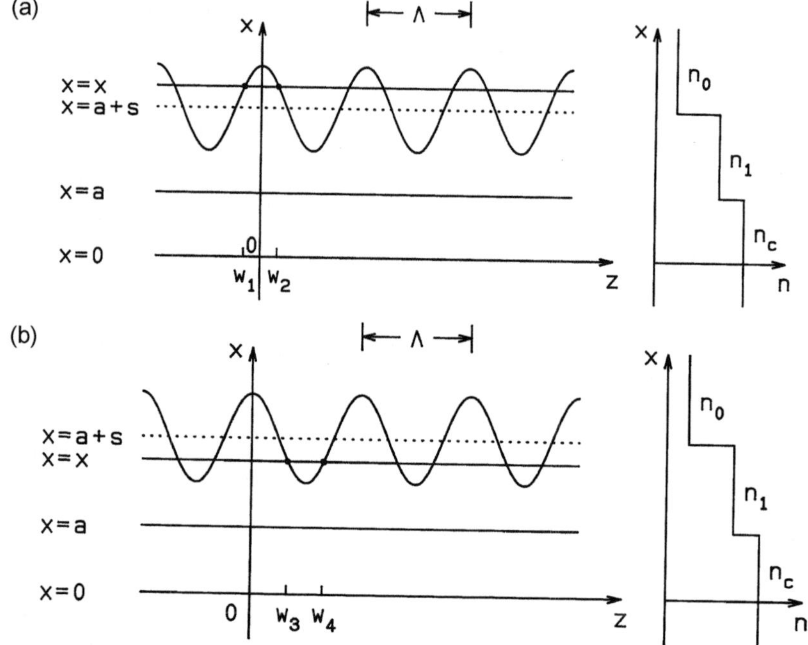

Figure 4.18 Coordinate systems in the calculation of $A_m(x)$ for (a) $x \geqslant a+s$ and (b) $x < a+s$.

Refractive-index perturbation $N^2(x,z) - N_2^2(x)$ is then given, from Eqs. (4.125)–(4.131), as

$$N^2 - N_2^2 = \begin{cases} 0 & \left(x > a+s+\dfrac{h}{2}\right) \\ \displaystyle\sum_{m=-\infty}^{\infty} \frac{n_1^2 - n_0^2}{\pi m} \sin\left(\frac{2\pi m}{\Lambda} w_2\right) \exp\left(-j\frac{2\pi m}{\Lambda} z\right) & \left(a+s \leqslant x \leqslant a+s+\dfrac{h}{2}\right) \\ -\displaystyle\sum_{m=-\infty}^{\infty} \frac{n_1^2 - n_0^2}{\pi m} \sin\left(\frac{2\pi m}{\Lambda} w_4\right) \exp\left(-j\frac{2\pi m}{\Lambda} z\right) & \left(a+s-\dfrac{h}{2} \leqslant x \leqslant a+s\right) \\ 0 & \left(x < a+s-\dfrac{h}{2}\right). \end{cases} \tag{4.132}$$

Integer m in this equation represents the diffraction order of the grating. The coupled mode equation for the mth diffraction order is given, from Eqs. (4.124) and (4.132), as

$$\frac{dA}{dz} = -j\kappa_G B \exp\left[j\left(2\beta - \frac{2\pi m}{\Lambda}\right)z\right], \tag{4.133a}$$

$$\frac{dB}{dz} = j\kappa_G A \exp\left[-j\left(2\beta - \frac{2\pi m}{\Lambda}\right)z\right], \tag{4.133b}$$

where

$$\kappa_G = \frac{k^2}{2\beta P}\frac{n_1^2 - n_0^2}{\pi m}\left[\int_{a+s}^{a+s+h/2} \sin\left(\frac{2\pi m}{\Lambda}w_2\right)|E_y|^2 dx - \int_{a+s-h/2}^{a+s} \sin\left(\frac{2\pi m}{\Lambda}w_4\right)|E_y|^2 dx\right], \tag{4.134}$$

$$P = \int_{-\infty}^{\infty} |E_y|^2 dx. \tag{4.135}$$

Let us obtain the electric field distribution E_y in the nonperturbed refractive-index profile $N_1(x)$ [or $N_2(x)$] in order to calculate κ_G. Here we assume the following practical parameters in the five-layer slab waveguide as shown in Fig. 4.19 [6]:

$$\begin{cases} n_c = 3.50,\ n_1 = 3.38,\ n_0 = 3.17 \\ 2a = 0.25\ \mu\text{m},\ s = 0.1\ \mu\text{m},\ h = 100 - 1500\text{Å}. \end{cases} \tag{4.136}$$

Under these waveguide parameters, the propagation constant β lies between kn_0 and $kn_1 (kn_0 < \beta < kn_1)$. The electric field distribution is then obtained as

$$E_y = \begin{cases} Q\cos(\eta x) & (0 \leqslant |x| \leqslant a) \\ H\cos[\gamma(x-a)] + C\sin[\gamma(x-a)] & (a \leqslant |x| \leqslant a+s) \\ D\exp[-\sigma(x-a-s)] & (|x| > a+s), \end{cases} \tag{4.137}$$

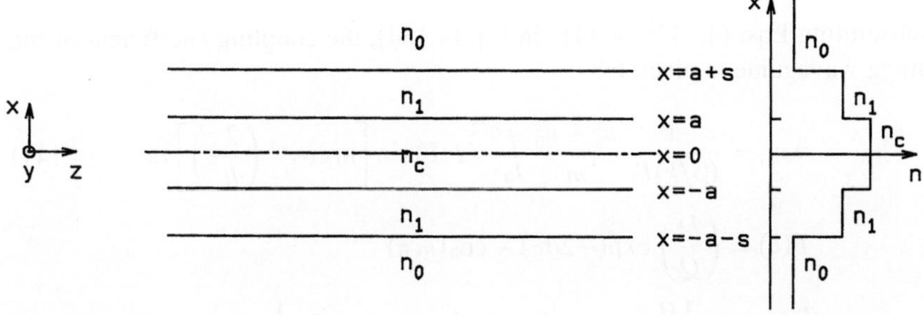

Figure 4.19 Nonperturbed refractive-index profile $N_1(x)$ or $N_2(x)$ before grating is formed.

where transverse wavenumbers are given by

$$\begin{cases} \eta = k\sqrt{n_c^2 - \left(\dfrac{\beta}{k}\right)^2} \\ \gamma = k\sqrt{n_1^2 - \left(\dfrac{\beta}{k}\right)^2} \\ \sigma = k\sqrt{\left(\dfrac{\beta}{k}\right)^2 - n_0^2}. \end{cases} \tag{4.138}$$

The eigenvalue equation for the TE mode is obtained by applying the continuity conditions for E_y and $H_x \propto dE_y/dx$:

$$\left[\frac{\gamma + \sigma\tan(\gamma s)}{\sigma - \gamma\tan(\gamma s)}\right]\eta\sin(\eta a) = \gamma\cos(\eta a). \tag{4.139}$$

Constants H, C, and D in Eq. (4.137) and optical power P in Eq. (4.135) are expressed in terms of Q as

$$\frac{H}{Q} = \cos(\eta a), \tag{4.140a}$$

$$\frac{C}{Q} = -\frac{\eta}{\gamma}\sin(\eta a), \tag{4.140b}$$

$$\frac{D}{Q} = \cos(\eta a)\cos(\gamma s) - \frac{\eta}{\gamma}\sin(\eta a)\sin(\gamma s), \tag{4.140c}$$

$$\begin{aligned} P_0 \equiv \frac{P}{Q^2} &= a + \frac{\sin(2\eta a)}{2\eta} + \left(\frac{D}{Q}\right)^2\frac{1}{\sigma} + \left(\frac{H}{Q}\right)^2\left[s + \frac{\sin(2\gamma s)}{2\gamma}\right] \\ &+ \frac{H}{Q}\frac{C}{Q}\frac{1}{\gamma}[1 - \cos(2\gamma s)] + \left(\frac{C}{Q}\right)^2\left[s - \frac{\sin(2\gamma s)}{2\gamma}\right]. \end{aligned} \tag{4.140d}$$

Substituting Eqs. (4.137)–(4.141) in Eq. (4.134), the coupling coefficient of the Bragg waveguide is given by

$$\lambda\kappa_G = \frac{1}{(\beta/k)P_0}\frac{n_1^2 - n_0^2}{m}\int_0^{h/2} F(\xi)\sin\left[m\cos^{-1}\left(\frac{2}{h}\xi\right)\right]d\xi \tag{4.141}$$

$$\begin{aligned} F(\xi) = &\left(\frac{D}{Q}\right)^2\exp(-2\sigma\xi) - \cos(m\pi) \\ &\times\left\{\frac{H}{Q}\cos[\gamma(s-\xi)] + \frac{C}{Q}\sin[\gamma(s-\xi)]\right\}. \end{aligned} \tag{4.142}$$

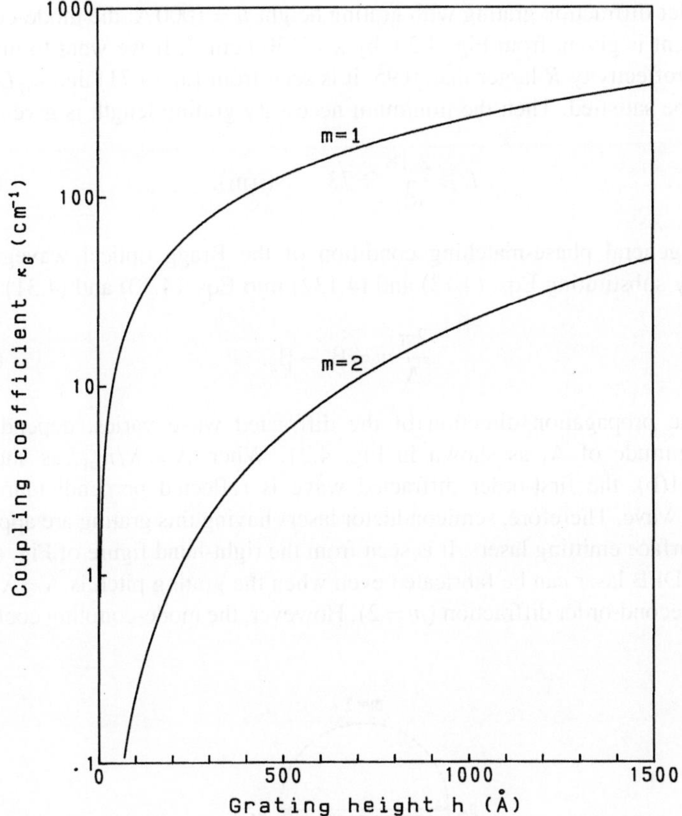

Figure 4.20 Coupling coefficient of the Bragg waveguide with respect to the grating height h.

Figure 4.20 shows the coupling coefficient κ_G of the TE mode in the Bragg waveguide with the parameters of Eq. (4.136). The effective index of the non-perturbed waveguide with the parameters of Eq. (4.136) is calculated to be

$$n_{\text{eff}} = \frac{\beta}{k} = 3.289136. \tag{4.143}$$

The phase-matching condition for the maximum mode coupling is given, from Eq. (4.65), as

$$\Lambda = m\frac{\lambda}{2n_{\text{eff}}} \cong 0.2356m \quad (\mu\text{m}) \qquad (m = 1, 2, \ldots). \tag{4.144}$$

It is seen from Eq. (4.144) that the grating pitch should be $\Lambda = 0.2356(\mu\text{m})$ in order to fabricate DFB lasers with first-order diffraction ($m = 1$). For the first-order diffraction grating with grating height $h = 1000\,\text{Å}$, the mode-coupling coefficient is given, from Fig. 4.20, by $\kappa_G \cong 300\ \text{cm}^{-1}$. If we want to make the grating reflectivity R larger than 0.95, it is seen from Eq. (4.71) that $\kappa_G L \geqslant 2.18$ should be satisfied. Then the minimum necessary grating length is given by

$$L \geqslant \frac{2.18}{\kappa_G} \cong 73 \qquad (\mu\text{m}). \tag{4.145}$$

The general phase-matching condition of the Bragg optical waveguide is given by substituting Eqs. (4.13) and (4.132) into Eqs. (4.30) and (4.31):

$$\frac{2\pi}{\Lambda} m = \beta_1 - \beta_2. \tag{4.146}$$

Then the propagation direction of the diffracted wave varies, depending on the magnitude of Λ, as shown in Fig. 4.21. When $\Lambda = \lambda / n_{\text{eff}}$, as shown in Fig. 4.21(b), the first-order diffracted wave is reflected perpendicular to the incident wave. Therefore, semiconductor lasers having this grating are applicable to the surface emitting lasers. It is seen from the right-hand figure of Fig. 4.21(b) that the DFB laser can be fabricated even when the grating pitch is $\Lambda = \lambda / n_{\text{eff}}$ if we use second-order diffraction ($m = 2$). However, the mode-coupling coefficient

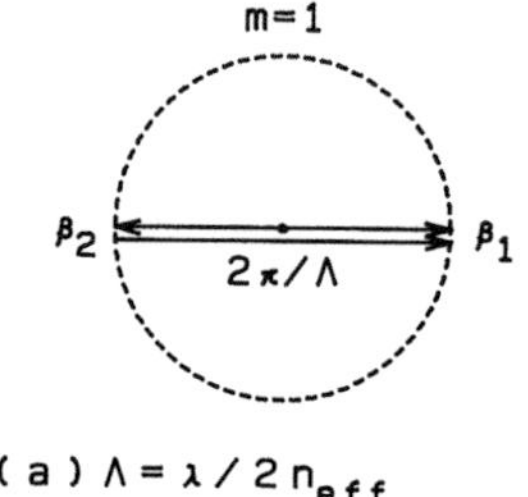

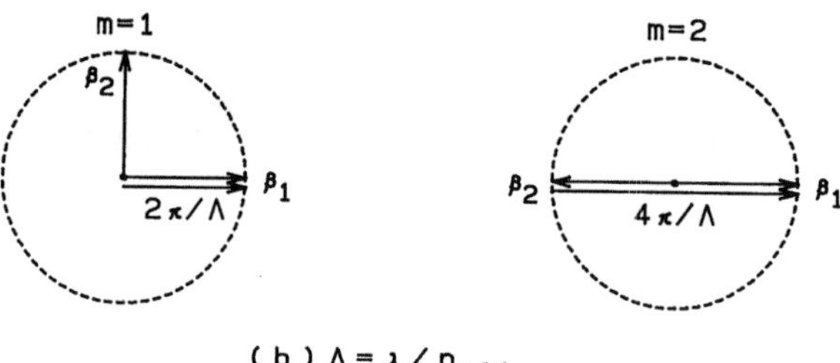

Figure 4.21 Relation of the propagation direction of a diffracted wave with the grating period Λ.

is $\kappa_G \cong 20\,\text{cm}^{-1}$ for the second-order diffraction wave at the grating height of $h = 1000\,\text{Å}$. Then the minimum grating length necessary to obtain the reflectivity of $R \geqslant 0.95$ becomes $L \geqslant 1.1$ (mm). Such a long grating is disadvantageous for lasers, since the chip size becomes large and propagation loss in the grating increases. It is well understood that the first-order grating is particularly important for DFB lasers.

4.5. OPTICAL WAVEGUIDE DEVICES USING DIRECTIONAL COUPLERS

Directional couplers are very important components in the fabrication of various optical devices. In this subsection, several optical devices utilizing directional couplers are described.

4.5.1. Mach–Zehnder Interferometers

We consider the case in which light is coupled into the upper waveguide of a Mach–Zehnder interferometer. Here we assume that both arms have the same waveguide structures; that is, we have $\delta = 0$ and $q = \kappa$ in Eqs. (4.36)–(4.38). Substituting $A(0) = A_0$ and $B(0) = 0$ in Eqs. (4.36) and (4.37), the outputs of the first directional coupler are given by

$$\begin{cases} A_1 = A_0 \cos(\kappa\ell) & (4.147\text{a}) \\ B_1 = -jA_0 \sin(\kappa\ell), & (4.147\text{b}) \end{cases}$$

where ℓ denotes the coupling length. It should be noted here that mode coupling takes place not only in the straight coupling region but also in the curved regions. Therefore, the coupling length ℓ in this subsection is an effective straight coupling length, which includes the entire mode-coupling effect in the straight and curved coupling regions [13]. When the first coupler is a 3-dB coupler with $\kappa\ell = \pi/4$, light-splitting ratios are $A_1 = A_0/\sqrt{2}$ and $B_1 = -jA_0/\sqrt{2}$. After passing through the interferometer straight arms, A_2 and B_2 become

$$\begin{cases} A_2 = A_1 \exp(-j\beta L) = \dfrac{A_0}{\sqrt{2}} \exp(-j\beta L) & (4.148\text{a}) \\ B_2 = B_1 \exp(-j\beta L + j\phi) = -j\dfrac{A_0}{\sqrt{2}} \exp(-j\beta L + j\phi), & (4.148\text{b}) \end{cases}$$

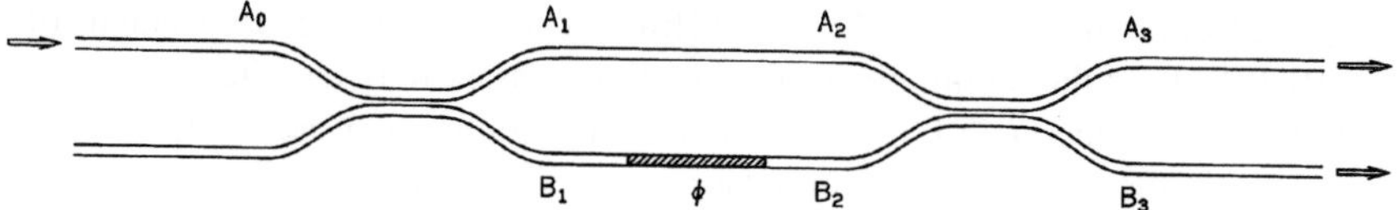

Figure 4.22 Mach–Zehnder optical interferometer.

where ϕ denotes excess phase shift in the lower arm, as shown in Fig. 4.22. Then the outputs of the interferometer are given by substituting Eq. (4.148) into Eqs. (4.36) and (4.37):

$$\begin{cases} A_3 = -jA_0 \sin\left(\frac{\phi}{2}\right) \exp\left(-j\beta L + \frac{j\phi}{2}\right) & (4.149a) \\ B_3 = -jA_0 \cos\left(\frac{\phi}{2}\right) \exp\left(-j\beta L + \frac{j\phi}{2}\right). & (4.149b) \end{cases}$$

Here we assumed that the second coupler is also a 3-dB coupler having $\kappa\ell = \pi/4$. The optical intensity in each output port is given by

$$\begin{cases} |A_3|^2 = |A_0|^2 \sin^2\left(\frac{\phi}{2}\right) & (4.150a) \\ |B_3|^2 = |A_0|^2 \cos^2\left(\frac{\phi}{2}\right). & (4.150b) \end{cases}$$

It is seen from these equations that light can be switched from port A to port B or vice versa by changing the phase ϕ from π to zero. When the Mach–Zehnder interferometer is used as an optical modulator, optical phase ϕ is modulated in proportion to the input signal. When phase ϕ is slightly modulated with $\delta\phi$, output intensity in Eqs. (4.150) becomes $|A_3|^2 \cong |A_0|^2(\delta\phi/2)^2$ and $|B_3|^2 \cong |A_0|^2$. It is shown that linear modulation is not obtained with the present condition. If we add the phase bias of $\pi/2$ and apply the phase modulation of $\delta\phi$, Eq. (4.150a) becomes

$$|A_3|^2 = |A_0|^2 \sin^2\left(\frac{\pi}{4} + \frac{\delta\phi}{2}\right) = \frac{1}{2}|A_0|^2[1 + \sin(\delta\phi)] \cong \frac{1}{2}[A_0]^2(1 + \delta\phi). \quad (4.151)$$

Then optical intensity becomes linearly dependent on the input signal $\delta\phi$.

4.5.2. Ring Resonators

The steady-state input–output relations of the optical ring resonator in Fig. 4.23 are expressed by

$$\begin{cases} A = (1-\gamma)^{1/2}[A_0 \cos(\kappa\ell) - jB_0 \sin(\kappa\ell)] & (4.152a) \\ B = (1-\gamma)^{1/2}[-jA_0 \sin(\kappa\ell) + B_0 \cos(\kappa\ell)], & (4.152b) \end{cases}$$

where κ, ℓ, and γ denote the mode-coupling coefficient of the directional coupler, the coupling length, and the intensity-insertion-loss coefficient, respectively [14]. In Eqs. (4.152), we assumed that input/output and resonator waveguides have the same propagation constant β. When we denote the intensity attenuation coefficient of the ring waveguide as ρ, B_0 is expressed by

$$B_0 = B \exp\left(-\frac{\rho}{2}L - j\beta L\right). \tag{4.153}$$

The amplitude transmittance of the optical ring resonator is then given, from Eqs. (4.152) and (4.153), by

$$\frac{A}{A_0} = (1-\gamma)^{1/2} \left[\frac{\cos(\kappa\ell) - (1-\gamma)^{1/2} \exp\left(-\frac{\rho}{2}L - j\beta L\right)}{1 - (1-\gamma)^{1/2} \cos(\kappa\ell) \exp\left(-\frac{\rho}{2}L - j\beta L\right)} \right]. \tag{4.154}$$

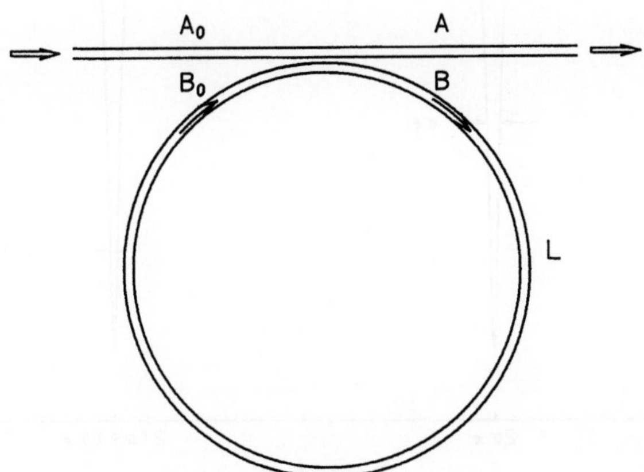

Figure 4.23 Optical ring resonator.

When we introduce new parameters x, y, and ϕ, defined by

$$\begin{cases} x = (1-\gamma)^{1/2}\exp\left(-\frac{\rho}{2}L\right) & (4.155a) \\ y = \cos(\kappa\ell) & (4.155b) \\ \phi = \beta L & (4.155c) \end{cases}$$

then the intensity transmittance of the optical ring resonator is obtained as

$$T(\phi) = \left|\frac{A}{A_0}\right|^2 = (1-\gamma)\left[1 - \frac{(1-x^2)(1-y^2)}{(1-xy)^2 + 4xy\sin^2(\phi/2)}\right]. \tag{4.156}$$

Figure 4.24 shows the transmission characteristics of the optical ring resonator as a function of ϕ. The maximum and minimum transmittances are given by

$$T_{\max} = (1-\gamma)\frac{(x+y)^2}{(1+xy)^2}, \tag{4.157}$$

$$T_{\min} = (1-\gamma)\frac{(x-y)^2}{(1-xy)^2}. \tag{4.158}$$

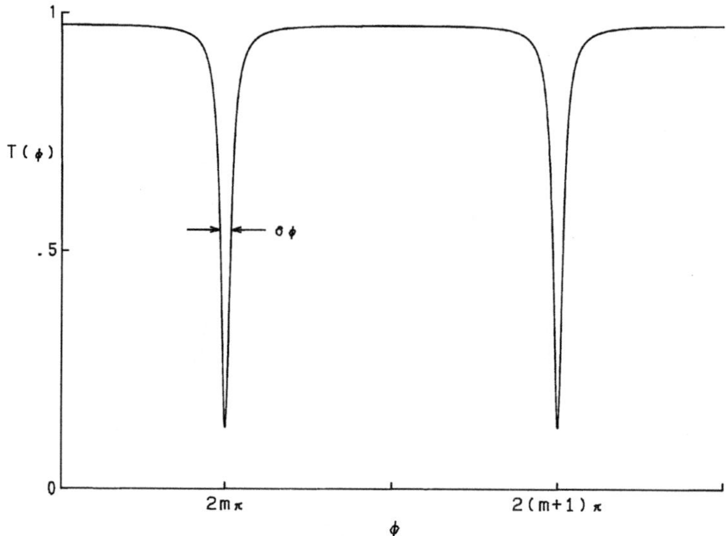

Figure 4.24 Transmission characteristics of the optical ring resonator.

It is seen from these equations that $x \cong y \cong 1$ should be satisfied in order to maximize T_{max} while minimizing T_{min} as much as possible. The full width at the half maximum (FWHM) $\delta\phi$ and the finesse F of the resonator are given by

$$\delta\phi = \frac{2(1-xy)}{\sqrt{xy}}. \tag{4.159}$$

$$F = \frac{2\pi}{\delta\phi} = \frac{\pi\sqrt{xy}}{(1-xy)}. \tag{4.160}$$

The resonance peak of T_{min} in Eq. (4.158) is obtained at

$$\phi = \beta L = 2m\pi. \tag{4.161}$$

Moreover, T_{min} becomes zero when $x = y$ or

$$\cos(\kappa\ell) = (1-\gamma)^{1/2}\exp\left(-\frac{\rho}{2}L\right) \tag{4.162}$$

is satisfied. For example, the best resonance characteristics are obtained at

$$\begin{cases} m = 20000 \\ \kappa\ell = 0.262 \end{cases} \tag{4.163}$$

in the ring resonator with the intensity insertion loss of the coupler 0.1 dB ($\gamma \cong 0.023$), ring resonator length $L = 2\,\text{cm}$, intensity attenuation coefficient of the waveguide 0.1 dB ($\rho \cong 0.023\,\text{cm}^{-1}$), wavelength of light $\lambda = 1.5\,\mu\text{m}$, and effective index of the core $n = 1.5(\beta = 2\pi \times 10^4\,\text{cm}^{-1})$. The finesse of the ring resonator is $F = 45$ at these conditions.

Let us next obtain the spacing of the two resonance peaks. We denote the wavenumber corresponding to $\phi = 2m\pi$ as k and that corresponding to $\phi = 2(m+1)\pi$ as $(k + \Delta k)$. Since m is very large, as shown in Eq. (4.163), the deviation of the wavenumber Δk is quite small with respect to k. In other words, we have $|\Delta k| \ll k$. The deviation in β caused by the slight variation of the wavenumber is obtained, from Eq. (4.161), as $[\beta(k+\Delta k) - \beta(k)] = 2\pi/L$. This is rewritten, by taking into account the relation $|\Delta k| \ll k$, as

$$\frac{d\beta}{dk}\Delta k = \frac{2\pi}{L}. \tag{4.164}$$

Substituting $\beta = kn$ (n is an effective index) into Eq. (4.164), we obtain

$$\frac{d\beta}{dk} = n + k\frac{dn}{dk} = n - \lambda\frac{dn}{d\lambda} \equiv N, \tag{4.165}$$

where N is a group index, given by Eq. (3.119). Since the frequency shift Δf and the wavelength shift $\Delta\lambda$ are related to the variation of the wavenumber Δk as $\Delta f = (c/2\pi)\Delta k$ and $\Delta\lambda = -(\lambda^2/2\pi)\Delta k$, resonance spacings in terms of the frequency and wavelength are given by

$$\Delta f = \frac{c}{NL}, \tag{4.166a}$$

$$\Delta\lambda = -\frac{\lambda^2}{NL}. \tag{4.166b}$$

The frequency spacing of the two resonance peaks is called a *free spectral range* (FSR). FWHMs in terms of frequency and wavelength at the resonance peaks are given, from Eqs. (4.160) and (4.161), by

$$\delta f = \frac{c}{FNL}, \tag{4.167a}$$

$$\delta\lambda = \frac{\lambda^2}{FNL}, \tag{4.167b}$$

where we used the relation $\delta\phi = \delta(\beta L) = (d\beta/dk)\delta k \cdot L = 2\pi/F$. For the previous parameters of ring resonator, the resonance peaks are

$$\begin{aligned} \Delta f &= 10\,\text{GHz}, \\ \Delta\lambda &= -0.075\,\text{nm}, \end{aligned} \tag{4.168}$$

and the FWHMs are

$$\begin{aligned} \delta f &= 222\,\text{MHz}, \\ \delta\lambda &= 0.0017\,\text{nm}. \end{aligned}$$

Here we assumed $N = n$ for simplicity.

4.5.3. Bistable Devices

Here we consider the open type of ring resonator, as shown in Fig. 4.25, consisting of the optical waveguide whose refractive index changes in accordance with optical intensity, that is, the Kerr medium [15]. The intensity transmittance of the open type of ring resonator is given, using the parameters of Eq. (4.155), by

$$T(\phi) = \left|\frac{E}{E_0}\right|^2 = \frac{P}{P_0} = (1-\gamma)\frac{x^2(1-y)^2}{(1-x^2y^2)^2 + 4x^2y^2\sin^2(\phi/2)}. \tag{4.169}$$

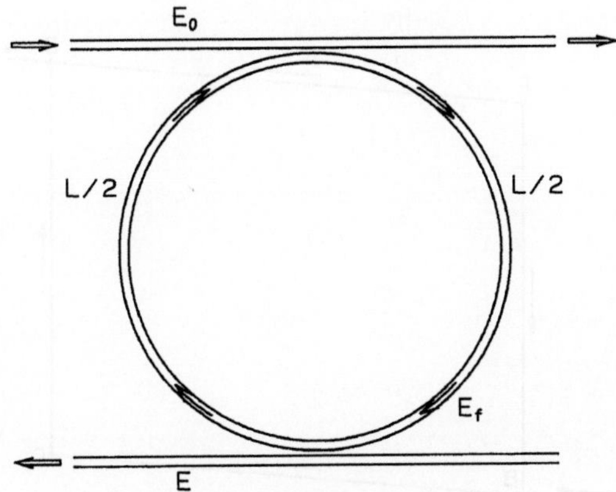

Figure 4.25 Open type of optical ring resonator.

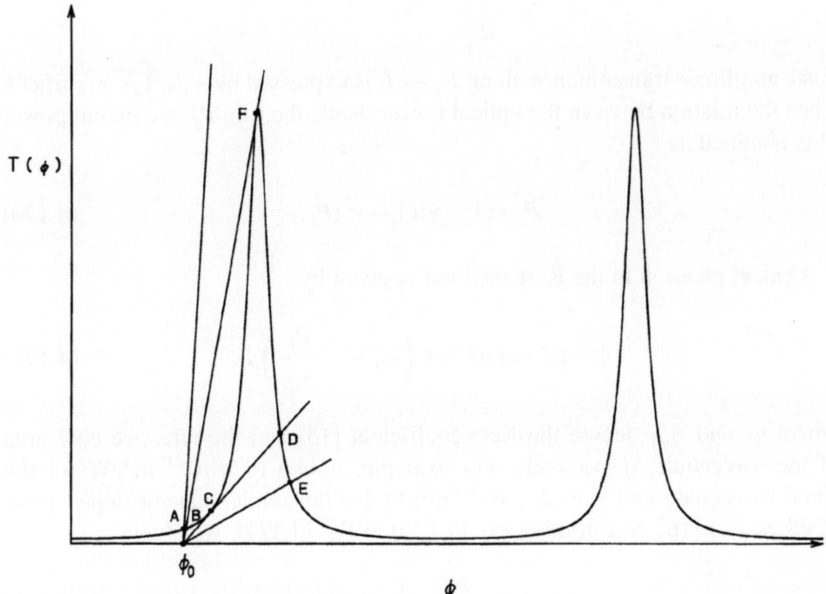

Figure 4.26 Graphical representation of the bistable optical device. Curved and straight lines represent Eqs. (4.169) and (4.171), respectively.

The dependence of intensity transmittance on optical phase ϕ is shown in Fig. 4.26. On the other hand, intensity transmittance along $P_f \rightarrow P$ is given by

$$(1-\gamma)\sin^2(\kappa\ell) = (1-\gamma)[1-\cos^2(\kappa\ell)] = (1-\gamma)(1-y^2)$$

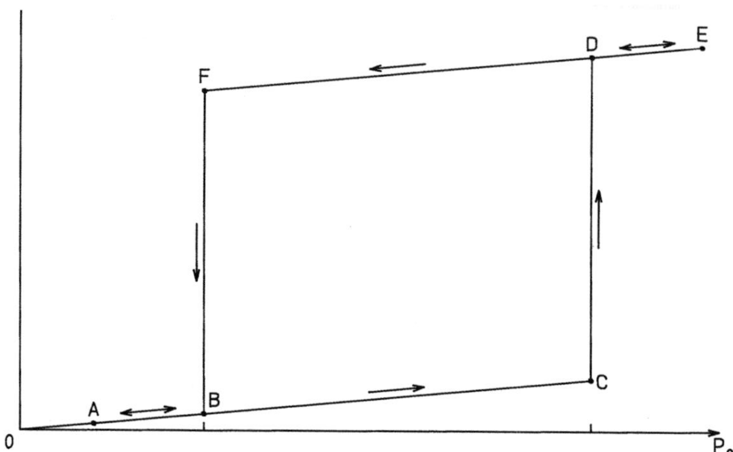

Figure 4.27 Hysteresis curve of the bistable optical device.

since amplitude transmittance along $E_f \to E$ is expressed by $-j\sqrt{1-\gamma}\cdot\sin(\kappa\ell)$. Then the relation between the optical power inside the ring P_f and output power P is obtained as

$$P = (1-\gamma)(1-y^2)P_f. \tag{4.170}$$

Optical phase ϕ in the Kerr medium is given by

$$\phi = \beta L = knL = k\left(n_0 + n_2\frac{P_f}{A_{\text{eff}}}\right)L, \tag{4.171}$$

where n_2 and A_{eff} denote the Kerr coefficient [15] and the effective core area of the waveguide, respectively. For example, $n_2 = 3.18 \times 10^{-20}\,\text{m}^2/\text{W}$ for the silica waveguide and $n_2 = 2 \times 10^{-14}\,\text{m}^2/\text{W}$ for the semiconductor doped glass (CdS_xSe_{1-x}) [16]. Substituting Eq. (4.170) in Eq. (4.171), we obtain

$$T(\phi) = \frac{P}{P_0} = \frac{S}{P_0}(\phi - \phi_0), \tag{4.172}$$

where

$$\phi_0 = kn_0L, \tag{4.173}$$

$$S = (1-\gamma)(1-y^2)\frac{A_{\text{eff}}}{kn_2L}. \tag{4.174}$$

Several straight lines in Fig. 4.26 show Eq. (4.172) for different input power P_0. When a constant optical phase ϕ_0, called a *detuning*, is properly set, as shown in Fig. 4.26, output power P varies along $A \to B \to C \to D \to E$ in accordance with the input power change, as shown in Fig. 4.27. In contrast, when input power decreases, output power varies along $E \to D \to F \to B \to A$. Therefore, a bistable condition is obtained for the same input power P_0 but for a different orientation.

4.6. FIBER BRAGG GRATINGS

A fiber Bragg grating, which has periodical perturbation of the refractive index in the fiber core, acts as a wavelength-selective reflection filter. UV (ultra violet) exposure causes a refractive-index change in germanium-doped silica glass [17, 18]. A fiber Bragg grating is fabricated by exposing a UV interference pattern to the fiber core from the transverse direction. Figure 4.28 shows the grating fabrication method using a phase mask. The wavelength of UV light is selected to correspond to the absorption band of germanium-related glass defects. Generally, a KrF excimer laser (248 nm) or an SHG A_r laser (244 nm) is used as a UV light source. Photosensitivity can be enhanced by increasing the germanium concentration or the hydrogen loading. In the case of hydrogen loading, a refractive-index change of more than 1×10^{-2} can be obtained.

The reflection spectrum of the fiber Bragg grating filter is given by Eqs. (4.67)–(4.69) and Fig. 4.8. If the grating is formed uniformly, as shown in Fig. 4.6 or Fig. 4.29(a), the sidelobe level of the reflection spectrum becomes rather high (about 0.2 in Fig. 4.8). For the applications to the bandpass or band rejection filters, the sidelobe level should be well below -30 dB. Weighting the amplitude of modulation by using a certain window function, generally called *apodization*, is effective for sidelobe suppression [19]. Figure 4.29(b) shows

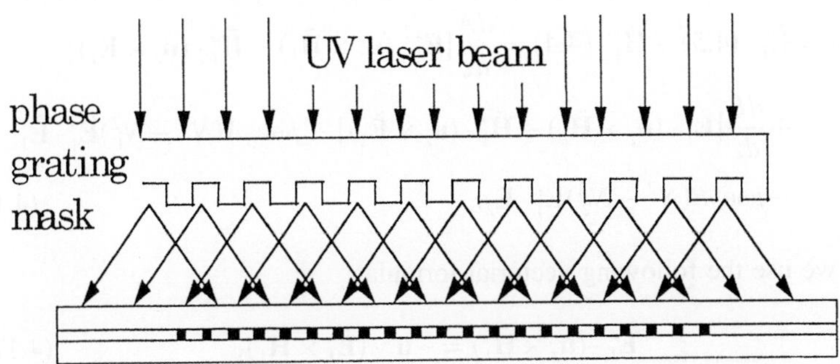

Figure 4.28 Fiber Bragg grating fabrication method using a phase mask.

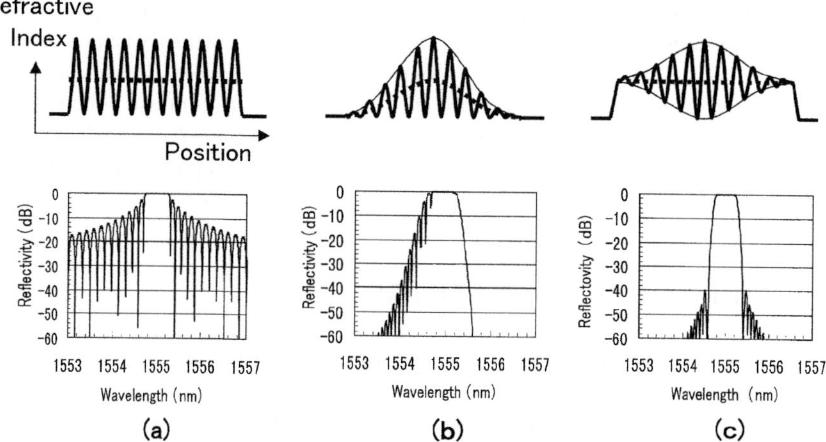

Figure 4.29 Refractive-index profiles and calculated reflection spectra for (a) uniform grating, (b) Gaussian apodized grating, and (c) Gaussian apodized grating with raised average refractive index. (After Ref. [20]).

a calculated reflection spectrum of a Gaussian apodized grating [20]. In this case, a nonuniformity of the average refractive index along the fiber causes a Fabry–Perot resonance ripple on the short-wavelength side of the reflection band. By correcting the nonuniformity of the average refractive index, a symmetrical and sidelobe-suppressed spectrum without ripple can be obtained, as shown in Fig. 4.29(c).

Appendix 4A Derivation of Equations (4.8) and (4.9)

The term in Eq. (4.6) to be integrated is expressed as

$$I_1 = \tilde{\mathbf{E}}_1^* \cdot (4.5) - \tilde{\mathbf{H}}_1^* \cdot (4.4) = \frac{dA}{dz}[\tilde{\mathbf{E}}_1^* \cdot (\mathbf{u}_z \times \tilde{\mathbf{H}}_1) - \tilde{\mathbf{H}}_1^* \cdot (\mathbf{u}_z \times \tilde{\mathbf{E}}_1)]$$
$$+\frac{dB}{dz}[\tilde{\mathbf{E}}_1^* \cdot (\mathbf{u}_z \times \tilde{\mathbf{H}}_2) - \tilde{\mathbf{H}}_1^* \cdot (\mathbf{u}_z \times \tilde{\mathbf{E}}_2)] - j\omega\varepsilon_0 A(N^2 - N_1^2)\tilde{\mathbf{E}}_1^* \cdot \tilde{\mathbf{E}}_1$$
$$-j\omega\varepsilon_0 B(N^2 - N_2^2)\tilde{\mathbf{E}}_1^* \cdot \tilde{\mathbf{E}}_2. \tag{4.175}$$

When we use the following vectorial formulas:

$$\tilde{\mathbf{E}}_1^* \cdot (\mathbf{u}_z \times \tilde{\mathbf{H}}_1) = -\mathbf{u}_z \cdot (\tilde{\mathbf{E}}_1^* \times \tilde{\mathbf{H}}_1), \tag{4.176a}$$
$$\tilde{\mathbf{H}}_1^* \cdot (\mathbf{u}_z \times \tilde{\mathbf{E}}_1) = \mathbf{u}_z \cdot (\tilde{\mathbf{E}}_1 \times \tilde{\mathbf{H}}_1^*), \tag{4.176b}$$

then Eq. (4.175) can be rewritten as

$$I_1 = -\frac{dA}{dz}\mathbf{u}_z \cdot [\tilde{\mathbf{E}}_1^* \times \tilde{\mathbf{H}}_1 + \tilde{\mathbf{E}}_1 \times \tilde{\mathbf{H}}_1^*] - \frac{dB}{dz}\mathbf{u}_z \cdot [\tilde{\mathbf{E}}_1^* \times \tilde{\mathbf{H}}_2 + \tilde{\mathbf{E}}_2 \times \tilde{\mathbf{H}}_1^*]$$
$$-j\omega\varepsilon_0 A(N^2 - N_1^2)\tilde{\mathbf{E}}_1^* \cdot \tilde{\mathbf{E}}_1 - j\omega\varepsilon_0 B(N^2 - N_2^2)\tilde{\mathbf{E}}_1^* \cdot \tilde{\mathbf{E}}_2. \quad (4.177)$$

In a similar manner, the term in Eq. (4.7) to be integrated is expressed as

$$I_2 = \tilde{\mathbf{E}}_2^* \cdot (4.5) - \tilde{\mathbf{H}}_2^*(4.4) = -\frac{dA}{dz}\mathbf{u}_z \cdot [\tilde{\mathbf{E}}_2^* \times \tilde{\mathbf{H}}_1 + \tilde{\mathbf{E}}_1 \times \tilde{\mathbf{H}}_2^*]$$
$$-\frac{dB}{dz}\mathbf{u}_z \cdot [\tilde{\mathbf{E}}_2^* \times \tilde{\mathbf{H}}_2 + \tilde{\mathbf{E}}_2 \times \tilde{\mathbf{H}}_2^*] - j\omega\varepsilon_0 A(N^2 - N_1^2)\tilde{\mathbf{E}}_2^* \cdot \tilde{\mathbf{E}}_1$$
$$-j\omega\varepsilon_0 B(N^2 - N_2^2)\tilde{\mathbf{E}}_2^* \cdot \tilde{\mathbf{E}}_2. \quad (4.178)$$

Appendix 4B Exact Solutions for the Coupled Mode Equations (4.26) and (4.27)

We assume the solutions of the coupled-mode equations (4.26) and (4.27) in the forms

$$A(z) = [a_1 e^{jQz} + a_2 e^{-jQz}] \exp\left[-j\delta z + j\frac{\alpha_a + \alpha_b}{2}z\right], \quad (4.179)$$

$$B(z) = [b_1 e^{jQz} + b_2 e^{-jQz}] \exp\left[j\delta z + j\frac{\alpha_a + \alpha_b}{2}z\right]. \quad (4.180)$$

Substituting these equations in Eqs. (4.26) and (4.27), the following relations are obtained:

$$\chi_a b_1 = -(Q - \hat{\delta})a_1, \quad (4.181)$$
$$\chi_a b_2 = (Q + \hat{\delta})a_2, \quad (4.182)$$
$$\chi_b a_1 = -(Q + \hat{\delta})b_1, \quad (4.183)$$
$$\chi_b a_2 = (Q - \hat{\delta})b_2, \quad (4.184)$$

where

$$\hat{\delta} = \delta + \frac{\alpha_a - \alpha_b}{2}. \quad (4.185)$$

In order that Eqs. (4.181)–(4.184) have nontrivial solutions except for $a_1 = a_2 = b_1 = b_2 = 0$, $Q(>0)$ should be given by

$$Q = \sqrt{\chi_a \chi_a + \hat{\delta}^2}. \quad (4.186)$$

Considering the boundary conditions at $z = 0$ as

$$a_1 + a_2 = A(0), \tag{4.187}$$

$$b_1 + b_2 = B(0), \tag{4.188}$$

coefficients a_1, a_2, b_1, and b_2 are given by

$$a_1 = \frac{1}{2}\left\{\left(1 + \frac{\hat{\delta}}{Q}\right)A(0) - \frac{\chi_a}{Q}B(0)\right\}, \tag{4.189}$$

$$a_2 = \frac{1}{2}\left\{\left(1 - \frac{\hat{\delta}}{Q}\right)A(0) + \frac{\chi_a}{Q}B(0)\right\}, \tag{4.190}$$

$$b_1 = \frac{1}{2}\left\{-\frac{\chi_b}{Q}A(0) + \left(1 - \frac{\hat{\delta}}{Q}\right)B(0)\right\}, \tag{4.191}$$

$$b_2 = \frac{1}{2}\left\{\frac{\chi_b}{Q}A(0) + \left(1 + \frac{\hat{\delta}}{Q}\right)B(0)\right\}. \tag{4.192}$$

Substituting Eqs. (4.189)–(4.192) in Eqs. (4.179) and (4.180), we obtain the strict solutions for the codirectional coupled-mode equations:

$$A(z) = \left\{\left[\cos(Qz) + j\frac{\hat{\delta}}{Q}\sin(Qz)\right]A(0) - j\frac{\chi_a}{Q}\sin(Qz)B(0)\right\} \times \exp[-j(\hat{\delta} - \alpha_a)z], \tag{4.193}$$

$$B(z) = \left\{-j\frac{\chi_b}{Q}\sin(Qz)A(0) + \left[\cos(Qz) - j\frac{\hat{\delta}}{Q}\sin(Qz)\right]B(0)\right\} \times \exp[j(\hat{\delta} - \alpha_b)z]. \tag{4.194}$$

REFERENCES

[1] Marcuse, D. 1972. *Light Transmission Optics*. New York: Van Nostrand Reinhold.

[2] Hardy, A., and W. Streifer. 1985. Coupled-mode theory of parallel waveguides. *IEEE J. Lightwave Tech.* LT-3:1135–1147.

[3] Marcatili, E. A. J. 1986. Improved coupled-mode equations for dielectric guides. *IEEE J. Quantum Electron.* QE-22:988–993.

[4] Yariv, A. 1985. *Introduction to Optical Electronics*. New York: Holt, Reinhart and Winston.

[5] Haus, H. A. 1984. *Waves and Fields in Optoelectronics*. Englewood Cliffs, NJ: Prentice-Hall.

[6] Koyama, F., Y. Suematsu, K. Kojima, and K. Furuya. 1984. 1.5 μm phase adjusted active distributed reflector laser for complete dynamic single-mode operation. *Electron. Lett.* 10:391–393.

[7] Utaka, K., S. Akiba, K. Sakai, and Y. Matsushita. 1984. Analysis of quarter-wave-shifted DFB laser. *Electron. Lett.* 20:326–327.

[8] Marcuse, D. 1974. *Theory of Dielectric Optical Waveguides*. New York: Academic Press.

[9] Marcuse, D. 1971. The coupling of degenerate modes in two parallel dielectric waveguides. *Bell. Syst. Tech. J.* 50:1791–1816.

[10] Snyder, A. W., and J. D. Love. 1983. *Optical Waveguide Theory*. London: Chapman and Hall.

[11] Watson, G. N. 1962. *Theory of Bessel Functions*. New York: Cambridge University Press.

[12] Streifer, W., D. R. Scifres, and R. D. Burnham. 1975. Coupling coefficients for distributed feedback single- and double-heterostructure diode lasers. *IEEE J. Quantum Electron.* QE-11:867–873.

[13] Takato, N., M. Kawachi, M. Nakahara, and T. Miyashita. 1989. Silica-based single-mode guided-wave devices. *Integrated Optics Optoelectronics* SPIE 1177:92–100.

[14] Stokes, L. F., M. Chodorow, and H. J. Shaw. 1982. All-single-mode fiber resonator. *Opt. Lett.* 7:288–290.

[15] Stegeman, G. I., E. M. Wright, N. Finlayson, R. Zanoni, and C. T. Seaton. 1988. Third order nonlinear integrated optics. *IEEE J Lightwave Tech.* LT-6:953–970.

[16] Ironside, C. N., J. F. Duffy, R. Hutchins, W. C. Bany, C. T. Seaton, and G. I. Stegeman. 1985. Waveguide fabrication in nonlinear semiconductor-doped glasses. *Proc. 11th European Conf. Opt. Commun.*, Venetia, Italy, 1985, pp. 237–240.

[17] Hill, K. O., Y. Fujii, D. C. Johnson, and B. S. Kawasaki. 1978. Photosensitivity in optical fiber waveguides: Application to reflection filter fabrication. *App. Phys. Lett.* 32:647–649.

[18] Meltz, G., W. W. Morey, and W. H. Glenn. 1989. Formation of Bragg gratings in optical fibers by a transverse holographic method. *Opt. Lett.* 14:823–825.

[19] Malo, B., S. Theriault, D. C. Johnson, F. Bilodeau, J. Albert, and K. O. Hill. 1995. Apodized in-fiber Bragg grating reflectors photoimprinted using a phase mask. *Electron. Lett.* 31:223–225.

[20] Inoue, A., T. Iwashima, T. Enomoto, S. Ishikawa, and H. Kanamori. 1998. Optimization of fiber Bragg grating for dense WDM transmission system. *IEICE Trans. Electron.* E81-C:1209–1218.

Chapter 5

Nonlinear Optical Effects in Optical Fibers

Though the nonlinearity of silica-based fiber is quite small, several nonlinear optical effects manifest themselves conspicuously owing to the fact that (a) the power density is very high because light is confined into a small cross-sectional area, (b) the interaction length between the light wave and fiber material is quite long due to the low-loss property of fibers, and (c) coherent interaction is possible since the modal field distribution and polarization are well prescribed and maintained over the long length [1]. Various nonlinear optical effects in fibers will be explained, such as optical solitons, stimulated Raman scattering, stimulated Brillouin scattering, and second-harmonic generation.

5.1. FIGURE OF MERIT FOR NONLINEAR EFFECTS

When 1 W of optical power is coupled into single-mode optical fiber with the core diameter of 10 μm, the optical power density exceeds $1\,\mathrm{MW/cm^2}$. Such high power density and very long interaction length are the features of nonlinear optical effects in optical fibers. The $I \cdot L$ product, which is important to evaluate the nonlinear interactions, is defined as the product of optical intensity I($I =$ optical power P/effective area of the beam) and the interaction length L. In the bulk optics, when the spot size (beam radius at which an electric field becomes $1/e$) at the focal point is W_0, the beam radius $w(z)$ at the distance z from the focal point is expressed by [2]

$$w(z) = w_0\sqrt{1+\left(\frac{\lambda z}{\pi n w_0^2}\right)^2}, \tag{5.1}$$

where λ and n denote the wavelength of light and the refractive index of the medium, respectively. The optical intensity at z is given by

$$I_B(z) = \frac{P}{\pi w(z)^2}, \tag{5.2}$$

Then $I \cdot L$ product of the bulk lens system is obtained as

$$[I \cdot L]_B = \int_{-\infty}^{\infty} I_B(z)dz = \pi\frac{nP}{\lambda}. \tag{5.3}$$

It is known that there is no other way than to increase the input power P in order to enhance the nonlinear effect in the bulk optics system. In contrast, the optical intensity of the fiber at distance z is given by

$$I_F(z) = \frac{P\exp(-\alpha z)}{\pi w_0^2}, \tag{5.4}$$

where α and w_0 denote the attenuation coefficient and spot size of the fiber, respectively. The $I \cdot L$ product of the fiber with length L is given by

$$[I \cdot L]_F = \int_{-\infty}^{\infty} I_F(z)dz = \frac{P}{\pi w_0^2}L_{\text{eff}}, \tag{5.5}$$

where L_{eff} denotes the effective interaction length, which is defined by

$$L_{\text{eff}} = \frac{[1 - \exp(-\alpha L)]}{\alpha}. \tag{5.6}$$

It is seen from Eq. (5.5) that the $I \cdot L$ product can be increased by using low-loss and small-core (high refractive-index difference) fibers. When fiber length L is sufficiently long, effective length can be approximated by $L_{\text{eff}} = 1/\alpha$. Then the ratio of the $I \cdot L$ product between bulk optics and optical fibers is expressed as

$$\frac{[1 \cdot L]_F}{[1 \cdot L]_B} = \frac{\lambda}{(\pi W_0)^2 n\alpha}. \tag{5.7}$$

For example, we have $[I \cdot L]_F/[I \cdot L]_B \approx 5 \times 10^7$ for the fiber parameters of $\lambda = 1\,\mu\text{m}$, $n = 1.5$, $\alpha = 2.3 \times 10^{-4}\,\text{m}^{-1}$ (loss of 1 dB/km) and $w_0 = 2.4\,\mu\text{m}$. It is known that 1 W of optical power is sufficient in optical fibers to generate the same level of nonlinear effects for which several megawatts was required.

5.2. OPTICAL KERR EFFECT

The optical Kerr effect is the phenomenon in which the refractive index of the medium changes when the electron orbit is deformed by the strong electric field [3]. The refractive index under the Kerr effect is expressed as $n_0 + n_2|E|^2$, where n_0 and n_2 denote linear refractive index and the Kerr coefficient, respectively. The Kerr coefficient in the silica glass fiber is typically given by $n_2 = 1.22 \times 10^{-22}\,\mathrm{m^2/V^2}$ [4]. It is expressed in the different unit systems as $n_2 = 3.18 \times 10^{-20}\,\mathrm{m^2/W}$ or $n_2 = 1.1 \times 10^{-13}$ (esu, or $\mathrm{cm^2/statvolt^2}$). The interesting and important nonlinear effects in optical fibers utilizing optical Kerr effect are (1) optical solitons, (2) optical pulse compression and (3) modulational instabilities.

5.2.1. Self-phase Modulation

When a high-intensity short pulse is coupled to optical fiber, the instantaneous phase of optical pulse rapidly changes through the optical Kerr effect. If we express the envelope of the optical pulse as E and the linear refractive index at the angular frequency ω_0 as $n(\omega_0)$, the effective index of the optical fiber is given by

$$n(\omega_0, |E|^2) = \frac{c\beta}{\omega_0} = n(\omega_0) + n_0|E|^2. \tag{5.8}$$

Since we define the optical phase as $\Phi = \omega_0 t - \beta z$, instantaneous angular frequency is given as the derivative of Φ with respect to time t:

$$\omega(t) = \frac{\partial \Phi}{\partial t} = \omega_0 - \frac{\omega_0 n_2}{c} z \frac{\partial |E|^2}{\partial t}. \tag{5.9}$$

Here we consider the variation of optical intensity in the medium at z during the passage of optical pulse. Therefore, time t progresses from right-hand side (preceding edge of the pulse) of Fig. 5.1 to the left-hand side (trailing edge). As shown in Fig. 5.1 we have $\partial|E|^2/\partial t > 0$ at the preceding edge of the pulse and $\partial|E|^2/\partial t < 0$ at the trailing edge. Then it is seen from Eq. (5.9) that the angular frequency decreases ($\omega < \omega_0$) at the preceding edge and increases ($\omega > \omega_0$) at the trailing edge of the pulse. This is schematically illustrated in Fig. 5.1(b). This phenomenon is called *self-phase modulation* (*SPM*), which causes the frequency chirping to the optical pulse.

As described in Section 3.6.4, wavelength dependencies of the group velocity for a 1.3-μm zero-dispersion fiber and a 1.55-μm zero-dispersion fiber (dispersion-shifted fiber, DSF) are shown in Fig. 5.2. The spectral region shorter than the zero-dispersion wavelength λ_0 is called a *normal dispersion region*, and that longer than λ_0 is called an *anomalous dispersion region*. In the anomalous dispersion region, the lower the frequency (the longer the wavelength), the smaller the group velocity. Then the group velocity at the preceding

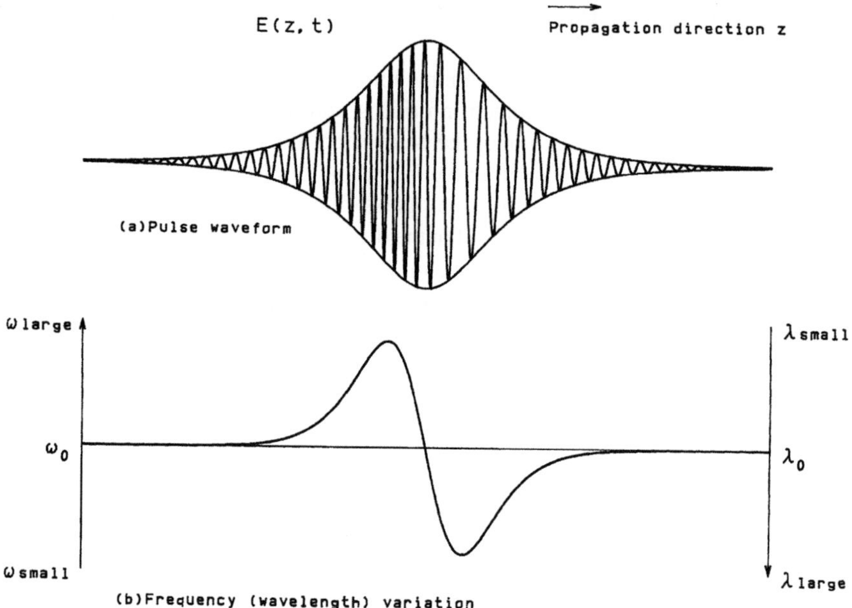

Figure 5.1 Self-phase modulation of optical pulse: (a) Pulse waveform and (b) instantaneous angular frequency (or wavelength) change.

edge of the optical pulse having a lower frequency becomes small. In contrast, the group velocity at the trailing edge of the optical pulse having a higher frequency becomes large. This compresses the optical pulse. If the compression of the optical pulse due to the self-phase modulation balances with and cancels the pulse broadening caused by the dispersion, the optical pulse propagates through the fiber while maintaining its original pulse shape. This is called an *optical soliton* (more precisely, a *bright optical soliton*) [5, 6]. The historically well-known solitary wave on the surface of shallow water and the nonlinear vibration of the one-dimensional lattice are solitons of the waves themselves. In the optical fiber, however, the envelope of the optical pulse becomes a solitary wave. Therefore a soliton in the fiber is called an *envelope soliton.*

In the normal dispersion region, the group velocity at the preceding edge of the optical pulse having a lower frequency becomes large and the group velocity at the trailing edge of the optical pulse having a higher frequency becomes small. Then the energy of the optical pulse is dispersed into preceding and trailing edges of the pulse and the pulse temporal shape becomes square. When such a frequency-chirped and square-shaped pulse is passed through an anomalous medium such as a grating pair, the optical pulse is compressed. This will be described in Section 5.4.

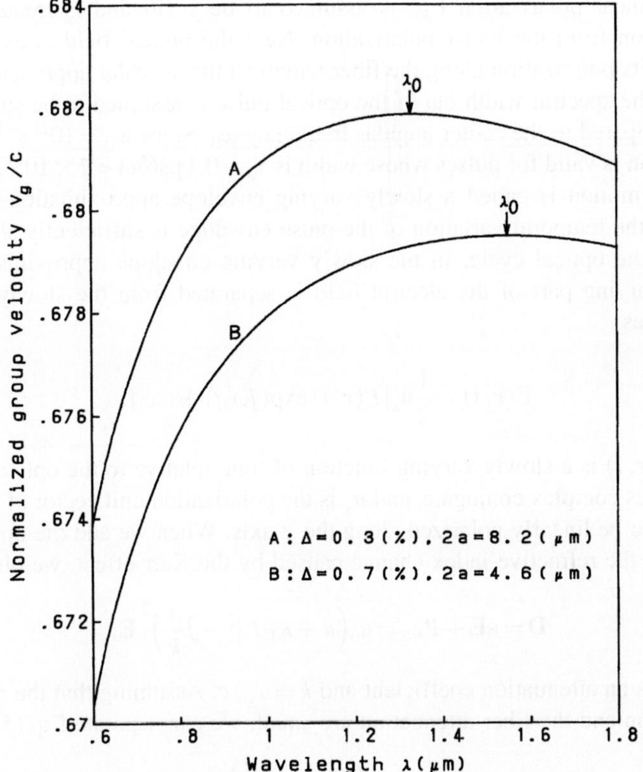

Figure 5.2 Wavelength dependencies of the group velocity op optical fibers. A: 1.3-μm zero-dispersion fiber; B: 1.55-μm zero-dispersion fiber (dispersion-shifted fiber, DSF).

In the normal dispersion region, a *dark soliton* exists. The dark soliton is also a solitary wave that is generated by cutting a portion of a continuous wave. Nonlinear chirping of the intensity dip in the continuous wave balances the group velocity dispersion of optical fiber in the normal region.

5.2.2. Nonlinear Schrödinger Equation

The wave equation in the medium with nonlinear electric polarization $\mathbf{F}_{NL}$ is expressed as

$$\nabla^2 \mathbf{E} = \mu_0 \frac{\partial^2 \mathbf{D}}{\partial t^2}, \tag{5.10}$$

$$\mathbf{D} = \varepsilon \mathbf{E} + \mathbf{P}_{NL}. \tag{5.11}$$

The nonlinear polarization F_{NL} is assumed to be small and is treated as the perturbation from the linear polarization. Next the optical field is assumed to maintain its polarization along the fiber length so that a scalar approach is valid. Thirdly, the spectral width $\delta\omega$ of the optical pulse is assumed to be sufficiently small compared to the center angular frequency ω_0. Since $\omega_0 \cong 10^{15}\,\mathrm{s}^{-1}$, the last assumption is valid for pulses whose width is $\tau_0 > 0.1\,\mathrm{ps}(\delta\omega < 2 \times 10^{13}\,\mathrm{s}^{-1})$. The third assumption is called a slowly varying envelope approximation (SVEA), in which the temporal variation of the pulse envelope is sufficiently slow compared to the optical cycle. In the slowly varying envelope approximation, the rapidly varying part of the electric field is separated from the slowly varying envelope as

$$\mathbf{E}(\mathbf{r}, t) = \frac{1}{2}\mathbf{u}_x[E(\mathbf{r}, t)\exp(j\omega_0 t) + \text{c.c.}], \tag{5.12}$$

where $E(\mathbf{r}, t)$ is a slowly varying function of time relative to the optical period, c.c. denotes complex conjugate, and $\mathbf{u}_x$ is the polarization unit vector of the light, assumed to be linearly polarized along the x-axis. When we add the optical loss or gain to the refractive-index change caused by the Kerr effect, we obtain [1]

$$\mathbf{D} = \varepsilon\mathbf{E} + \mathbf{P}_{NL} = \varepsilon_0\left(n + n_2|E|^2 - j\frac{\alpha}{k}\right)^2 \mathbf{E}, \tag{5.13}$$

where α is an attenuation coefficient and $k = \omega_0/c$. Assuming that the nonlinear polarization and the fiber attenuation are small, we can separate Eq. (5.13) into

$$\varepsilon\mathbf{E} = \varepsilon_0\left(n^2 - j2n\frac{\alpha}{k}\right)\mathbf{E}, \tag{5.14}$$

$$\mathbf{P}_{NL} = 2\varepsilon_0 n n_2 |E|^2 \mathbf{E}. \tag{5.15}$$

The envelope function of the electric field $E(\mathbf{r}, t)$ is expressed as the product of the transverse field distribution $R(r, \theta)$ and the axial amplitude variation $A(z, t)\exp(-j\beta_0 z)$:

$$E(\mathbf{r}, t) = R(r, \theta)A(z, t)\exp(-j\beta_0 z), \tag{5.16}$$

where β_0 denotes the propagation constant in the absence of the Kerr effect. Substituting Eqs. (5.12) and (5.16) in Eq. (5.10), $\nabla^2\mathbf{E}$ is given by

$$\nabla^2\mathbf{E} = \mathbf{u}_x\nabla^2 e_x = \mathbf{u}_x\left(\frac{\partial^2}{\partial r^2} + \frac{1}{r^2}\frac{\partial}{\partial r} + \frac{1}{r^2}\frac{\partial^2}{\partial\theta^2} + \frac{\partial^2}{\partial z^2}\right)e_x, \tag{5.17}$$

where

$$e_x = \frac{1}{2}R(r, \theta)A(z, t)\exp[j(\omega_0 t - \beta_0 z)] + \text{c.c.} \tag{5.18}$$

Since the variation of $A(z, t)$ along the z-direction is much slower than that of $\exp(-j\beta_0 z)$, we can assume $|\partial^2 A/\partial z^2| \ll \beta_0^2|A|$. Taking this into account, Eq. (5.17) is reduced to

$$\nabla^2\mathbf{E} = \frac{1}{2}\mathbf{u}_x\left\{\left[A(z,t)\left(\frac{\partial^2 R}{\partial r^2} + \frac{1}{r}\frac{\partial R}{\partial r} + \frac{1}{r^2}\frac{\partial^2 R}{\partial \theta^2}\right)\right.\right.$$
$$\left.\left. + R(r,\theta)\left(-j2\beta_0\frac{\partial A}{\partial z} - \beta_0^2 A\right)\right]\exp[j(\omega_0 t - \beta_0 z)] + \text{c. c.}\right\}. \quad (5.19)$$

The right-hand side of Eq. (5.10) is calculated by substituting Eqs. (5.11)–(5.16) in it and using the slowly-varying envelope approximation:

$$\mu_0\frac{\partial^2(\varepsilon\mathbf{E})}{\partial t^2} = -\frac{1}{2}\mathbf{u}_x k^2\left(n^2 - j2n\frac{\alpha}{k}\right)$$
$$\times\{R(r,\theta)A(z,t)\exp[j(\omega_0 t - \beta_0 z)] + \text{c.c.}\}, \quad (5.20)$$

$$\mu_0\frac{\partial^2\mathbf{P}_{NL}}{\partial t^2} = -\mathbf{u}_x k^2 n n_2|\mathbf{E}|^2\{R(r,\theta)A(z,t)\exp[j(\omega_0 t - \beta_0 z)] + \text{c.c.}\}. \quad (5.21)$$

From Eqs. (5.19)–(5.21), Eq. (5.10) reduces to

$$\left[\frac{\partial^2 R}{\partial r^2} + \frac{1}{r}\frac{\partial R}{\partial r} + \frac{1}{r^2}\frac{\partial^2 R}{\partial\theta^2} + (k^2 n^2 - \beta_0^2)R\right]A$$
$$+\left(-j2\beta_0\frac{\partial A}{\partial z} - j2kn\alpha A + 2k^2 n n_2|\mathbf{E}|^2 A\right)R = 0. \quad (5.22)$$

Strictly speaking, the transvere mode profile of the optical fiber under Kerr effect nonlinearity becomes different from the unperturbed profile $R(r, \theta)$. Based on first-order perturbation theory, however, the electric field profile $R(r, \theta)$ can be approximated to be the same as that of the linear state, although the propagation constant becomes different as $\beta_0 \to \beta(\omega)$. Then the electric field $R(r, \theta)$ satisfies the wave equation

$$\frac{\partial^2 R}{\partial r^2} + \frac{1}{r}\frac{\partial R}{\partial r} + \frac{1}{r^2}\frac{\partial^2 R}{\partial\theta^2} + (k^2 n^2 - \beta^2)R = 0. \quad (5.23)$$

Substitution of Eq. (5.23) in Eq. (5.22) gives

$$(\beta^2 - \beta_0^2)RA + \left(-j2\beta_0\frac{\partial A}{\partial z} - j2kn\alpha A + 2k^2 n n_2|R|^2|A|^2 A\right)R = 0. \quad (5.24)$$

Multiplying this last equation by R^* and integrating it over the cross-sectional area, we have

$$(\beta^2 - \beta_0^2)A - j2\beta_0\frac{\partial A}{\partial z} - j2kn\alpha A + 2k^2 n n_2\eta|A|^2 A = 0. \quad (5.25)$$

where η is defined by

$$\eta = \frac{\int_0^{2\pi} \int_0^{\infty} |R|^4 r\, dr\, d\theta}{\int_0^{2\pi} \int_0^{\infty} |R^2| r\, dr\, d\theta}. \tag{5.26}$$

Figure 5.3 shows the variation of η with the normalized frequency v for the HE_{11} mode in the step-index fiber, where the transversel electric fields in the core and cladding are given by $J_0(ur/a)$ and $[J_0(u)/K_0(w)]K_0(wr/a)$, respectively [refer to Eqs. (3.94) and (3.95) or (4.109) and (4.110)]. It is seen from Fig. 5.3 that we can approximate as $\eta \cong 1/2$ under the normal operating condition of the optical fibers ($v = 1.5$–2.4). Based on the weakly guiding approximation, we approximate $\beta \cong \beta_0 \cong kn$ in Eq. (5.25). Dividing Eq. (5.25) by $2kn$, we obtain

$$(\beta - \beta_0)A - j\frac{\partial A}{\partial z} - j\alpha A + \frac{1}{2}kn_2|A|^2 A = 0. \tag{5.27}$$

Propagation constant $\beta(\omega)$ is approximated by the Taylor series expansion:

$$\beta(\omega) - \beta_0 = (\omega - \omega_0)\beta' + \frac{1}{2}(\omega - \omega_0)^2\beta'' + \cdots. \tag{5.28}$$

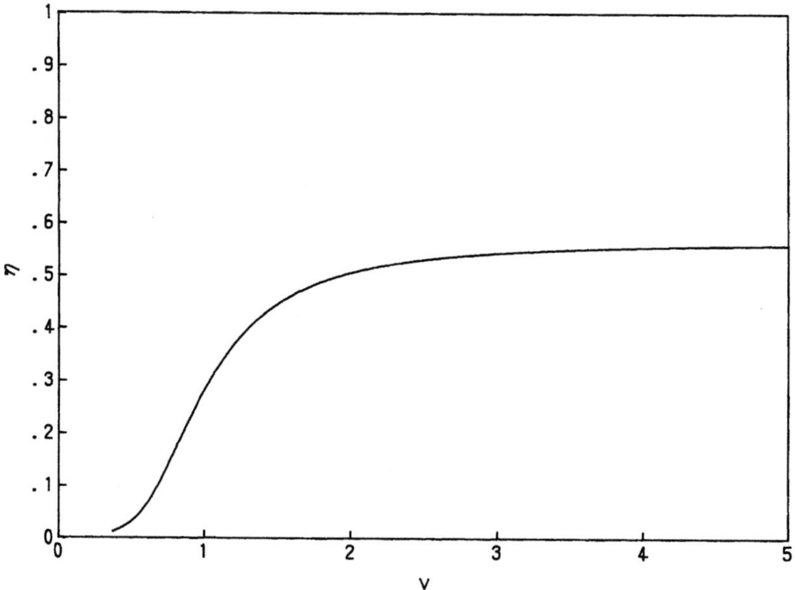

Figure 5.3 Dependency of η on the normalized frequency v for the HE_{11} mode in the step-index fiber.

Substitution of this equation into Eq. (5.27) gives

$$j\frac{\partial A}{\partial z} - (\omega - \omega_0)\beta' A - \frac{1}{2}(\omega - \omega_0)^2\beta'' A + j\alpha A - \frac{1}{2}kn_2|A|^2 A = 0. \tag{5.29}$$

We notice here the Fourier transformation formula for the differential equation:

$$\int_{-\infty}^{\infty} \frac{\partial A}{\partial t} \exp[-j(\omega - \omega_0)t]\, dt$$
$$= [A(z,t)\exp\{-j(\omega - \omega_0)t\}]_{-\infty}^{\infty} + \int_{-\infty}^{\infty} j(\omega - \omega_0) A \exp[-j(\omega - \omega_0)t]\, dt$$
$$= \int_{-\infty}^{\infty} j(\omega - \omega_0) A \exp[-j(\omega - \omega_0)t]\, dt, \tag{5.30a}$$

$$\int_{-\infty}^{\infty} \frac{\partial^2 A}{\partial t^2} \exp[-j(\omega - \omega_0)t]\, dt = \int_{-\infty}^{\infty} -(\omega - \omega_0)^2 A \exp[-j(\omega - \omega_0)t]\, dt. \tag{5.30b}$$

Comparing both terms in Eqs. (5.30a) and (5.30b), we see that the following substitution relations hold:

$$j(\omega - \omega_0)A \rightarrow \frac{\partial A}{\partial t}, \tag{5.31a}$$

$$-(\omega - \omega_0)^2 A \rightarrow \frac{\partial^2 A}{\partial t^2}. \tag{5.31b}$$

Then Eq. (5.29) is rewritten, by using Eq. (5.31), as

$$j\left[\frac{\partial A}{\partial z} + \beta'\frac{\partial A}{\partial t} + \alpha A\right] = -\frac{1}{2}\beta''\frac{\partial^2 A}{\partial t^2} + \frac{1}{2}kn_2|A|^2 A. \tag{5.32}$$

This is the nonlinear Schrödinger equation that governs the envelope function of the optical pulse $A(z, t)$ under Kerr effect nonlinearity and loss (or gain) in the optical fibers.

5.3. OPTICAL SOLITONS

We first solve the nonlinear Schrödinger equation under the ideal case of lossless fiber and examine the optical soliton.

5.3.1. Fundamental and Higher-Order Solitons

When loss of the optical fiber is zero, Eq. (5.32) is expressed as

$$j\left(\frac{\partial A}{\partial z} + \frac{1}{v_g}\frac{\partial A}{\partial t}\right) = -\frac{1}{2}\beta''\frac{\partial^2 A}{\partial t^2} + \frac{1}{2}kn_2|A|^2 A, \tag{5.33}$$

where $v_g(=1/\beta')$ is a group velocity given by Eq. (3.108). In order to investigate the progress of optical pulse shape, we change the fixed coordinate system to the moving coordinate at the velocity v_g:

$$\begin{cases} A(z,t) = \phi(z,\tau) & (5.34a) \\ \tau = t - \dfrac{z}{v_g}. & (5.34b) \end{cases}$$

Partial derivatives of A with respect to z and t are then given by

$$\frac{\partial A}{\partial z} = \frac{\partial \phi}{\partial \tau}\frac{\partial \tau}{\partial z} + \frac{\partial \phi}{\partial z} = -\frac{1}{v_g}\frac{\partial \phi}{\partial \tau} + \frac{\partial \phi}{\partial z}, \tag{5.35a}$$

$$\frac{\partial A}{\partial t} = \frac{\partial \phi}{\partial \tau}\frac{\partial \tau}{\partial t} = \frac{\partial \phi}{\partial \tau}, \tag{5.35b}$$

$$\frac{\partial^2 A}{\partial t^2} = \frac{\partial^2 \phi}{\partial \tau^2}\frac{\partial \tau}{\partial t} = \frac{\partial^2 \phi}{\partial \tau^2}. \tag{5.35c}$$

Substituting Eq. (5.35) into Eq. (5.33), we obtain

$$j\frac{\partial \phi}{\partial z} = -\frac{1}{2}\beta''\frac{\partial^2 \phi}{\partial \tau^2} + \frac{1}{2}kn_2|\phi|^2\phi. \tag{5.36}$$

The fundamental solution of Eq. (5.36) is given by [6]

$$\phi(z,\tau) = \phi_p \exp\left(j\frac{\beta''}{2t_0^2}z\right)\operatorname{sech}\left(\frac{\tau}{t_0}\right), \tag{5.37}$$

where t_0 is related to the FWHM (full width at the half maximum) width of the optical intensity τ_0 by

$$t_0 = \frac{\tau_0}{2\cosh^{-1}\sqrt{2}} \cong 0.567\tau_0. \tag{5.38}$$

As is confirmed by substituting Eq. (5.37) into Eq. (5.36), the peak amplitude of the electric field ϕ_p should satisfy

$$|\phi_p|^2 = \frac{-2\beta''}{t_0^2 kn_2}. \tag{5.39}$$

Since $\beta'' = \partial v_g^{-1}/\partial\omega \propto \partial v_g/\partial\lambda$, optical soliton is generated in the anomalous region ($\partial v_g/\partial\lambda < 0$), where the signal wavelength is longer than the zero-dispersion wavelength, as shown in Section 5.2.1. β'' represents the dispersion of the group velocity with respect to the wavelength and is called the *group velocity dispersion (GVD)*.

We next express the soliton condition of Eq. (5.39) in terms of the optical power. The electromagnetic fields of HE_{11}^x mode is expressed by (refer to Section 3.5)

$$\begin{cases} H_y = n_1 \varepsilon_0 c E_x \\ E_y = H_x = 0, \end{cases}$$

where we assumed $\beta = kn_1$. The instantaneous peak power of the HE_{11}^x mode is then given by

$$P = \int_0^{2\pi} \int_0^{\infty} (E_x H_y^* - E_y H_x^*) r\, dr\, d\theta = n_1 \varepsilon_0 c \int_0^{2\pi} \int_0^{\infty} |E_x|^2 r\, dr\, d\theta. \tag{5.40}$$

Substituting $E_x = R(r, \theta)\phi(z, 0)$ to Eq. (5.40), we obtain

$$P = n_1 \varepsilon_0 c |\phi_p|^2 \int_0^{2\pi} \int_0^{\infty} |R|^2 r\, dr\, d\theta. \tag{5.41}$$

Equation (5.41) is also obtained for the HE_{11}^y mode. Here we introduce the new parameter defined by [7]

$$A_{\mathrm{eff}} = \frac{\left[\int_0^{2\pi} \int_0^{\infty} |R|^2 r\, dr\, d\theta\right]^2}{\int_0^{2\pi} \int_0^{\infty} |R|^4 r\, dr\, d\theta}. \tag{5.42}$$

A_{eff} represents the cross-sectional area occupied by the substantial part of the light field and is called the *effective area*. Using Eq. (5.26) and (5.42), Eq. (5.41) is rewritten as

$$P = \eta n_1 \varepsilon_0 c |\phi_p|^2 A_{\mathrm{eff}} \cong \frac{1}{2} n_1 \varepsilon_0 c |\phi_p|^2 A_{\mathrm{eff}}, \tag{5.43}$$

where η is assumed to be 0.5. Figure 5.4 shows the dependence of A_{eff}/core area on the normalized frequency v for the HE_{11} mode of the step-index fiber. Substitution of Eq. (5.39) in Eq. (5.43) gives the power condition to generate the fundamental optical soliton. We should note here that the Kerr coefficient n_2 of Eq. (5.39) is in units of m^2/V^2. In order to obtain the power condition of the optical soliton, the Kerr constant in $m^2/V^2 (n_2 = 1.22 \times 10^{-22} m^2/V^2)$ should be transformed into units of $m^2/W (n_2 = 3.18 \times 10^{-20} m^2/W)$. The transformation relation is given by

$$n_2[m^2/V^2] = n_2[m^2/W] \cdot n_1 \varepsilon_0 c, \tag{5.44}$$

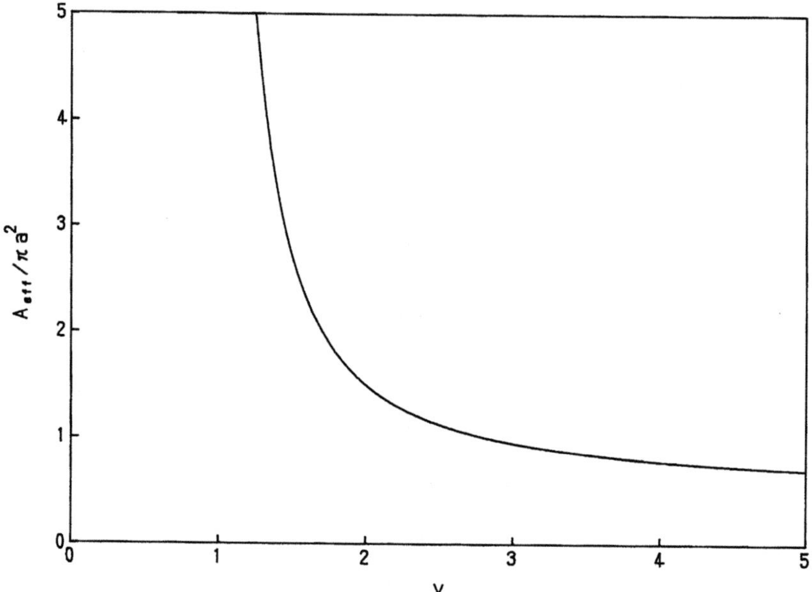

Figure 5.4 Dependence of A_{eff}/core area on the normalized frequency ν for the HE_{11} mode in the step-index fiber.

where $\varepsilon_0 = 8.854 \times 10^{-12}$ F/m and $n_1 = 1.45$. Substituting Eqs. (5.38), (5.39) and (5.44) into Eq. (5.43) and using the chromatic dispersion relation of $\beta'' = -(\lambda^2/2\pi c)\sigma$ [Eq. (3.143)], the peak power to generate the fundamental soliton is obtained:

$$P = \frac{0.7768\lambda^3 A_{\mathrm{eff}}|\sigma|}{\pi^2 c n_2 \tau_0^2}. \tag{5.45}$$

In order to simplify this last equation, we express the chromatic dispersion σ in units of ps/km · nm, wavelength λ in units of μm, and the core diameter as $d(\mu\mathrm{m})$ and define, $\xi = A_{\mathrm{eff}}/\pi(d/2)^2$. The power condition is then given by

$$P\tau_0^2 = 6.48 \times 10^{-3}\xi d^2\lambda^3|\sigma| \qquad [W \cdot \mathrm{ps}^2]. \tag{5.46}$$

Figure 5.5 shows the dependence of $P\tau_0^2$ on the chromatic dispersion σ at a 1.55-μm wavelength for the effective area parameter $\xi = 1.5(v = 2.0)$. When, for example, chromatic dispersion of the fiber is $\sigma = 2$ ps/km · nm and the core diameter $d = 5\,\mu$m, we obtain $P\tau_0^2 = 1.81$. Therefore, peak power is known to be $P = 18.1$ mW in order to generate the optical soliton with the FWHM pulse

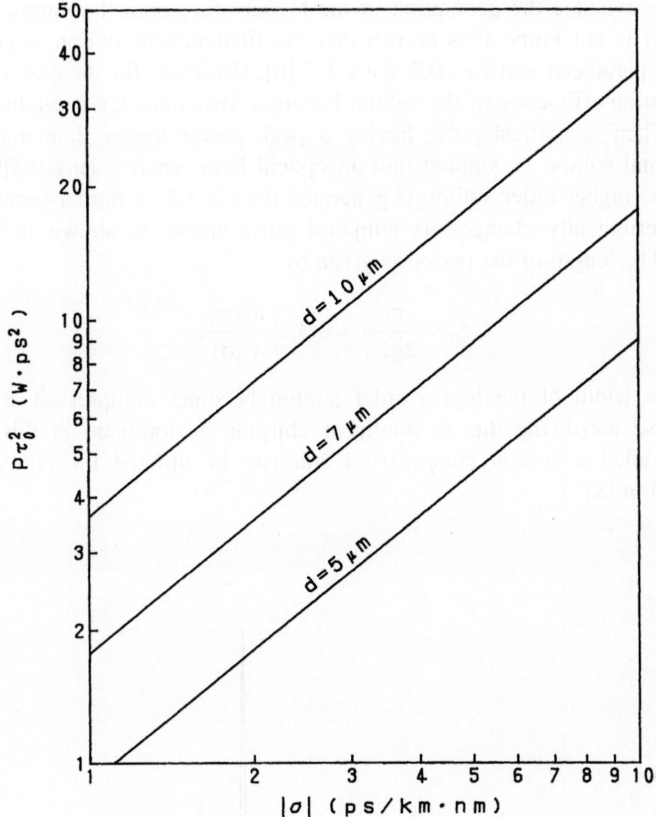

Figure 5.5 Dependence of $P\tau_0^2$ on the chromatic dispersion σ at 1.55-μm wavelength.

width of $\tau_0 = 10\,\text{ps}$. When the bitrate of the pulse (pulse repetition rate) is B, the average power of the soliton is obtained by

$$P_{av} = B\int_{-1/2B}^{1/2B}\left[P^{1/2}\text{sech}\left(\frac{\tau}{t_0}\right)\right]^2 d\tau \cong BP\int_{-\infty}^{\infty}\text{sech}^2\left(\frac{\tau}{t_0}\right)d\tau$$

$$= t_0BP\left[\tanh\left(\frac{\tau}{t_0}\right)\right]_{-\infty}^{\infty} = 2t_0BP = \frac{\tau_0BP}{\cosh^{-1}\sqrt{2}} \cong 1.135\tau_0BP. \qquad (5.47)$$

Then the average power of the $B = 10$-Gbit/s optical pulse is about $P_{av} = 2.1\,\text{mW}$.

Generally, the parameter

$$\nu = |\phi_p|t_0\sqrt{\frac{kn_2}{-2\beta''}} \qquad (5.48)$$

is used to evaluate the generation of the higher-order optical solitons. Even if Eq. (5.48) is not unity, it is known that the fundamental soliton is generated when the parameter satisfies $0.5 \leqslant \nu \leqslant 1.5$ [6]. However, for the case of $\nu \neq 1$, the excitation efficiency of the soliton becomes low, since the nonsoliton wave exists. When an optical pulse having a peak power higher than that of the fundamental soliton is coupled into an optical fiber, an $N = [\nu + 0.5]$th (N is an integer) higher-order soliton is generated for $\nu \geqslant 1.5$. A higher-order optical soliton periodically changes its temporal pulse shape, as shown in Fig. 5.6 ($\nu = 3$). The length of the period is given by

$$z_0 = \frac{\pi t_0^2}{2|\beta''|} = 0.322 \frac{\pi^2 c \tau_0^2}{\lambda^2 |\sigma|}. \tag{5.49}$$

The pulse width of the higher-order soliton becomes compressed at $z < z_0$, since pulse narrowing due to nonlinear chirping is dominant in this region. This is called a *soliton compression* and can be utilized for optical pulse compression [8].

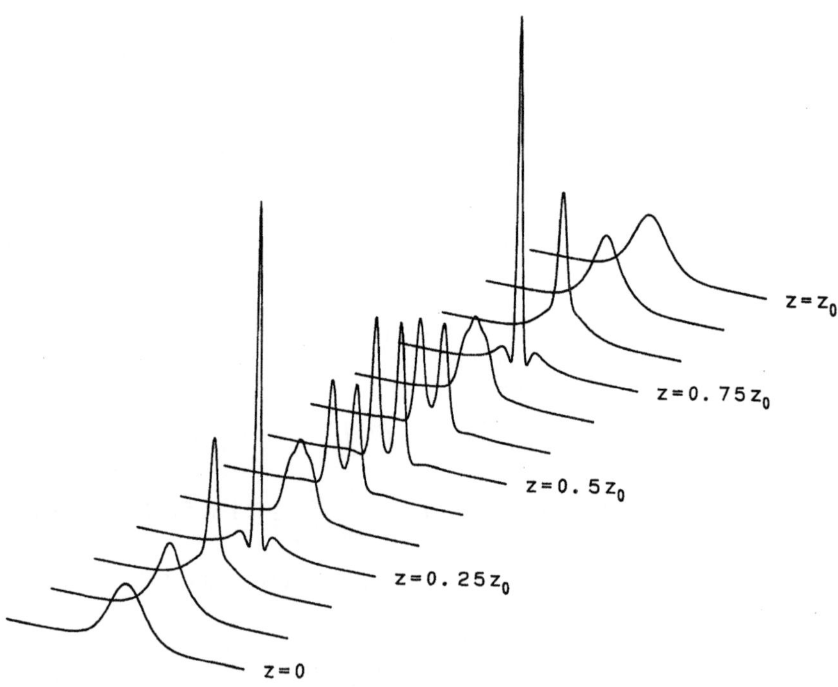

Figure 5.6 Periodic variation of the temporal pulse shape for the third-order ($\nu = 3$) optical soliton.

5.3.2. Fiber Loss Compensation by Optical Amplification

The optical soliton is an ideal signal waveform for the ultrahigh-bitrate long-distance optical communications, since it does not suffer from signal waveform distortion by the chromatic dispersion of optical fiber. However, we have neglected fiber loss in the preceding discussions. When loss exists in the fiber, pulse peak power decreases and pulse width becomes broadened, since pulse narrowing caused by nonlinear chirping is weakened. Figure 5.7 shows the variation of temporal pulse waveform calculated by using the beam propagation method (BPM) when the optical pulse with the peak power $P = 18\,\text{mW}$ and FWHM width $\tau_0 = 9.4\,\text{ps}$ is coupled to optical fiber having an attenuation of 0.18 dB/km at a 1.55-μm wavelength. Numerical simulation by BPM will be described in Chapter 7.

When signal loss becomes larger than about 3 dB (propagation distance over about 15 km in Fig. 5.7), optical soliton loses its narrowing effect and is governed by chromatic dispersion. In order to compensate for the optical loss, the optical soliton should be amplified directly in the optical stage. Stimulated Raman scattering in optical fiber [9] and an Er-doped optical amplifier [10] can be utilized for the direct optical amplification of optical solitons. Stimulated Raman scattering is a phenomenon observed when strong monochromatic light irradiates the material [11]. Coherent light is scattered with the specific wavelength shift through the interaction between the optical phonon of the material and the excitation light field. The wavenumber shift in silica glass is about $440\,\text{cm}^{-1}$. For example, when we use light at $\lambda_p = 1.45\,\mu\text{m}(1.45 \times 10^{-4}\,\text{cm})$ as a pumping light, we can amplify the signal light directly at $\lambda_s = 1.55\,\mu\text{m}(1.55 \times 10^{-4}\,\text{cm} : 1/\lambda_s = 1/\lambda_p - 440\,\text{cm}^{-1})$ through the interaction with the optical phonon. An Er-doped fiber amplifier is a

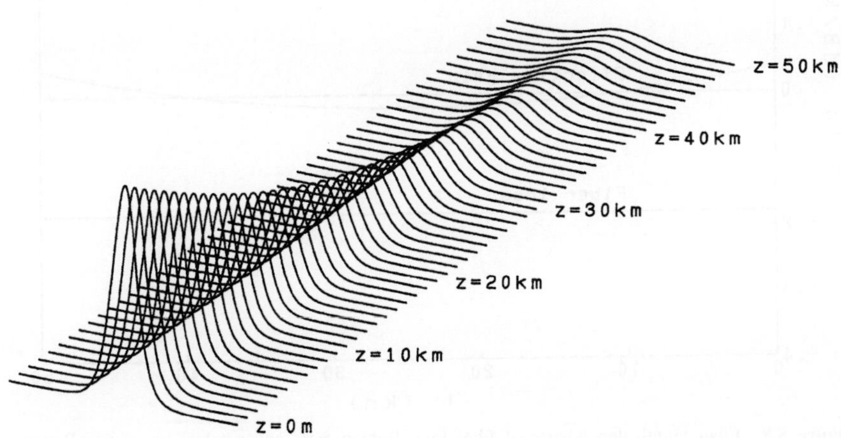

Figure 5.7 Variation of pulse waveform of the fundamental soliton in the optical fiber with loss.

fiber in which Er^{3+} ion is doped in the core, at several hundred parts per million. When it is pumped by the light at a wavelength of 0.98 μm or 1.48 μm, the optical signal in the wavelength region of 1.53–1.55 μm is amplified through the stimulated emission between the transition lines ${}^4I_{13/2} \rightarrow {}^4I_{15/2}$. In the following, amplification of optical soliton by using stimulated Raman scattering will be described.

It is shown by the numerical simulation that an optical soliton with signal wavelength $\lambda_s = 1.55\,\mu m$, FWHM pulse width $\tau_0 = 9.4\,ps$, and peak power $P = 18\,mW$ can be transmitted at 10 Gbit/s over several thousands of kilometers of fiber with chromatic dispersion $\sigma = 2\,ps/km \cdot nm$, effective area $A_{eff} = 25\,\mu m^2$ (core diameter $\cong 5\,\mu m$), loss at the signal wavelength of 0.18 dB/km, and loss at the pump wavelength $\lambda_p = 1.45\,\mu m$ of 0.29 dB/km when it is amplified by a pumping light of 50-mW (CW) fiber coupled power with a period of 50 km [12]. Figure 5.8 shows fiber length dependence of fiber loss, Raman gain, and net loss or gain with the preceding parameters. Figure 5.9 shows the variation of pulse waveform along one optical amplifier span calculated by BPM. It is shown that the fundamental soliton can be transmitted over a long fiber by direct optical amplification.

In the experiment on soliton transmission by Raman amplification, the signal from the F-center laser at 1.60 μm (FWHM pulse width of 55 ps, peak power

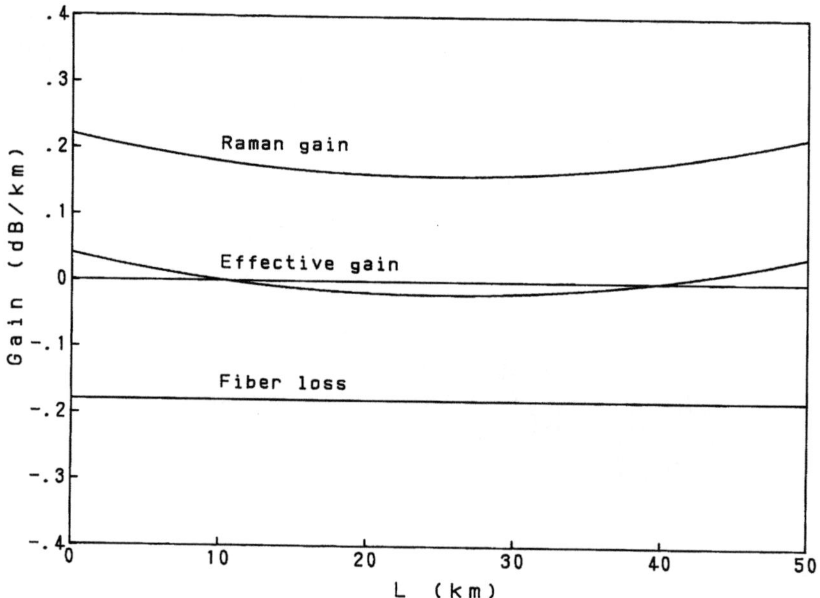

Figure 5.8 Fiber length dependence of fiber loss, Raman gain, and net loss or gain in Raman amplification.

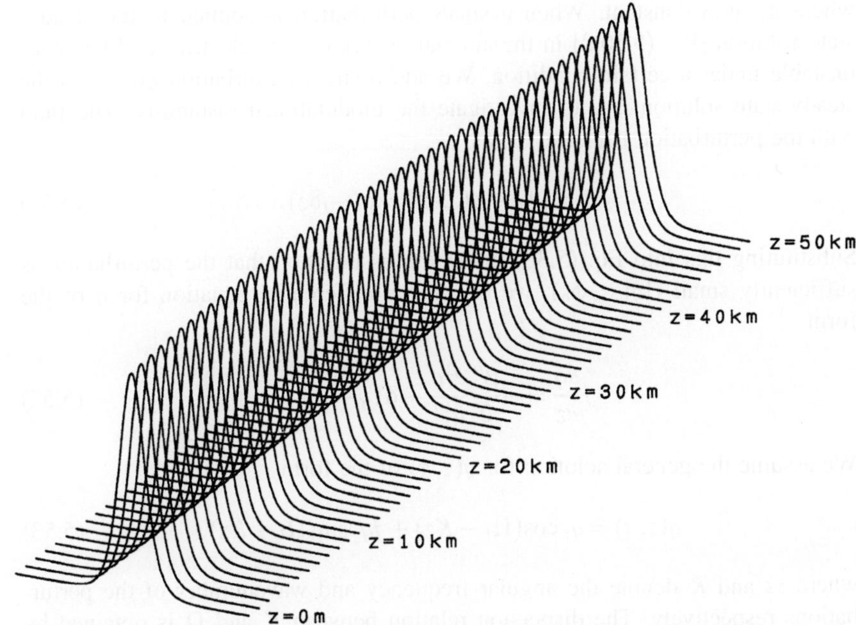

Figure 5.9 Variation of temporal pulse waveform along one optical amplifier span.

of 15 mW, and repetition rate of 100 MHz) was recirculated in the fiber loop of length 41.7 km (total length of 4000 km) by using F-center laser pump light at 1.50 μm [13]. As the transmission experiment using an Er-doped fiber amplifier, an MQW-DFB laser oscillating at 1.52 μm (FWHM pulse width of 20 ps, peak power of 4–6 mW, and signal bitrate of 20 Gbit/s) was transmitted over 200 km by amplifying the signal with a period of 25 km using a 1.48-μm semiconductor laser as the pump source [14].

5.3.3. Modulational Instability

Modulational instability (MI) is a phenomenon observed in a nonlinear dispersive medium in which the side-band component of the amplitude-modulated light grows exponentially when a certain condition is satisfied [15]. The steady-state solution of the nonlinear Schrödinger equation (5.36) (continuous-wave solution under the condition of $\partial\phi/\partial\tau = 0$) is given by

$$\phi_{cw} = \phi_0 \exp(-j\delta z), \tag{5.50a}$$

$$\delta = \frac{kn_2}{2} |\phi_0|^2, \tag{5.50b}$$

where ϕ_0 is a constant. When a small perturbation is applied to the steady-state solution [Eq. (5.50a)] in the anomalous region, the electric field becomes unstable under a certain condition. We add a small perturbation $q(z, \tau)$ to the steady-state solution ϕ_{cw} to investigate the modulational instability. The field with the perturbation is expressed as

$$\phi = [\phi_0 + q(z, \tau)] \exp(-j\delta z). \tag{5.51}$$

Substituting this into Eq. (5.36) under the assumption that the perturbation is sufficiently small ($|q| \ll \phi_0$), we obtain the differential equation for q of the form

$$j\frac{\partial q}{\partial z} = -\frac{\beta''}{2}\frac{\partial^2 q}{\partial \tau^2} + \delta\,(q + q^*). \tag{5.52}$$

We assume the general solution for $q(z, \tau)$ of the form

$$q(z, \tau) = q_1 \cos(\Omega t - Kz) + jq_2 \sin(\Omega t - Kz), \tag{5.53}$$

where Ω and K denote the angular frequency and wavenumber of the perturbations respectively. The dispersion relation between K and Ω is obtained by substituting Eq. (5.53) into Eq. (5.52):

$$K^2 = \left(\frac{\beta''\Omega}{2}\right)^2 \left[\Omega^2 + \frac{2kn_2}{\beta''}|\phi_0|^2\right]. \tag{5.54}$$

It is seen from Eq. (5.54) that K becomes a pure imaginary number when the following conditions are satisfied:

$$\frac{n_2}{\beta''} < 0 \tag{5.55}$$

$$\Omega < \Omega_c \equiv \left[\frac{2kn_2}{-\beta''}|\phi_0|\right]^{1/2}. \tag{5.56}$$

Then q grows exponentially. Of course, we have the exponentially decaying solution. But it is not important here. If the perturbation is the amplitude modulation, this phenomenon implies that the modulation depth grows exponentially. Therefore, such a phenomenon is called the *modulational instability*.

The angular frequency at which the growth rate of the perturbation becomes the maximum is given by $\Omega = \pm\Omega_c/\sqrt{2}$. Here the growth rate of q is expressed by $\exp(kn_2 \cdot |\phi_0|^2/2)z$.

Even when there is no perturbation feeding, the seed of the perturbation may originate in the thermally activated phonon. Figure 5.10 shows the experimental

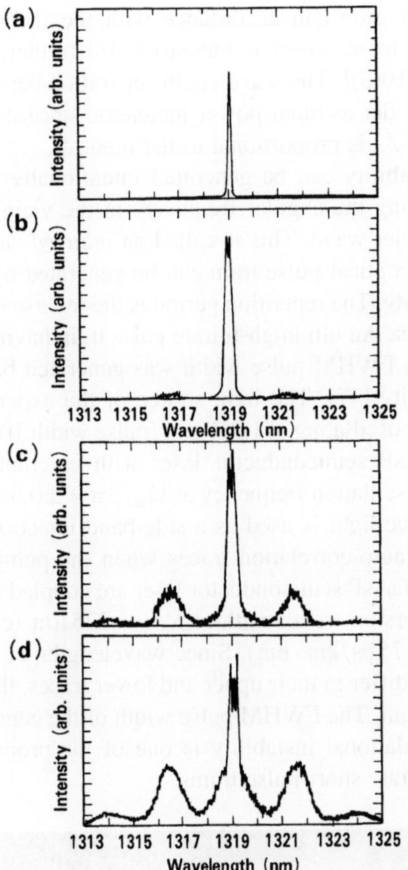

Figure 5.10 Growth of side-band components by the modulational instability in optical fiber. Input power: (a) low, (b) 5.5 W, (c) 6.1 W, and (d) 7.1 W. (After Ref. [16]).

observation of the growth of side-band components by the modulational instability in optical fiber [16]. The light source in the experiment was a mode-locked Nd:YAG laser with a 100-MHz repetition rate and a 100-ps pulse width. The reason why a 100-ps pulse was used instead of using CW light was to suppress the stimulated Brillouin scattering (refer to Section 5.7). The parameters of the fiber used in the experiment were chromatic dispersion $\sigma = 2.4\,\text{ps/km}\cdot\text{nm}$, length of fiber $L = 1\,\text{km}$, effective core area $A_{\text{eff}} = 60\,\mu\text{m}^2$, and fiber loss of 0.67 dB/km. Figure 5.10(a) shows the output spectrum for low input power. The output spectrum at this power level coincides with that of the input spectrum. When input power is increased to (b) 5.5 W, (c) 6.1 W, and (d) 7.1 W, a side band is generated from the thermally excited phonon at angular frequency $\Omega_c/\sqrt{2}$

[Fig. 5.10(b)], and it grows in accordance with the increase of input power [Fig. 5.10(c)]. When input power is increased still further, a higher-order side band appears [Fig. 5.10(d)]. The wavelength separation between pump light and side band becomes wider as input power increases, since the angular frequency of the side band $\Omega_c/\sqrt{2}$ is proportional to the input ϕ_0.

Modulational instability can be generated intentionally by injecting a side-band component having the angular frequency in the vicinity of $\Omega_m = \Omega_c/\sqrt{2}$ together with the carrier wave. This is called an *induced modulational instability*. A high-repetition optical pulse train can be generated by using this induced modulational instability. The repetition period is the inverse of the given modulation frequency $\Omega_m/2\pi$. An ultrahigh-bitrate pulse train having about a 0.34-THz repetition with 0.5-ps FWHM pulse width was generated based on the induced modulational instability [17]. The light source of the experiment was a mode-locked Nd:YAG laser oscillating at 1.319 μm (pulse width 100 ps and peak power 3 W), and an InGaAsP semiconductor laser with external cavity (cw output 0.5 mW) having the oscillation frequency at $\Omega_m/2\pi \cong \pm 0.34$ THz (1.8 nm) apart from that of the source light is used as a side-band injection light. Figure 5.11 shows the measured auto-correlation traces when the pumping Nd:YAG laser and the side-band InGaAsP semiconductor laser are coupled to single-mode fiber having the zero-dispersion wavelength at $\lambda_0 = 1.275$ μm (chromatic dispersion at 1.319 μm is $\sigma = 3.75$ ps/km · nm). Since wavelengths of side-band InGaAsP semiconductor lasers differ in their upper and lower traces, the repetition angular frequencies are different. The FWHM pulse width of the generated pulse is about 0.5 ps. Induced modulational instability is one of the promising techniques to generate ultrahigh-bitrate short-pulse trains.

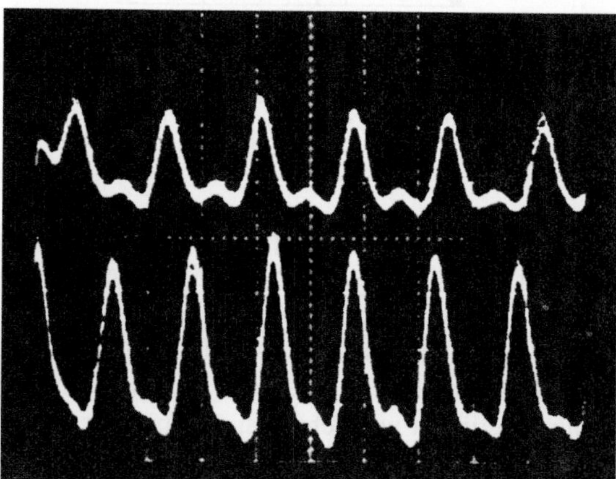

Figure 5.11 Auto-correlation traces of pulse trains generated by the induced modulational instability. Wavelengths of side-band InGaAsP semiconductor lasers differ in their upper and lower traces. (After Ref. [17]).

5.3.4. Dark Solitons

A bright soliton cannot exist in the normal dispersion region in which $\beta'' > 0$. However, a dark soliton, which is an amplitude dip in the continuous wave, can exist in this normal dispersion region [18]. The solution of Eq. (5.36) under the condition of $\beta'' > 0$ is given by

$$\phi(z, \tau) = \phi_p \exp\left(-j\frac{\beta''}{2t_0^2}z\right) \tanh\left(\frac{\tau}{t_0}\right), \tag{5.57}$$

where the definition of t_0 is the same as for Eq. (5.38). The condition for the peak electric field ϕ_p is given by

$$|\phi_p|^2 = \frac{2\beta''}{t_0^2 k n_2}. \tag{5.58}$$

Figure 5.12 shows the pulse waveform and chirping property of a dark soliton. The phase of the dark soliton jumps at the minimum amplitude point. Experimental observation of the dark soliton is already reported [19].

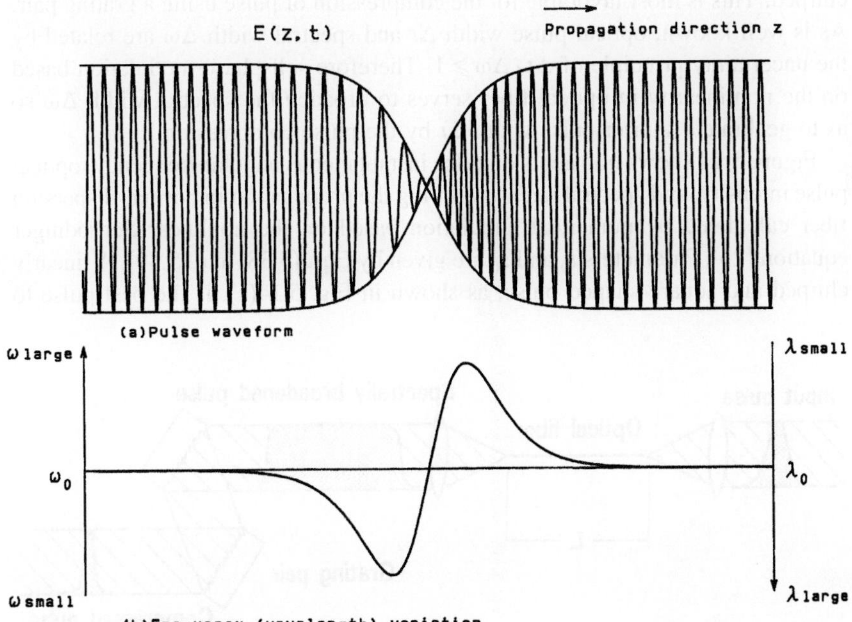

Figure 5.12 Pulse waveform and chirping property of a dark soliton.

5.4. OPTICAL PULSE COMPRESSION

Ultrashort optical pulses are indispensable for research into ultrafast phenomena. An oscillating optical pulse width of 27 fs from a colliding pulse-mode-locked dye laser is reported by compensating the group velocity dispersion (GVD) in the laser cavity with prism chains [20]. However, from a practical standpoint, the technique of generating ultrashort light pulses from the laser itself is rather disadvantageous, since the wavelength region of laser oscillation is limited. The optical pulse compression technique [21] based on, for example, the combination of single-mode fiber (chirping medium) and grating pair (dispersive medium) is able to cover a wide spectral range, since pulse compression is done outside of the laser cavity.

An optical pulse of 50-fs width from the colliding pulse-mode-locked dye laser oscillating at 620 nm was compressed down to 6 fs by the pulse compression technique [22]. So far this is the shortest optical pulse. Figure 5.13 shows the schematics of optical pulse compression using fiber and grating pair. Transients of the optical pulse waveform propagating in single-mode fiber is described by Eq. (5.32). In the normal dispersion region, in which the longer-wavelength component at the preceding edge of the pulse travels faster than the shorter one in the trailing edge, the pulse waveform becomes square shaped and linearly chirped. This is most favorable for the compression of pulse using a grating pair. As is well known, optical pulse width Δt and spectral width $\Delta\omega$ are related by the uncertainty principle of $\Delta t \cdot \Delta\omega \geqslant 1$. Therefore self-phase modulation based on the nonlinearity in optical fiber serves to broaden the spectral width $\Delta\omega$ so as to generate a shorter pulse width Δt by the pulse compression.

Figure 5.14 shows transients of pulse instantaneous angular frequency, optical pulse intensity, and spectral intensity during the propagation in normal-dispersion fiber calculated by numerical simulation based on the nonlinear Schrödinger equation [23]. Parameters t_0 and z_0 are given by Eqs. (5.38) and (5.49). A linearly chirped and square-shaped pulse, as shown in Fig. 5.14(c), is the best pulse to

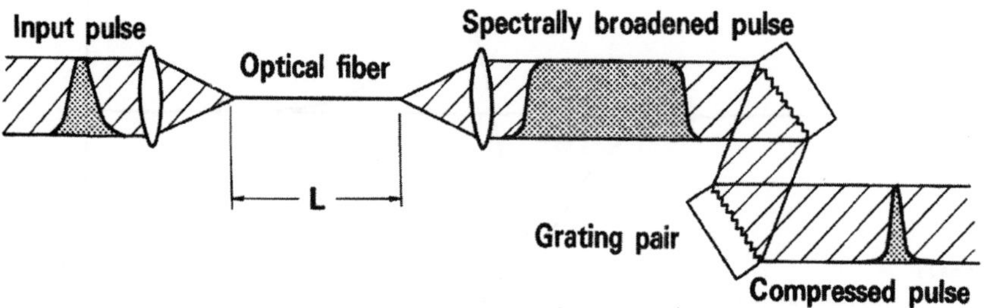

Figure 5.13 Schematic configuration of optical pulse compression using fiber and grating pair.

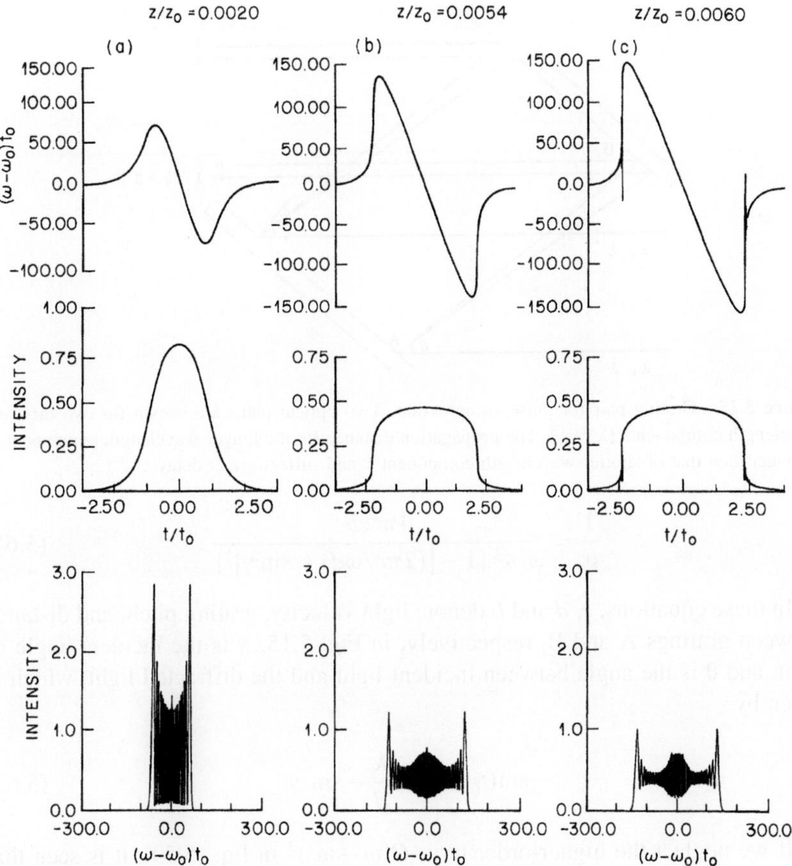

Figure 5.14 Numerical simulations of pulse instantaneous angular frequency (top row), optical pulse intensity (center row) and spectral intensity (bottom row) during propagation in normal-dispersion fiber. (After Ref. [23]).

compress by using a grating pair [24]. The wavelength (frequency-) dependent delay time of the grating pair, as shown in Fig. 5.15, is expressed by

$$\tau = \tau_G - \frac{\omega - \omega_0}{\mu} + O(\omega - \omega_0)^2, \tag{5.59}$$

where τ_G and μ are given by

$$\tau_G = \left(\frac{b}{c}\right)(1 + \cos\theta), \tag{5.60}$$

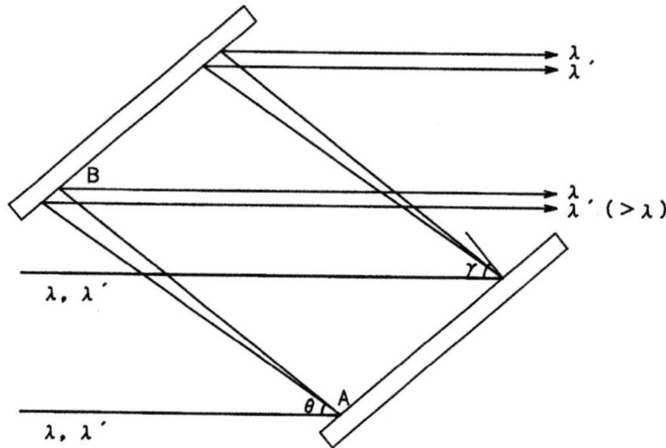

Figure 5.15 Grating pair for pulse compression. Two optical paths are shown for two different wavelength components ($\lambda' > \lambda$). The propagation distance for the longer-wavelength component λ' is longer than that of shorter-wavelength component λ and suffers grater delay.

$$\frac{1}{\mu} = \frac{4\pi^2 cb}{\omega^3 d^2 \{1 - [(2\pi c/\omega d) - \sin\gamma]^2\}}. \tag{5.61}$$

In these equations, c, d and b denote light velocity, grating pitch, and distance between gratings A and B, respectively, in Fig. 5.15. γ is the incident angle of light, and θ is the angle between incident light and the diffracted light, which is given by

$$\sin(\gamma - \theta) = \frac{\lambda}{d} - \sin\gamma. \tag{5.62}$$

If we neglect the higher-order term $O(\omega - \omega_0)^2$ in Eq. (5.59), it is seen that the grating pair is a medium in which the higher-frequency (shorter-wavelength) component has shorter delay time (larger group velocity). This is equivalent to the single-mode optical fiber in the anomalous region. It is also confirmed from Eq. (5.61) that the delay-time difference can be increased by enlarging the distance b of the grating pair.

A prism pair can also be utilized as the anomalous medium for pulse compression [25]. In this case, the distance between the two prisms should be large, since the dispersion effect of the prisms is smaller than that of the grating pair. However, the insertion loss of the prism pair can be reduced by adjusting the angle of the prism to Brewster's angle. Therefore, prism pair is quite advantageous in the area of subpicosecond pulse generation.

So far we have neglected the influence of the third term in Eq. (5.59). However, this higher-order term cannot be neglected in the pulse generation of the order of 10 fs. In order to compensate for the third term in Eq. (5.59), a compression scheme has been devised that combines the prism pair inside the grating pair. A ultrashort light pulse of 6 fs was generated with this configuration. Considering that one cycle of light at $\lambda = 0.62\,\mu$m is $T = 2.1$ fs$(T = \lambda/c)$, we see that optical pulse compression technologies are approaching to its ultimate stage.

5.5. LIGHT SCATTERING IN ISOTROPIC MEDIA

Generally, when light in the visible region is injected into a transparent material, some part of the light is scattered nonelastically. When we observe the scattered light, there is Rayleigh-scattered light having the same wavelength as the input (excitation) light and also new light having a longer or shorter wavelength than that of the excitation light [26]. This effect is generally called the *Raman effect*. When scattered new light is generated through the interaction of excitation light with molecular vibration, optical phonons of the solid, and other elementary excitations, such as impurity, plasma and polariton, the scattering is called *Raman scattering*. On the otherhand, if scattered light is generated by the interaction of the excitation field with acoustical phonons of the liquid or solid, it is called *Brillouin scattering*.

Spontaneous Raman or Brillouin scattering is the phenomenon in which Stokes light with angular frequency $\omega_S = \omega_L - \omega_F$ and anti-Stokes light with angular frequency $\omega_A = \omega_L + \omega_F$ are emitted, where ω_L and ω_F denote angular frequencies of excitation light and optical or acoustical phonon, respectively. Stokes and anti-Stokes waves are generated through the modulation of electric polarization $\mathbf{P}$ by the polarizability α as $\mathbf{P} = \alpha \mathbf{E} \cos(\omega_L t)$, since polarizability α varies with the specific angular frequency of the phonon as $\alpha = \alpha_0 + (\partial\alpha/\partial k)k \cos(\omega_F \mathrm{t})$. When the excitation field is small, scattered light is incoherent, since each lattice vibration is random in phase. However, when the excitation field becomes strong, the lattice vibration is coherently excited at the angular frequency $(\omega_L - \omega_S)$ by the nonlinear interaction between the incident light and the Stokes light. The coupling of the coherent lattice vibration with the input light field causes third-order nonlinear polarization and generates stimulated scattering of the Stokes light. This is the origin of stimulated Raman scattering (SRS) and stimulated Brillouin scattering (SBS).

5.5.1. Vibration of One-Dimensional Lattice

A phonon is a quantized state of the lattice vibration. Let us consider the vibration of a one-dimensional lattice consisting of two kinds of atoms so as to obtain the physical image of a phonon. We consider the linear lattice in which two different atoms having masses M and m are aligned alternately as shown in Fig. 5.16 and obtain the dispersion relation for the vibrational wave

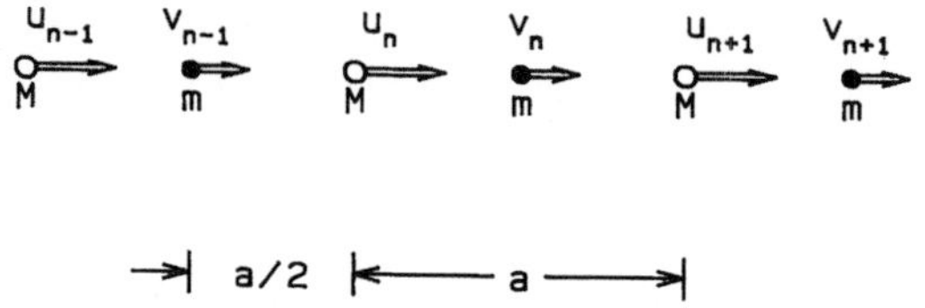

Figure 5.16 One-dimensional lattice consisting of two different atoms.

propagating along the linear direction. The displacements of the atoms from the static positions are expressed as u_n and v_n for the nth atoms M and m, where the positions of the two atoms are denoted by $x_n = na$ and $s_n = x_n + (1/2)a$ for the nth atoms M and m. Here a is a periodicity of the atom (or unit cell). If we assume that each atom is forced only by the adjacent atoms and that it obeys Hooke's law, we obtain the following equation of motion for the pair of nth atoms:

$$M\frac{d^2u_n}{dt^2} = -q(u_n - v_n) - q(u_n - v_{n-1}) = -q(2u_n - v_n - v_{n-1}), \quad (5.63a)$$

$$m\frac{d^2v_n}{dt^2} = -q(v_n - u_{n+1}) - q(v_n - u_n) = -q(2v_n - u_{n+1} - u_n), \quad (5.63b)$$

where q denotes the Hooke's constant. Since we are interested in the traveling vibrational wave, we express u_n and v_n in the following forms:

$$u_n = A\exp j(\omega t - kx_n), \quad (5.64a)$$

$$v_n = B\exp j\left(\omega t - k\left(x_n + \frac{1}{2}a\right)\right). \quad (5.64b)$$

Substitution of Eqs. (5.64) in Eqs. (5.63) gives

$$(-M\omega^2 + 2q)u_n = q(1 + e^{jka})v_n, \quad (5.65a)$$

$$q(1 + e^{-jka})u_n = (-m\omega^2 + 2q)v_n. \quad (5.65b)$$

Solution of these simultaneous equation gives ω^2 as

$$\omega^2 = q\left(\frac{1}{M} + \frac{1}{m}\right) \pm q\sqrt{\left(\frac{1}{M} + \frac{1}{m}\right)^2 - \frac{4\sin^2(ka/2)}{Mm}}. \quad (5.66)$$

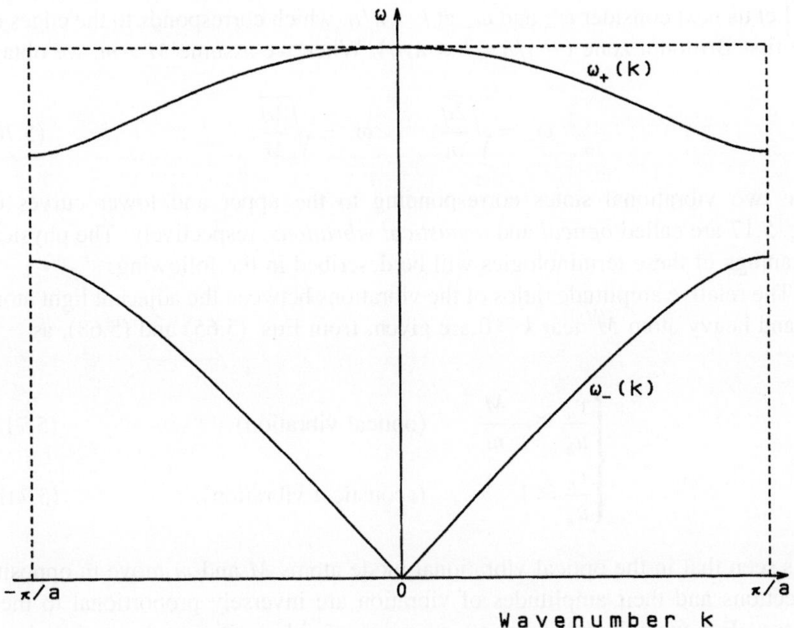

Figure 5.17 Dispersion relations of ω_+ and ω_- with respect to the wavenumber k.

Among the four possible solutions of Eq. (5.66), two positive solutions ω_+ and ω_- give the traveling wave solutions. Dispersion relations of ω_+ and ω_- with respect to wavenumber k are shown in Fig. 5.17. We have

$$\omega_+ = \sqrt{2q\left(\frac{1}{M} + \frac{1}{m}\right)}, \qquad \omega_- = 0, \tag{5.67}$$

for $k = 0$. For small k, where we can approximate $\sin(ka/2) \cong ka/2$, we obtain

$$\omega_+ = \omega_{+0}\left[1 - \frac{mM(ka)^2}{8(M+m)^2}\right], \tag{5.68a}$$

$$\omega_- = ka\sqrt{\frac{q}{2(M+m)}}, \tag{5.68b}$$

where ω_{+0} is defined by

$$\omega_{+0} = \sqrt{2q\left(\frac{1}{M} + \frac{1}{m}\right)}. \tag{5.69}$$

Let us next consider ω_+ and ω_- at $k = \pi/a$, which corresponds to the edges of the first Brillouin zone ($-\pi/a \leqslant k \leqslant \pi/a$). When we assume $M > m$, we obtain

$$\omega_+ = \sqrt{\frac{2q}{m}}, \qquad \omega_- = \sqrt{\frac{2q}{M}}. \tag{5.70}$$

The two vibrational states corresponding to the upper and lower curves of Fig. 5.17 are called *optical* and *acoustical vibrations*, respectively. The physical meanings of these terminologies will be described in the following.

The relative amplitude ratios of the vibrations between the adjacent light atom m and heavy atom M near $k \cong 0$ are given, from Eqs. (5.65) and (5.68), as

$$\begin{cases} \dfrac{v_n}{u_n} \cong -\dfrac{M}{m} & \text{(optical vibration)} \qquad (5.71\text{a}) \\ \dfrac{v_n}{u_n} \cong 1 & \text{(acoustical vibration).} \qquad (5.71\text{b}) \end{cases}$$

It is seen that in the optical vibrational mode atoms M and m move in opposite directions and their amplitudes of vibration are inversely proportional to their masses. For example, when two atoms are ions with positive and negative signs, such as Na^+ and Cl^-, optical vibration corresponds to the vibration of electric polarization and strongly interacts with the light field. Therefore it is called *optical vibrational mode*. On the other hand, in the acoustical vibrational mode, the directions of vibration for the two atoms are the same and their amplitudes are also the same. Since such a vibration is observed when an acoustic wave propagates in the crystal, it is called *acoustical vibrational mode*.

Generally, there exist transverse and longitudinal modes for the waves. Then there are four possible vibrational modes for each wavenumber k, as shown in Fig. 5.18: transverse optic (TO), longitudinal optic (LO), transverse acoustic (TA), and longitudinal acoustic (LA) modes. Moreover, there are two orthogonal vibrations (x- and y-directions) for the transverse mode, TA and TO vibrations are twofold degenerated.

5.5.2. Selection Rules for Light Scattering by Phonons

Figure 5.19 shows the dispersion relations of optical and acoustical phonons and a light (electromagnetic) wave $\omega = ck$. The intersection points between the phonons and light give the selection condition for the interaction between phonon and light. Since the speed of light c is very large compared to that of an optical phonon wave, the dispersion curve of light ($\omega = ck$) intersects with that of the optical branch close to ω_{+0}. The energy of an optical phonon

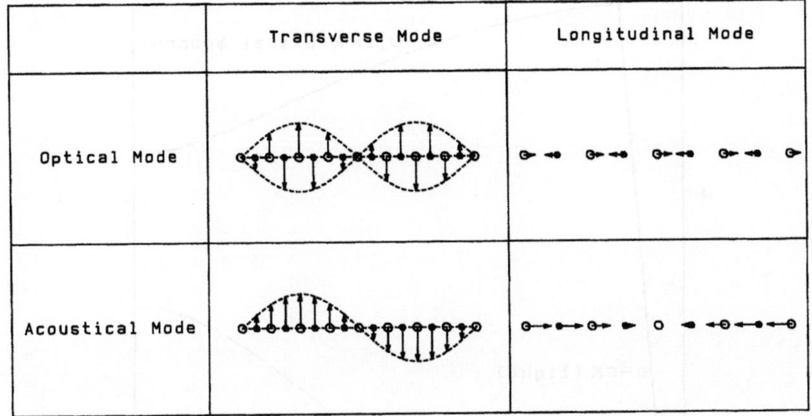

Figure 5.18 Displacements of atoms in the optical and acoustical vibrations.

is about $\hbar\omega_{+0} \cong 10^{-2}$ eV, where $\hbar = h/2\pi$ and Planck's constant $h = 6.626 \times 10^{-34}$ J · s. Then angular frequency ω_{+0} is seen to be $\omega_{+0} \cong 1.5 \times 10^{13}\,\text{s}^{-1}$, which corresponds to the electromagnetic wave with a wavelength of 120 μm. The wavenumber k at the intersection point between optical branch and light is given by $k = \omega_{+0}/c = 1.5\times10^{13}/3 \times 10^{10} \cong 500\,\text{cm}^{-1}$. This wavenumber is quite small when compared to the wavenumber $k_{\max} = \pi/a \cong 10^{8}\,\text{cm}^{-1}$ at the edge of the Brillouin zone [27], where the lattice constant is assumed to be $a = 3 \times 10^{-8}$ cm. Therefore, the wavenumber at which the optical phonon interacts with light is considered to be $k/k_{\max} \cong 0$.

First-order selection rules between phonon and light are given by

$$\omega_s = \omega_p \pm \omega_f, \tag{5.72}$$

$$\mathbf{k}_s = \mathbf{k}_p \pm \mathbf{k}_f, \tag{5.73}$$

where $(\omega_p, \mathbf{k}_p)$, $(\omega_s, \mathbf{k}_s)$ and $(\omega_f, \mathbf{k}_f)$ are sets of angular frequencies and wave vectors of pump light, scattered light, and phonon, respectively. Equations (5.72) and (5.73) represent the energy conservation rule and the momentum conservation rule respectively. The plus-or-minus sign in Eqs. (5.72) and (5.73) correspond to anti-Stokes or Stokes scattering. When the refractive indices of the medium for the pump and scattered light are expressed as n_p and n_s, respectively, we obtain

$$\frac{k_p c}{\omega_p} = n_p, \tag{5.74a}$$

$$\frac{k_s c}{\omega_s} = n_s, \tag{5.74b}$$

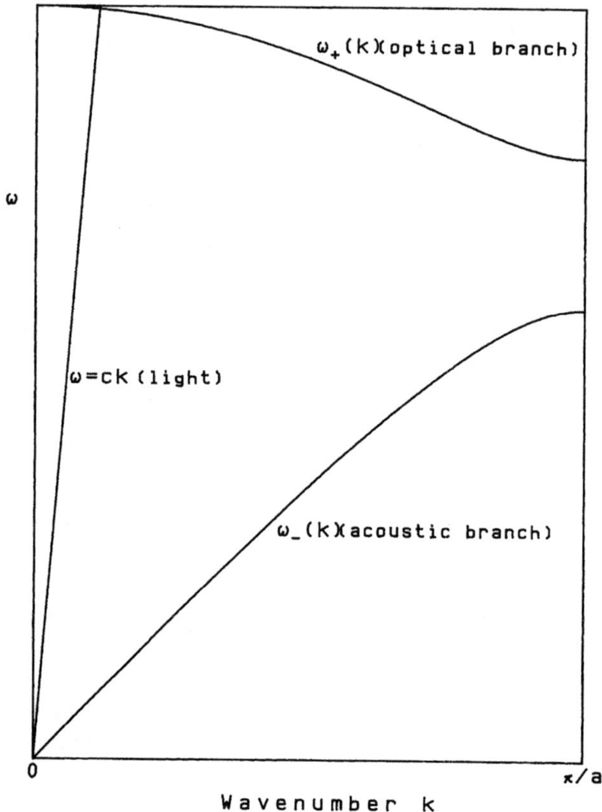

Figure 5.19 Dispersion relations between optical and acoustical phonons and a light (electromagnetic) wave.

where $k_p = |\mathbf{k}_p|$ and $k_s = |\mathbf{k}_s|$. Since the angular frequency of phonon ω_f is quite small $[\omega_p \cong \omega_s (\cong 10^{15}\, s^{-1}) \gg \omega_f (\cong 10^{13}\, s^{-1})]$, we obtain, from Eqs. (5.74):

$$k_s = \frac{n_s}{n_p} k_p. \tag{5.75}$$

If the medium is isotropic and refractive-index dispersion is small $(n_s \cong n_p)$, we can assume $k_s \cong k_p$. Figure 5.20(a) shows the relation of the wave vectors between pump and scattered light and phonon. When we consider the Stokes scattering $(\mathbf{k}_s = \mathbf{k}_p - \mathbf{k}_f)$, the scattering diagram is represented by Fig. 5.20(b), where θ denotes the scattering angle. The wavenumber of the phonon $\mathbf{k}_f = |k_f|$

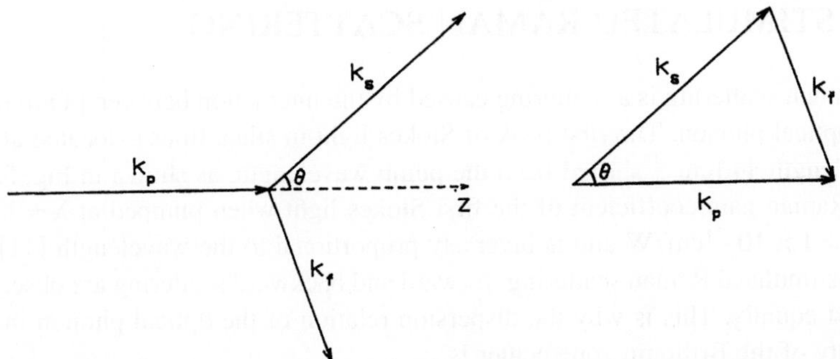

Figure 5.20 Relation of the wave vectors between pump and scattered light and phonon.

is obtained, from Eqs. (5.72) and (5.74), as

$$k_f^2 = k_p^2 + k_s^2 - 2k_p k_s \cos\theta = \left(\frac{n_p}{c}\right)^2 \left[(\omega_p - \omega_s)^2 + 4\omega_p\omega_s \sin^2\left(\frac{\theta}{2}\right)\right]$$
$$= \left(\frac{n_p}{c}\right)^2 \left[\omega_f^2 + 4\omega_p(\omega_p - \omega_f)\sin^2\left(\frac{\theta}{2}\right)\right], \quad (5.76)$$

where we assumed $n_s \cong n_p$. The above equation gives the relation between the angle θ of the scattered light and the amplitude of the phonon wave vector k_f contributing the scattering. When we assume $n_s \cong n_p$ and $\omega_p \gg \omega_f$ in Eq. (5.76) we obtain the following relationships for θ and k_f:

$$\begin{cases} \theta = 0^\circ & \text{(forwardscattering)} & k_f = \dfrac{n_p\omega_f}{c} \\ \theta = 90^\circ & \text{(right-angle scattering)} & k_f = \sqrt{2}\dfrac{n_p\omega_p}{c} = \sqrt{2}k_p \\ \theta = 180^\circ & \text{(backward scattering)} & k_f = 2\dfrac{n_p\omega_p}{c} = 2k_p. \end{cases} \quad (5.77)$$

The wavenumber of the pump light is of the order of $k_p = 4 \times 10^4$–$10^5\,\text{cm}^{-1}$. This is quite small when compared with the wavenumber at the edge of the first Brillouin zone $k_{\max} = 10^8\,\text{cm}^{-1}$ by about 10^{-4}–10^{-3}. Therefore, k_f's in Eqs. (5.77) lie in the vicinity of the center of the Brillouin zone and we have, irrespective of the following relation: scattering angle θ

$$k_f / k_{\max} \cong 0 \quad (5.78)$$

Especially, k_f for the forward scattering is extremely small, since $\omega_f(\cong 10^{13} s^{-1}) \ll \omega_p(\cong 10^{15} s^{-1})$.

5.6. STIMULATED RAMAN SCATTERING

Raman scattering is a scattering caused by the interaction between pump light and optical phonon. The first peak of Stokes light in silica fiber is located at the wavelength $440\,\text{cm}^{-1}$ shifted from the pump wavelength, as shown in Fig. 5.21. The Raman gain coefficient of the first Stokes light when pumped at $\lambda = 1\,\mu\text{m}$ is $g_R = 1 \times 10^{-11}\text{cm/W}$ and is inversely proportional to the wavelength [11].

In stimulated Raman scattering, forward and backward scattering are observed almost equally. This is why the dispersion relation of the optical phonon in the vicinity of the Brillouin zone center is

$$\omega_+(k_f) \cong \text{constant}$$

as shown in Eq. (5.68a) and Fig. 5.17. In other words, although the phonon wavenumber k_f contributing to the forward or backward scattering is different in the momentum conservation rule [Eq. (5.73)], the energy conservation rule is satisfied for any scattering angle, since $\omega + (k_f)$ is almost constant.

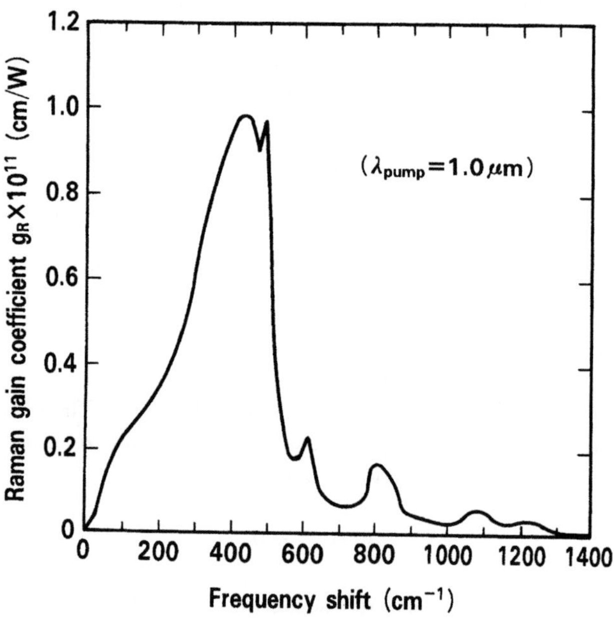

Figure 5.21 Raman gain spectrum of silica glass. (After Ref. [11]).

The progress of pump light intensity I_p and Stokes light intensity I_s in stimulated Raman scattering is described by the following coupled equations:

$$\frac{dI_s}{dz} = g_R I_p I_s - \alpha_s I_s, \tag{5.79a}$$

$$\frac{dI_p}{dz} = -\frac{\omega_p}{\omega_s} g_R I_p I_s - \alpha_p I_p, \tag{5.79b}$$

where α_p and α_s denote fiber losses at the wavelengths of pump and Stokes light, respectively. When we ignore the pump depletion and assume $I_p = I_0 \exp(-\alpha_p z)$ (I_0 is the pump intensity at $z = 0$), Eq. (5.79a) reduces to

$$\frac{dI_s}{dz} = g_R I_s I_0 \exp(-\alpha_p z) - \alpha_s I_s. \tag{5.80}$$

The solution of Eq. (5.80) is given by

$$I_s(L) = I_s(0) \exp(g_R I_0 L_{\text{eff}} - \alpha_s L), \tag{5.81}$$

where the effective fiber length L_{eff} is defined by

$$L_{\text{eff}} = \frac{1 - \exp(-\alpha_p L)}{\alpha_p}. \tag{5.82}$$

When the seed of the Stokes light $I_s(0)$ is not injected at $z = 0$, stimulated Raman scattering builds up from the spontaneous Raman scattering. In this case, the critical pump power at which Stokes power becomes equal to the pump power is obtained as [28]

$$P_c = \frac{16 A_{\text{eff}}}{g_R L_{\text{eff}}}. \tag{5.83}$$

Here the effective core area A_{eff} is approximately given by Eq. (5.42). However, strictly speaking we should take into account the wavelength difference between pump and Stokes light. Then strict expression of the effective area is given by

$$A_{\text{eff}} = \frac{\int_0^{2\pi} \int_0^{\infty} |R_p|^2 r\, dr\, d\theta \int_0^{2\pi} \int_0^{\infty} |R_s|^2 r\, dr\, d\theta}{\int_0^{2\pi} \int_0^{\infty} |R_p|^2 |R_s|^2 r\, dr\, d\theta}, \tag{5.84}$$

where $R_p(r)$ and $R_s(r)$ represent electric field distributions of pump and Stokes light, respectively. The critical power for the single-mode fiber with $A_{\text{eff}} = 50\,\mu\text{m}^2$, $\alpha_p = 0.2\,\text{dB/km}(4.6 \times 10^{-5}\,\text{m}^{-1})$, $L \gg 1/\alpha_p(\approx 22\,\text{km})$, and $g_R = 0.6 \times 10^{-11}\,\text{cm/W}(\lambda = 1.55\,\mu\text{m})$ is obtained as $P_c = 600\,\text{mW}$.

Next we obtain the gain coefficient by SRS when the Stokes seed $I_s(0)$ (signal to be amplified by SRS) is injected in Eq. (5.81). When we assume $\alpha_p = \alpha_s = 0$ for simplicity, the gain coefficient is obtained as

$$G = \frac{I_s(L)}{I_s(0)} = \exp(g_R I_0 L). \tag{5.85}$$

If the pump power $P_0 = I_0 A_{\text{eff}} = 4\,\text{W}$ in the fiber having $g_R = 0.6 \times 10^{-11}\,\text{cm/W}$ and $A_{\text{eff}} = 50\,\mu\text{m}^2$, 21-dB gain is obtained at the fiber length of 1 km. Figure 5.22 shows the bit error rate (BER) characteristics of the fiber Raman amplification experiment (signal and pump propagate in the opposite direction) when a 1.57-μm-wavelength DFB laser is used as the signal and a 1.47-μm-wavelength F-center laser is used as pump [29]. Signal bit rate and fiber length are 1 Gbit/s and 45 km, respectively. The gain coefficient at 100 mW pump power is about 3.5 dB, and the maximum gain is 5.8 dB. The dotted lines in the figure represent the theoretical values for the BERs. Any difference from the theoretical value is attributed to the fluctuation of the pump light and to its back scattering.

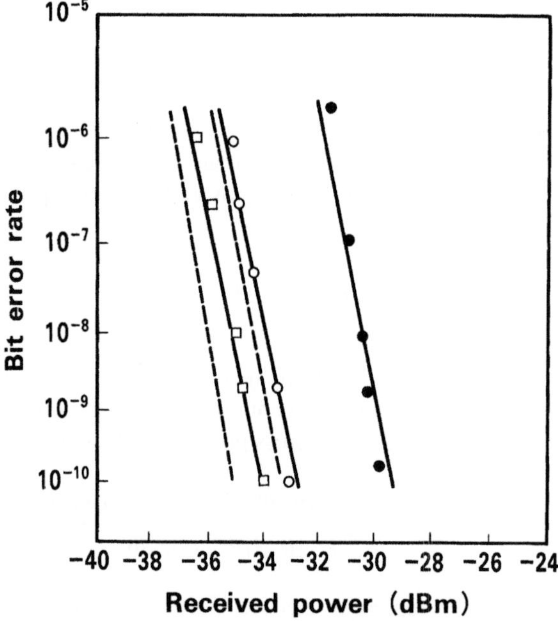

Figure 5.22 Bit error rate characteristics of the optical amplification experiment using SRS. Filled circles represent no pump light, and open circles and open rectangles represent 3.9 dB and 5.8 dB gain, respectively. (After Ref. [29]).

5.7. STIMULATED BRILLOUIN SCATTERING

Stimulated Brillouin scattering is a scattering caused by the interaction between pump light and acoustical phonon. Since the angular frequency of an acoustical phonon satisfies the linear dispersion relation with the wavenumber in the center of the Brillouin zone [Eq. (5.68b)], only the backward scattering occurs strongly.

Stimulated Brillouin scattering can be described by classical mechanics as the parametric interaction between the pump, Stokes and acoustical waves [30]. First, the pump light $E_p \exp j(\omega_p t - \mathbf{k}_p \cdot \mathbf{r})$ is spontaneously scattered by the thermally excited acoustical phonon in the medium and generates the scattered light $E_s \exp j(\omega_s t - \mathbf{k}_s \cdot \mathbf{r})$. Then the electric fields of the pump and scattered light create the density fluctuations through the electrostriction. The density fluctuation is a traveling wave permitivity grating, which is expressed by $\exp \pm j(\Omega t - \mathbf{q} \cdot \mathbf{r})$. Here Ω and $\mathbf{q}$ are given by

$$\Omega = \omega_p - \omega_s, \tag{5.86a}$$

$$\mathbf{q} = \mathbf{k}_p - \mathbf{k}_s. \tag{5.86b}$$

This permitivity grating scatters the pump light and generates the Stokes light, which results in the stimulated Brillouin scattering. The variance of the relative permitivity $\delta\varepsilon_s$ for the Stokes light is caused by the permitivity grating is given by

$$\delta\varepsilon_s = \rho_0 \left(\frac{\partial\varepsilon}{\partial\rho}\right)^2 \frac{|E_p|^2}{16\pi} \frac{q^2}{(\Omega_B^2 - \Omega^2 - j2\Omega\Gamma)}. \tag{5.87}$$

Here, ρ_0 is the density of the medium, $\partial\varepsilon/\partial\rho$ is the rate of change in the relative permitivity with respect to the unit density change, and Γ is the FWHM spectral width of the permitivity given by $\Gamma = 1/\tau_A$, where τ_A is the decay relaxation time of the acoustical wave. Ω_B is the angular frequency of the acoustical phonon, which is given by

$$\Omega_B = |\mathbf{q}| v_A = q v_A, \tag{5.88}$$

where v_A is the velocity of a longitudinal acoustic wave. In silica glass, we have $\rho_0 = 2.2\,\mathrm{g/cm^3}$, $\tau_A = 20\,\mathrm{ns}$ at $\lambda = 1.55\,\mu\mathrm{m}$, and $v_A = 5940\,\mathrm{m/s}$ [31, 32]. From Eq. (5.87), the refractive index for the Stokes light n_s is obtained as

$$n_s = \left(n_0^2 + \delta\varepsilon_s\right)^{1/2} \cong n_0 + \frac{\partial\varepsilon_s}{2n_0}, \tag{5.89}$$

where n_0 denotes the original refractive index. When we ignore the attenuation of the Stokes wave, its amplitude variation is expressed by

$$E_s(L) = E_s(0)\exp(-jk_s n_s L) = E_s(0)\exp\left(-jk_s n_0 L - \frac{jk_s \delta\varepsilon_s L}{2n_0}\right). \tag{5.90}$$

It is seen from this last equation that the imaginary part of $\delta\varepsilon_s$ gives the gain of the Stokes light. Equation (5.90) is rewritten into the intensity form as

$$I_s(L) = I_s(0)\exp\left(\frac{k_s}{n_0} Im[\delta\varepsilon_s]L\right). \tag{5.91}$$

We should note here that the relation between optical intensity (= power/effective area) and electric field amplitude is expressed in MKS units as

$$I_s = \frac{1}{2} n_0 \varepsilon_0 c |E_s|^2 \qquad [\mathrm{W/m^2}], \tag{5.92a}$$

and in cgs units is expressed as

$$I_s = \frac{n_0 c}{8\pi}|E_s|^2 \qquad [\mathrm{erg\cdot s^{-1}/cm^2}], \tag{5.92b}$$

When we consider the Stokes light near the resonance angular frequency $\Omega \approx \Omega_B (= qv_A)$, Eq. (5.87) reduces to

$$Im[\delta\varepsilon_s] = \frac{n_0^7 p_{12}^2}{4c\rho_0 v_A} \frac{q\Gamma}{[(\Omega - \Omega_B)^2 + \Gamma^2]} I_0, \tag{5.93}$$

where $I_0 = (n_0 c/8\pi)|E_p|^2$ in cgs unit and the following relation has been used:

$$\rho_0 \left(\frac{\partial\varepsilon}{\partial\rho}\right) = n_0^4 p_{12}. \tag{5.94}$$

The Photoelastic coefficient p_{12} for silica glass is $p_{12} = 0.27$. The gain coefficient of SBS is then given, from Eqs. (5.91) and (5.93), as

$$g_B = \frac{n_0^6 p_{12}^2}{2c\lambda\rho_0 v_A \Delta\nu_B} q \frac{(\Delta\nu_B/2)^2}{[(\nu - \nu_B)^2 + (\Delta\nu_B/2)^2]}. \tag{5.95}$$

Here ν is a frequency of Stokes light ($\nu = \Omega/2\pi$), ν_B is a frequency shift of the Stokes light and $\Delta\nu_B$ is the FWHM width of Brillouin gain, which is obtained by $\Delta\nu_B = \Gamma/\pi = 1/\pi\tau_A$. Since $q = |\mathbf{k}_p - \mathbf{k}_s| \approx 0$ for forward scattering [Eq. (5.77)], the Brillouin gain is almost zero for forward Brillouin scattering [33]. In contrast,

q becomes the maximum $q = |\mathbf{k}_p - \mathbf{k}_s| \approx 2|\mathbf{k}_p| \approx 4\pi n_0/\lambda$ for backward scattering. Then the Brillouin gain also becomes the maximum

$$g_{B0} = \frac{2\pi n_0^7 p_{12}^2}{c\lambda^2 \rho_0 v_A \Delta\nu_B} \tag{5.96}$$

for backward scattering. Since the FWHM width of the Brillouin gain depends on the wavelength as ($\Delta\nu_B \propto 1/\lambda^2$), the Brillouin gain itself is almost wavelength independent. The frequency shift ν_B of the Stokes light becomes the maximum for backward scattering and is given by

$$\nu_B = \frac{\Omega_B}{2\pi} = \frac{q v_A}{2\pi} = \frac{2n_0 v_A}{\lambda}. \tag{5.97}$$

The frequency shift ν_B of the Stokes light at $\lambda = 1.55\,\mu\text{m}$ is $\nu_B = 11.1\,\text{GHz}$. Since the relaxation time τ_A of the acoustical phonon at $\lambda = 1.55\,\mu\text{m}$ is about $\tau_A \cong 20\,\text{ns}$, the FWHM spectral width of the Brillouin gain is given by $\Delta\nu_B = 1/\pi\tau_A \cong 16\,\text{MHz}$. At the $\lambda = 1.3\,\mu\text{m}$ wavelength region, $\nu_B = 13.3\,\text{GHz}$ and $\Delta\nu_B \cong 23\,\text{MHz}$.

The Brillouin gain g_{B0} at $\lambda = 1.55\,\mu\text{m}$ wavelength region is obtained, from Eq. (5.96) by $g_{B0} = 4.1 \times 10^{-9}\,\text{cm/W}$, where we assumed $n_0 = 1.45$. The gain of the stimulated Brillouin scattering is about 400 times larger than that of the SRS ($g_R = 0.6 \times 10^{-11}\,\text{cm/W}$). The Brillouin gain spectrum has a Lorentz shape, as shown in Eq. (5.95). When the spectrum of the pump light also has Lorentz shape with an FWHM of $\Delta\nu_p$, Brillouin gain coefficient is given by the convolution integral of the two spectral distributions as [34]:

$$g_B = \frac{\Delta\nu_B}{\Delta\nu_B + \Delta\nu_p} g_{B0}. \tag{5.98}$$

When the pump light has a rather narrow spectral width compared to the Brillouin gain width ($\Delta\nu_p \ll \Delta\nu_B$), the SBS gain becomes $g_B \cong g_{B0}$. However, if the pump light has a wide spectral width compared to the Brillouin gain width ($\Delta\nu_p \gg \Delta\nu_B$), the SBS gain becomes small and inversely proportional to $\Delta\nu_p$ as $g_B \cong (\Delta\nu_B/\Delta\nu_p) g_{B0}$. Therefore it is seen that a pump light source with a narrow spectral width is necessary to generate SBS efficiently.

Variation of Stokes light in the SBS process is obtained in a manner similar to that in SRS. When we consider that Stokes light travels in a direction opposite to that of the pump light, we obtain

$$I_s(0) = I_s(L) \exp(g_B I_0 L_{\text{eff}} - \alpha L), \tag{5.99}$$

where we assumed $\alpha_p \approx \alpha_s \approx \alpha$. Stimulated Brillouin scattering builds up from the thermally excited spontaneous Brillouin scattering. The critical input power

P_c at which Stokes light power becomes equal to the pump power is obtained by [28]

$$P_c = \frac{21A_{\text{eff}}}{g_B L_{\text{eff}}} = \frac{\Delta\nu_B + \Delta\nu_p}{\Delta\nu_B}\frac{21A_{\text{eff}}}{g_{B0}L_{\text{eff}}}. \tag{5.100}$$

In single-mode optical fiber with $A_{\text{eff}} = 50\,\mu\text{m}^2$, $\alpha = 0.2\,\text{dB/km}$ $(4.6\times10^{-5}\,\text{m}^{-1})$ at 1.55-μm wavelength, $L \gg 1/\alpha(\approx 22\,\text{km})$ and $g_{B0} = 4.1\times10^{-9}\,\text{cm/W}$, the critical power is $P_c = 1.2\,\text{mW}$ for a narrow pump line width $(\Delta\nu_p \ll \Delta\nu_B)$ and is $P_c = (\Delta\nu_p/\Delta\nu_B)\times 1.2\,\text{mW}$ for a wider pump line width.

A single-longitudinal-mode Ar laser and YAG laser with narrow spectral width have been utilized for the generation of SBS [31]. However, after the development of narrow spectral line width (less than 10 MHz) and high-power single-mode semiconductor lasers, experimental observation of SBS [35] and signal amplification by SBS [36] using the semiconductor laser as pump light have been reported. Figure 5.23 shows the measurement of the SBS threshold power using a 1.3-μm-wavelength DFB laser having spectral width of 15 MHz [35]. The attenuation and the length of the single-mode fiber are 0.46 dB/km at 1.3 μm and 30 km, respectively. It is known that the threshold input power for SBS is about 10 mW. It means that light with more than about 10 mW of power cannot be transmitted in single-mode fiber, since it is reflected back even if we increase the input power level.

The gain bandwidth of SBS can be enlarged up to about several hundred mega hertz by connecting different kinds of fibers, since the Brillouin shift frequency of doped-silica glass differs slightly depending on the dopant material. Figure 5.24 shows the result of a signal amplification experiment by SBS using single-mode fibers with a broadened gain spectrum [36]. The signal and pump lasers are semiconductor lasers with external cavity oscillating at 1.5 μm (spectral width of 15 kHz and tuning range of 1.42–1.52 μm). The average loss of fibers is 0.27 dB/km, and the total fiber length is 37.5 km. The amplification gain with respect to 1 mW pump power is 4.3 dB, which is far more efficient than that of stimulated Raman scattering. However, since the gain bandwidth of SBS is at most several hundred megahertz, it cannot amplify broadband (high bit-rate) signal or ultrashort optical pulses.

5.8. SECOND-HARMONIC GENERATION

Generally, second-harmonic generation (SHG) is believed to be impossible in centerosymmetric materials such as silica glass. However, SHG with relatively high efficiency in single-mode optical fibers has been reported. Figure 5.25 shows the growth of SHG power when mode-locked and Q-switched Nd:YAG

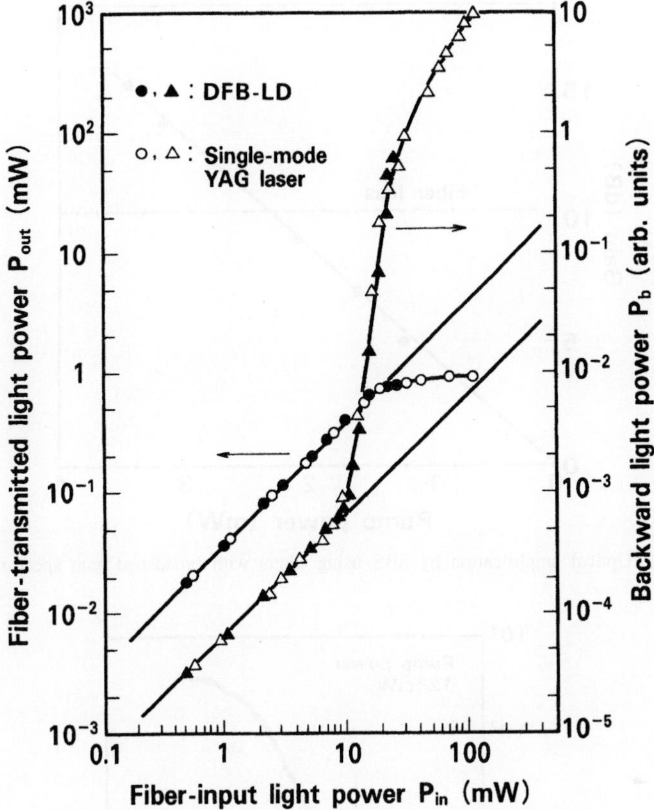

Figure 5.23 Transmitted and reflected light power by SBS. (After Ref. [35]).

laser pulses at 1.06-μm wavelength (pulse width of 100–130 ps and average power of 125 mW) are propagated through a 1-m-long single-mode fiber [37]. The second-harmonic power grows almost exponentially with time, and the maximum conversion efficiency of 3% was obtained.

The physical mechanisms to explain second-harmonic generation are not fully understood. However, it is recognized that the origin of high-efficiency SHG may be due to the formation of periodic color centers or defects [38]. First, small higher-order nonlinearities exist to generate weak second harmonics even in optical fibers; they are: nonlinearities at the core–cladding interface and nonlinearities resulting from quadrupole and magnetic-dipole moments [39]. When the pump wavelength is $\lambda_p = 1.06\,\mu\text{m}$, the period of the beat component generated by the pump light and the SHG light ($\lambda_s = 0.53\,\mu\text{m}$) is about $\Lambda_c = 2\pi/\Delta k \cong 30-40\,\mu\text{m}$, by taking into account the dispersion effect [40]. Here $\Delta k = k_s - 2k_p$, where k_p

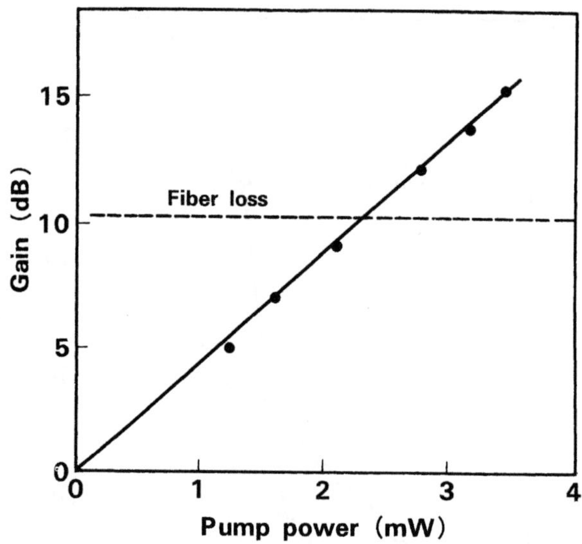

Figure 5.24 Optical amplification by SBS using fibers with broadened gain spectrum. (After Ref. [36]).

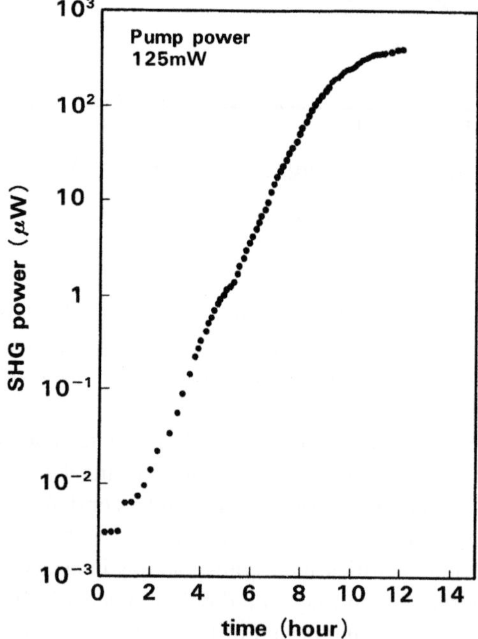

Figure 5.25 Second-harmonic power generated in a silica fiber as a function of time. (After Ref. [37]).

and k_s denote the wavenumbers of pump and SHG light, respectively. In the normal SHG, the variation of the SHG power is given by [2]

$$P_s(z) \propto \frac{\sin^2(\Delta k z/2)}{(\Delta k)^2}. \tag{5.101}$$

When the phase-matching condition ($\Delta k = 0$) is satisfied, the SHG power increases with increase in propagation distance z. However, the SHG power does not grow when the phase-matching condition is not satisfied ($\Delta k \neq 0$).

In contrast to normal SHG, the phase-matching condition is automatically satisfied when photoinduced defects are generated periodically in optical fiber. As shown in Fig. 5.26(a), the pump and SHG light adds up or cancel each other at the positions where they are in phase or out of phase, respectively. Then photoinduced defects and also $\chi^{(2)}$ are created at positions where the beat intensity is strong. The resulting distribution of $\chi^{(2)}$ in the fiber becomes a grating with a period of Λ_c. Since second harmonics are generated only where the pump and SHG light are in phase, the SHG light grows [Fig. 5.26(c)] in proportion to the propagation distance. The back-coupling from the SHG light to the pump light, which is observed in normal SHG, is prohibited, since there is no $\chi^{(2)}$ where SHG and pump light are out of phase (negligibly small $\chi^{(2)}$ exists caused by higher-order nonlinearity such as quadrupole moment). SHG in single-mode fibers is quite interesting for the nonlinear optical effects, since the phase-matching condition is automatically satisfied and the transverse modes are also well preserved throughout the interaction.

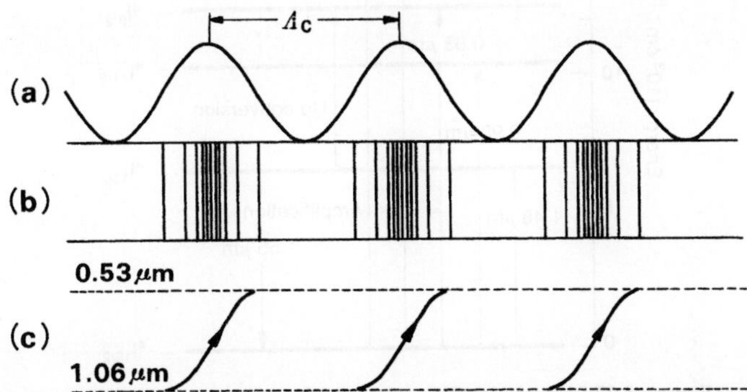

Figure 5.26 Schematics to explain SHG in optical fiber: (a) Beat wave created by pump and SHG light, (b) $\chi^{(2)}$ grating caused by photoinduced defects, and (c) efficient SHG at positions where pump and SHG light get in phase.

5.9. ERBIUM-DOPED FIBER AMPLIFIER

The erbium-doped fiber amplifier (EDFA) had a great impact on optical fiber communication systems [10, 41]. EDFA has a broad gain bandwidth around the 1.55-μm-wavelength region that coincides with the low-loss transmission wavelength of the silica glass fibers.

Erbium ions have the energy level diagram as shown in Fig. 5.27. Three states, i.e., the ground state ($^4\mathbf{I}_{15/2}$), the first excited state ($^4\mathbf{I}_{13/2}$), and one of the other higher excited states, participate and act as a three-level laser in the amplification of 1.55-μm-wavelength light, except for the 1.48-μm pumping scheme. In the case of 1.48-μm pumping, the upper portion of the $^4\mathbf{I}_{15/2}$ state, which has a certain bandwidth, as described later, is used as a pumping level, and the Er ions are operated as a quasi-three-level laser. The energy difference between the $^4\mathbf{I}_{13/2}$ state and the $^4\mathbf{I}_{15/2}$ state corresponds to the 1.55-μm-wavelength band. When an incident signal photon comes into an Er ion in the $^4\mathbf{I}_{13/2}$ excited state, the Er ion emits a photon with a certain probability and returns to the ground state through the stimulated emission process. The photon generated by the stimulated emission has exactly the same frequency and phase as the incident photon, thus enabling signal amplification. Even if the incident photon does not exist, the $^4\mathbf{I}_{13/2}$ level decays to the ground state, accompanied by a spontaneous emission.

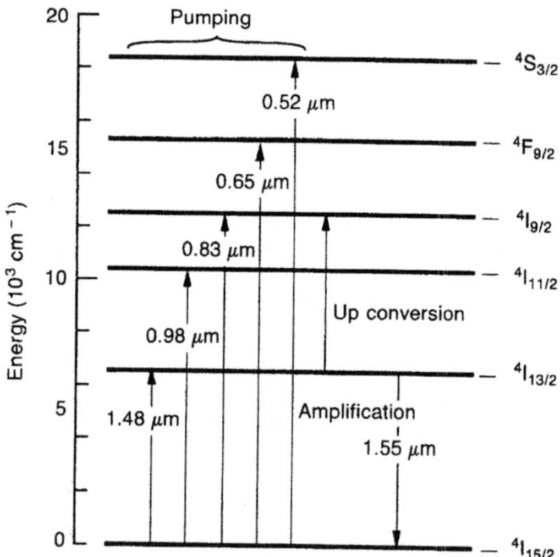

Figure 5.27 Energy level diagram of the triply ionized erbium ion.

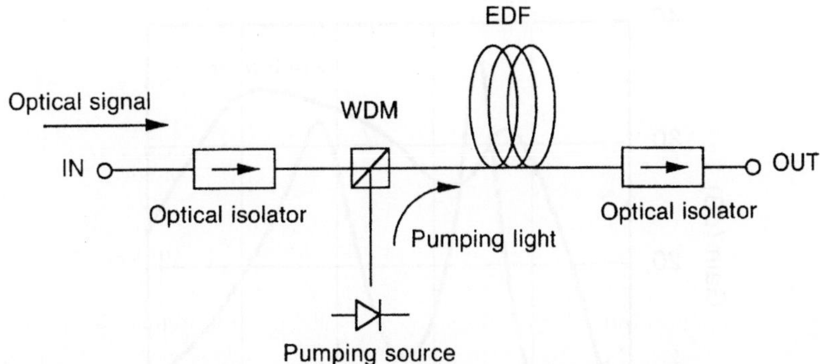

Figure 5.28 Amplifier configuration using Er-doped fiber.

Since spontaneous emission light has no correlation with the incident light in terms of frequency and phase, the amplified spontaneous emission (ASE) light becomes a noise source of optical fiber amplifiers. EDFA basically consists of an Er-doped fiber, a pumping light source, an optical coupler that combines signal and pump light, and optical isolators to reject the unwanted back-scattered light, as shown in Fig. 5.28. A fused-taper fiber WDM coupler or a dichroic mirror with dielectric multilayer is used for multiplexing pump and signal lights. The pump propagation direction is not necessarily the same as the direction of the signal. A better noise figure (NF) can be obtained by the copropagating pump scheme as compared to that of counter-propagating pump. However, the counterpropagating scheme is suitable as a booster application, since a higher conversion efficiency is obtained with this scheme. A bandpass filter is added in the output path to eliminate the ASE light.

In order to realize high gain and a low pumping threshold in the EDFA, it is essential to reduce the mode field diameter of the Er-doped fiber at the pump wavelength. Er-doped fiber generally has a high refractive-index difference and a small core to reduce the mode field diameter. A high doping concentration of Er-ion is desirable to shorten the fiber length and to reduce the amplifier size. However, there is a limitation on the available maximum doping concentration due to the cooperative up-conversion process. The maximum Er concentration may be less than 100 wt.ppm for the Ge/Er doped fibers, while a concentration of up to 1000 wt.ppm is allowed for the Ge/Er/Al-doped fibers. Aluminum codoping is effective for increasing the allowable Er concentration. The aluminum codoping also offers an advantage in broadening and smoothing the signal gain spectrum.

Figure 5.29 shows a comparison between the gain spectra of Er-doped fibers with and without aluminum codoping. The gain spectrum of Er-doped fiber with

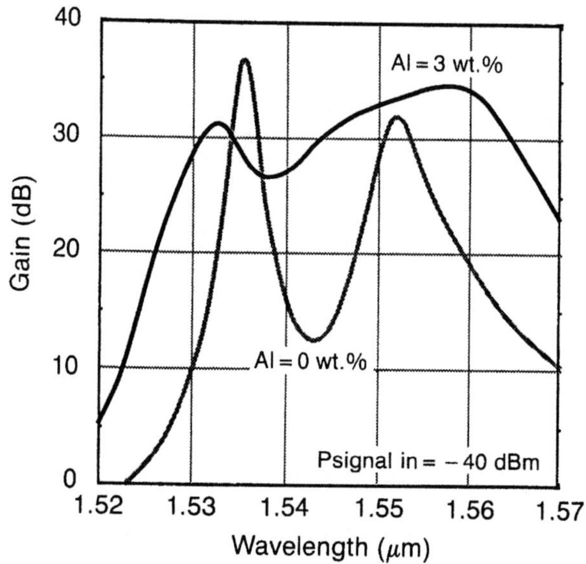

Figure 5.29 Gain spectrum of Er-doped fibers with different aluminum doping concentrations.

30,000 wt.ppm of Al is considerably flat and broad compared with that of fiber without Al.

The EDFA amplifies the optical signal directly, and thus transmission rate of the system can be changed even after the construction of the system. The EDFA is rapidly penetrating in long-haul terrestrial and submarine transmission systems.

5.10. FOUR-WAVE MIXING IN OPTICAL FIBER

The four-wave mixing (FWM) phenomenon is one of the important nonlinearities in optical fibers [42]. In FWM interactions, a fourth wavelength light is generated from three lights of different wavelengths. This phenomenon causes system degradation in multichannel transmission systems such as wavelength division multiplexing (WDM) system [43]. Contrary to it, FWM could be utilized for new frequency generation [44]. The efficiency of this nonlinear interaction strongly depends on phase matching conditions. The efficiency of the newly generated waves in the FWM process depends on the channel frequency separation, chromatic dispersion of fiber and fiber length.

Through an FWM process, three waves of frequencies f_i, f_j and $f_k (j \neq k)$ generate the frequency $f_{ijk} = f_i + f_j - f_k$ (subscripts i, j and k select 1, 2 and 3).

The time-averaged optical power P_{ijk} generated through the FWM process for the frequency component f_{ijk} is written as [42]

$$P_{ijk}(L) = \frac{1024\pi^6}{n^4\lambda^2c^2}\left(D\chi_{1111}^{(3)}\right)^2 \frac{P_iP_jP_k}{A_{\text{eff}}^2}\left|\frac{e^{(j\Delta\beta-\alpha)L}-1}{j\Delta\beta-\alpha}\right|^2 \cdot e^{-\alpha L}, \tag{5.102}$$

where L is the fiber length, n is the refractive index of the core, λ is the wavelength of light, c is the light velocity in vacuum, $D=3$ for two-tone products and 6 for three-tone products, $\chi_{1111}^{(3)}(=4\times10^{-15}\,\text{esu})$ is the third-order nonlinear susceptibility, A_{eff} is the effective area for the guided HE_{11} mode, P_i, P_j and P_k are the input powers launched into a single-mode fiber, α is the fiber attenuation coefficient and $\Delta\beta$ is the propagation constant difference defined by

$$\Delta\beta = \beta_{ijk} + \beta_k - \beta_i - \beta_j. \tag{5.103}$$

The third-order nonlinear susceptibility $\chi_{1111}^{(3)}$ can be expressed in terms of the nonlinear index of refraction n_2, in the case of a single polarization, as [45]

$$\chi_{1111}^{(3)}[\text{esu}] = \frac{cn^2}{480\pi^2} n_2[\text{m}^2/\text{W}]. \tag{5.104}$$

β is expressed by a Taylor series expansion around the angular frequency ω_0 as

$$\begin{aligned}\beta(\omega) &= \beta(\omega_0) + (\omega-\omega_0)\left(\frac{d\beta}{d\omega}\right)_{\omega=\omega_0} + \frac{(\omega-\omega_0)^2}{2}\left(\frac{d^2\beta}{d\omega^2}\right)_{\omega=\omega_0} \\ &\quad + \frac{(\omega-\omega_0)^3}{6}\left(\frac{d^3\beta}{d\omega^3}\right)_{\omega=\omega_0} \\ &= \beta(\omega_0) + \frac{\omega-\omega_0}{v_g} - \frac{(\omega-\omega_0)^2}{\omega_0^2}\pi c\sigma + \frac{(\omega-\omega_0)^3}{\omega_0^3}\frac{\pi c\lambda_0}{3}\left(\frac{2\sigma}{\lambda_0}+\rho\right),\end{aligned} \tag{5.105}$$

where Eqs. (3.108) and (3.143) are used for the expression of group velocity v_g and chromatic dispersion σ. In the above equation, ρ is a dispersion slope which is defined by

$$\rho = \frac{d\sigma}{d\lambda}. \tag{5.106}$$

$\Delta\beta$ is then given from Eqs. (5.103) and (5.105) as

$$\begin{aligned}\Delta\beta &= \frac{\pi\lambda_0^2\sigma}{c}\{(f_i - f_0)^2 + (f_j - f_0)^2 - (f_k - f_0)^2 - (f_{ijk} - f_0)^2\} \\ &\quad + \frac{\pi\lambda_0^4}{3c^2}\left(\frac{2\sigma}{\lambda_0} + \rho\right)\{(f_{ijk} - f_0)^3 + (f_k - f_0)^3 - (f_i - f_0)^3 - (f_j - f_0)^3\} \\ &= \frac{2\pi\lambda_0^2\sigma}{c}(f_i - f_k)(f_k - f_j) \\ &\quad + \frac{\pi\lambda_0^4}{c^2}\left(\frac{2\sigma}{\lambda_0} + \rho\right)(f_i + f_j - 2f_0)(f_i - f_k)(f_j - f_k),\end{aligned} \tag{5.107}$$

where $f_\ell = \omega_\ell/2\pi$ and phase-matching condition $f_{ijk} = f_i + f_j - f_k$ has been used. Here we choose f_0 as the fiber zero-dispersion frequency ($\sigma(f_0) = 0$). When signal frequencies f_i, f_j, f_k and f_{ijk} are close to the zero-dispersion frequency, σ becomes almost zero. In this case, Eq. (5.107) reduces to

$$\Delta\beta = \frac{\pi\lambda_0^4}{c^2}\rho(f_i + f_j - 2f_0)(f_i - f_k)(f_j - f_k). \tag{5.108}$$

It is known that the phase-matching condition ($\Delta\beta = 0$) is always satisfied when the fiber zero-dispersion frequency is located at the middle of the two signals with frequency f_i and $f_j (f_0 = (f_i + f_j)/2)$. Since $f_{ijk} = f_i + f_j - f_k = 2f_0 - f_k$, we then obtain the relation for the frequency of FWM light as

$$f_0 - f_{ijk} = f_k - f_0. \tag{5.109}$$

Thus, FWM light is generated at the opposite side of f_k with equal frequency separation to the zero-dispersion frequency. Frequency arrangement of this phase-matching condition is shown in Fig. 5.30(a). When two of the three lights are degenerate as $f_i = f_j$, Eq. (5.108) can be rewritten as

$$\Delta\beta = \frac{\pi\lambda_0^4\rho}{c^2}2(f_i - f_0)(f_i - f_k)^2. \tag{5.110}$$

It is noted from Eq. (5.110) that the phase-matching condition is always satisfied when f_i coincides with the zero-dispersion frequency ($f_i = f_0$). Frequency arrangement for this phase-matching condition is illustrated in Fig. 5.30(b).

Efficiency of the generated wave η with respect to phase mismatch $\Delta\beta \cdot L$ can be obtained by

$$\eta = \frac{P_{ijk}(L, \Delta\beta)}{P_{ijk}(L, \Delta\beta = 0)} = \frac{\alpha^2}{\alpha^2 + (\Delta\beta)^2} \cdot \left[1 + \frac{\sin^2(\Delta\beta \cdot L/2)}{\sinh^2(\alpha L/2)}\right]. \tag{5.111}$$

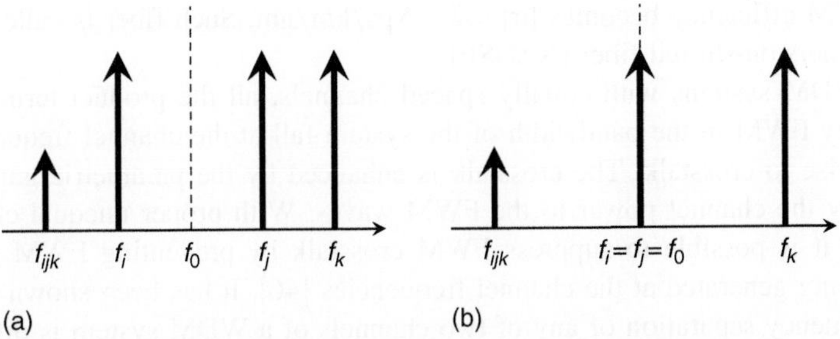

Figure 5.30 Signal frequency arrangement satisfying the phase-matching condition in the zero-dispersion region in (a) nondegenerate case and, (b) partially degenerate case.

P_{ijk} of Eq. (5.102) is given for two cases of frequency arrangement by using the efficiency η as

$$P_{ijk} = \eta \frac{1024\pi^6}{n^4\lambda^2c^2}\left(6\chi_{1111}^{(3)}\right)^2\left(\frac{L_{\text{eff}}}{A_{\text{eff}}}\right)^2 P_iP_jP_k \cdot e^{-\alpha L} \quad (f_i \neq f_j \neq f_k) \quad (5.112a)$$

and

$$P_{iik} = \eta \frac{1024\pi^6}{n^4\lambda^2c^2}\left(3\chi_{1111}^{(3)}\right)^2\left(\frac{L_{\text{eff}}}{A_{\text{eff}}}\right)^2 P_i^2P_k \cdot e^{-\alpha L} \quad (f_i = f_j \neq f_k), \quad (5.112b)$$

where L_{eff} is the effective interaction length (Eq. (5.6)).

Figure 5.31 shows the generated wave efficiency η for a two-tone product $(f_i = f_j \neq f_k)$ as a function of channel spacing Δf in WDM by substituting Eq. (5.107) into (5.111). $\Delta\beta$ for the two-tone product case is obtained from Eq. (5.107) as

$$\Delta\beta = -\frac{2\pi\lambda_0^2}{c}(f_k - f_i)^2\left\{\sigma + \frac{\lambda_0^2}{c}\left(\frac{2\sigma}{\lambda_0} + \rho\right)(f_0 - f_i)\right\}. \quad (5.113)$$

Parameters that are used in the calculation are $\lambda_0 = 1.55\,\mu\text{m}$, $\alpha = 0.2\,\text{dB/km}(4.6 \times 10^{-5}\,\text{m}^{-1})$, $L = 100\,\text{km}$ and $\rho = 0.06\,\text{ps/km/nm}$. In the case of $\sigma = 0$, one of the two tones f_k is coincident with the fiber zero-dispersion frequency f_0, and the mixing product farthest from the zero-dispersion frequency is considered. It is noted from Fig. 5.31 that FWM efficiency is quite high for DSF ($\sigma = 0\,\text{ps/km/nm}$) when channel spacing Δf is less than 100 GHz. Slight increase in $|\sigma|$ dramatically decreases the FWM efficiency as shown in the plot of $\sigma = 2\,\text{ps/km/nm}$. Chromatic dispersion should be as small as possible since the signal bandwidth B is inversely proportional to $\sqrt{\sigma}$ (Eq. (3.213)) or σ (Eq. (3.214)). Then the optimum dispersion value σ while keeping sufficiently low FWM efficiency becomes $|\sigma| = 2 \sim 5$ ps/km/nm. Such fiber is called non-zero dispersion-shifted fiber (NZDSF).

In WDM systems with equally spaced channels, all the product terms generated by FWM in the bandwidth of the system fall at the channel frequencies, giving rise to crosstalk. The crosstalk is enhanced by the parametric gain provided by the channel power to the FWM waves. With proper unequal channel spacing it is possible to suppress FWM crosstalk by preventing FWM waves from being generated at the channel frequencies [46]. It has been shown that if the frequency separation of any of two channels of a WDM system is different from that of any other pair of channels, no FWM waves will be generated at any of the channel frequencies. Therefore, unequal-channel-spacing signal allocation is quite advantageous especially for WDM systems using DSF. The effectiveness of unequal channel spacing in keeping mixing products outside the channel frequency slots is shown in Fig. 5.32(b), where the number of FWM waves generated in each frequency slot is plotted for the case of an eight-channel system. Arrows show channel locations. It can be observed that all equal-channel-spaced (Fig. 5.32(a)) mixing products in the bandwidth of the system are located in slots occupied by the channels, generating maximum interference. Figure 5.32(b) shows the effect of using proper unequal spacing [46]. The frequency slots dedicated to channels are free from mixing products. The mixing products are all evenly distributed in slots between the channels and they can be filtered out by the filter [47].

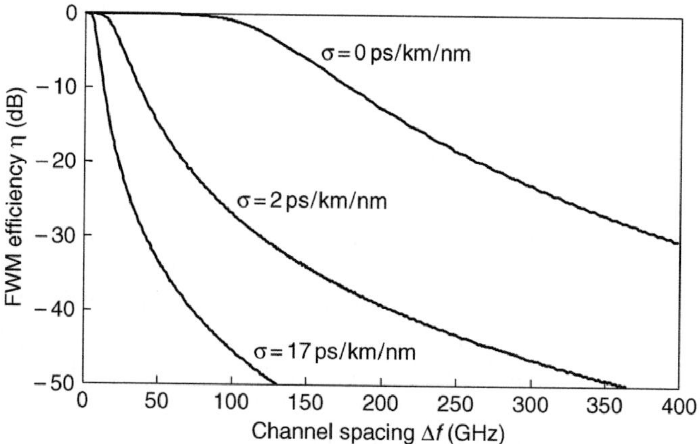

Figure 5.31 Generated wave efficiency η for a two-tone product ($f_i = f_j \neq f_k$) as a function of channel spacing Δf in WDM.

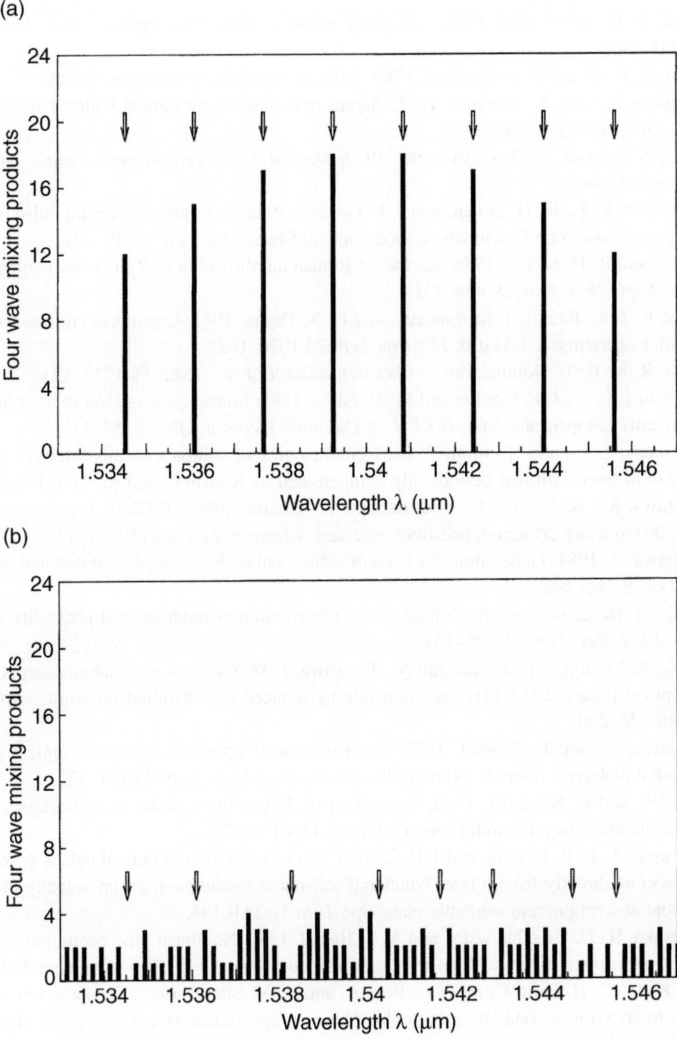

Figure 5.32 Number of FWM waves generated in the case of an eight-channel WDM system with (a) equal and (b) unequal channel spacing. Arrows indicate channel centers.

REFERENCES

[1] Agrawal, G. P. 1989. *Nonlinear Fiber Optics*. San Diego: Academic Press.

[2] Yariv, A. 1977. *Introduction to Optical Electronics*. New York: Holt, Rinehart and Winston.

[3] Hellwarth, R. W. 1977. Third-order optical susceptibilities of liquids and solids. *Prog. Quantum Electron*. 5:1–68.

[4] Stolen, R. H. and C. Lin. 1978. Self-phase-modulation in silica optical fibers. *Phys. Rev. A* 17:1448–1453.

[5] Bullough, R. K. and P. J. Caudrey. 1980. *Solitons*. Heidelberg: Springer-Verlag.

[6] Hasegawa, A. and Y. Kodama. 1981. Signal transmission by optical solitons in monomode fiber. *Proc. IEEE* 69:1445–1450.

[7] Miller, S. E., and A. G. Chynoweth. 1979. *Optical Fiber Telecommunications*. New York: Academic Press.

[8] Mollenauer, L. F., R. H. Stolen, and J. P. Gordon. 1983. Extreme picosecond pulse narrowing by means of soliton effect in single-mode optical fibers. *Opt. Lett.* 8:289–291.

[9] Lin, C., and R. H. Stolen. 1976. Backward Raman amplification and pulse steepening in silica fibers. *Appl. Phys. Lett.* 29:428–431.

[10] Mears, R. J., L. Reekie, I. M. Jauncey, and D. N. Payne. 1987. Low-noise erbium-doped fiber amplifier operating at 1.54 μm. *Electron Lett.* 23:1026–1028.

[11] Stolen, R. H. 1980. Nonlinearity in fiber transmission. *Proc. IEEE* 68:1232–1236.

[12] Mollenauer, L. F., J. P. Gordon and M. N. Islam. 1986. Soliton propagation in long fibers with periodically compensated loss. *IEEE J. of Quantum Electron.* QE-22:157–173.

[13] Mollenauer, L. F., and K. Smith. 1988. Demonstration of soliton transmission over more than 4000 km in fiber with loss periodically compensated by Raman gain. *Opt. Lett.* 13:657–677.

[14] Nakazawa, M., K. Suzuki, K. Yamada, and Y. Kimura. 1990. 20 Gbit/s soliton transmission over 200 km using erbium-doped fiber repeaters. *Electron. Lett.* 26:1592–1593.

[15] Hasegawa, A. 1984. Generation of a train of soliton pulses by induced modulational instability. *Opt. Lett.* 9:288–290.

[16] Tai, K., A. Hasegawa, and A. Tomita. 1986. Observation of modulational instability in optical fibers. *Phys. Rev. Lett.* 56:135–138.

[17] Tai, K., A. Tomita, J. L. Jewell, and A. Hasegawa. 1986. Generation of subpicosecond soliton-like optical pulses at 0.3 THz repitition rate by induced modulational instability. *Appl. Phys. Lett.* 49:236–238.

[18] Hasegawa, A., and F. Tappert. 1973. Transmission of stationary nonlinear optical pulses in dispersive dielectric fibers II. Normal dispersion. *Appl. Phys. Lett.* 23:171–172.

[19] Zhao, W., and E. Bourkoff. 1990. Generation of dark solitons under a cw background using waveguide electro-optic modulators. *Opt. Lett.* 15:405–407.

[20] Valdmanis, J. A., R. L. Fork, and J. P. Gordon. 1985. Generation of optical pulses as short as 27 femtosecond directly from a laser balancing self-phase modulation, group-velocity dispersion, saturable absorption, and saturable gain. *Opt. Lett.* 10:131–133.

[21] Nakatsuka, H., D. Grischkowsky, and A. C. Balant. 1981. Nonlinear picosecond-pulse propagation through optical fibers with positive group velocity dispersion. *Phys. Rev. Lett.* 47:910–913.

[22] Fork, R. L., C. H. Brito Cruz, P. C. Becker, and C. V. Shank. 1987. Compression of optical pulses to six femtoseconds by using cubic phase compensation. *Opt. Lett.* 12:483–485.

[23] Tomlinson, W. J., R. H. Stolen, and A. M. Johnson. 1985. Optical wave breaking of pulses in nonlinear optical fibers. *Opt. Lett.* 10:457–459.

[24] Treacy, E. B. 1969. Optical pulse compression with diffraction gratings. *IEEE J. Quantum Electron.* QE-5:454–458.

[25] Kafka, J. D., and T. Baer. 1987. Prism-pair dispersive delay lines in optical pulse compression. *Opt. Lett.* 12:401–403.

[26] Cardona, M., and G. Ed. Guntherodt. 1982. *Light Scattering in Solids III*. Berlin: Springer-Verlag.

[27] Grindlay, J., and R. Howard. 1965. *Lattice Dynamics*. New York: Pergamon Press.

[28] Smith, R. G. 1972. Optical power handling capability of low loss optical fibers as determined by stimulated Raman and Brillouin scattering. *Appl. Opt.* 11:2489–2494.

[29] Hegarty, J., N. A. Olsson, and L. Goldner. 1985. CW pumped Raman preamplifier in a 45 km-long fiber transmission system operating at 1.5 μm and 1 Gbit/s. *Electron. Lett.* 21:290–292.

[30] Zel'dovich, B. Y., N. F. Pilipetsky, and V. V. Shkunov. 1985. *Principles of Phase Conjugation.* Berlin: Springer-Verlag.

[31] Lagakos, N., J. A. Bucaro, and R. Hughes. 1980. Acoustic sensitivity predictions of single-mode optical fibers using Brillouin scattering. *Appl. Opt.* 19:3668–3670.

[32] Schroeder, J., L. G. Hwa, M. C. Shyong, G. A. Floudas, D. A. Thompson, and M. G. Drexhage. 1987. Brillouin scattering and phonon attenuation in halide glasses—Stimulated Brillouin emission. *Electron. Lett.* 23:1128–1130.

[33] Shelby, R. M., M. D. Levenson, and P. W. Bayer. 1985. Resolved forward Brillouin scattering in optical fibers. *Phys. Rev. Lett.* 54:939–942.

[34] Denariez, M., and G. Bret. 1968. Investigation of Rayleigh wings and Brillouin-stimulated scattering in liquids. *Phys. Rev.* 171:160–171.

[35] Aoki, Y., K. Tajima, and I. Mito. 1986. Observation of stimulated Brillouin scattering in single-mode fibers with DFB-LD pumping and its suppression by FSK modulation. *Tech. Digest of CLEO '86*, San Francisco, Post Deadline Paper no. ThU4.

[36] Olsson, N. A., and J. P. van der Ziel. 1986. Cancellation of fiber loss by semiconductor laser pumped Brillouin amplification at 1.5 μm. *Appl. Phys. Lett.* 48:1329–1330.

[37] Österberg, U., and W. Margulis. 1986. Dye laser pumped by Nd:YAG laser pulses frequency doubled in a glass optical fiber. *Opt. Lett.* 11:516–518.

[38] Gabriagues, J. M., and H. Fevrier. 1987. Analysis of frequency-doubling processes in optical fibers using Raman spectroscopy. *Opt. Lett.* 12:720–722.

[39] Bethune, D. S. 1981. Quadrupole second-harmonic generation for a focused beam of arbitrary transverse structure and polarization. *Opt. Lett.* 6:287–289.

[40] Farries, M. C., P. St. J. Russell, M. E. Fermann, and D. N. Payne. 1987. Second-harmonic generation in an optical fiber by self-written $\chi^{(2)}$ grating. *Electron. Lett.* 23:322–324.

[41] Snitzer, E. 1961. Optical maser action of Nd^{3+} in a barium crown glass. *Phys. Rev. Lett.* 7:444–446.

[42] Hill, K. O., D. C. Johnson, B. S. Kawasaki and R. I. MacDonald. 1978. CW three-wave mixing in single-mode optical fibers. *J. Appl. Phys.* 49:5098–5106.

[43] Shibata, N., K. Nosu, K. Iwashita, and Y. Azuma. 1990. Transmission limitation due to four-wave mixing in single-mode optical fibers. *IEEE J. Select. Area Commun.* 8:1068–1077.

[44] Lin, C., W. A. Reed, A. D. Pearson, and H. T. Shang. 1982. Designing single-mode fibers for near-IR (1.1 mm–1.7 mm) frequency generation by phase-matched four-wave mixing in the minimum chromatic dispersion region. *Electron. Lett.* 18:87–88.

[45] Tkach, R. W., A. R. Chraplyvy, F. Forghieri, A. H. Gnauck, and R. M. Derosier. 1995. Four-photon mixing and high-speed WDM systems. *IEEE J. of Lightwave Tech.* 13:841–849.

[46] Forghieri, F., R. W. Tkach, A. R. Chraplyvy, and D. Marcuse. 1994. Reduction of four-wave mixing crosstalk in WDM systems using unequally spaced channels. *IEEE Photonics Tech. Lett.* 6:754–756.

[47] Okamoto, K., M. Ishii, Y. Hibino, Y. Ohmori, and H. Toba. 1995. Fabrication of unequal channel spacing arrayed-waveguide grating multiplexer modules. *Electron. Lett.* 31:1464–1465.

Chapter 6

Finite Element Method

The waveguide analyses described in Chapters 2 and 3 are restricted in applicability to the homogeneous-core (step-index) planar optical waveguides and optical fibers, except for the WKB (Wentzel–Kramers–Brillouin) method described in Section 3.7.2. However, inhomogeneous-core (graded-index) planar waveguides and fibers are utilized in many practical fields. Therefore, analysis techniques capable of solving the wave equations for inhomogeneous-core planar waveguides and fibers are quite important. As shown in Section 2.2.4, Ridge waveguides, which have a homogeneous core but complicated cross-sectional waveguide geometries, are often used for semiconductor optical devices, The finite element method (FEM) is suitable for the mode analysis of optical waveguides having arbitrary refractive-index profiles and complicated waveguide structures. Needless to say, FEM is also applicable to the stress analysis of optical waveguides. In this chapter, FEM mode analyses of slab waveguides, rectangular waveguides, and optical fibers are first presented. Then stress analysis of waveguides and the combination of stress analysis with mode analysis are explained.

6.1. INTRODUCTION

In the variational method, the boundary-value problem (the problem given in the form of a differential equation in a certain domain, which should be solved under the given boundary conditions) is transformed into the equivalent variational problem and is solved by applying the variational principle [1–4]. In the finite element method, the domain of the problem is discretized into small elements. The solution of the problem is approximated in each element and it is connected at the nodal points to form the solution model in the entire analysis domain. Therefore, FEM is applicable to the complicated domain structures and to problems in which electromagnetic fields are localized. In classical analytical procedures without subdivision processes, the system is modeled using analytical functions defined over the whole region of interest, and therefore these procedures generally are applicable only to simple geometries and materials. One of the simplest method that employs the discretization procedure is the finite difference method (FDM). In FDM, the domain is discretized into small lattice regions using regular rectangular grids. However, a rectangular grid is not suitable for curved boundaries or interfaces, because they intersect gridlines obliquely at points other than the nodes. Moreover, a regular grid is not suitable for problems with very steep variations of fields. In FEM, a simple form of function is adopted to approximate the field in each element. The possible error in the solution is alleviated by increasing the number of elements and thus reducing the element size. All of the element contributions to the system are assembled to form the functional. The functional essentially consists of the field values at the n nodes and boundary conditions at the peripheral nodes; that is, n-th order linear simultaneous equations are obtained. The solutions of the simultaneous equations give the unknown field values to be determined.

In this chapter, FEM waveguide analyses for slab waveguide, optical fibers, and three-dimensional waveguides and also FEM stress analyses in optical waveguide devices are described. Waveguide analysis and stress analysis are totally different problems. However, the discretization procedures and the formulation of the functionals are rather similar in both problems. Such versatility in the mathematical procedures is the great advantage of FEM.

6.2. FINITE ELEMENT METHOD ANALYSIS OF SLAB WAVEGUIDES

6.2.1. Variational Formulation

In this section, the formulation of FEM is described, taking the TE mode as an example in the inhomogeneous slab waveguide. As shown in Fig. 6.1, the transverse region $0 \leqslant x \leqslant A$ which has an inhomogeneous refractive-index profile, is denoted as the core, and refractive indices in the cladding and the substrate are assumed to be constant. The maximum refractive index in the core is n_1, and the refractive indices in cladding and the substrate are n_0 and n_s, respectively. Here we assume $n_s \geqslant n_0$. The wave equation for the TE mode is given, by Eq. (2.5) as

$$\frac{d^2E_y}{dx^2} + (k^2n^2 - \beta^2)E_y = 0. \tag{6.1}$$

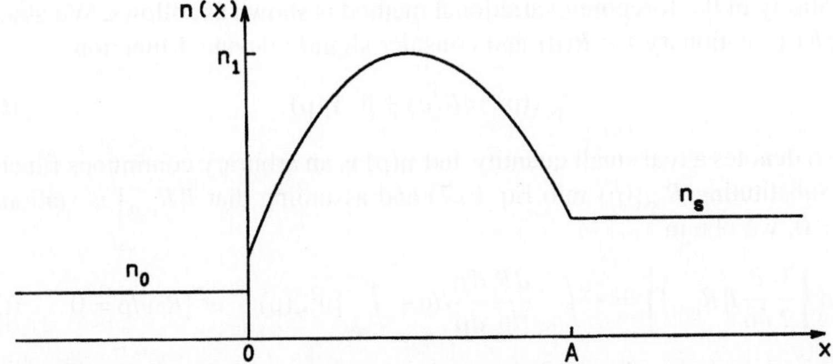

Figure 6.1 Refractive-index distribution of the inhomogeneous slab optical waveguide.

The boundary conditions require the continuity of E_y and

$$H_z = \frac{j}{\omega\mu_0}\frac{dE_y}{dx} \tag{6.2}$$

at $x = 0$ and $x = A$. Before transforming the wave equation (6.1) and boundary condition (6.2) into the variational problem, the parameters are normalized as

$$\rho = x/a, \; E_y(x) = R(\rho), \; D = A/a. \tag{6.3}$$

The wave equation and boundary condition are then rewritten as

$$\frac{d^2R}{d\rho^2} + [v^2 q(\rho) - w^2]R = 0, \tag{6.4}$$

$$R(\rho) \text{ and } dR(\rho)/d\rho \text{ are continuous at } \rho = 0 \text{ and } \rho = D. \tag{6.5}$$

Here normalized transverse wavenumber w, normalized frequency v and normalized refractive-index distribution $q(\rho)$ are defined by

$$w = a\sqrt{\beta^2 - k^2 n_s^2}, \tag{6.6a}$$

$$v = ka\sqrt{n_1^2 - n_s^2}, \tag{6.6b}$$

$$q(\rho) = \frac{n^2 - n_s^2}{n_1^2 - n_s^2}. \tag{6.6c}$$

The solution of the wave equation (6.4) under the constraints of the boundary condition (6.5) is obtained as the solution of the variational problem which satisfies the stationary condition of the functional

$$I[R] = -\int_{-\infty}^{\infty}\left(\frac{dR}{d\rho}\right)^2 d\rho + \int_{-\infty}^{\infty}[v^2 q(\rho) - w^2]R^2 \, d\rho. \tag{6.7}$$

The validity of the foregoing variational method is shown as follows. We assume that $I[R]$ is stationary for $R(\rho)$ and consider slightly deviated function

$$R_{\text{pert}}(\rho) = R(\rho) + \delta \cdot \eta(\rho), \tag{6.8}$$

where δ denotes a real small quantity and $\eta(\rho)$ is an arbitrary continuous function of ρ. Substituting $R_{\text{pert}}(\rho)$ into Eq. (6.7) and assuming that $I[R_{\text{pert}}]$ is stationary for $\delta = 0$, we obtain

$$\lim_{\delta \to 0} \left\{ \frac{1}{2} \frac{\partial}{\partial \delta} I[R_{\text{pert}}] \right\} = -\int_{-\infty}^{\infty} \frac{dR}{d\rho} \frac{d\eta}{d\rho} d\rho + \int_{-\infty}^{\infty} [v^2 q(\rho) - w^2] R \eta d\rho = 0. \tag{6.9}$$

By partial integration, Eq. (6.9) is rewritten as

$$-\left[\eta \frac{dR}{d\rho} \right]_{-\infty}^{\infty} + \int_{-\infty}^{\infty} \left\{ \frac{d^2 R}{d\rho^2} + [v^2 q(\rho) - w^2] R \right\} \eta(\rho) d\rho = 0. \tag{6.10}$$

Since $\eta(\rho)$ is arbitrary function of ρ, the first and the second terms of Eq. (6.10) should be zero independently. Then $R(\rho)$ satisfies the wave equation (6.4) and the boundary conditions of

$$\frac{dR}{d\rho} \text{ is continuous and } \lim_{\rho \to \pm\infty} \frac{dR}{d\rho} = 0. \tag{6.11}$$

The second condition is a natural boundary condition that states that the solution decays at the infinity (electromagnetic field is confined in the waveguide). It is then proved that the function $R(\rho)$ that makes the functional (6.7) stationary satisfies the wave equation (6.4) and the boundary condition (6.5) simultaneously.

6.2.2. Discretization of the Functional

In order to simplify calculation of the functional, the field profile in the core is discretized and expressed as

$$R(\rho) = \begin{cases} R_0 \exp(w_0 \rho) & (\rho < 0) \\ \sum_{i=0}^{N} R_i \phi_i(\rho) & (0 \leqslant \rho \leqslant D) \\ R_N \exp[-w(\rho - D)] & (\rho > D), \end{cases} \tag{6.12}$$

where $R_0 - R_N$ are field values at the sampling points and

$$w_0 = a\sqrt{\beta^2 - k^2 n_0^2}, \tag{6.13a}$$

$$R_i = R(\rho_i) \quad (i = 0 - N), \tag{6.13b}$$

$$\rho_i = i\frac{D}{N} \quad (i = 0 - N). \tag{6.13c}$$

The solutions in the cladding and the substrate are given by the analytical functions. The sampling function $\phi_i(\rho)$ becomes unity at $\rho = \rho_i$, becomes zero at the neighboring sampling points $\rho = \rho_{i-1}$ and $\rho = \rho_{i+1}$ and is zero throughout all other regions, as shown in Fig. 6.2. The precise expressions of $\phi_i(\rho)$ are given by

$$\phi_o(\rho) = \begin{cases} \dfrac{N}{D}(\rho_1 - \rho) & (0 \leqslant \rho \leqslant \rho_1) \\ 0 & \text{all other areas} \end{cases} \tag{6.14a}$$

$$\phi_i(\rho) = \begin{cases} \dfrac{N}{D}(\rho - \rho_{i-1}) & (\rho_{i-1} \leqslant \rho \leqslant \rho_i) \\ \dfrac{N}{D}(\rho_{i+1} - \rho) & (\rho_i \leqslant \rho \leqslant \rho_{i+1}) \\ 0 & \text{all other areas} \end{cases} \tag{6.14b}$$

$$\phi_N(\rho) = \begin{cases} \dfrac{N}{D}(\rho - \rho_{N-1}) & (\rho_{N-1} \leqslant \rho \leqslant \rho_N) \\ 0 & \text{all other areas.} \end{cases} \tag{6.14c}$$

Since the sampling function here is a linear function of ρ, Eq. (6.12) means that the continuous function $R(\rho)$ is approximated by the broken lines. The normalized refractive-index distribution $q(\rho)$ is also approximated, by using the

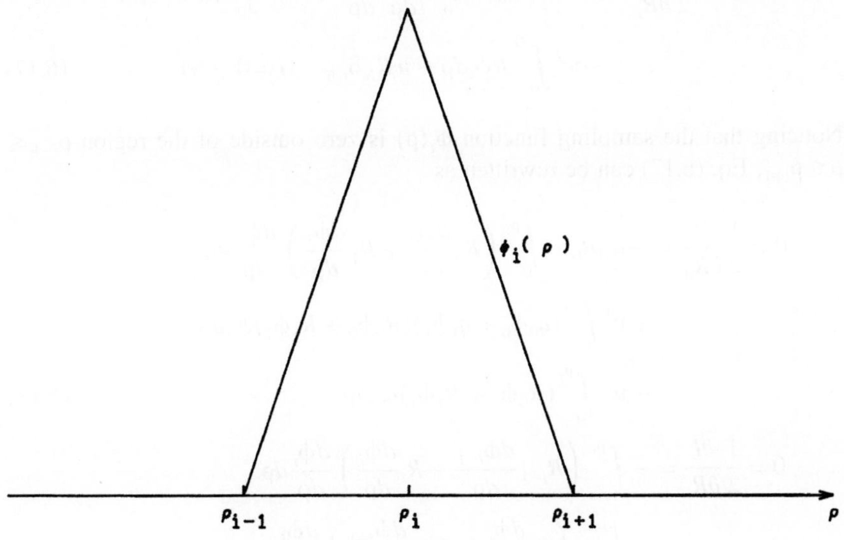

Figure 6.2 Sampling function $\phi_i(\rho)$.

sampling function, as

$$q(\rho) = \sum_{i=0}^{N} q_i \phi_i(\rho) \tag{6.15a}$$

$$q_i = \frac{n^2(\rho_i) - n_s^2}{n_1^2 - n_s^2} \tag{6.15b}$$

in order to deal with the waveguides having arbitrary inhomogeneous refractive-index profiles. Substituting Eq. (6.12) into Eq. (6.7), we obtain the functional

$$I = -w_0 R_0^2 - \int_0^D \left(\frac{dR}{d\rho}\right)^2 d\rho + \int_0^D [v^2 q(\rho) - w^2] R^2 \, d\rho - w R_N^2. \tag{6.16}$$

6.2.3. Dispersion Equation Based on the Stationary Condition

The stationary condition of the functional (6.16) is given, by the partial differentiation with respect to $R_i (i = 0 - N)$, as

$$0 = \frac{1}{2}\frac{\partial I}{\partial R_i} = -w_0 R_0 \delta_{i,o} - \int_0^D \frac{dR}{d\rho}\frac{d\phi_i}{d\rho} d\rho + v^2 \int_0^D q(\rho) R \phi_i d\rho$$
$$- w^2 \int_0^D R\phi_i d\rho - w R_N \delta_{i,N} \quad (i = 0 - N). \tag{6.17}$$

Noticing that the sampling function $\phi_i(\rho)$ is zero outside of the region $\rho_{i-1} \leqslant \rho \leqslant \rho_{i+1}$, Eq. (6.17) can be rewritten as

$$0 = \frac{1}{2}\frac{\partial I}{\partial R_0} = -w_0 R_0 - \int_0^{\rho_1} \left(R_0 \frac{d\phi_0}{d\rho} + R_1 \frac{d\phi_1}{d\rho}\right) \frac{d\phi_0}{d\rho} d\rho$$
$$+ v^2 \int_0^{\rho_1} (q_0\phi_0 + q_1\phi_1)(R_0\phi_0 + R_1\phi_1)\phi_0 d\rho$$
$$- w^2 \int_0^{\rho_1} (R_0\phi_0 + R_1\phi_1)\phi_0 d\rho. \tag{6.18}$$

$$0 = \frac{1}{2}\frac{\partial I}{\partial R_i} = -\int_{\rho_{i-1}}^{\rho_i} \left(R_{i-1}\frac{d\phi_{i-1}}{d\rho} + R_i \frac{d\phi_i}{d\rho}\right)\frac{d\phi_i}{d\rho} d\rho$$
$$- \int_{\rho_i}^{\rho_{i+1}} \left(R_i \frac{d\phi_i}{d\rho} + R_{i+1}\frac{d\phi_{i+1}}{d\rho}\right)\frac{d\phi_i}{d\rho} d\rho$$

$$+v^2\int_{\rho_{i-1}}^{\rho}(q_{i-1}\phi_{i-1}+q_i\phi_i)(R_{i-1}\phi_{i-1}+R_i\phi_i)\phi_i d\rho$$
$$+v^2\int_{\rho_i}^{\rho_{i+1}}(q_i\phi_i+q_{i+1}\phi_{i+1})(R_i\phi_i+R_{i+1}\phi_{i+1})\phi_i d\rho$$
$$-w^2\int_{\rho_{i-1}}^{\rho_i}(R_{i-1}\phi_{i-1}+R_i\phi_i)\phi_i d\rho$$
$$-w^2\int_{\rho_i}^{\rho_{i+1}}(R_i\phi_i+R_{i+1}\phi_{i+1})\phi_i d\rho,\quad (i=1-N-1) \tag{6.19}$$

$$0=\frac{1}{2}\frac{\partial I}{\partial R_N}=-\int_{\rho_{N-1}}^{\rho_N}\left(R_{N-1}\frac{d\phi_{N-1}}{d\rho}+R_N\frac{\phi_N}{d\rho}\right)\frac{d\phi_N}{d\rho}d\rho$$
$$+v^2\int_{\rho_{N-1}}^{\rho_N}(q_{N-1}\phi_{N-1}+q_N\phi_N)(R_{N-1}\phi_{N-1}+R_N\phi_N)\phi_N d\rho$$
$$-w^2\int_{\rho_{N-1}}^{\rho_N}(R_{N-1}\phi_{N-1}+R_N\phi_N)\phi_N d\rho-w\,R_N. \tag{6.20}$$

The integral of the sampling functions, which appears in Eqs. (6.18) and (6.19), is given by

$$\int_{\rho_{i-1}}^{\rho_i}\frac{d\phi_{i-1}}{d\rho}\frac{d\phi_i}{d\rho}d\rho=-\frac{N}{D}\qquad(i=1-N) \tag{6.21a}$$
$$\int_{\rho_{i-1}}^{\rho_i}\left(\frac{d\phi_i}{d\rho}\right)^2 d\rho=\frac{N}{D}\qquad(i=1-N) \tag{6.21b}$$
$$\int_{\rho_i}^{\rho_{i+1}}\left(\frac{d\phi_i}{d\rho}\right)^2 d\rho=\frac{N}{D}\qquad(i=0-N-1) \tag{6.21c}$$
$$\int_{\rho_{i-1}}^{\rho_i}\phi_{i-1}^2\phi_i\,d\rho=\frac{1}{12}\frac{D}{N}\qquad(i=1-N) \tag{6.21d}$$
$$\int_{\rho_{i-1}}^{\rho_i}\phi_{i-1}\phi_i^2\,d\rho=\frac{1}{12}\frac{D}{N}\qquad(i=1-N) \tag{6.21e}$$
$$\int_{\rho_{i-1}}^{\rho_i}\phi_i^3\,d\rho=\frac{1}{4}\frac{D}{N}\qquad(i=1-N) \tag{6.21f}$$
$$\int_{\rho_i}^{\rho_{i+1}}\phi_i^3\,d\rho=\frac{1}{4}\frac{D}{N}\qquad(i=0-N-1) \tag{6.21g}$$
$$\int_{\rho_{i-1}}^{\rho_i}\phi_{i-1}\phi_i\,d\rho=\frac{1}{6}\frac{D}{N}\qquad(i=1-N) \tag{6.21h}$$
$$\int_{\rho_{i-1}}^{\rho_i}\phi_i^2\,d\rho=\frac{1}{3}\frac{D}{N}\qquad(i=1-N) \tag{6.21i}$$
$$\int_{\rho_i}^{\rho_{i+1}}\phi_i^2\,d\rho=\frac{1}{3}\frac{D}{N}\qquad(i=0-N-1). \tag{6.21j}$$

Substituting Eq. (6.21) in Eqs. (6.18)–(6.20), we obtain

$$-\frac{1}{2}\frac{D}{N}\frac{\partial I}{\partial R_0}=R_0\left\{1-(3q_0+q_1)\frac{v^2}{12}\left(\frac{D}{N}\right)^2+\frac{w^2}{3}\left(\frac{D}{N}\right)^2+w_0\frac{D}{N}\right\}$$

$$+R_1\left\{-1-(q_0+q_1)\frac{v^2}{12}\left(\frac{D}{N}\right)^2+\frac{w^2}{6}\left(\frac{D}{N}\right)^2\right\}=0, \quad (6.22a)$$

$$-\frac{1}{2}\frac{D}{N}\frac{\partial I}{\partial R_i}=R_{i-1}\left\{-1-(q_{i-1}+q_i)\frac{v^2}{12}\left(\frac{D}{N}\right)^2+\frac{w^2}{6}\left(\frac{D}{N}\right)^2\right\}$$

$$+R_i\left\{2-(q_{i-1}+6q_i+q_{i+1})\frac{v^2}{12}\left(\frac{D}{N}\right)^2+\frac{2w^2}{3}\left(\frac{D}{N}\right)^2\right\}$$

$$+R_{i+1}\left\{-1-(q_i+q_{i+1})\frac{v^2}{12}\left(\frac{D}{N}\right)^2\right.$$

$$\left.+\frac{w^2}{6}\left(\frac{D}{N}\right)^2\right\}=0 \qquad (i=1-N-1) \quad (6.22b)$$

$$-\frac{1}{2}\frac{D}{N}\frac{\partial I}{\partial R_N}=R_{N-i}\left\{-1-(q_{N-1}+q_N)\frac{v^2}{12}\left(\frac{D}{N}\right)^2+\frac{w^2}{6}\left(\frac{D}{N}\right)^2\right\}$$

$$+R_N\left\{1-(q_{N-1}+3q_N)\frac{v^2}{12}\left(\frac{D}{N}\right)^2+\frac{w^2}{3}\left(\frac{D}{N}\right)^2+w\frac{D}{N}\right\}=0. \quad (6.22c)$$

Equation (6.22) is a set of $(N+1)$th order simultaneous equations having R_0-R_N as the unknown values. In order that Eq. (6.22) have nontrivial solutions except for $R_0=R_1=\cdots=R_N=0$, the determinant of the matrix **C** should be

$$\det(\mathbf{C})=0. \quad (6.23)$$

The matrix elements of **C** are given by

$$c_{0,0}=1-(3q_0+q_1)\frac{v^2}{12}\delta^2+\frac{w^2}{3}\delta^2+w_0\delta, \quad (6.24a)$$

$$c_{i,i}=2-(q_{i-1}+6q_i+q_{i+1})\frac{v^2}{12}\delta^2+\frac{2w^2}{3}\delta^2 \quad (i=1-N-1), \quad (6.24b)$$

$$c_{i,i+1}=c_{i+1,i}=-1-(q_i+q_{i+1})\frac{v^2}{12}\delta^2+\frac{w^2}{6}\delta^2 \quad (i=0-N-1), \quad (6.24c)$$

$$c_{N,N}=1-(q_{N-1}+3q_N)\frac{v^2}{12}\delta^2+\frac{w^2}{3}\delta^2+w\delta, \quad (6.24d)$$

where discretization step δ is given by

$$\delta = \frac{D}{N}. \tag{6.25}$$

Equation (6.23) is a dispersion equation (eigenvalue equation) for the TE modes in the arbitrary refractive-index profiles. When the refractive-index distribution $q(\rho)$ of the waveguide and the normalized frequency v are given, the propagation constant β (implicitly contained in w and w_0) is calculated from Eqs. (6.23) and (6.24). When we set $w = 0(\beta = kn_s)$ in Eq. (6.24), the solution of Eq. (6.23) gives the cutoff v-value of the waveguide.

6.2.4. Dispersion Characteristics of Graded-index Slab Waveguides

Next FEM analysis for the TM mode in slab waveguides with an arbitrary refractive-index profile will be described. The wave equation for the TM mode is given, from Eq. (2.6), as

$$\frac{d}{dx}\left(\frac{1}{n^2}\frac{dH_y}{dx}\right) + \left(k^2 - \frac{\beta^2}{n^2}\right)H_y = 0. \tag{6.26}$$

From the boundary conditions, the continuity of H_y and

$$E_z = -\frac{j}{\omega\varepsilon_0 n^2}\frac{dH_y}{dx} \tag{6.27}$$

at $x = 0$ and $x = A$ are required. Employing the same normalization of variables, Eqs. (6.3) and (6.6), as in the TE mode and transforming the wave equation (6.26) and boundary condition (6.27) into a variational problem, the functional of the problem is expressed as

$$I[R] = -\int_{-\infty}^{\infty}\frac{n_s^2}{n^2(\rho)}\left(\frac{dR}{d\rho}\right)^2 d\rho + \int_{-\infty}^{\infty}\frac{n_s^2}{n^2(\rho)}[v^2\, q(\rho) - w^2]R^2\, d\rho. \tag{6.28}$$

In this functional, constant n_s^2 has been multiplied in order to have consistency between the TE and TM modes. Substituting the discretized field distribution (6.12) into the functional and applying the stationary condition, the dispersion equation for the TM mode is obtained. The elements of matrix $\mathbf{C}$ for the TM mode are slightly different from those for the TE mode. But if we use the following notations:

$$\eta_i = \begin{cases} 1 & \text{TE mode} \\ n_s^2/n^2(\rho_i) & \text{TM mode} \end{cases} \tag{6.29a}$$

$$\eta_{s_0} = \begin{cases} 1 & \text{TE mode} \\ n_s^2/n_0^2 & \text{TM mode,} \end{cases} \tag{6.29b}$$

the matrix elements for the TE and TM modes are expressed in the unified form as

$$c_{0,0} = \eta_0 - (3q_0 + q_1)\eta_0 \frac{v^2}{12}\delta^2 + \eta_0 \frac{w^2}{3}\delta^2 + \eta_{s0} w_0 \delta, \tag{6.30a}$$

$$c_{i,i} = (\eta_{i-1} + \eta_i) - (q_{i-1}\eta_{i-1} + 3q_i\eta_{i-1} + 3q_i\eta_i + q_{i+1}\eta_i)\frac{v^2}{12}\delta^2$$
$$+(\eta_{i-1} + \eta_i)\frac{w^2}{3}\delta^2 \quad (i = 1 - N - 1) \tag{6.30b}$$

$$c_{i,i+1} = c_{i+1,i} - \eta_i - (q_i + q_{i+1})\eta_i \frac{v^2}{12}\delta^2 + \eta_i \frac{w^2}{6}\delta^2 \quad (i = 0 - N - 1) \tag{6.30c}$$

$$c_{N,N} = \eta_{N-1} - (q_{N-1} + 3q_N)\eta_{N-1}\frac{v^2}{12}\delta^2 + \eta_{N-1}\frac{w^2}{3}\delta^2 + w\delta. \tag{6.30d}$$

When eigenvalue β of the matrix **C** is obtained, the corresponding eigen vector $R_0, R_1, \ldots, R_N$ is calculated by the matrix operation. Actually however, the relative value of $R_i(i = 1 - N)$ with respect, for example, to $R_0(\neq 0)$ is obtained and R_0 is still unknown. R_0 can be determined when we specify the optical power P carried by the mode. Power flow in the waveguide for the TE and TM modes are given, from Eqs. (2.31) and (2.39), as

$$P = \frac{\beta}{2\omega\mu_0}\int_{-\infty}^{\infty} |E_y|^2 dx \qquad \text{TE mode,} \tag{6.31a}$$

$$P = \frac{\beta}{2\omega\varepsilon_0}\int_{-\infty}^{\infty} \frac{1}{n^2}|H_y|^2 dx \quad \text{TE mode.} \tag{6.31b}$$

Substituting Eqs. (6.3), (6.12) and (6.29) in Eq. (6.31), we obtain

$$P = P_{\text{core}} + P_{\text{clad}}, \tag{6.32}$$

$$P_{\text{core}} = \frac{C}{3}\delta \sum_{i=0}^{N-1} \eta_i (R_i^2 + R_i\, R_{i+1} + R_{i+1}^2), \tag{6.33a}$$

$$P_{\text{clad}} = \frac{C}{2}\left(\eta_{s0}\frac{R_0^2}{w_0} + \frac{R_N^2}{w}\right), \tag{6.33b}$$

where C is defined by

$$C = \begin{cases} \dfrac{\beta a}{2\omega\mu_0} & \text{TE mode} \\[2ex] \dfrac{\beta a}{2\omega\varepsilon_0 n_s^2} & \text{TM mode.} \end{cases} \tag{6.34}$$

R_0 is then determined from Eqs. (6.32) and (6.33) when optical power P is given.

Figures 6.3–6.5 show the results of FEM analyses for the TE modes in the α-power refractive-index profiles given by

$$n^2(x) = \begin{cases} n_s^2 & (x < 0) \\ n_1^2 - (n_1^2 - n_s^2)\left|\dfrac{x}{a} - 1\right|^\alpha & (0 \leqslant x \leqslant 2a) \\ n_s^2 & (x > 2a). \end{cases} \tag{6.35}$$

Here $2a(= A)$ is a full core width and the number of divisions in the core $N = 100$. The Step-index slab waveguide is also analyzed by setting $\alpha = \infty$ in Eq. (6.35). Figures 6.3–6.5 show the cutoff normalized frequency v_c, normalized propagation constant b for the TE_0 mode, and the confinement factor Γ of slab

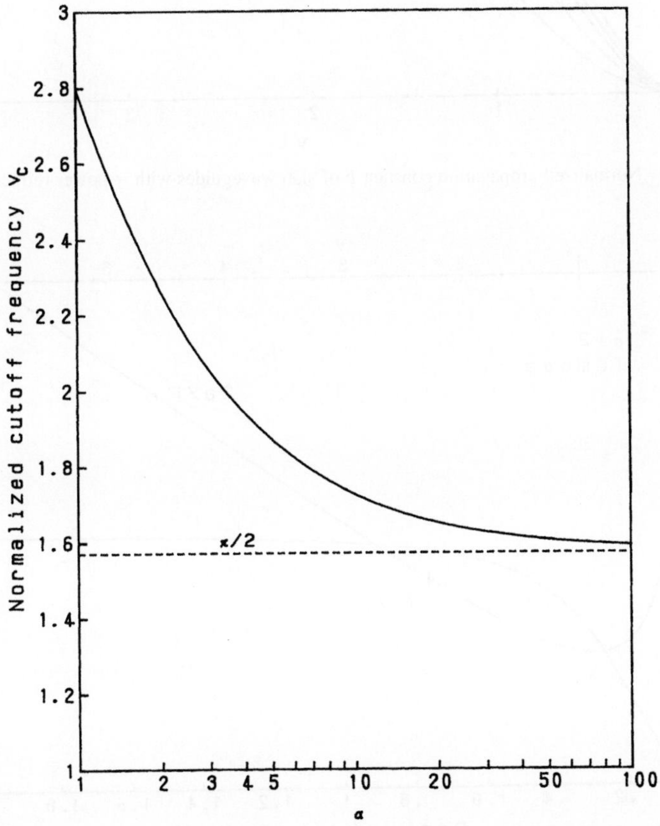

Figure 6.3 Cutoff normalized frequency v_c of slab waveguides with α-power refractive-index profiles.

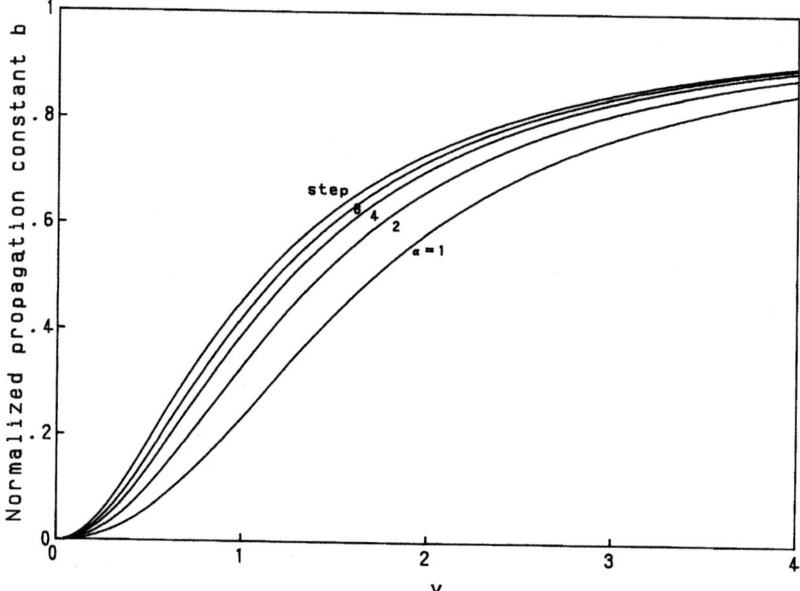

Figure 6.4 Normalized propagation constant b of slab waveguides with α-power refractive-index profiles.

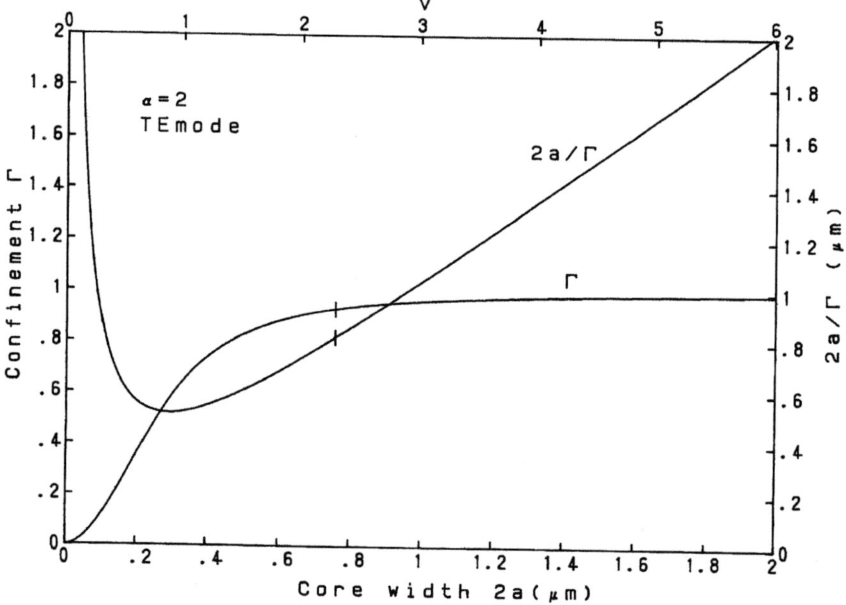

Figure 6.5 Confinement factor Γ of slab waveguides with α-power refractive-index profiles.

Table 6.1

Numerical error in FEM analysis with respect to the number of devisions N

Number of divisions N	Cutoff v-value	Error (%)
10	1.57726369	0.412
20	1.57241173	0.103
30	1.57151416	0.046
40	1.57120009	0.026
50	1.57120009	0.026
60	1.57105473	0.016
70	1.57097577	0.011
80	1.570928160	0.008
90	1.570876077	0.005
100	1.570860924	0.004

waveguides with α-power refractive-index profiles, respectively. The power-confinement factor, which is defined by

$$\Gamma = \frac{P_{\text{core}}}{P}, \tag{6.36}$$

can be calculated using Eqs. (6.32) and (6.33). Here we assumed $n_1 = 3.5$ and $n_s = 3.17$.

As described in Eq. (2.26b), the cutoff normalized frequency for the TE_1 mode in step-index slab waveguide is given by $v_{c0} = \pi/2$. Table 6.1 shows the dependencies of the numerical error $(v_c - v_{c0})/v_{c0} \times 100(\%)$ for the cutoff normalized frequency with respect to the number of core divisions N in FEM analysis. It is known that the numerical error becomes less than 0.05% for $N > 30$.

6.3. FINITE ELEMENT METHOD ANALYSIS OF OPTICAL FIBERS

6.3.1. Variational Formulation

In this section, FEM analysis of HE_{11} mode in optical fiber having an arbitrary refractive-index profile will be described. The core is defined as the region $0 \leqslant r \leqslant A$, where the refractive index is inhomogeneous, as shown in Fig. 6.6. The maximum refractive index of the core is denoted as n_1 and that in the

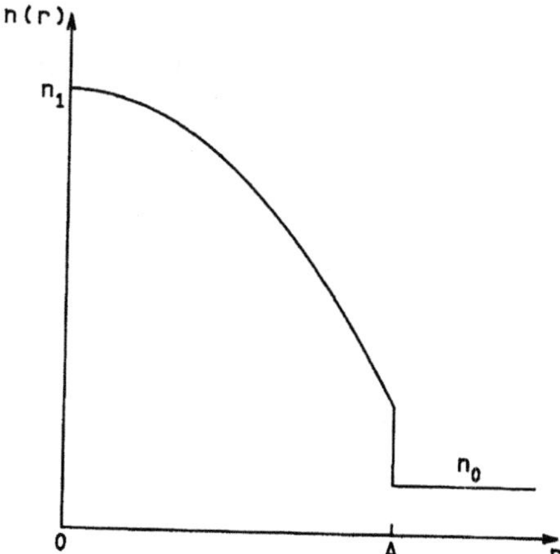

Figure 6.6 Refractive-index distribution of inhomogeneous optical fiber.

cladding as n_0. The wave equation for the HE_{11} mode is given, by Eq. (3.169) with $m = 0$, as

$$\frac{1}{r}\frac{d}{dr}\left(r\frac{dE_t}{dr}\right) + (k^2n^2 - \beta^2)E_t = 0, \tag{6.37}$$

where $E_t (t = x$ or $y)$ denotes the transverse electric field. The boundary condition is given by the continuity for E_t and dE_t/dr at $r = A$. Before transforming Eq. (6.37) into variational expression, the waveguide parameters are normalized:

$$\rho = r/a, \ \ E_t(r) = R(a), \ \ D = A/a. \tag{6.38}$$

Using this normalization, the wave equation and the boundary condition are rewritten as

$$\frac{1}{\rho}\frac{d}{d\rho}\left(\rho\frac{dR}{d\rho}\right) + [v^2q(\rho) - w^2]R = 0, \tag{6.39}$$

$$R(\rho) \text{ and } dR(\rho)/d\rho \text{ are continuous at } \rho = D. \tag{6.40}$$

Here the transverse wavenumber w, the normalized frequency v and the normalized refractive-index profile $q(\rho)$ are given by

$$w = a\sqrt{\beta^2 - k^2n_0^2}, \tag{6.41a}$$

$$v = ka\sqrt{n_1^2 - n_0^2}, \tag{6.41b}$$

$$q(\rho) = \frac{n^2 - n_0^2}{n_1^2 - n_0^2}. \tag{6.41c}$$

The solution of the wave equation (6.39) under the constraint of the boundary condition (6.40) can be obtained as the solution of the variational problem that makes the functional stationary:

$$I[R] = -\int_0^\infty \left(\frac{dR}{d\rho}\right)^2 \rho d\rho + \int_0^\infty [v^2 q(\rho) - w^2] R^2 \rho d\rho. \qquad (6.42)$$

The validity of Eq. (6.42) is proved in the similar manner as that in Section 6.2.1.

6.3.2. Discretization of the Functional

In order to simplify the calculation of the functional (6.42), the field profile in the core is discretized and expressed as

$$R(\rho) = \begin{cases} \sum_{i=0}^{N} R_i \phi_i(\rho) & (0 \leqslant \rho \leqslant D) \qquad (6.43a) \\ \dfrac{R_N}{K_0(wD)} K_0(w\rho) & (\rho > D), \qquad (6.43b) \end{cases}$$

where $R_0 - R_N$ are field values at the sampling points to be solved and K_0 is 0-th order modified Bessel function. The definitions of $R_i = R(\rho_i)$ and ρ_i are the same as those in Eqs. (6.13b) and (6.13c), and the sampling function $\phi_i(\rho)$ is given by Eq. (6.14). The normalized refractive-index distribution $q(\rho)$ is also approximated by using the sampling function as

$$q(\rho) = \sum_{i=0}^{N} q_i \phi_i(\rho) \qquad (6.44a)$$

$$q_i = \frac{n^2(\rho_i) - n_0^2}{n_1^2 - n_0^2}. \qquad (6.44b)$$

Substituting Eq. (6.43) in Eq. (6.42), we obtain the functional

$$I = -\int_0^D \left(\frac{dR}{d\rho}\right)^2 \rho d\rho + \int_0^D [v^2 q(\rho) - w^2] R^2 \rho d\rho - \frac{wDK_1(wD)}{K_0(wD)} R_N^2. \qquad (6.45)$$

6.3.3. Dispersion Equation Based on the Stationary Condition

The stationary condition of the functional (6.45) is given, by partial differentiation with respect to $R_i (i = 0 - N)$ as

$$0 = -\frac{1}{2}\frac{\partial I}{\partial R_i} = -\int_0^D \frac{dR}{d\rho}\frac{d\phi}{d\rho} \rho d\rho + v^2 \int_0^D q(\rho) R \phi_i \rho d\rho - w^2 \int_0^D R\phi_i \rho d\rho$$
$$- \frac{wDK_1(wD)}{K_0(wD)} R_N \delta_{i,N} \quad (i = 0 - N). \qquad (6.46)$$

Substituting Eq. (6.44) in Eq. (6.46) and calculating the stationary conditions in the same way as those in Section 6.2.3, $(N+1)$th order simultaneous equations are obtained:

$$R_0\left\{\frac{1}{2}-(3q_0+2q_1)\frac{v^2}{60}\left(\frac{D}{N}\right)^2+\frac{w^2}{12}\left(\frac{D}{N}\right)^2\right\}$$

$$+R_1\left\{-\frac{1}{2}-(2q_0+3q_1)\frac{v^2}{60}\left(\frac{D}{N}\right)^2+\frac{w^2}{12}\left(\frac{D}{N}\right)^2\right\}=0 \tag{6.47a}$$

$$R_{i-1}\left\{-\frac{2i-1}{2}-[(5i-3)q_{i-1}+(5i-2)q_i]\frac{v^2}{60}\left(\frac{D}{N}\right)^2+\frac{2i-1}{12}w^2\left(\frac{D}{N}\right)^2\right\}$$

$$+R_i\left\{2i-[(5i-2)q_{i-1}+30iq_i+(5i+2)q_{i+1}]\frac{v^2}{60}\left(\frac{D}{N}\right)^2+\frac{2i}{3}w^2\left(\frac{D}{N}\right)^2\right\}$$

$$+R_{i+1}\left\{-\frac{2i+1}{2}-[(5i+2)q_i+(5i+3)q_{i+1}]\frac{v^2}{60}\left(\frac{D}{N}\right)^2\right.$$

$$\left.+\frac{2i+1}{12}w^2\left(\frac{D}{N}\right)^2\right\}=0\quad(i=1-N-1) \tag{6.47b}$$

$$R_{N-1}\left\{-\frac{2N-1}{2}-[(5N-3)q_{N-1}+(5N-2)q_N]\frac{v^2}{60}\left(\frac{D}{N}\right)^2+\frac{2N-1}{12}w^2\left(\frac{D}{N}\right)^2\right\}$$

$$+R_N\left\{\frac{2N-1}{2}-[(5N-2)q_{N-1}+3(5N-1)q_N]\frac{v^2}{60}\left(\frac{D}{N}\right)^2\right.$$

$$\left.+\frac{4N-1}{12}w^2\left(\frac{D}{N}\right)^2+\frac{wDK_1(wD)}{K_0(wD)}\right\}=0. \tag{6.47c}$$

We should note here that the integration for the products of sampling functions in cylindrical coordinates is slightly different from that in Cartesian coordinates. For example, the integral of $\phi_{i-1}\phi_i$ is given by

$$\int_{\rho_{i-1}}^{\rho_i}\phi_{i-1}\phi_i\rho d\rho=\frac{2i-1}{12}\left(\frac{D}{N}\right)^2.$$

In order that Eqs. (6.47) have nontrivial solutions except for $R_0=R_1=\cdots=R_N=0$, the determinant of the matrix $\mathbf{C}$ should be

$$\det(\mathbf{C})=0. \tag{6.48}$$

The matrix elements of **C** are given by

$$c_{0,0} = \frac{1}{2} - (3q_0 + 2q_1)\frac{v^2}{60}\delta^2 + \frac{w^2}{12}\delta^2, \tag{6.49a}$$

$$c_{i,i} = 2i - [(5_i - 2)q_{i-1} + 30iq_i + (5i+2)q_{i+1}]\frac{v^2}{60}\delta^2$$
$$+\frac{2i}{3}w^2\delta^2, \quad (i = 1 - N - 1) \tag{6.49b}$$

$$c_{i,i+1} = c_{i+1,i} = -\frac{2i+1}{2} - [(5i+2)q_i + (5i+3)q_{i+1}]\frac{v^2}{60}\delta^2$$
$$+\frac{(2i+1)}{12}w^2\delta^2, \quad (i = 0 - N - 1) \tag{6.49c}$$

$$c_{N,N} = \frac{2N-1}{2} - [(5N-2)q_{N-1} + 3(5N-1)q_N]\frac{v^2}{60}\delta^2 + \frac{4N-1}{12}w^2\delta^2$$
$$+\frac{wDK_1(wD)}{K_0(wD)}, \tag{6.49d}$$

where discretization step δ is given by $\delta = D/N$. When refractive-index distribution $q(\rho)$ of the optical fiber and the normalized frequency v are given, the propagation constant β (implicitly contained in w) is calculated from Eqs. (6.48) and (6.49).

6.3.4. Single-mode Conditions of Graded-index Fibers

In order to know the single-mode condition of optical fiber, the cutoff v-value of the $TE_{01}(LP_{11})$ mode should be calculated. The wave equation of the TE mode is given, by putting $m = 1$ in Eq. (3.169), as

$$\frac{1}{r}\frac{d}{dr}\left(r\frac{dE_\theta}{dr}\right) + \left(k^2n^2 - \beta^2 - \frac{1}{r^2}\right)E_\theta = 0. \tag{6.50}$$

Applying the same normalization of the parameters as for Eqs. (6.38) and (6.41) and noting that $w = 0$ at the mode cutoff, Eq. (6.50) can be rewritten as

$$\frac{1}{\rho}\frac{d}{d\rho}\left(\rho\frac{dR_c}{d\rho}\right) + \left[v^2q(\rho) - \frac{1}{\rho^2}\right]R_c = 0, \tag{6.51}$$

where $R_c = E_\theta(a\rho)$. The functional that has Eq. (6.51) as an Euler equation is expressed by

$$I[R_c] = -\int_0^\infty \left(\frac{dR_c}{d\rho}\right)^2 \rho d\rho + \int_0^\infty \left[v^2q(\rho) - \frac{1}{\rho^2}\right]R_c^2\rho\, d\rho. \tag{6.52}$$

When we discretize the electric field profile R_c, we should note that $R_c = 0$ at $\rho = 0$ for the TE mode. Then R_c can be expressed as

$$R_c(\rho) = \begin{cases} \sum_{i=1}^{N} R_{c,i}\phi_i(\rho) & (0 \leqslant \rho \leqslant D) \quad (6.53a) \\ R_{c,N}\dfrac{D}{\rho} & (\rho > D). \quad (6.53b) \end{cases}$$

Summation starts from $i = 1$ in Eq. (6.53a). Since $q(\rho) = 0$ in the cladding, the field distribution is given by constant t/ρ as shown in Eq. (6.53b). Substituting Eqs. (6.53) into Eq. (6.52), the functional is reduced to

$$I = -\int_0^D \left(\frac{dR_c}{d\rho}\right)^2 \rho\, d\rho + \int_0^D \left[v^2 q(\rho) - \frac{1}{\rho^2}\right] R_c^2 \rho\, d\rho - R_{c,N}^2. \quad (6.54)$$

Integrating the functional (6.54) in each discretization interval and applying the partial differentiation with respect to $R_{c,i} (i = 1 - N)$, N-th order simultaneous equations are obtained:

$$R_{c,1}\left\{-4\ell n2 + (3q_0 + 30q_1 + 7q_2)\frac{v^2}{60}\delta^2\right\} + R_{c,2}\left\{2\ell n2 + (7q_1 + 8q_2)\frac{v^2}{60}\delta^2\right\} = 0, \quad (6.55a)$$

$$R_{c,i-1}\left\{i(i-1)\ell n\frac{i}{i-1} + [(5i-3)q_{i-1} + (5i-2)q_i]\frac{v^2}{60}\delta^2\right\} + R_{c,i}\left\{-(i-1)^2\ell n\frac{i}{i-1} - (i+1)^2\ell n\frac{i+1}{i} + [(5i-2)q_{i-1} + 30iq_i + (5i+2)q_{i+1}]\frac{v^2}{60}\delta^2\right\} + R_{c,i+1}\left\{i(i+1)\ell n\frac{i+1}{i} + [(5i+2)q_i + (5i+3)q_{i+1}]\frac{v^2}{60}\delta^2\right\} = 0 \ (i = 2 - N-1), \quad (6.55b)$$

$$R_{c,N-1}\left\{N(N-1)\ell n\frac{N}{N-1} + [(5N-3)q_{N-1} + (5N-2)q_N]\frac{v^2}{60}\delta^2\right\} + R_{c,N}\left\{-2 - (N-1)^2\ell n\frac{N}{N-1} + [(5N-2)q_{N-1} + 3(5N-1)q_N]\frac{v^2}{60}\delta^2\right\} = 0. \quad (6.55c)$$

In order that Eq. (6.22) has nontrivial solutions except for $R_1 = \cdots = R_N = 0$, the determinant of the matrix **H** should be

$$\det(\mathbf{H}) = 0. \tag{6.56}$$

Elements of the matrix **H** are obtained as

$$h_{1,1} = -4\ell n2 + (3q_0 + 30q_1 + 7q_2)\frac{v^2}{60}\delta^2, \tag{6.57a}$$

$$h_{i,i} = -(i-1)^2 \ell n\frac{i}{i-1} - (i+1)^2 \ell n\frac{i+1}{i}$$
$$+ [(5i-2)q_{i-1} + 30iq_i + (5i+2)q_{i+1}]\frac{v^2}{60}\delta^2 \quad (i = 2 - N - 1) \tag{6.57b}$$

$$h_{i,i+1} = h_{i+1,i} = i(i+1)\ell n\frac{i+1}{i}$$
$$+ [(5i+2)q_i + (5i+3)q_{i+1}]\frac{v^2}{60}\delta^2 \quad (i = 1 - N - 1) \tag{6.57c}$$

$$h_{N,N} = -2 - (N-1)^2 \ell n\frac{N}{N-1}$$
$$+ [(5N-2)q_{N-1} + 3(5N-1)q_N]\frac{v^2}{60}\delta^2. \tag{6.57d}$$

In the foregoing equations, $\delta = D/N$. Solution of Eqs. (6.56) and (6.57) gives the cutoff normalized frequency for the TE_{01} (LP_{11}) mode and determines the single-mode condition.

6.3.5. Variational Expression for the Delay Time

When $E_t(r)$ is the solution of the wave equation (6.37) for HE_{11} mode satisfying the boundary condition,

$$\beta^2 = \frac{-\int_0^\infty \left(\frac{dE_t}{dr}\right)^2 r\,dr + \int_0^\infty k^2 n^2(r) E_t^2(r) r\,dr}{\int_0^\infty E_t^2(r) r\,dr}, \tag{6.58}$$

is stationary with respect to small variations of $E_t(r)$. The proof is obtained in the same way as shown for Eqs. (6.8)–(6.11). Based on this variational expression of β, the first derivative of β is obtained [5] (see Appendix 6A at the end of this chapter)

$$\frac{\beta}{k}\frac{d\beta}{dk} = \frac{\int_0^\infty n^2(r) E_t^2(r) r\,dr}{\int_0^\infty E_t^2(r) r\,dr}. \tag{6.59}$$

Using the normalization of parameters as shown in Eqs. (6.38) and (6.41) and noting $q(\rho)=0$ in the cladding $\rho > D$, we obtain

$$\frac{\beta}{k}\frac{d\beta}{dk} = n_0^2 + (n_1^2 - n_0^2)\frac{\int_0^D q(\rho)R^2(\rho)\rho\, d\rho}{\int_0^\infty R^2(\rho)\rho\, d\rho}. \tag{6.60}$$

Substituting Eqs. (6.43) and (6.44) into Eq. (6.60), the denominator and numerator of the right-hand term of Eq. (6.60) are given by

$$\int_0^\infty R^2(\rho)\rho\, d\rho = \frac{\delta^2}{12}\sum_{i=0}^{N-1}[(4i+1)R_i^2 + 2(2i+1)R_i\, R_{i+1} + (4i+3)R_{i+1}^2] + \left[\frac{K_1^2(wD)}{K_0^2(wD)} - 1\right]\frac{D^2R_N^2}{2}, \tag{6.61}$$

$$\int_0^D q(\rho)R^2(\rho)\rho\, d\rho = \frac{\delta^2}{12}\sum_{i=0}^{N-1}\left[\left(3i+\frac{3}{5}\right)q_iR_i^2 + \left(i+\frac{2}{5}\right)(2q_i\, R_{i+1} + q_{i+1}R_i)R_i + \left(i+\frac{3}{5}\right)(q_i\, R_{i+1} + 2q_{i+1}R_i)R_{i+1} + \left(3i+\frac{12}{5}\right)q_{i+1}R_{i+1}^2\right]. \tag{6.62}$$

When propagation constant β is obtained from the dispersion equation (6.48), electric field amplitudes at the sampling points $R_0, R_1, \ldots, R_N$ are readily calculated by the matrix operations. Then substituting $R_0, R_1, \ldots, R_N$ into Eqs. (6.60)–(6.62), delay time τ, which is defined by

$$\tau = \frac{d\beta}{d\omega} = \frac{1}{c}\frac{d\beta}{dk}, \tag{6.63}$$

is obtained for optical fibers with arbitrary refractive-index distributions.

Figures 6.7–6.11 show the results of FEM analyses for optical fibers having α-power refractive-index profiles given by

$$n^2(r) = \begin{cases} n_1^2 - (n_1^2 - n_0^2)\left(\dfrac{r}{a}\right)^\alpha & (0 \leqslant r \leqslant a) \\ n_0^2 & (r > a). \end{cases} \tag{6.64}$$

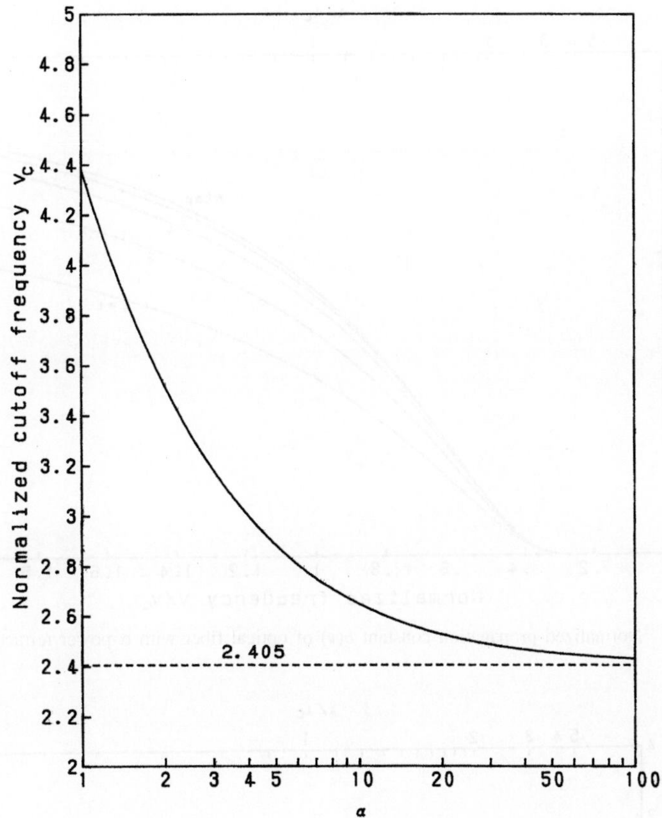

Figure 6.7 Cutoff normalized frequency v_c of optical fiber with α-power refractive-index profiles.

Here $a(=A)$ is a core radius and number of divisions in the core $N = 100$. Step-index optical fiber corresponds to $\alpha = \infty$ in Eq. (6.64). Figure 6.7 shows the cutoff normalized frequency v_c. The cutoff normalized frequency of the quadratic index profile ($\alpha = 2$), is $v_c = 3.51816$. As α large, v_c approaches that of the step-index fiber $v_c = 2.405$. Figures 6.8–6.10 show the normalized propagation constant $b(v)$, the normalized delay $d(vb)/dv$ and normalized waveguide dispersion $vd^2(vb)/dv^2$, respectively. When we obtain $d(vb)/dv$ and $vd^2(vb)/dv^2$ for arbitrary refractive-index profiles, we can calculate the chromatic dispersion characteristics for any kinds of fibers using Eqs. (3.138) and (3.142).

Figure 6.11 shows relative effective core areas $A_{\text{eff}}/\pi a^2$ [refer to Eq. (5.42)] of optical fibers with the α-power index profiles. Effective core area A_{eff} is very important in the investigation of nonlinear effects in optical fibers.

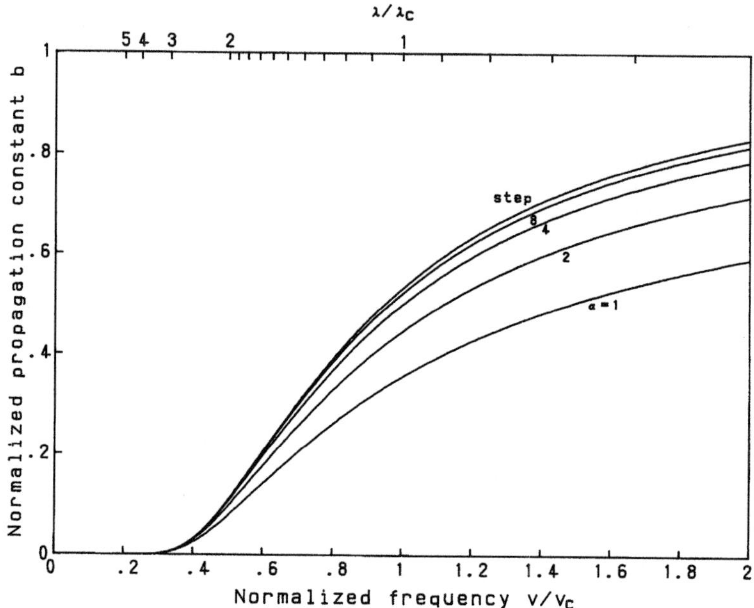

Figure 6.8 Normalized propagation constant $b(v)$ of optical fiber with α-power refractive-index profiles.

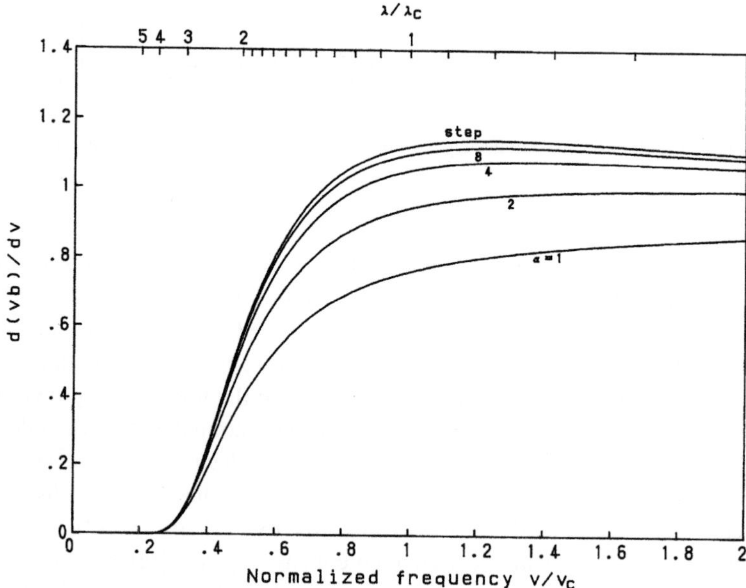

Figure 6.9 Normalized delay $d(vb)/dv$ of optical fiber with α-power refractive-index profiles.

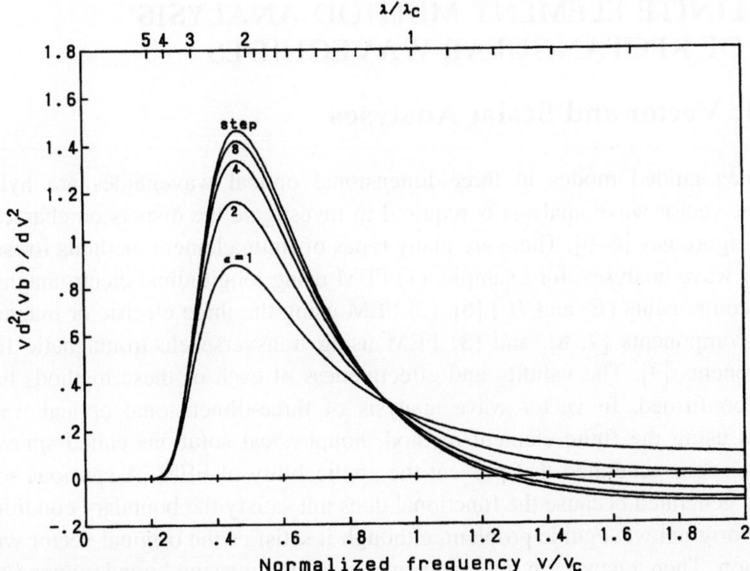

Figure 6.10 Normalized waveguide dispersion $vd^2(vb)/dv^2$ of optical fiber with α-power refractive-index profiles.

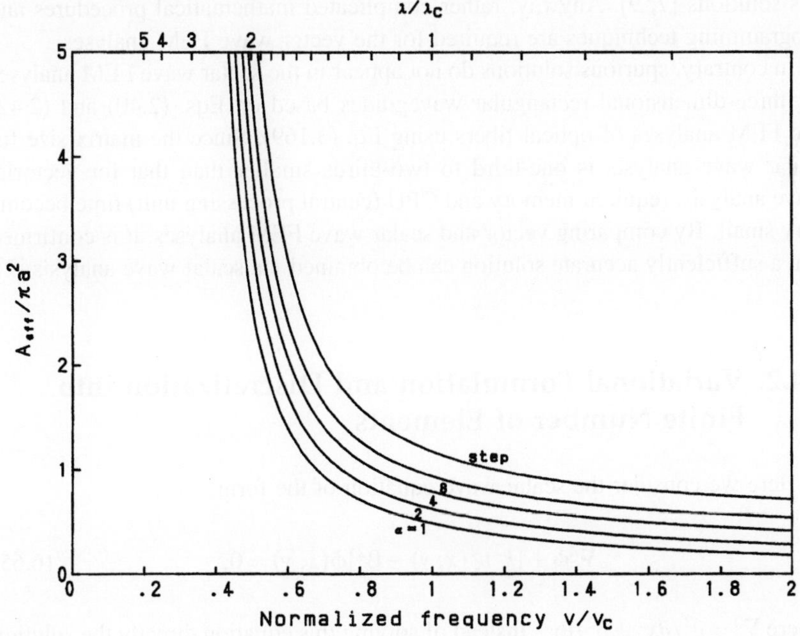

Figure 6.11 Relative effective areas $A_{\mathrm{eff}}/\pi a^2$ of optical fiber with α-power refractive-index profiles.

6.4. FINITE ELEMENT METHOD ANALYSIS OF RECTANGULAR WAVEGUIDES

6.4.1. Vector and Scalar Analyses

Since guided modes in three-dimensional optical waveguides are hybrid modes, vector wave analysis is required to investigate the dispersion characteristics rigorously [6–9]. There are many types of finite element methods for such vector wave analyses, for example, (1) FEM using longitudinal electromagnetic field components (E_z and H_z) [6], (2) FEM using the three electric or magnetic field components [7, 8], and (3) FEM using transverse electromagnetic field components [9]. The validity and effectiveness of each of these methods have been confirmed. In vector wave analysis of three-dimensional optical waveguides using the finite element method, nonphysical solutions called *spurious solutions* are generated that prevent the applicability of FEM. A spurious solution is generated because the functional does not satisfy the boundary conditions in the original waveguide problem, although it satisfies the original vector wave equation. Then a new term that compensates for the missing boundary condition must be added in the functional to eliminate the spurious solutions. Various kinds of techniques have been developed to suppress and eliminate the spurious solutions [7, 9]. Anyway, rather complicated mathematical procedures and programming techniques are required for the vector wave FEM analyses.

In contrary, spurious solutions do not appear in the scalar wave FEM analyses for three-dimensional rectangular waveguides based on Eqs. (2.40) and (2.42) and FEM analyses of optical fibers using Eq. (3.169). Since the matrix size for scalar wave analysis is one-third to two-thirds smaller than that for vectorial wave analysis, required memory and CPU (central processing unit) time become very small. By comparing vector and scalar wave FEM analyses, it is confirmed that a sufficiently accurate solution can be obtained via scalar wave analysis [2].

6.4.2. Variational Formulation and Discretization into Finite Number of Elements

Here we consider the scalar wave equation of the form

$$\nabla^2\phi + [k^2n^2(x, y) - \beta^2]\phi(x, y) = 0, \tag{6.65}$$

where $\nabla^2 = \partial^2/\partial x^2 + \partial^2/\partial y^2$. Instead of solving this equation directly the solution of the wave equation can be obtained as the solution of the variational problem that makes the following functional stationary:

$$I[\phi] = \frac{1}{2}\int_{-\infty}^{\infty}\int_{-\infty}^{\infty}\left[\left(\frac{\partial\phi}{\partial x}\right)^2 + \left(\frac{\partial\phi}{\partial y}\right)^2 - (k^2n^2 - \beta^2)\phi^2\right] dx\, dy. \qquad (6.66)$$

The proof is given in Appendix 6B at the end of this chapter.

In calculating the functional, the entire region of the problem is divided into small regions (generally a triangular region). The electric field $\phi(x, y)$ in each region is approximated by simple analytical functions and is connected at the nodal points (vertexes of triangle). Here we consider three-dimensional rib waveguide shown in Fig. 6.12 and analyze the propagation characteristics using the finite element method. Since the waveguide geometry is symmetrical with respect to the y-axis, it is sufficient to analyze only right-hand side of Fig. 6.12, taking into account the even or odd symmetry of the electric field distribution. Figure 6.13 shows an example of element division. The number of triangular elements is $N = 280$, and the number of nodes is $n = 165$. The boundaries at positive x-direction and the positive and negative y-directions are called *fictitious boundaries*, which should be far enough from the center of the core that the electromagnetic field amplitude becomes almost zero. Of course, we do not know the electromagnetic field distributions before carrying out FEM analysis, so we cannot fully determine the fictitious boundary. Therefore, we first take the fictitious boundary sufficiently far from the core center and calculate the eigenvalue (propagation constant) and electromagnetic field distribution. Then we check the convergence of the eigenvalue by changing the width of the fictitious boundary. If the variation of the eigenvalue becomes small even when the width of the fictitious boundary is changed, the boundary is considered appropriate.

The electric field $\phi(x, y)$ in element $e(e = 1 - N)$ is approximated by a linear function of x and y:

$$\phi(x, y) = p_0^e + p_1^e x + p_2^e y, \qquad (6.67)$$

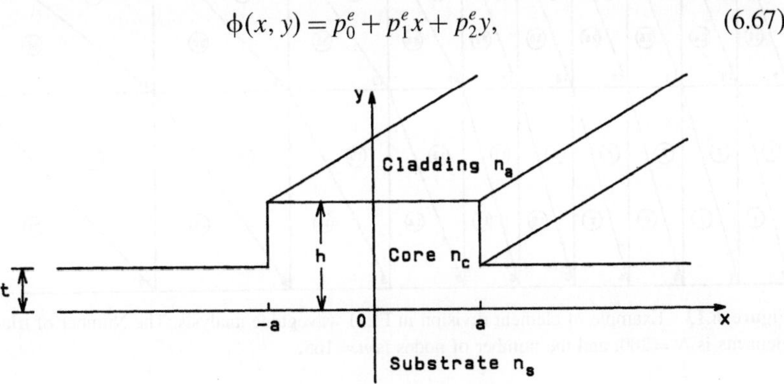

Figure 6.12 Rib-type optical waveguide.

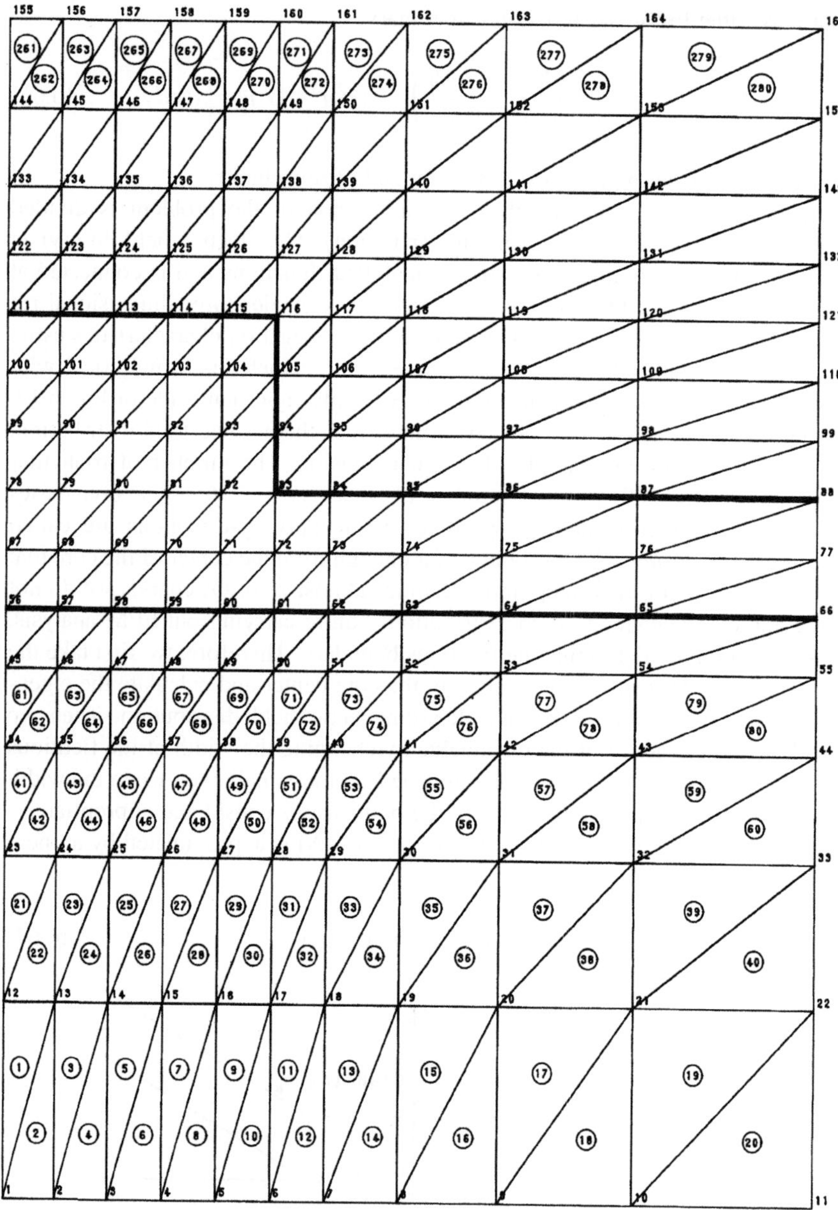

Figure 6.13 Example of element division in FEM waveguide analysis. The Number of triangular elements is $N = 280$, and the number of nodes is $n = 165$.

where p_0^e, p_1^e and p_2^e are constants. Nodal points around the element e are labeled i, j, and k, as shown in Fig. 6.14, and their coordinates are denoted $(x_m, y_m)(m = i,\ j, \text{ and } k)$. Here, the numbering of the nodal points goes in counter-clockwise direction. For example, the nodal points of element $e = 50$ in Fig. 6.13 are $i = 27$, $j = 28$, and $k = 39$. The electric field amplitude at each nodal point is expressed in a simplified manner as

$$\begin{cases} \phi_i = \phi(x_i,\ y_i) = p_0^e + p_1^e x_i + p_2^e y_i \\ \phi_j = \phi(x_j,\ y_j) = p_0^e + p_1^e x_j + p_2^e y_j \\ \phi_k = \phi(x_k,\ y_k) = p_0^e + p_1^e x_k + p_2^e y_k. \end{cases} \tag{6.68}$$

The expansion coefficients p_0^e, p_1^e, and p_2^e of electric field in the eth element are given by

$$\begin{aligned} \begin{pmatrix} p_0^e \\ p_1^e \\ p_2^e \end{pmatrix} &= \begin{pmatrix} 1 & x_i & y_i \\ 1 & x_j & y_j \\ 1 & x_k & y_k \end{pmatrix}^{-1} \begin{pmatrix} \phi_i \\ \phi_j \\ \phi_k \end{pmatrix} \\ &= \frac{1}{2s_e} \begin{bmatrix} (x_j y_k - x_k y_j) & (x_k y_i - x_i y_k) & (x_i y_j - x_j y_i) \\ (y_j - y_k) & (y_k - y_i) & (y_i - y_j) \\ (x_k - x_j) & (x_i - x_k) & (x_j - x_i) \end{bmatrix} \begin{pmatrix} \phi_i \\ \phi_j \\ \phi_k \end{pmatrix}. \end{aligned} \tag{6.69}$$

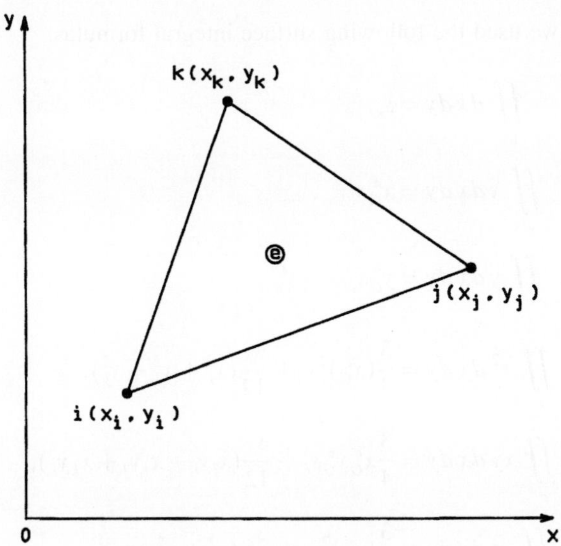

Figure 6.14 Coordinates of eth element.

Here, s_e is an area of element e which is given by

$$S_e = \frac{1}{2}[(x_j - x_i)(y_k - y_i) - (x_k - x_i)(y_j - y_i)]. \tag{6.70}$$

When we calculate the functional of Eq. (6.66), we divide the integral into each element. Then the integral in the eth element is obtained by using Eqs. (6.67) and (6.68):

$$\begin{aligned}
I^e &= \frac{1}{2}\iint_e \left[\left(\frac{\partial\phi}{\partial x}\right)^2 + \left(\frac{\partial\phi}{\partial y}\right)^2 - (k^2n^2 - \beta^2)\phi^2\right] dx\,dy \\
&= \frac{1}{2}\iint_e \left[(p_1^e)^2 + (p_2^e)^2 - (k^2n_e^2 - \beta^2)(p_0^e + p_1^e x + p_2^e y)^2\right] dx\,dy \\
&= \frac{1}{2}\left[(p_1^e)^2 + (p_2^e)^2\right] s_e - \frac{(k^2n_e^2 - \beta^2)s_e}{2}\left\{(p_0^e)^2 + 2p_0^e p_1^e x_G^e + 2p_0^e p_2^e y_G^e\right. \\
&\quad + \frac{3}{4}(p_1^e)^2\left[(x_G^e)^2 + \frac{1}{9}(x_i^2 + x_j^2 + x_k^2)\right] + \frac{3}{2}p_1^e p_2^e\left[x_G^e y_G^e + \frac{1}{9}(x_i y_i + x_j y_j + x_k y_k)\right] \\
&\quad \left. + \frac{3}{4}(p_2^e)^2\left[(y_G^e)^2 + \frac{1}{9}(y_i^2 + y_j^2 + y_k^2)\right]\right\}.
\end{aligned} \tag{6.71}$$

Here $\iint_e dx\,dy$ represents the integral inside the eth element. In the derivation of Eq. (6.71), we used the following surface integral formulas:

$$\iint_e dx\,dy = s_e, \tag{6.72a}$$

$$\iint_e x\,dx\,dy = x_G^e s_e, \tag{6.72b}$$

$$\iint_e y\,dx\,dy = y_G^e s_e, \tag{6.72c}$$

$$\iint_e x^2\,dx\,dy = \frac{3}{4}(x_G^e)^2 s_e + \frac{s_e}{12}(x_i^2 + x_j^2 + x_k^2), \tag{6.72d}$$

$$\iint_e xy\,dx\,dy = \frac{3}{4}x_G^e y_G^e s_e + \frac{s_e}{12}(x_i y_i + x_j y_j + x_k y_k), \tag{6.72e}$$

$$\iint_e y^2\,dx\,dy = \frac{3}{4}(y_G^e)^2 s_e + \frac{s_e}{12}(y_i^2 + y_j^2 + y_k^2). \tag{6.72f}$$

Here, x_G^e and y_G^e denote the median centers of eth element, which are given by

$$\begin{cases} x_G^e = \dfrac{1}{3}(x_i + x_j + x_k) \\ y_G^e = \dfrac{1}{3}(y_i + y_j + y_k). \end{cases} \tag{6.73}$$

Substituting Eq. (6.69) in Eq. (6.71) and using the surface integration formulas of Eqs. (6.72), we obtain

$$\begin{aligned} I^e = &\frac{1}{8s_e}\left[(y_j - y_k)\phi_i + (y_k - y_i)\phi_j + (y_i - y_j)\phi_k\right]^2 \\ &+ \frac{1}{8s_e}\left[(x_k - x_j)\phi_i + (x_i - x_k)\phi_j + (x_j - x_i)\phi_k\right]^2 \\ &- \frac{(k^2 n_e^2 - \beta^2)s_e}{12}(\phi_i^2 + \phi_j^2 + \phi_k^2 + \phi_i\phi_j + \phi_j\phi_k + \phi_k\phi_i). \end{aligned} \tag{6.74}$$

The functional of Eq. (6.66) is then given by

$$I = 2\sum_{e=1}^{N} I^e. \tag{6.75}$$

6.4.3. Dispersion Equation Based on the Stationary Condition

In order to express the functional in normalized and dimensionless form, we introduce the following parameters:

$$n_1 = \max[n(x, y)], \tag{6.76a}$$

$$v = ka\sqrt{n_1^2 - n_s^2}, \tag{6.76b}$$

$$q^e = \frac{n_e^2 - n_s^2}{n_1^2 - n_s^2}, \tag{6.76c}$$

$$b = \frac{(\beta/k)^2 - n_s^2}{n_1^2 - n_s^2}, \tag{6.76d}$$

$$\begin{cases} \xi_m = x_m/a \\ \eta_m = y_m/a, \end{cases} \tag{6.77}$$

$$\sigma_e = \frac{s_e}{a^2} = \frac{1}{2}\left[(\xi_j - \xi_i)(\eta_k - \eta_i) - (\xi_k - \xi_i)(\eta_j - \eta_i)\right], \tag{6.78}$$

where n_s denotes the refractive index in the substrate. Substituting Eqs. (6.76)–(6.78) in Eq. (6.75), the functional is expressed by

$$I=\sum_{e=1}^{N}\left\{\frac{1}{4\sigma_e}\left[(\eta_j-\eta_k)\phi_i+(\eta_k-\eta_i)\phi_j+(\eta_i-\eta_j)\phi_k\right]^2\right.$$
$$+\frac{1}{4\sigma_e}\left[(\xi_k-\xi_j)\phi_i+(\xi_i-\xi_k)\phi_j+(\xi_j-\xi_i)\phi_k\right]^2$$
$$\left.-\frac{v^2(q^e-b)\sigma_e}{6}(\phi_i^2+\phi_j^2+\phi_k^2+\phi_i\phi_j+\phi_j\phi_k+\phi_k\phi_i)\right\}. \tag{6.79}$$

The stationary condition of Eq. (6.79) is obtained by the partial differenciation with respect to $\phi_\ell(\ell=1-n)$:

$$\frac{\partial I}{\partial\phi_\ell}=\sum_{m=1}^{n}c_{\ell m}\phi_m=0 \quad (\ell=1-n). \tag{6.80}$$

These simultaneous equations expressed in matrix form as

$$\mathbf{C}\{\phi\}=\{0\}, \tag{6.81}$$

where $\mathbf{C}$ is an $n\times n$ matrix and $\{\phi\}$ and $\{0\}$ are column vector of the electric field distribution $\phi_1-\phi_n$ and zero vector, respectively. For Eq. (6.81) to have a nontrivial solution other than $\{\phi\}=\{0\}$, the determinant of the matrix $\mathbf{C}$ should be zero; that is,

$$\det(\mathbf{C})=0. \tag{6.82}$$

Equation (6.82) is a dispersion (eigenvalue) equation for the wave equation (6.65). The eigenvalue of Eq. (6.82) gives the propagation constant β, and column vector $\{\phi\}$ gives the electric field distribution of the mode corresponding to β.

It is very important to calculate matrix element $c_{\ell m}(\ell, m=1-n)$ in the practical procedures of FEM. Calculation of $c_{\ell m}$ is done in each element, as described in the following. Combining Eqs. (6.75) and (6.80), the stationary condition can be written by

$$\frac{\partial I}{\partial\phi_\ell}=2\sum_{e=1}^{N}\frac{\partial I^e}{\partial\phi_\ell}=2\sum_{e=1}^{N}\left(\frac{\partial I^e}{\partial\phi_i}+\frac{\partial I^e}{\partial\phi_j}+\frac{\partial I^e}{\partial\phi_k}\right). \tag{6.83}$$

Partial differentiation of element functional I^e with respect to $\phi_\ell(\ell=1-n)$ has a nonzero value only for values ϕ_i, ϕ_j, and ϕ_k, since I^e is given by

Eq. (6.74). For example, the nodal points of element $e = 50$ in Fig. 6.13 are $i=27$, $j=28$, and $k=39$. Then, among n differential terms in $e(=50)$th element, only $\partial I^{50}/\partial\phi_{27}$, $\partial I^{50}/\partial\phi_{28}$, and $\partial I^{50}/\partial\phi_{39}$ remain to be nonzero. Summing up these terms, nth-order linear simultaneous equation are constructed. Next, it is important to contain the components in the eth element matrix in the global matrix component $c_{\ell m}$. The detailed expressions of partial differentiation in Eq. (6.83) are:

$$\begin{aligned}\frac{\partial I^e}{\partial\phi_i} &= \left\{\frac{1}{\sigma_e}[(\eta_j-\eta_k)^2+(\xi_k-\xi_j)^2]-\frac{2}{3}v^2(q^e-b)\sigma_e\right\}\phi_i \\ &+\left\{\frac{1}{\sigma_e}[(\eta_j-\eta_k)+(\eta_k-\eta_i)+(\xi_k-\xi_j)(\xi_i-\xi_k)]-\frac{1}{3}v^2(q^e-b)\sigma_e\right\}\phi_j \\ &+\left\{\frac{1}{\sigma_e}[(\eta_j-\eta_k)(\eta_i-\eta_j)+(\xi_k-\xi_j)(\xi_j-\xi_i)]-\frac{1}{3}v^2(q^e-b)\sigma_e\right\}\phi_k,\end{aligned} \tag{6.84a}$$

$$\begin{aligned}\frac{\partial I^e}{\partial\phi_j} &= \left\{\frac{1}{\sigma_e}[(\eta_k-\eta_i)(\eta_j-\eta_k)+(\xi_i-\xi_k)(\xi_k-\xi_j)]-\frac{1}{3}v^2(q^e-b)\sigma_e\right\}\phi_i \\ &+\left\{\frac{1}{\sigma_e}[(\eta_k-\eta_i)^2+(\xi_i-\xi_k)^2]-\frac{2}{3}v^2(q^e-b)\sigma_e\right\}\phi_j \\ &+\left\{\frac{1}{\sigma_e}[(\eta_k-\eta_i)(\eta_i-\eta_j)+(\xi_i-\xi_k)(\xi_j-\xi_i)]-\frac{1}{3}v^2(q^e-b)\sigma_e\right\}\phi_k,\end{aligned} \tag{6.84b}$$

$$\begin{aligned}\frac{\partial I^e}{\partial\phi_k} &= \left\{\frac{1}{\sigma_e}[(\eta_i-\eta_j)(\eta_j-\eta_k)+(\xi_j-\xi_i)(\xi_k-\xi_j)]-\frac{1}{3}v^2(q^e-b)\sigma_e\right\}\phi_i \\ &+\left\{\frac{1}{\sigma_e}[(\eta_i-\eta_j)(\eta_k-\eta_i)+(\xi_j-\xi_i)(\xi_i-\xi_k)]-\frac{1}{3}v^2(q^e-b)\sigma_e\right\}\phi_j \\ &+\left\{\frac{1}{\sigma_e}[(\eta_i-\eta_j)^2+(\xi_j-\xi_i)^2]-\frac{2}{3}v^2(q^e-b)\sigma_e\right\}\phi_j.\end{aligned} \tag{6.84c}$$

It should be noted here that component $c_{\ell m}$ of the global matrix $\mathbf{C}$ is a coefficient of ϕ_m when functional I is partially differentiated by ϕ_ℓ. Then it is seen that the coefficients for ϕ_i, ϕ_j, and ϕ_k in Eq. (6.84a) are contained in $c_{i,i}$, $c_{i,j}$, and $c_{i,k}$, respectively. Similarly, the coefficients for ϕ_i, ϕ_j, and ϕ_k in Eq. (6.84b) are contained in $c_{j,i}$, $c_{j,j}$, and $c_{j,k}$ and coefficients for ϕ_i, ϕ_j, and ϕ_k in Eq. (6.84c) are contained in $c_{k,i}$, $c_{k,j}$, and $c_{k,k}$. In our earlier example for $e(=50)$th element, where $i=27$, $j=28$, and $k=39$, the coefficients for $\phi_i(=\phi_{27})$, $\phi_j(=\phi_{28})$, and $\phi_k(=\phi_{39})$ in Eq. (6.84a) are contained into $c_{27,27}$, $c_{27,28}$, and $c_{27,39}$, respectively.

Summing up all contributions from each element, the component $c_{\ell,m}$ of the global matrix **C** is calculated.

It is seen from Eq. (6.84) that component $c_{i,j}$ of the global matrix **C** can be rewritten as

$$c_{i,j} = p_{i,j} - b \cdot r_{i,j}, \tag{6.85}$$

where $p_{i,j}$ and $r_{i,j}$ are constants that are independent of eigenvalue b (normalized propagation constant). Then Eq. (6.81) can be rewritten as

$$\mathbf{C}\{\phi\} = (\mathbf{P} - b\mathbf{R})\{\phi\} = \{0\}, \tag{6.86}$$

where **P** and **R** are $n \times n$ matrices whose components are given by $p_{i,j}$ and $r_{i,j}$. Equation (6.86) is further rewritten as

$$\mathbf{A}\{\phi\} = b\{\phi\}, \tag{6.87}$$

$$\mathbf{A} = \mathbf{R}^{-1}\mathbf{P}. \tag{6.88}$$

Equation (6.87) is an eigenvalue problem of matrix **A**. Eigenvalue b and the column vector of the electric field distribution $\{\phi\}$ can easily be obtained via numerical calculation libraries such as Jacobi's method and Householder's method [10].

Figure 6.15 shows optical intensity distribution of E_{11} mode (the E^x_{11} and E^y_{11} modes cannot be discriminated in scalar wave analysis) in the rib waveguide shown in Fig. 6.12. The waveguide parameters of the waveguide are $n_c = 3.38$, $n_s = 3.17$, $n_a = 1.0$, $2a = 1.5$ μm, $h = 0.75$ μm, $t = 0.3$ μm, and wavelength of light is $\lambda = 1.55$ μm. The width of the fictitious boundaries are ± 7.5 μm in the x-axis direction and $+3$ μm and -4.5 μm in y-axis direction. The number of divisions are 20 for the span of $x = 0 - a$, 20 for $x = a - 7.5$ μm, 20 for $y = -4.5 - 0$ μm, 20 for $y = 0 - h$, and 10 for $y = h - 3$ μm. Then the total number of triangular elements is $N = 4000$ and that of nodal points is $n = 2091$. The effective index of E_{11} mode is $\beta/k = 3.271198$.

Figure 6.16 shows the optical intensity distribution of the E_{11} mode in the ridge (rib-loaded) waveguide (the definition of the waveguide parameters is shown in Fig. 2.15). Ridge waveguides are very important in the fabrication of semiconductor lasers and passive semiconductor waveguides. The waveguide parameters of the waveguide are $n_c = 3.38$, $n_s = 3.17$, $n_r = n_s$, $n_a = 1.0$, core width $2a = 2$ μm, core thickness $d = 0.2$ μm, rib height in the center $h = 1$ μm, rib height in the peripheral region $t = 0.1$ μm, and wavelength of light is $\lambda =$ 1.55 μm. The effective index of E_{11} mode is $\beta/k = 3.194346$.

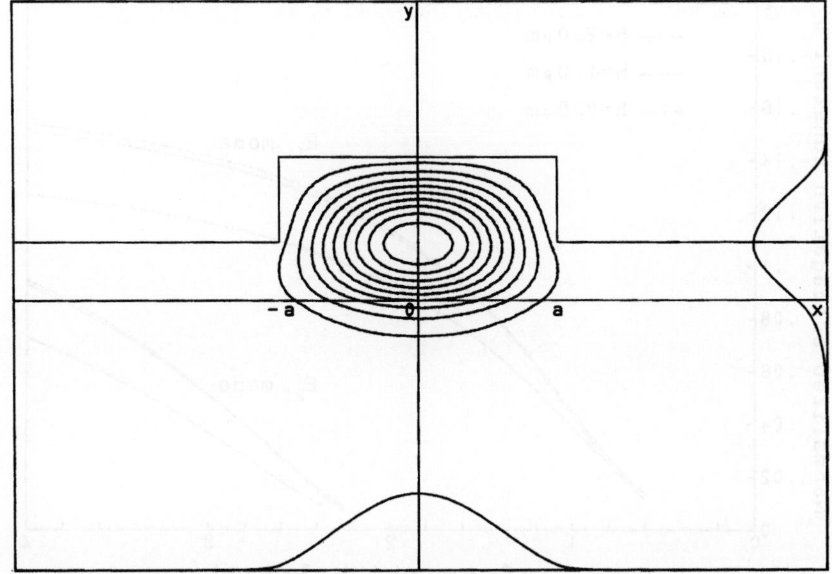

Figure 6.15 Optical intensity distribution of E_{11} mode in the rib waveguide. $n_c = 3.38$, $n_s = 3.17$, $n_a = 1.0$, $2a = 1.5$ µm, $h = 0.75$ µm, $t = 0.3$ µm and $\lambda = 1.55$ µm.

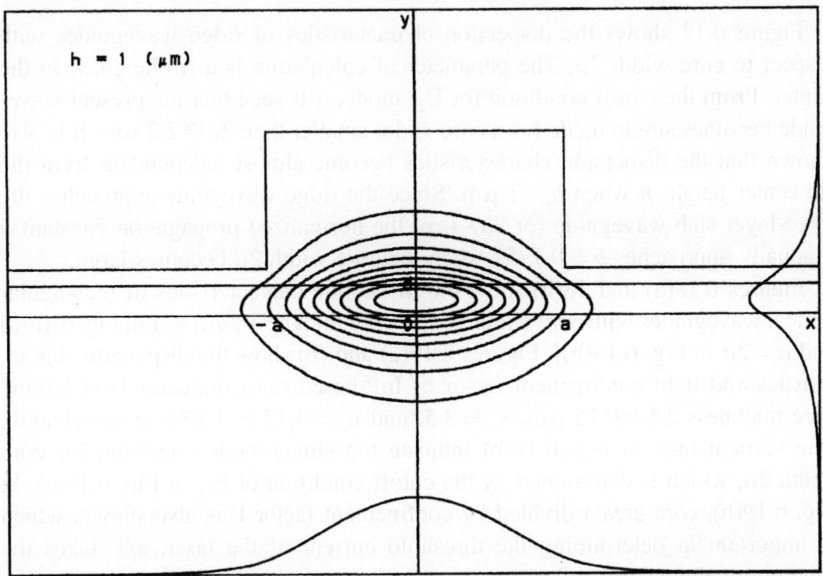

Figure 6.16 Optical intensity distribution of the E_{11} mode in the ridge waveguide, $n_c = 3.38$, $n_s = 3.17$, $n_r = n_s$, $n_a = 1.0$, $2a = 2$ µm, $d = 0.2$ µm, $h = 1$ µm, $t = 0.1$ µm and $\lambda = 1.55$ µm.

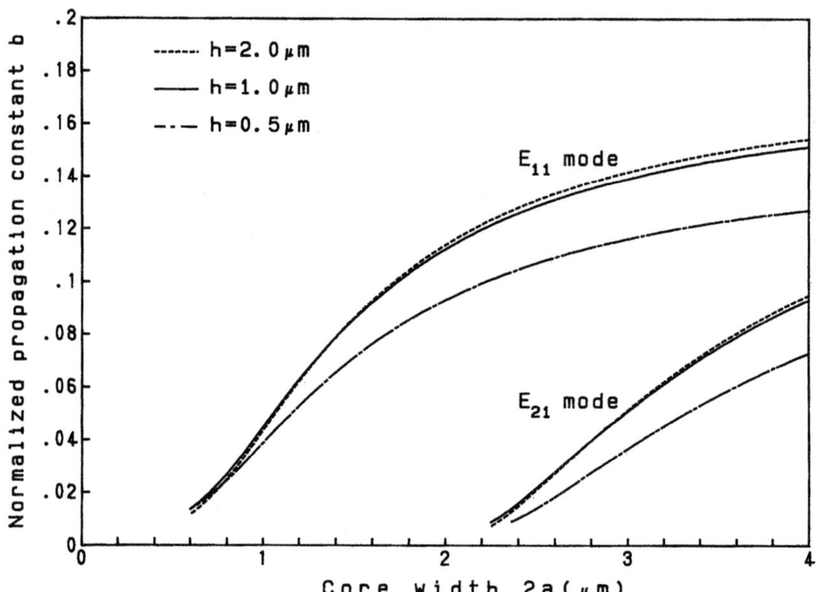

Figure 6.17 Dispersion characteristics of ridge waveguides.

Figure 6.17 shows the dispersion characteristics of ridge waveguides with respect to core width $2a$. The parameter of calculation is a rib height h in the center. From the cutoff condition for E_{21} mode, it is seen that the present waveguide becomes single mode for a core width smaller than $2a \cong 2.2$ μm. It is also known that the dispersion characteristics become almost independent from the rib center height h when $h > 1$ μm. Since the ridge waveguide approaches the three-layer slab waveguide for $2a \to \infty$, the normalized propagation constant b gradually approaches $b = 0.1751$ when the core width $2a$ becomes large.

Figures 6.18(a) and 18(b) show the dispersion characteristics of rectangular optical waveguides with core width $2a$ and core thickness $2d[a = d$ in Fig. 6.18(a) and $a = 2d$ in Fig. 6.18(b)]. Figures 6.19(a) and (b) show the dispersion characteristics and light confinement factor of InP-based semiconductor laser having core thickness $2d = 0.15$ μm, $n_c = 3.5$, and $n_s = 3.17$ at 1.55-μm wavelength. The vertical bars in Fig. 6.19(b) indicate the single-mode condition for core width $2a$, which is determined by the cutoff condition of E_{21} in Fig. 6.19(a). In Fig. 6.19(b), core area s divided by confinement factor Γ is also shown, which is important in determining the threshold current of the laser. s/Γ takes the minimum value of $s/\Gamma = 0.693$ at $2a = 0.82$ μm.

Next, FEM analysis of the coupling efficiency between a rectangular waveguide and optical fiber will be described. Here we assume that the waveguide

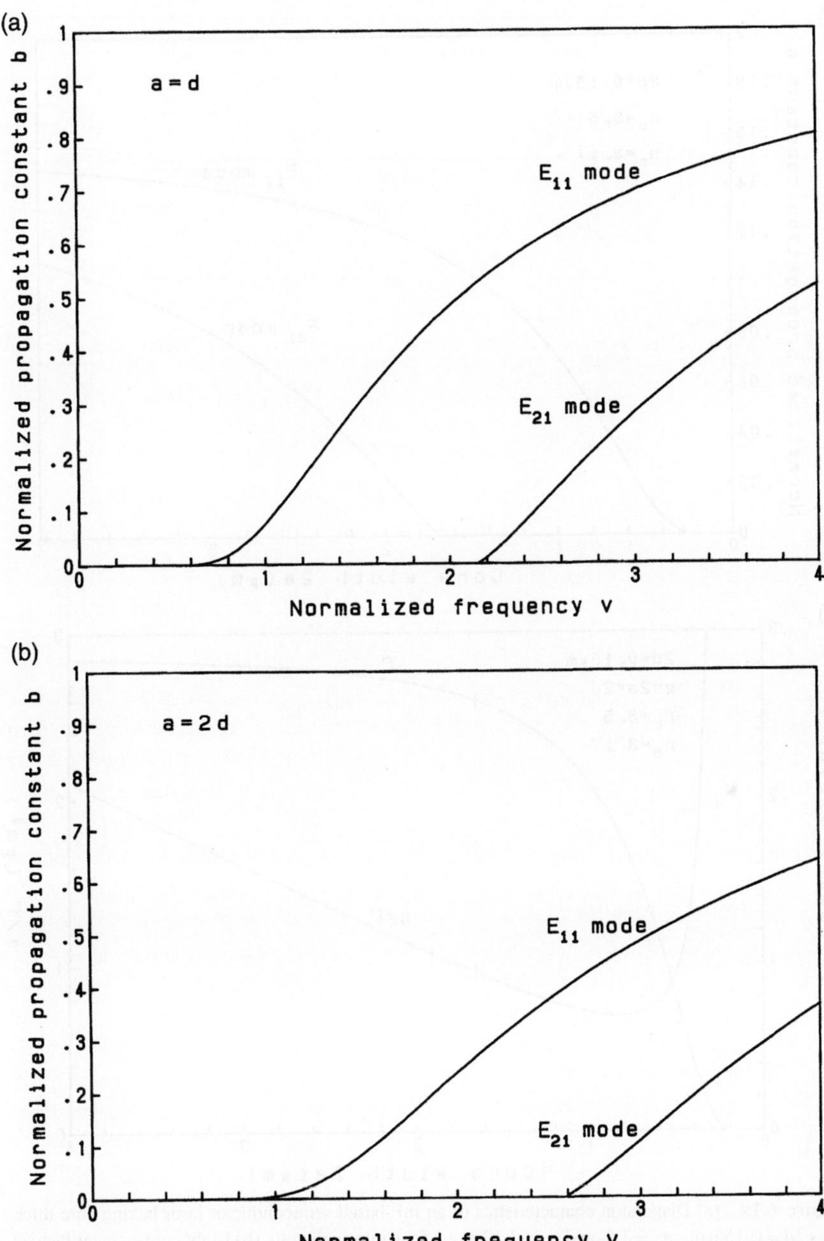

Figure 6.18 Dispersion characteristics of rectangular optical waveguides with core width $2a$ and core thickness $2d$. (a) $a = d$; (b) $a = 2d$.

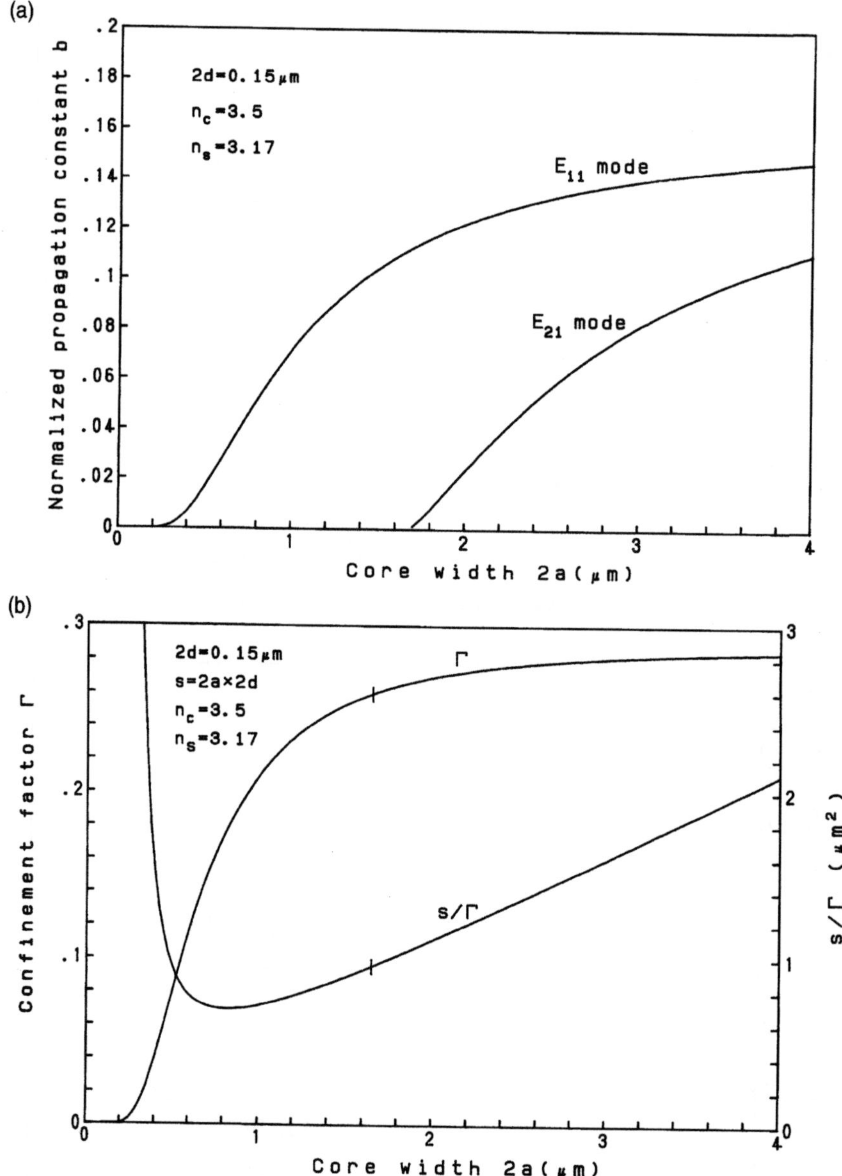

Figure 6.19 (a) Dispersion characteristics of an InP-based semiconductor laser having core thickness $2d = 0.15$ μm, $n_c = 3.5$, and $n_s = 3.17$ at a 1.55-μm wavelength. (b) Light confinement factor Γ and core area/Γ of an InP-based semiconductor laser having core thickness $2d = 0.15$ μm, $n_c = 3.5$ and, $n_s = 3.17$ at a 1.55-μm wavelength.

parameters of optical fiber are fixed at core diameter $2a = 9$ μm and relative refractive-index difference $\Delta = 0.3\%$. In the rectangular waveguide, the core thickness and refractive-index difference are fixed at $2d = 6$ μm and $\Delta = 0.75\%$. Then the dependency of the coupling coefficient on the core width $2a$ at $\lambda =$ 1.55 μm is calculated. The coupling coefficient between optical fiber and the rectangular waveguide is given by [11]

$$C_{AMP} = \frac{\iint f(x, y)g(x, y)dx\,dy}{[\iint f^2\, dx\,dy]^{1/2}[\iint g^2\, dx\,dy]^{1/2}}, \tag{6.89}$$

where $f(x, y)$ and $g(x, y)$ denote the electric field distributions of the optical fiber and the rectangular waveguide, respectively. The power-coupling coefficient is then given by

$$c = |c_{AMP}|^2. \tag{6.90}$$

Figure 6.20 shows the power-coupling coefficient between the rectangular waveguide and optical fiber when the core width of the waveguide $2a$ is varied. The coupling coefficient of a square waveguide with a core width $2a = 6$ μm is $c =$ 0.932(−0.31 dB loss), since the mismatch of the fields between the waveguide

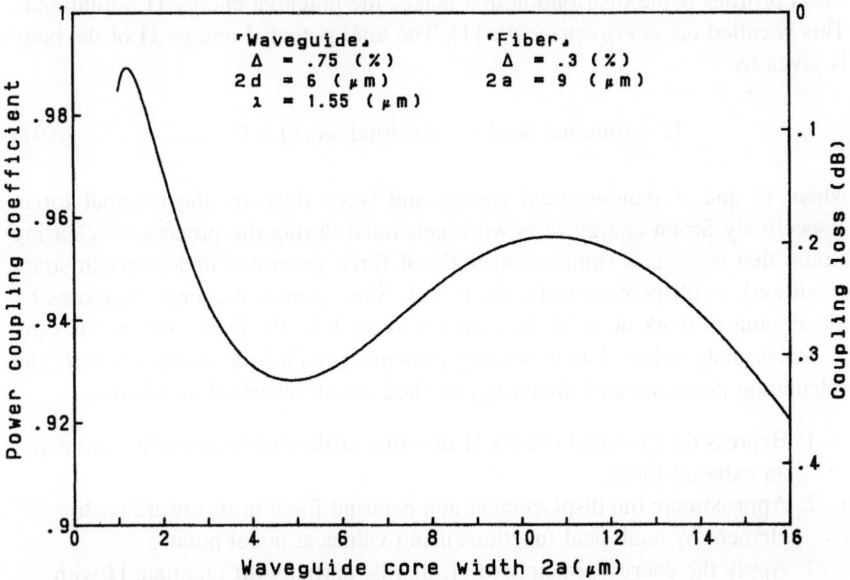

Figure 6.20 Power-coupling coefficient between a rectangular waveguide and optical fiber when the core width of the waveguide $2a$ is varied.

and the fiber is rather large. There are two core widths at which the coupling coefficient has a local maximum. One is $2a = 1.2\,\mu$m; the other is $2a = 10.7\,\mu$m. The coupling coefficients are $c = 0.989(-0.05\,\text{dB}$ loss) at $2a = 1.2\,\mu$m and $c = 0.956(-0.2\,\text{dB}$ loss) at $2a = 10.7\,\mu$m. The highest coupling coefficient is obtained when the core width $2a$ is quite small. Figure 6.21 shows light intensity distributions of rectangular waveguides for (a) $2a = 1.2\,\mu$m, (b) $2a = 6\,\mu$m, and (c) $2a = 10.7\,\mu$m. Figure 6.21(d) shows the intensity distribution of optical fiber with a core diameter $2a = 9\,\mu$m and a refractive-index difference $\Delta = 0.3\%$. Since the electric field profile is almost uniformly expanded in Fig. 6.21(a), the highest coupling coefficient with optical fiber is obtained.

6.5. STRESS ANALYSIS OF OPTICAL WAVEGUIDES

6.5.1. Energy Principle

The finite element method was originally developed for the stiffness analysis of airplane [12]. Consequently, stress analysis is the most typical application of FEM. Generally, it is well known that the total potential energy Π should be a minimum when thermal stress and/or an external force is applied to the body. In other words, the strain distribution that is actually generated among all possible strain profiles is the distribution that makes the potential energy Π a minimum. This is called the *energy principle* [1]. The total potential energy Π of the body is given by

$$\Pi = (\text{internal work}) - (\text{external work}) = U - V, \tag{6.91}$$

where U and V denote strain energy and work done by the external force; respectively Strain energy U is work generated during the process of releasing strain; that is, U is a summation of {local force generated under certain strain condition} $\times$ {displacement by the force}. Since potential energy decreases by the amount of work done by the external force, V in Eq. (6.91) has minus sign.

Stress analysis based on the energy principle is called the *energy method*. The calculation procedures of the energy method are summarized as follows:

1. Express the potential energy Π in terms of the displacement by strain and an external force.
2. Approximate the displacement and external force in or toward each element by analytical functions using values at nodal points.
3. Apply the energy principle to Π; that is, partially differentiate Π with respect to the displacement and obtain an equilibrium equation (linear simultaneous equation).

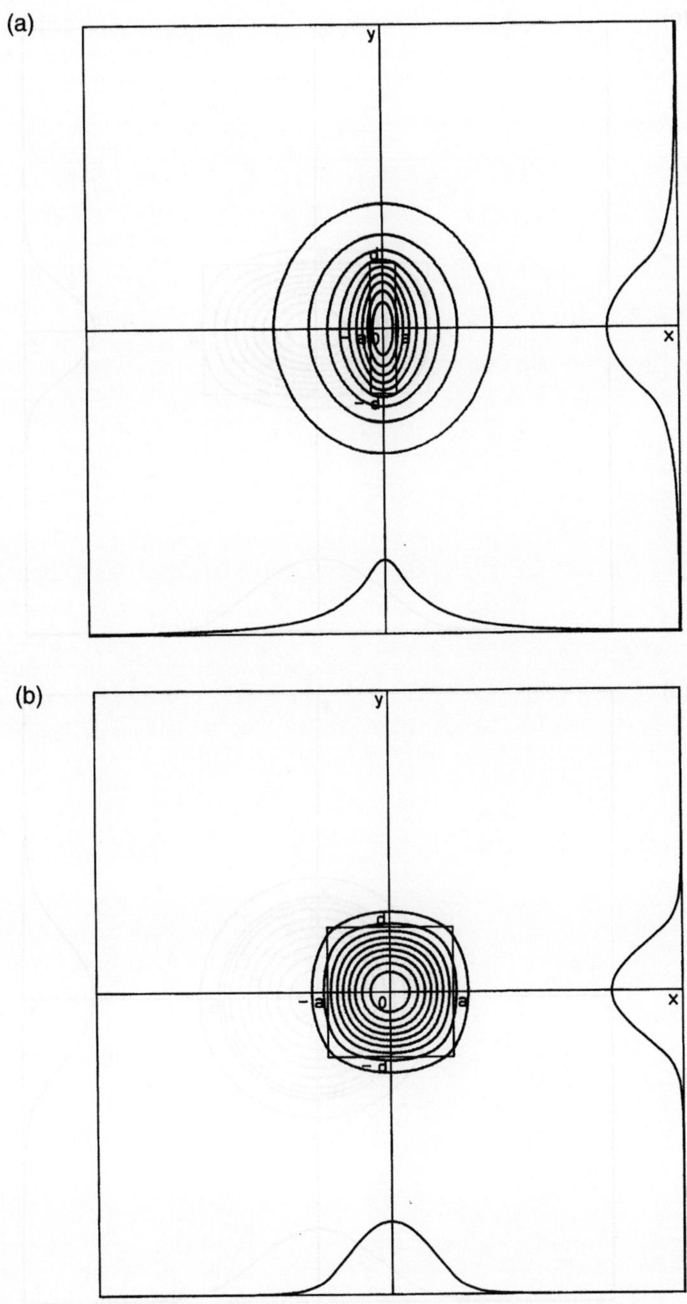

Figure 6.21 Light intensity distributions of rectangular waveguides for (a) $2a = 1.2\,\mu\text{m}$,

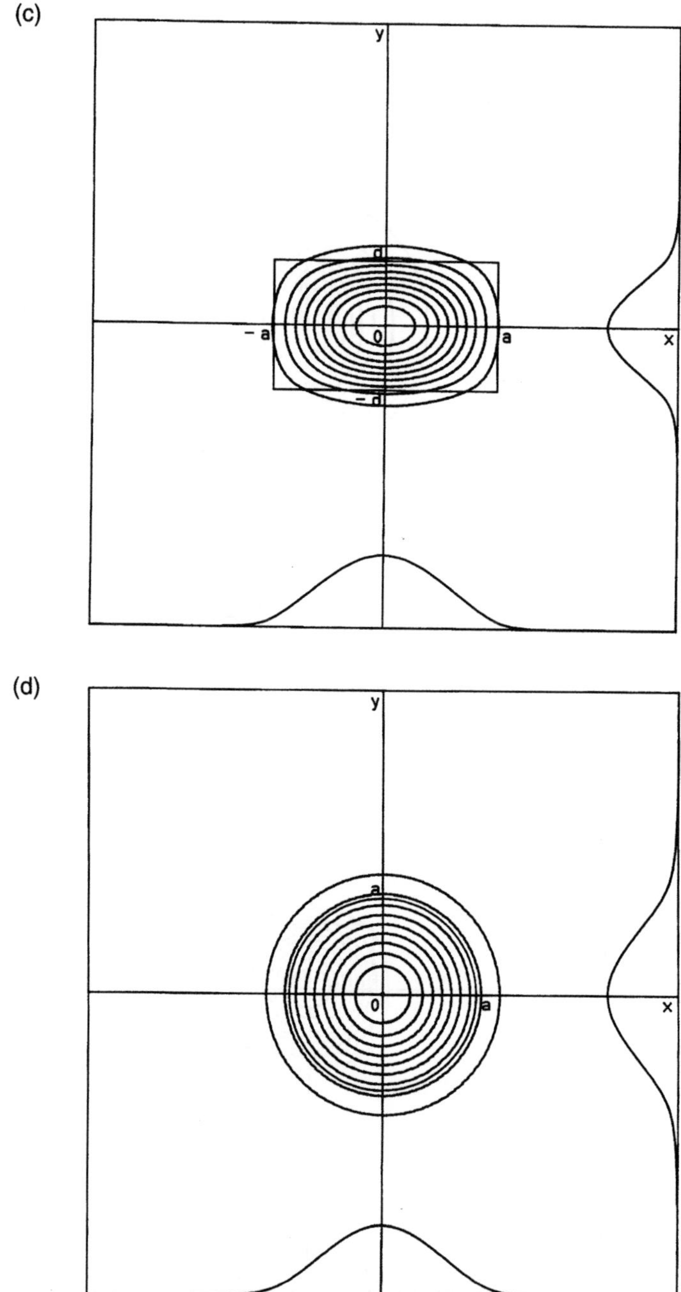

Figure 6.21 (*Continued*) (b) $2a = 6$ μm, and (c) $2a = 10.7$ μm. (d) is an intensity distribution of optical fiber with a core diameter $2a = 9$ μm and a refractive-index difference $\Delta = 0.3\%$.

4. Solve the simultaneous equation and determine the displacement at each nodal point.
5. The strain and stress in each element are calculated by using the displacements at the nodes surrounding the element.

6.5.2. Plane Strain and Plane Stress

Generally, three-dimensional FEM analysis requires a large computer memory and a long CPU time for calculation. Therefore, two-dimensional analysis is often used for the three-dimensional body, using an appropriate assumption for each problem.

First, let us consider a body that is long along its z-axis direction compared to its cross-sectional area, such as optical fibers and waveguides. In this case, strain in the body along z-axis direction ε_z is considered to be zero, except at both ends. Then we can assume

$$\varepsilon_z = 0. \tag{6.92}$$

Stress analysis based on this assumption is called a *plane strain problem.* On the other hand, when a body is quite thin compared to its cross-sectional area, the stress component σ_z normal to the plane is considered to be zero; that is,

$$\sigma_z = 0. \tag{6.93}$$

Stress analysis based on this assumption is called a *plane stress problem.*

In the following sections, stress analyses of optical waveguides based on the plane strain approximation will be described.

6.5.3. Basic Equations for Displacement, Strain and Stress

The definitions of the parameters in stress analysis are:

u and v:	Displacements along the x- and y-axis directions, respectively
ε_x, ε_y and ε_z:	Principal strains along x-, y- and z-axis directions, respectively
γ_{xy}:	Shear strain in the x–y plane
σ_x, σ_y and σ_z:	Principal stress along the x-, y- and z-axis directions, respectively
τ_{xy}:	Shear stress in the x–y plane
f and g:	External forces along x- and y-axis directions, respectively
E and ν:	Young's modulus and Poisson's ratio, respectively.

The relationship between displacement and strain is given by [13]

$$\varepsilon_x = \frac{\partial u}{\partial x}, \tag{6.94a}$$

$$\varepsilon_y = \frac{\partial v}{\partial y}, \tag{6.94b}$$

$$\gamma_{xy} = \frac{\partial v}{\partial x} + \frac{\partial u}{\partial y}. \tag{6.94c}$$

Next, the relationship between stress and strain is generally is expressed as

$$\varepsilon_x = \frac{1}{E}\left[\sigma_x - \nu(\sigma_y + \sigma_z)\right] + \alpha\Delta T, \tag{6.95a}$$

$$\varepsilon_y = \frac{1}{E}\left[\sigma_y - \nu(\sigma_z + \sigma_x)\right] + \alpha\Delta T, \tag{6.95b}$$

$$\varepsilon_z = \frac{1}{E}\left[\sigma_z - \nu(\sigma_x + \sigma_y)\right] + \alpha\Delta T, \tag{6.95c}$$

$$\gamma_{xy} = \frac{\tau_{xy}}{G} = \frac{2(1+\nu)}{E}\tau_{xy}, \tag{6.96}$$

where G, α and ΔT denote shear modulus, thermal expansion coefficient and temperature change (negative for cooling), respectively. Substituting Eq. (6.92) in Eq. (6.95), the relationship between stress and strain in the plane strain problem is given by

$$\sigma_x = \frac{E}{(1+\nu)(1-2\nu)}[(1-\nu)\varepsilon_x + \nu\varepsilon_y] - \frac{\alpha E\Delta T}{(1-2\nu)}, \tag{6.97a}$$

$$\sigma_y = \frac{E}{(1+\nu)(1-2\nu)}[\nu\varepsilon_x + (1-\nu)\varepsilon_y] - \frac{\alpha E\Delta T}{(1-2\nu)}, \tag{6.97b}$$

$$\sigma_z = \nu(\sigma_x + \sigma_y) - \alpha E\Delta T. \tag{6.97c}$$

In contrast, the relationship between stress and strain in the plane stress problem is given by substituting Eq. (6.93) into (6.95), as

$$\sigma_x = \frac{E}{(1-\nu^2)}[\varepsilon_x + \nu\varepsilon_y] - \frac{\alpha E\Delta T}{(1-\nu)}, \tag{6.98a}$$

$$\sigma_y = \frac{E}{(1-\nu^2)}[\nu\varepsilon_x + \varepsilon_y] - \frac{\alpha E\Delta T}{(1-\nu)}. \tag{6.98b}$$

In the following section, FEM stress analysis for the rib optical waveguide, whose FEM waveguide analysis has already been shown in Section 6.4.2, will be described based on the plane strain problem.

6.5.4. Formulation of the Total Potential Energy

The components of stress, strain, and initial strain due to thermal strain are expressed in the vector form as

$$\{\sigma\} = \begin{pmatrix} \sigma_x \\ \sigma_y \\ \tau_{xy} \end{pmatrix}, \tag{6.99}$$

$$\{\varepsilon\} = \begin{pmatrix} \varepsilon_x \\ \varepsilon_y \\ \gamma_{xy} \end{pmatrix}, \tag{6.100}$$

$$\{\varepsilon_0\} = (1+\nu)\alpha\Delta T \begin{pmatrix} 1 \\ 1 \\ 0 \end{pmatrix}. \tag{6.101}$$

The relationship between stress and strain in Eqs. (6.96) and (6.97) of the plane strain problem is expressed by using Eqs. (6.99)–(6.101):

$$\{\sigma\} = \mathbf{D}[\{\varepsilon\} - \{\varepsilon_0\}], \tag{6.102}$$

where 3×3 matrix $\mathbf{D}$ is given by

$$\mathbf{D} = \frac{E}{(1+\nu)(1-2\nu)} \begin{bmatrix} (1-\nu) & \nu & 0 \\ \nu & (1-\nu) & 0 \\ 0 & 0 & (1-2\nu)/2 \end{bmatrix}. \tag{6.103}$$

Strain energy per unit length is obtained by

$$(\text{strain energy}) = \frac{1}{2}\iint (\text{stress}) \cdot [(\text{strain}) - (\text{initial strain})]dx\, dy.$$

Then U is expressed by using Eqs. (6.99)–(6.101):

$$U = \frac{1}{2}\iint \{\sigma\}^t[\{\varepsilon\} - \{\varepsilon_0\}]dx\, dy, \tag{6.104}$$

where $\{\ \}^t$ represents the transpose of the vector and $\{\sigma\}^t = [\sigma_x,\ \sigma_y,\ \tau_{xy}]$ is a raw vector of σ. The entire rib waveguide structure (actually a half of the structure, since it is symmetrical with respect to the y-axis) is divided into small elements, as shown in Fig. 6.22, and the integral of Eq. (6.104) is carried out in

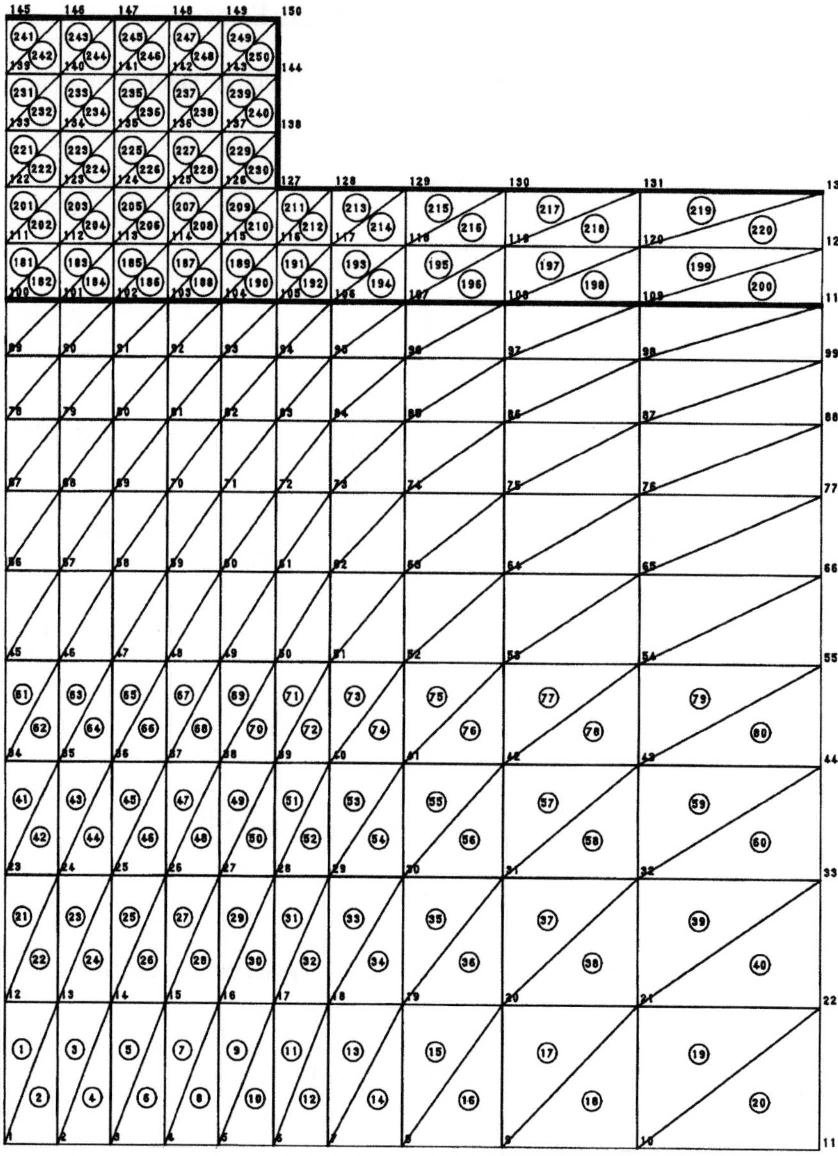

Figure 6.22 Example of element division in FEM stress analysis. The Number of triangular elements is $N = 250$, and the number of nodes is $n = 150$.

each element. In contrast to the FEM waveguide analysis in Section 6.4.2, the actual boundary of the body becomes the boundary in FEM stress analysis, since strain and stress do not penetrate into the air region. The number of triangular elements in Fig. 6.22 is $N = 250$ and number of nodes is $n = 150$. The strain $u(x, y)$ and $v(x, y)$ along x- and y-axis directions in the eth ($e = 1 - N$) element is approximated by the linear function of x and y:

$$\begin{cases} u(x, y) = p_0^e + p_1^e x + p_2^e y & (6.105a) \\ v(x, y) = q_0^e + q_1^e x + q_2^e y, & (6.105b) \end{cases}$$

where p_0^e, p_1^e, p_2^e and q_0^e, q_1^e, q_2^e are constants. The numbers of nodal points in element e are denoted, as shown in Fig. 6.14, by i, j, and k and the coordinates of the nodal point are expressed as $(x_m, y_m)(m = i, j, k)$. Assuming that the displacements at nodal points i, j and k in the eth element are given by (u_i, v_i), (u_j, v_j) and (u_k, v_k), the expansion coefficients p_0^e, p_1^e, p_2^e and q_0^e, q_1^e, q_2^e are obtained by

$$\begin{pmatrix} p_0^e \\ p_1^e \\ p_2^e \end{pmatrix} = \mathbf{C}_e \begin{pmatrix} u_i \\ u_j \\ u_k \end{pmatrix}, \tag{6.106a}$$

$$\begin{pmatrix} q_0^e \\ q_1^e \\ q_2^e \end{pmatrix} = \mathbf{C}_e \begin{pmatrix} v_i \\ v_j \\ v_k \end{pmatrix}. \tag{6.106b}$$

Here, element matrix $\mathbf{C}_e$ is given by

$$\boldsymbol{C}_e = \frac{1}{2s_e} \begin{bmatrix} (x_j y_k - x_k y_j) & (x_k y_i - x_i y_k) & (x_i y_j - x_j y_i) \\ (y_j - y_k) & (y_k - y_i) & (y_i - y_j) \\ (x_k - x_j) & (x_i - x_k) & (x_j - x_i) \end{bmatrix}. \tag{6.107}$$

Cross-sectional area s_e is given by Eq. (6.70). Substituting Eqs. (6.105) and (6.106) in Eq. (6.94), the strain components in the eth element are obtained as

$$\begin{pmatrix} \varepsilon_x \\ \varepsilon_y \\ \gamma_{xy} \end{pmatrix} = \frac{1}{2s_e} \begin{bmatrix} (y_j - y_k) & 0 & (y_k - y_i) & 0 & (y_i - y_j) & 0 \\ 0 & (x_k - x_j) & 0 & (x_i - x_k) & 0 & (x_j - x_i) \\ (x_k - x_j) & (y_j - y_k) & (x_i - x_k) & (y_k - y_i) & (x_j - x_i) & (y_i - y_j) \end{bmatrix} \begin{pmatrix} u_i \\ v_i \\ u_j \\ v_j \\ u_k \\ v_k \end{pmatrix}. \tag{6.108}$$

This is rewritten in matrix form as

$$\{\varepsilon^e\} = \mathbf{B}_e \{d^e\}, \tag{6.109}$$

where $\mathbf{B}_e$ is a 3×6-element matrix in the right-hand side of Eq. (6.108) and $\{d^e\} = [u_i,\ v_i\ u_j,\ v_j\ u_k,\ v_k]^t$ is a 6×1 raw vector representing displacements. The strain energy in the eth element is then expressed as

$$U^e = \frac{1}{2} \iint_e \{\sigma^e\}^t [\{\varepsilon^e\} - \{\varepsilon_0^e\}] dx\, dy, \tag{6.110}$$

where $\{\sigma^e\}^t$ is expressed, by using Eqs. (6.102) and (6.109), as

$$\{\sigma^e\}^t = [\{\varepsilon^e\}^t - \{\varepsilon_0^e\}^t]\mathbf{D}_e = [\{d^e\}^t \mathbf{B}^t{}_e - \{\varepsilon_0^e\}^t]\mathbf{D}_e. \tag{6.111}$$

In the above equation, element matrix $\mathbf{D}_e$ may be different in each element, since Young's modulus and Poisson's ratio are different in the core and substrate regions. Substitution of Eq. (6.111) in Eq. (6.110) gives

$$\begin{aligned} U^e &= \frac{1}{2} \iint_e [\{d^e\}^t \mathbf{B}_e^t \mathbf{D}_e \mathbf{B}_e \{d^e\} - 2\{d^e\}^t \mathbf{B}_e^t \mathbf{D}_e \{\varepsilon_0^e\} + \{\varepsilon_0^e\}^t \mathbf{D}_e \{\varepsilon_0^e\}]\, dx\, dy \\ &= \frac{s_e}{2} [\{d^e\}^t \mathbf{B}_e^t \mathbf{D}_e \mathbf{B}_e \{d^e\} - 2\{d^e\}^t \mathbf{B}_e^t \mathbf{D}_e \{\varepsilon_0^e\} + \{\varepsilon_0^e\}^t \mathbf{D}_e \{\varepsilon_0^e\}]. \end{aligned} \tag{6.112}$$

The last term in this equation, $\{\varepsilon_0^e\}^t\ \mathbf{D}_e\ \{\varepsilon_0^e\}$, is expressed by using Eqs. (6.101) and (6.103), as

$$\{\varepsilon_0^e\}^t \mathbf{D}_e \{\varepsilon_0^e\} = \frac{2(1+\nu_e)E_e}{(1-2\nu_e)} (\alpha_e \Delta T)^2. \tag{6.113}$$

Since Eq. (6.113) is always positive, it can be neglected in the minimization of potential energy. Then strain energy U^e in the eth element is expressed as

$$U^e = \frac{1}{2}\{d^e\}^t \mathbf{A}_e \{d^e\} - \{d^e\}^t \{h^e\}. \tag{6.114}$$

Here $\mathbf{A}_e$ is a 6×6-element stiffness matrix and $\{h^e\}$ is a 6×1 thermal stress vector, which are given by

$$\mathbf{A}_e = s_e \mathbf{B}_e^t \mathbf{D}_e \mathbf{B}_e, \tag{6.115a}$$

$$\{h^e\} = s_e \mathbf{B}_e^t \mathbf{D}_e \{\varepsilon_0^e\}. \tag{6.115b}$$

The total strain energy is obtained by summing the element strain energy:

$$U = \sum_{e=1}^{N} U^e = \frac{1}{2}\{d\}^t \mathbf{A}\{d\} - \{d\}^t\{H\}, \tag{6.116}$$

where $\{d\}$, $\mathbf{A}$ and $\{H\}$ are $2n \times 1$ global strain vector, the $2n \times 2n$ global stiffness matrix, and the $2n \times 1$ global thermal stress vector, respectively. The algorithm by which components of the element stiffness matrix $\mathbf{A}_e$ and thermal stress vector $\{h^e\}$ are contained in the global stiffness matrix $\mathbf{A}$ and the thermal stress vector $\{H\}$ is shown in Table 6.2.

An external force applied to the body is approximated by the force concentrated at the node on the surface of the body. Then the vector of the external force is expressed by

$$\{f_L\} = \begin{pmatrix} f_1 \\ g_1 \\ f_2 \\ g_2 \\ \vdots \\ f_n \\ g_n \end{pmatrix} \quad (n: \text{number of nodes}), \tag{6.117}$$

where f_i and g_i denote the x- and y-axis components of the external force applied to nodal point i. When a displacement $(u_i,\ v_i)$ is generated by the external force $(f_i,\ g_i)$, the work done by the force is $u_i f_i + v_i g_i$. The total work done by the external force is then given by

$$V = \{d\}^t \{f_L\}. \tag{6.118}$$

Table 6.2

Relationship between components of hte element and those of the global matrix

Component of the e-th element matrix → component of global matrix	Component of the e-th element matrix → component of global matrix
$a^e_{11} \to A_{2i-1,2i-1}$	$a^e_{33} \to A_{2j-1,2j-1}$
$a^e_{12} \to A_{2i-1,2i}$	$a^e_{34} \to A_{2j-1,2j}$
$a^e_{13} \to A_{2i-1,2j-1}$	$a^e_{35} \to A_{2j-1,2k-1}$
$a^e_{14} \to A_{2i-1,2j}$	$a^e_{36} \to A_{2j-1,2k}$
$a^e_{15} \to A_{2i-1,2k-1}$	$a^e_{44} \to A_{2j,2j}$
$a^e_{16} \to A_{2i-1,2k}$	$a^e_{45} \to A_{2j-1,2k-1}$
$a^e_{22} \to A_{2i,2i}$	$a^e_{46} \to A_{2j,2k}$
$a^e_{23} \to A_{2i,2j-1}$	$a^e_{55} \to A_{2k-1,2k-1}$
$a^e_{24} \to A_{2i,2j}$	$a^e_{56} \to A_{2k-1,2k}$
$a^e_{25} \to A_{2i,2k-1}$	$a^e_{66} \to A_{2k,2k}$
$a^e_{26} \to A_{2i,2k}$	
$h^e_1 \to H_{2i-1}$	$h^e_2 \to H_{2i}$
$h^e_3 \to H_{2j-1}$	$h^e_4 \to H_{2j}$
$h^e_5 \to H_{2k-1}$	$h^e_6 \to H_{2k}$

Substituting Eqs. (6.116) and (6.118) into (6.91), the total potential energy Π is given by

$$\Pi = \frac{1}{2}\{d\}^t\mathbf{A}\{d\} - \{d\}^t[\{H\} + \{f_L\}]. \tag{6.119}$$

In the thermal stress analyses of birefringent fibers and waveguides without external force, we simply make $\{f_L\} = \{0\}$ in Eq. (6.119).

6.5.5. Solution of the Problem by the Stationary Condition

Potential energy Π in Eq. (6.119) should be a minimum by the energy principle. Therefore, the partial derivative of Π with respect to the displacement of each nodal point should be zero. We then have $2n$th-order linear simultaneous equation:

$$\mathbf{A}\{d\} = \{H\} + \{f_L\}. \tag{6.120}$$

The solution of the displacement vector is easily obtained:

$$\{d\} = \mathbf{A}^{-1}[\{H\} + \{f_L\}]. \tag{6.121}$$

The stress in each element is calculated, by using Eqs. (6.102) and (6.109), as

$$\{\sigma^e\} = \mathbf{D}_e[\mathbf{B}_e\{d^e\} - \{\varepsilon_0^e\}] \quad (e = 1 - N). \tag{6.122}$$

In the symmetrical structure shown in Fig. 6.22, displacement on the y-axis is directed along the y-axis direction. Therefore, displacement on the y-axis along the x-axis direction should be zero. These boundary conditions, which are not considered in the element level, are taken into account during the process of solving the simultaneous equations (6.120). But it is not preferable to change the matrix size of $\mathbf{A}$ for the boundary conditions, because the number of boundary conditions is different in each problem. In practical FEM stress analysis procedures, boundary conditions are treated as follows. We rewrite $2n$th-order linear simultaneous equation as

$$\begin{bmatrix} A_{1,1} & A_{1,2} & \cdots & A_{1,2i-2} & A_{1,2i-1} & A_{1,2i} & \cdots & A_{1,2n-1} & A_{1,2n} \\ A_{2,1} & A_{2,2} & \cdots & A_{2,2i-2} & A_{2,2i-1} & A_{2,2i} & \cdots & A_{2,2n-1} & A_{2,2n} \\ \vdots & \vdots & \ddots & \vdots & \vdots & \vdots & \ddots & \vdots & \vdots \\ A_{2i-2,1} & A_{2i-2,2} & \cdots & A_{2i-2,2i-2} & A_{2i-2,2i-1} & A_{2i-2,2i} & \cdots & A_{2i-2,2n-1} & A_{2i-2,2n} \\ A_{2i-1,1} & A_{2i-1,2} & \cdots & A_{2i-1,2i-2} & A_{2i-1,2i-1} & A_{2i-1,2i} & \cdots & A_{2i-1,2n-1} & A_{2i-1,2n} \\ A_{2i,1} & A_{2i,2} & \cdots & A_{2i,2i-2} & A_{2i,2i-1} & A_{2i,2i} & \cdots & A_{2i,2n-1} & A_{2i,2n} \\ \vdots & \vdots & \ddots & \vdots & \vdots & \vdots & \ddots & \vdots & \vdots \\ A_{2n-1,1} & A_{2n-1,2} & \cdots & A_{2n-1,2i-2} & A_{2n-1,2i-1} & A_{2n-1,2i} & \cdots & A_{2n-1,2n-1} & A_{2n-1,2n} \\ A_{2n,1} & A_{2n,2} & \cdots & A_{2n,2i-2} & A_{2n,2i-1} & A_{2n,2i} & \cdots & A_{2n,2n-1} & A_{2n,2n} \end{bmatrix} \begin{pmatrix} u_1 \\ v_1 \\ \vdots \\ v_{i-1} \\ u_i \\ v_i \\ \vdots \\ u_n \\ v_n \end{pmatrix} = \begin{pmatrix} F_1 \\ F_2 \\ \vdots \\ F_{2i-2} \\ F_{2i-1} \\ F_{2i} \\ \vdots \\ F_{2n-1} \\ F_{2n} \end{pmatrix} \tag{6.123}$$

where $\{F\} = \{H\} + \{f_L\}$. We consider, for example, the boundary condition in which displacement along x-axis direction of the ith nodal point u_i is specified as zero. In this case, the contribution of u_i to Eq. (6.123) or [Eq. (6.120)] can be made zero by setting the matrix element $A_{m,2i-1} = 0$ for $m = 1$ to $2n$. However, we should have one equation which specifies $u_i = 0$. This condition is accomplished by setting $A_{2i-1,2i-1} = 1$, $F_{2i-1} = 0$ and $A_{2i-1,k} = 0$ for $k = 1$ to $2n$ except for $k = 2i - 1$. Then we obtain the following matrix expression in which the boundary condition of $u_i = 0$ is automatically included:

$$\begin{bmatrix} A_{1,1} & A_{1,2} & \cdots & A_{1,2i-2} & 0 & A_{1,2i} & \cdots & A_{1,2n-1} & A_{1,2n} \\ A_{2,1} & A_{2,2} & \cdots & A_{2,2i-2} & 0 & A_{2,2i} & \cdots & A_{2,2n-1} & A_{2,2n} \\ \vdots & \vdots & \ddots & \vdots & \vdots & \vdots & \ddots & \vdots & \vdots \\ A_{2i-2,1} & A_{2i-2,2} & \cdots & A_{2i-2,2i-2} & 0 & A_{2i-2,2i} & \cdots & A_{2i-2,2n-1} & A_{2i-2,2n} \\ 0 & 0 & \cdots & 0 & 1 & 0 & \cdots & 0 & 0 \\ A_{2i,1} & A_{2i,2} & \cdots & A_{2i,2i-2} & 0 & A_{2i,2i} & \cdots & A_{2i,2n-1} & A_{2i,2n} \\ \vdots & \vdots & \ddots & \vdots & \vdots & \vdots & \ddots & \vdots & \vdots \\ A_{2n-1,1} & A_{2n-1,2} & \cdots & A_{2n-1,2i-2} & 0 & A_{2n-1,2i} & \cdots & A_{2n-1,2n-1} & A_{2n-1,2n} \\ A_{2n-1} & A_{2n,2} & \cdots & A_{2n,2i-2} & 0 & A_{2n,2i} & \cdots & A_{2n,2n-1} & A_{2n,2n} \end{bmatrix} \begin{pmatrix} u_1 \\ v_1 \\ \vdots \\ v_{i-1} \\ u_i \\ v_i \\ \vdots \\ u_n \\ v_n \end{pmatrix} = \begin{pmatrix} F_1 \\ F_2 \\ \vdots \\ F_{2i-2} \\ 0 \\ F_{2i} \\ \vdots \\ F_{2n-1} \\ F_{2n} \end{pmatrix} \tag{6.124}$$

Here, the component of load vector F_{2i-1} corresponding to u_i is also set to zero. It is readily understood that the solution u_i in above Eq. (6.123) becomes zero, as specified by the boundary condition. Boundary conditions to other nodal points are treated in the same manner as just described above.

Another important boundary condition in FEM stress analysis is that one of the nodal points (for example, nodal point 1 in Fig. 6.22) should be fixed so as to prevent motion of the rigid body. Therefore, displacements of nodal point 1 along the x- and y-axis directions should be zero. These boundary conditions are also taken into account in global matrix **A**.

6.5.6. Combination of Finite-Element Waveguide and Stress Analysis

As described in Section 3.9 for stress-induced birefringent optical fibers, it is important to consider the refractive-index change due to the photoelastic effect in order to investigate the propagation characteristics of optical waveguides under stress or strain. Here we describe the combined FEM stress analysis and FEM waveguide analysis for the ridge waveguide consisting of GaAlAs semiconductor core and GaAs substrate and an oxide strip loaded on the GaAlAs core film as shown in Fig. 6.23. Different from the perturbation method analysis described in Section 3.10.2, in the combined FEM analysis refractive-index change is first obtained by FEM stress analysis, and it is taken into account into FEM waveguide analysis. The waveguide parameters of the oxide-strip-loaded semiconductor ridge waveguide in Fig. 6.23 are as follows: thickness and total width of the GaAlAs core are $d = 0.2\,\mu\text{m}$ and $100\,\mu\text{m}$, respectively, the thickness and total width of the GaAs substrate are both $100\,\mu\text{m}$, and the thickness and width of the oxide strip are $h = 0.4\,\mu\text{m}$ and $2a = 3\,\mu\text{m}$, respectively. The material parameters for each region are given in Table 6.3; the difference between room temperature

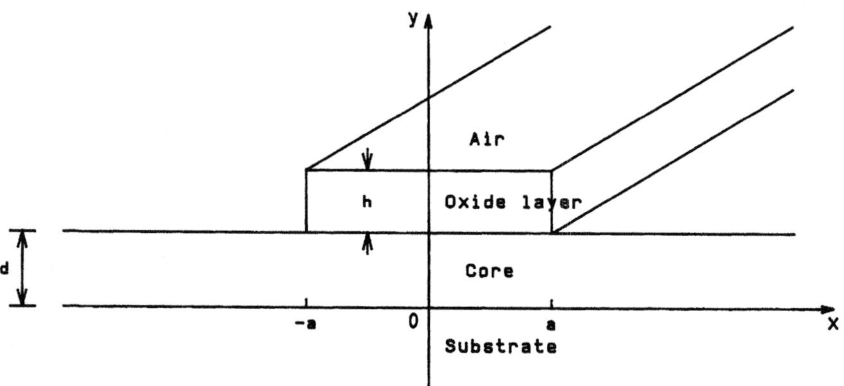

Figure 6.23 Oxide strip loaded a semiconductor ridge waveguide.

Table 6.3

Material parameters of substrate, core, and oxide strip

Material	Young's modulus kg/mm^2	Poisson's ratio ratio	Thermal expansion coefficient (°C^{-1})	Refractive index
GaAs	8700	0.31	6.4×10^{-6}	3.37
GaA1As	8620	0.315	5.8×10^{-6}	3.36
SiO_2	7830	0.186	5.4×10^{-7}	1.444

and growth temperature is assumed to be $\Delta T = -700\,°\mathrm{C}$ [14 – 16]. Contour plots of principal stress σ_x and σ_y calculated by FEM stress analysis are shown in Figs. 6.24(a) and 6.24(b). The curve plots at the bottom edges of Figs. 6.24(a) and (b) are the principal stress distributions along lines parallel to the x-axis that pass the points of maximum principal stress σ_x. and σ_y. The curve plots at the right-hand edges in Figs. 6.24(a) and (b) are the principal stress distributions along the y-axis. The Positive and negative values of the principal stress represent the tensile and compressive force, respectively.

When we consider the photoelastic effect, the refractive indices for x- and y-polarized lights are expressed by

$$\begin{aligned} n_x(x,y) &= n_{x0}(x,y) - C_1\sigma_x(x,y) \\ &\quad - C_2[\sigma_y(x,y) + \sigma_z(x,y)] \quad \text{(for } x\text{-polarization)} \qquad (6.125a) \\ n_y(x,y) &= n_{y0}(x,y) - C_1\sigma_y(x,y) \\ &\quad - C_2[\sigma_z(x,y) + \sigma_x(x,y)] \quad \text{(for } y\text{-polarization).} \qquad (6.125b) \end{aligned}$$

Here n_{x0} and n_{y0} are refractive indices without stress and C_1 and C_2 are photoelastic constants. The photoelastic constants of GaAs and SiO_2 are given [15, 16] by

$$\begin{cases} C_1 = -1.72 \times 10^{-4} & [\mathrm{mm^2/kg}] \\ C_2 = -1.0 \times 10^{-4} & [\mathrm{mm^2/kg}] \end{cases} \quad \text{(GaAs)} \qquad (6.126a)$$

$$\begin{cases} C_1 = 7.42 \times 10^{-6} & [\mathrm{mm^2/kg}] \\ C_2 = 4.102 \times 10^{-5} & [\mathrm{mm^2/kg}] \end{cases} \quad (\mathrm{SiO_2}). \qquad (6.126b)$$

Photoelastic constants C_1 and C_2 are related with Pockels coefficient p_{11} and p_{12} by the following relationship [17]:

$$\begin{cases} C_1 = \dfrac{n^3}{2E}(p_{11} - 2\nu p_{12}), \\ C_2 = \dfrac{n^3}{2E}[-\nu p_{11} + (1-\nu)p_{12}]. \end{cases} \qquad (6.127)$$

where E, v and n denote Young's modulus, Poisson's ratio, and the refractive index, respectively. Substituting principal stress σ_x and σ_y into Eq. (6.125), stress-induced refractive-index change $n_x - n_x0$ and $n_y - n_y0$ are plotted as shown in Fig. 6.25. It is known from the bottom plots in Figs. 6.25(a) and (b) that the refractive indices for both polarizations decrease markedly at the edges of the SiO_2 strip (0.016 for x-polarization and 0.014 for y-polarization). Figures 6.26(a) and (b) show light intensity distributions for x- and y-polarizations calculated by FEM

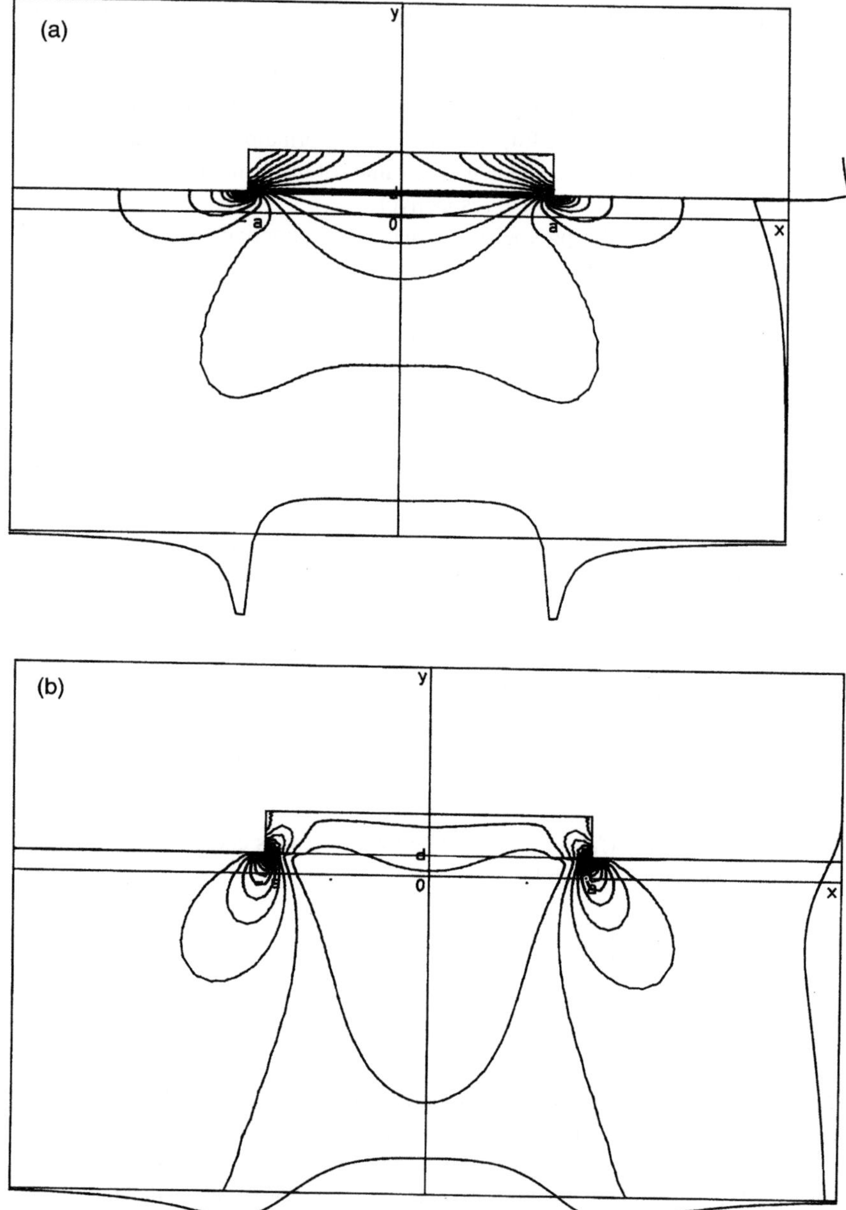

Figure 6.24 Contour plots of principal stress (a) σ_x and (b) σ_y calculated by FEM stress analysis.

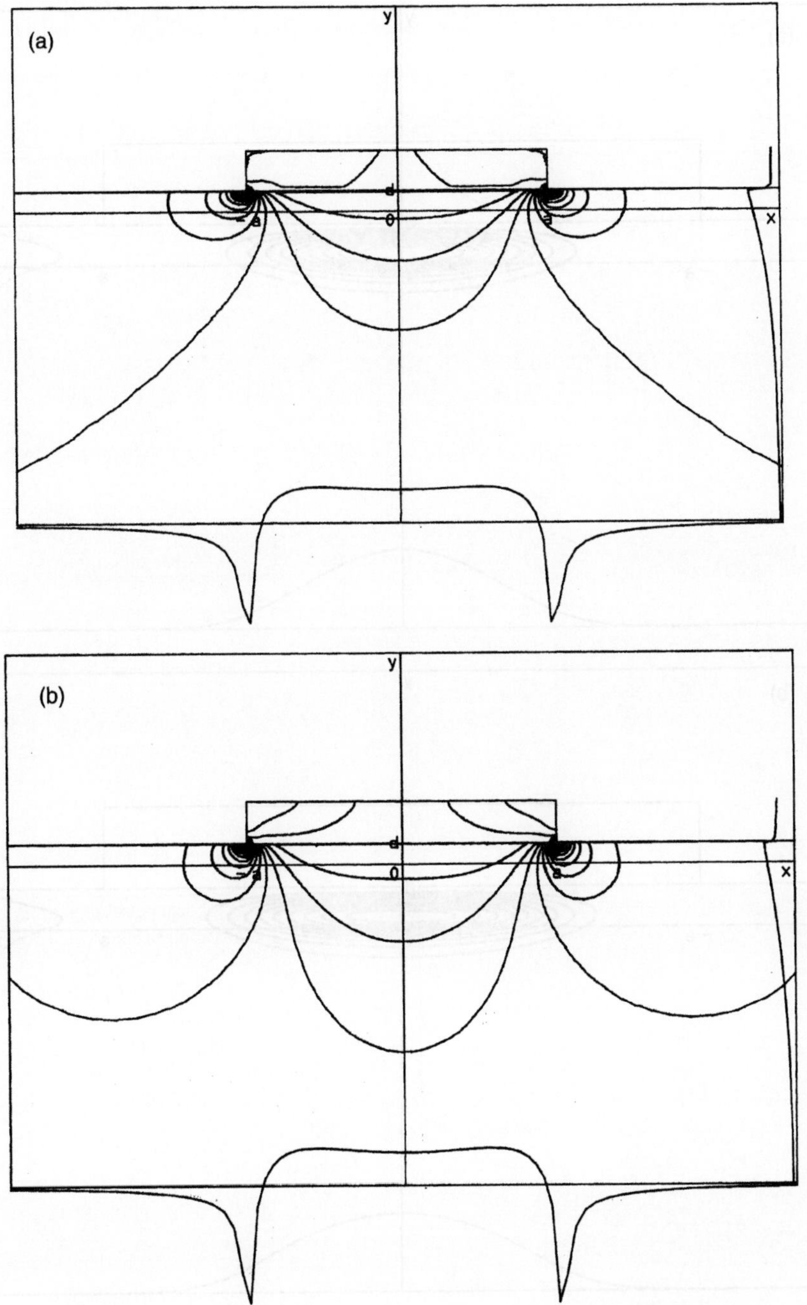

Figure 6.25 Stress-induced refractive-index change (a) $n_x - n_{x0}$ and (b) $n_y - n_{y0}$.

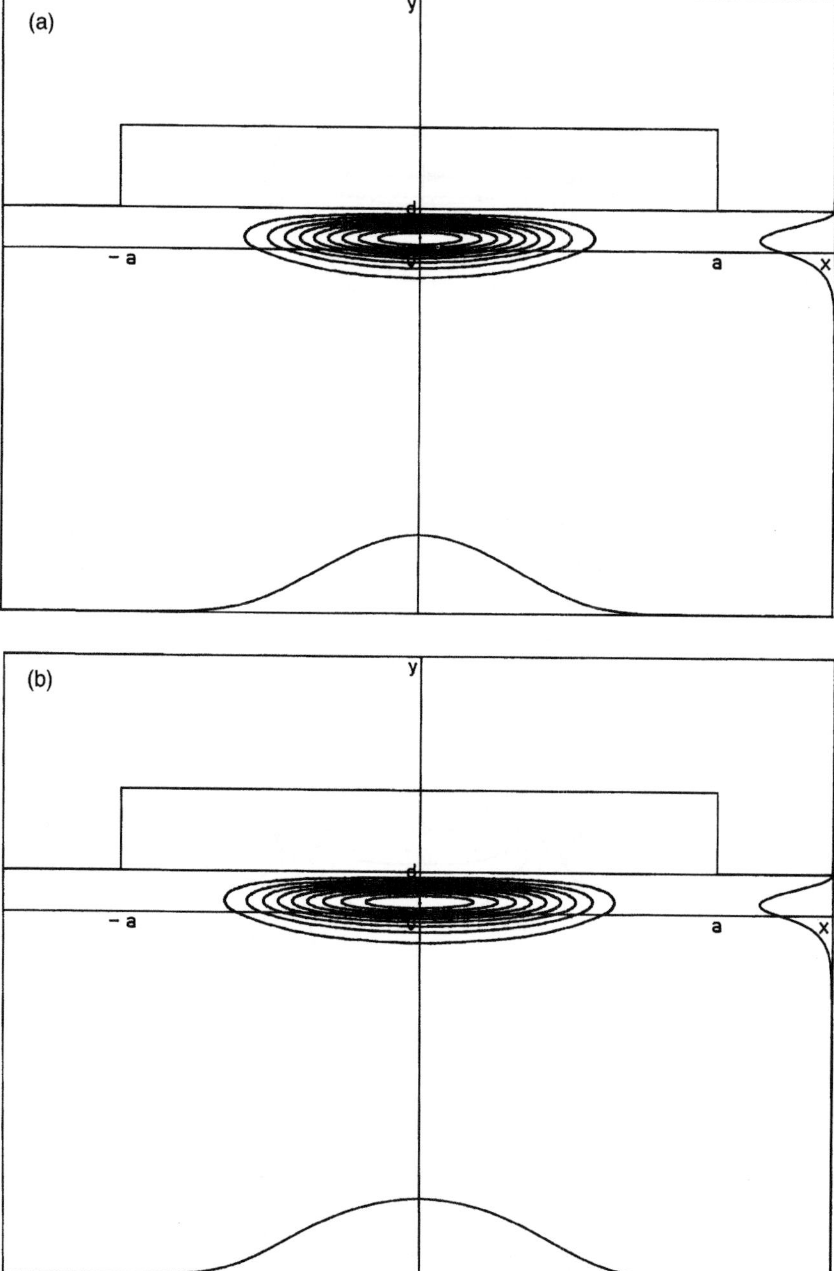

Figure 6.26 Light intensity distributions for (a) x-polarization and (b) y-polarizations calculated by FEM waveguide analysis.

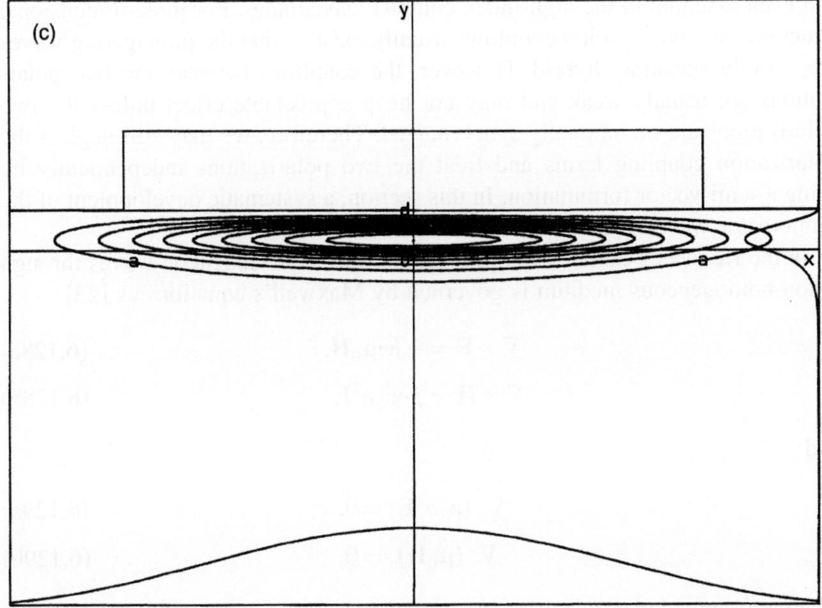

Figure 6.26 (*Continued*) (c) Intensity distribution without considering stress-induced refractive-index change.

waveguide analysis. Normalized propagation constants for x- and y-polarizations are $\beta_x/k = 3.36688$ and $\beta_y/k = 3.36612$, respectively. Figure 6.26(c) shows the light intensity distribution without considering stress-induced refractive-index change. It is seen from the comparison of Figs. 6.26(a) and (b) with (c) that light confinement effect becomes tighter due to the refractive-index decrease at both edges of SiO_2 strip.

6.6. SEMI-VECTOR FEM ANALYSIS OF HIGH-INDEX CONTRAST WAVEGUIDES

Extremely high-index contrast (EH-Δ) waveguides with Δ range 10–40% have attracted attention as regards the fabrication of ultra-compact waveguide devices [18–22]. Among them, silicon optical waveguides have emerged as the enabling technology for a new generation of optoelectronic circuits. Silicon optical waveguides can utilize the mature material processing technology and extensive electronic functionality of silicon.

So far, we have mainly treated a scalar FEM which is applicable to waveguides with low index difference. However, vector properties may become important and even essential in the high-index contrast waveguides. For three-dimensional structures, the polarization couplings usually exist so that the propagating waves are, strictly speaking, hybrid. However, the couplings between the two polarizations are usually weak and may not have appreciable effect unless the two polarizations are intentionally synchronized. Therefore, we may still neglect the polarization coupling terms and treat the two polarizations independently by using a semi-vector formulation. In this section, a systematic development of the semi-vector wave equations is described.

In the frequency domain, the propagation of electro-magnetic waves through a non-homogeneous medium is governed by Maxwell's equations as [23]

$$\nabla \times \mathbf{E} = -j\omega\mu_0 \mathbf{H}, \tag{6.128a}$$

$$\nabla \times \mathbf{H} = j\omega\varepsilon_0 n^2 \mathbf{E} \tag{6.128b}$$

and

$$\nabla \cdot (\varepsilon_0 n^2 \mathbf{E}) = 0, \tag{6.129a}$$

$$\nabla \cdot (\mu_0 \mathbf{H}) = 0, \tag{6.129b}$$

where refractive index $n(x, y, z)$ is assumed to be isotropic. A system of coupled vector wave equations for either the transverse electric or magnetic fields can be derived from the above equations.

6.6.1. E-field Formulation

The vector wave equation for the electric fields is obtained from Eqs. (6.128a) and (6.128b) as

$$\nabla \times (\nabla \times \mathbf{E}) = \nabla(\nabla \cdot \mathbf{E}) - \nabla^2 \mathbf{E} = \omega^2 \varepsilon_0 \mu_0 n^2 \mathbf{E} = k^2 n^2 \mathbf{E}, \tag{6.130}$$

where $k = \omega\sqrt{\varepsilon_0\mu_0}$ is the wave number in free space. Furthermore, Eq. (6.129a) gives

$$\nabla \cdot (n^2 \mathbf{E}) = \nabla_t \cdot (n^2 \mathbf{E}_t) + \frac{\partial (n^2 E_z)}{\partial z} = \nabla_t \cdot (n^2 \mathbf{E}_t) + \frac{\partial n^2}{\partial z} E_z + n^2 \frac{\partial E_z}{\partial z} = 0, \tag{6.131}$$

where $\nabla_t = \mathbf{u}_x \partial/\partial_x + \mathbf{u}_y \partial/\partial_y$. The term $(\partial n^2/\partial z) E_z$ in the above equation can be neglected since E_z is normally much smaller than the transversal components E_x and E_y and also the refractive index generally varies slowly along z-axis. Equation (6.131) is then approximated by

$$\frac{\partial E_z}{\partial z} = -\frac{1}{n^2} \nabla_t \cdot (n^2 \mathbf{E}_t) = -\frac{\partial E_x}{\partial x} - \frac{\partial E_y}{\partial y} - \frac{1}{n^2} \frac{\partial n^2}{\partial x} E_x - \frac{1}{n^2} \frac{\partial n^2}{\partial y} E_y. \tag{6.132}$$

$\nabla \cdot \mathbf{E}$ in (6.130) is expressed by

$$\nabla \cdot \mathbf{E} = \frac{\partial E_x}{\partial x} + \frac{\partial E_y}{\partial y} + \frac{\partial E_z}{\partial z} = -\frac{1}{n^2}\frac{\partial n^2}{\partial x}E_x - \frac{1}{n^2}\frac{\partial n^2}{\partial y}E_y. \quad (6.133)$$

Substituting Eq. (6.133) into (6.130), we obtain

$$\nabla_t^2 E_x + k^2 n^2 E_x + \frac{\partial^2 E_x}{\partial z^2} + \frac{\partial}{\partial x}\left(\frac{1}{n^2}\frac{\partial n^2}{\partial x}E_x + \frac{1}{n^2}\frac{\partial n^2}{\partial y}E_y\right) = 0, \quad (6.134)$$

$$\nabla_t^2 E_y + k^2 n^2 E_y + \frac{\partial^2 E_y}{\partial z^2} + \frac{\partial}{\partial y}\left(\frac{1}{n^2}\frac{\partial n^2}{\partial x}E_x + \frac{1}{n^2}\frac{\partial n^2}{\partial y}E_y\right) = 0. \quad (6.135)$$

The couplings between the two polarizations

$$\frac{\partial}{\partial x}\left(\frac{1}{n^2}\frac{\partial n^2}{\partial y}E_y\right)$$

in (6.134) and

$$\frac{\partial}{\partial y}\left(\frac{1}{n^2}\frac{\partial n^2}{\partial x}E_x\right)$$

in (6.135) are usually weak. Then we can neglect these coupling terms and treat Eqs. (6.134) and (6.135) independently as

$$\frac{\partial}{\partial x}\left[\frac{1}{n^2}\frac{\partial(n^2 E_x)}{\partial x}\right] + \frac{\partial^2 E_x}{\partial y^2} + \frac{\partial^2 E_x}{\partial z^2} + k^2 n^2 E_x = 0, \quad (6.136)$$

$$\frac{\partial^2 E_y}{\partial x^2} + \frac{\partial}{\partial y}\left[\frac{1}{n^2}\frac{\partial(n^2 E_y)}{\partial y}\right] + \frac{\partial^2 E_y}{\partial z^2} + k^2 n^2 E_y = 0. \quad (6.137)$$

These are called semi-vector equations based on the E-field formulation. Electric field modes obtained from Eqs. (6.136) and (6.137) are denoted as Quasi-TE mode and Quasi-TM mode, respectively.

6.6.2. H-field Formulation

Similar to the semi-vector wave equations for the electric fields, the equations for the magnetic fields are obtained as

$$\nabla \times \left(\frac{1}{n^2}\nabla \times \mathbf{H}\right) = \omega^2 \varepsilon_0 \mu_0 \mathbf{H} = k^2 \mathbf{H}. \quad (6.138)$$

$\nabla \times [(1/n^2)\nabla \times \mathbf{H}]$ is expressed by using vector formula (10.77) as

$$\nabla \times \left(\frac{1}{n^2}\nabla \times \mathbf{H}\right) = \nabla\left(\frac{1}{n^2}\right) \times (\nabla \times \mathbf{H}) + \frac{1}{n^2}\nabla \times (\nabla \times \mathbf{H}). \quad (6.139)$$

For the calculation of the semi-vector equation to H_y (Quasi-TE mode: E_x and H_y are the dominant fields) in the above equation, the term $[\partial(1/n^2)/\partial z](\partial H_z/\partial y)$ can be neglected since H_z is normally much smaller than the transversal components H_x and H_y and also the refractive index generally varies slowly along z-axis. Then equation for the Quasi-TE mode is expressed by

$$n^2 \frac{\partial}{\partial x}\left(\frac{1}{n^2}\frac{\partial H_y}{\partial x}\right) + \frac{\partial^2 H_y}{\partial y^2} + \frac{\partial^2 H_y}{\partial z^2} + n^2 \frac{\partial(1/n^2)}{\partial z}\frac{\partial H_y}{\partial z} + k^2 n^2 H_y = 0. \quad (6.140)$$

Here polarization coupling term has been neglected. Semi-vector equation for the Quasi-TM mode (E_y and H_x are the dominant fields) is calculated in the similar manner as

$$\frac{\partial^2 H_x}{\partial x^2} + n^2 \frac{\partial}{\partial y}\left(\frac{1}{n^2}\frac{\partial H_x}{\partial y}\right) + \frac{\partial^2 H_x}{\partial z^2} + n^2 \frac{\partial(1/n^2)}{\partial z}\frac{\partial H_x}{\partial z} + k^2 n^2 H_x = 0. \quad (6.141)$$

The term $[\partial(1/n^2)/\partial z](\partial H_z/\partial x)$ and polarization coupling term have been neglected in the derivation of the above equation.

Equations (6.140) and (6.141) are called as semi-vector equations based on the H-field formulation. Magnetic field modes obtained from (6.140) and (6.141) are denoted as Quasi-TE mode and Quasi-TM mode, respectively.

6.6.3. Steady State Mode Analysis

If the waveguide geometry and refractive index does not vary along the propagation direction z, semi-vector equations based on the E-field formulation reduce to

$$\frac{\partial}{\partial x}\left[\frac{1}{n^2}\frac{\partial(n^2\phi_x)}{\partial x}\right] + \frac{\partial^2 \phi_x}{\partial y^2} + (k^2 n^2 - \beta^2)\phi_x = 0, \quad \text{Quasi-TE Mode} \quad (6.142)$$

$$\frac{\partial^2 \phi_y}{\partial x^2} + \frac{\partial}{\partial y}\left[\frac{1}{n^2}\frac{\partial(n^2\phi_y)}{\partial y}\right] + (k^2 n^2 - \beta^2)\phi_y = 0, \quad \text{Quasi-TE Mode} \quad (6.143)$$

where $E_x = \phi_x(x, y)\exp(-j\beta z)$ and $E_y = \phi_y(x, y)\exp(-j\beta z)$ have been assumed. Boundary conditions for the transverse electric fields are built into the above equations. Transverse electric fields E_x and E_y are not continuous across the internal interfaces normal to the x- and y-axis, respectively. However, continuity of the electric displacement vectors $n^2 E_x$ and $n^2 E_y$, at internal interfaces normal to the x- and y-axis, are satisfied in the above equations.

If the refractive-index contrast is small (weakly guiding), terms containing $\partial n^2/\partial x$ and $\partial n^2/\partial y$ can be neglected. Under the scalar approximation, Eqs. (6.142) and (6.143) reduce to Eq. (6.65).

Similar to the E-field formulation, if the waveguide geometry and refractive index does not vary along the propagation direction z, semi-vector equations based on the H-field formulation reduce to

$$n^2\frac{\partial}{\partial x}\left(\frac{1}{n^2}\frac{\partial\psi_y}{\partial x}\right)+\frac{\partial^2\psi_y}{\partial y^2}+(k^2n^2-\beta^2)\psi_y=0,\quad \text{Quasi-TE Mode} \tag{6.144}$$

$$\frac{\partial^2\psi_x}{\partial x^2}+n^2\frac{\partial}{\partial y}\left(\frac{1}{n^2}\frac{\partial\psi_x}{\partial y}\right)+(k^2n^2-\beta^2)\psi_x=0,\quad \text{Quasi-TE Mode} \tag{6.145}$$

where $H_x = \psi_x(x, y)\exp(-j\beta z)$ and $\mathrm{H}_y = \psi_y(x, y)\exp(-j\beta z)$ have been assumed.

When we directly apply Galerkin's method to Eq. (6.144) or (6.145), numerical differentiation of n^2 becomes necessary. The numerical differentiation is not desirable since it normally causes error in the analysis.

Semi-vector equations (6.144) and (6.145) based on the H-field formulation can be expressed in a different form as

$$\begin{gathered}\frac{\partial}{\partial x}\left(\frac{1}{n^2}\frac{\partial\psi_y}{\partial x}\right)+j\beta\frac{1}{n^2}\frac{\partial\psi_z}{\partial y}+\left(k^2-\frac{\beta^2}{n^2}\right)\psi_y=0,\\ j\beta\psi_z=\frac{\partial\psi_z}{\partial y},\quad \text{Quasi-TE Mode}\end{gathered} \tag{6.146}$$

$$\begin{gathered}j\beta\frac{1}{n^2}\frac{\partial\psi_z}{\partial x}+\frac{\partial}{\partial y}\left(\frac{1}{n^2}\frac{\partial\psi_x}{\partial y}\right)+\left(k^2-\frac{\beta^2}{n^2}\right)\psi_x=0,\\ j\beta\psi_z=\frac{\partial\psi_x}{\partial x},\quad \text{Quasi-TE Mode}\end{gathered} \tag{6.147}$$

where $H_z = \psi_z(x, y)e^{-j\beta z}$ has been assumed. In the following paragraphs, finite-element formulation for the Quasi-TE mode will be described in detail. The finite-element formulation for the Quasi-TM mode is obtained in a similar manner to the Quasi-TE mode.

By applying the Galerkin's method [24] to Eq. (6.146), we obtain [25, 26]

$$\begin{aligned}I_1 = &-\sum_{e=1}^{N}\{u\}^T\iint_e \frac{1}{n^2}\frac{\partial[N]}{\partial x}\frac{\partial[N]^T}{\partial x}\,dx\,dy\cdot\{u\}\\ &-\sum_{e=1}^{N}\{u\}^T\beta\iint_e \frac{1}{n^2}[N]\frac{\partial[N]^T}{\partial y}\,dx\,dy\cdot\{v\}\\ &+\sum_{e=1}^{N}\{u\}^Tk^2\iint_e [N][N]^T\,dx\,dy\cdot\{u\}\\ &-\sum_{e=1}^{N}\{u\}^T\beta^2\iint_e \frac{1}{n^2}[N][N]^T\,dx\,dy\cdot\{u\}=0\end{aligned} \tag{6.148}$$

and

$$I_2 = -\sum_{e=1}^{N}\{u\}^T \iint_e [N]\frac{\partial [N]^T}{\partial y}\, dx\, dy \cdot \{u\} + \sum_{e=1}^{N}\{u\}^T \beta \iint_e [N][N]^T\, dx\, dy \cdot \{v\} = 0, \tag{6.149}$$

where $N(x, y)$ is a weight function which is defined in the triangular element (Fig. 6.14) as

$$[N(x, y)] = \begin{pmatrix} L_i \\ L_j \\ L_k \end{pmatrix}, \tag{6.150}$$

$$L_i = \frac{1}{2s_e}\left[(x_j y_k - x_k y_j) + (y_j - y_k)x + (x_k - x_j)y\right], \tag{6.151a}$$

$$L_i = \frac{1}{2s_e}\left[(x_k y_i - x_i y_k) + (y_k - y_i)x + (x_i - x_k)y\right], \tag{6.151b}$$

$$L_k = \frac{1}{2s_e}\left[(x_i y_j - x_j y_i) + (y_i - y_j)x + (x_j - x_i)y\right]. \tag{6.151c}$$

In Eqs. (6.148) and (6.149), $\{u\} = (u_i, u_j, u_k)^t$ and $\{v\} = (v_i, v_j, v_k)^t$ represent ψ_y and $-j\psi_z$, respectively, in the element as follows:

$$\psi_y = \sum_{\ell=1}^{3} L_\ell u_\ell, \tag{6.152}$$

$$-j\psi_z = \sum_{\ell=1}^{3} L_\ell v_\ell, \tag{6.153}$$

where $(\ )^t$ denotes the transpose of the vector. The functional I_1 and I_2 in Eqs. (6.148) and (6.149) are expressed in the matrix form as

$$I_1 = -\sum_{e=1}^{N}\{u\}^t[\mathbf{G}_e\{u\} + \mathbf{H}_e\{v\}] = \{U\}^t[\mathbf{G}\{U\} + \mathbf{H}\{V\}] = 0, \tag{6.154}$$

$$I_2 = -\sum_{e=1}^{N}\{u\}^t[\mathbf{R}_e\{u\} + \mathbf{T}_e\{v\}] = \{U\}^t[\mathbf{R}\{U\} + \mathbf{T}\{\mathbf{V}\}] = 0, \tag{6.155}$$

where $\mathbf{G}_e$, $\mathbf{H}_e$, $\mathbf{R}_e$ and $\mathbf{T}_e$ are 3×3 element matrices and $\{U\}$ and $\{\mathbf{V}\}$ are $N \times 1$ global column vectors representing ψ_y and $-j\psi_z$, respectively. Matrix elements of $\mathbf{G}_e$, $\mathbf{H}_e$, $\mathbf{R}_e$ and $\mathbf{T}_e$ are given by

$$\begin{cases} g_{11} = -\dfrac{1}{n_e^2} \iint\limits_e \dfrac{\partial L_i}{\partial x} \cdot \dfrac{\partial L_i}{\partial x} dx\,dy + \left(k^2 - \dfrac{\beta^2}{n_e^2}\right) \iint\limits_e L_i \cdot L_i \, dx\,dy \\ g_{12} = -\dfrac{1}{n_e^2} \iint\limits_e \dfrac{\partial L_i}{\partial x} \cdot \dfrac{\partial L_j}{\partial x} dx\,dy + \left(k^2 - \dfrac{\beta^2}{n_e^2}\right) \iint\limits_e L_i \cdot L_j \, dx\,dy = g_{21} \\ g_{13} = -\dfrac{1}{n_e^2} \iint\limits_e \dfrac{\partial L_i}{\partial x} \cdot \dfrac{\partial L_k}{\partial x} dx\,dy + \left(k^2 - \dfrac{\beta^2}{n_e^2}\right) \iint\limits_e L_i \cdot L_k \, dx\,dy = g_{31} \\ g_{22} = -\dfrac{1}{n_e^2} \iint\limits_e \dfrac{\partial L_j}{\partial x} \cdot \dfrac{\partial L_j}{\partial x} dx\,dy + \left(k^2 - \dfrac{\beta^2}{n_e^2}\right) \iint\limits_e L_j \cdot L_j \, dx\,dy \\ g_{23} = -\dfrac{1}{n_e^2} \iint\limits_e \dfrac{\partial L_j}{\partial x} \cdot \dfrac{\partial L_k}{\partial x} dx\,dy + \left(k^2 - \dfrac{\beta^2}{n_e^2}\right) \iint\limits_e L_j \cdot L_k \, dx\,dy = g_{32} \\ g_{33} = -\dfrac{1}{n_e^2} \iint\limits_e \dfrac{\partial L_k}{\partial x} \cdot \dfrac{\partial L_k}{\partial x} dx\,dy + \left(k^2 - \dfrac{\beta^2}{n_e^2}\right) \iint\limits_e L_k \cdot L_k \, dx\,dy \end{cases} \tag{6.156}$$

$$\begin{cases} h_{11} = -\dfrac{\beta}{n_e^2} \iint\limits_e L_i \cdot \dfrac{\partial L_i}{\partial y} dx\,dy \\ h_{12} = -\dfrac{\beta}{n_e^2} \iint\limits_e L_i \cdot \dfrac{\partial L_j}{\partial y} dx\,dy \\ h_{13} = -\dfrac{\beta}{n_e^2} \iint\limits_e L_i \cdot \dfrac{\partial L_k}{\partial y} dx\,dy \\ h_{21} = -\dfrac{\beta}{n_e^2} \iint\limits_e L_j \cdot \dfrac{\partial L_i}{\partial y} dx\,dy \\ h_{22} = -\dfrac{\beta}{n_e^2} \iint\limits_e L_j \cdot \dfrac{\partial L_j}{\partial y} dx\,dy \\ h_{23} = -\dfrac{\beta}{n_e^2} \iint\limits_e L_j \cdot \dfrac{\partial L_k}{\partial y} dx\,dy \\ h_{31} = -\dfrac{\beta}{n_e^2} \iint\limits_e L_k \cdot \dfrac{\partial L_i}{\partial y} dx\,dy \\ h_{32} = -\dfrac{\beta}{n_e^2} \iint\limits_e L_k \cdot \dfrac{\partial L_j}{\partial y} dx\,dy \\ h_{33} = -\dfrac{\beta}{n_e^2} \iint\limits_e L_k \cdot \dfrac{\partial L_k}{\partial y} dx\,dy \end{cases} \tag{6.157}$$

$$\begin{cases} r_{11} = \iint\limits_e L_i \cdot \dfrac{\partial L_i}{\partial y} dx\,dy \\ r_{12} = \dfrac{1}{2} \iint\limits_e L_i \cdot \dfrac{\partial L_j}{\partial y} dx\,dy + \dfrac{1}{2} \iint\limits_e L_j \cdot \dfrac{\partial L_i}{\partial y} dx\,dy = r_{21} \\ r_{13} = \dfrac{1}{2} \iint\limits_e L_i \cdot \dfrac{\partial L_k}{\partial y} dx\,dy + \dfrac{1}{2} \iint\limits_e L_k \cdot \dfrac{\partial L_i}{\partial y} dx\,dy = r_{31} \\ r_{22} = \iint\limits_e L_j \cdot \dfrac{\partial L_j}{\partial y} dx\,dy \\ r_{23} = \dfrac{1}{2} \iint\limits_e L_j \cdot \dfrac{\partial L_k}{\partial y} dx\,dy + \dfrac{1}{2} \iint\limits_e L_k \cdot \dfrac{\partial L_j}{\partial y} dx\,dy = r_{32} \\ r_{33} = \iint\limits_e L_k \cdot \dfrac{\partial L_k}{\partial y} dx\,dy \end{cases} \tag{6.158}$$

$$\begin{cases} t_{11} = \beta \iint\limits_e L_i \cdot L_i \; dx\,dy \\ t_{12} = \beta \iint\limits_e L_i \cdot L_j \; dx\,dy = t_{21} \\ t_{13} = \beta \iint\limits_e L_i \cdot L_k \; dx\,dy = t_{31} \\ t_{22} = \beta \iint\limits_e L_j \cdot L_j \; dx\,dy \\ t_{23} = \beta \iint\limits_e L_j \cdot L_k \; dx\,dy = t_{32} \\ t_{33} = \beta \iint\limits_e L_k \cdot L_k \; dx\,dy. \end{cases} \tag{6.159}$$

Eliminating $\{\mathbf{V}\}$ from Eqs. (6.154) and (6.155), simultaneous equations for $\{\mathbf{U}\}$ is obtained as

$$[\mathbf{G} - \mathbf{H}\mathbf{T}^{-1}\mathbf{R}]\{U\} = \{0\}, \tag{6.160}$$

where $\mathbf{G}$, $\mathbf{H}$, $\mathbf{R}$ and $\mathbf{T}$ are $N \times N$ global matrices containing $\mathbf{G}_e$, $\mathbf{H}_e$, $\mathbf{R}_e$ and $\mathbf{T}_e$. For Eq. (6.160) to have a nontrivial solution other than $\{U\} = \{0\}$, the determinant of the matrix should be zero; that is,

$$\det[\mathbf{G} - \mathbf{H}\mathbf{T}^{-1}\mathbf{R}] = 0. \tag{6.161}$$

Equation (6.161) is the dispersion (eigenvalue) equation for the Quasi-TE mode.

The finite-element formulation for the Quasi-TM mode is obtained in a similar manner to the Quasi-TE mode. By applying the Galerkin's method to Eq. (6.147), we obtain the functional I_1 and I_2 as

$$I_1 = \sum_{e=1}^{N} \{u\}^t [\mathbf{G}_e\{u\} + \mathbf{H}_e\{\mathbf{v}\}] = \{U\}^t [\mathbf{G}\{U\} + \mathbf{H}\{\mathbf{V}\}] = 0, \tag{6.162}$$

$$I_2 = \sum_{e=1}^{N} \{u\}^t [\mathbf{R}_e\{u\} + \mathbf{T}_e\{\mathbf{v}\}] = \{U\}^t [\mathbf{R}\{U\} + \mathbf{T}\{\mathbf{V}\}] = 0, \tag{6.163}$$

where $\{u\} = (u_i, u_j, u_k)^t$ and $\{\mathbf{v}\} = (\mathbf{v}_i, \mathbf{v}_j, \mathbf{v}_k)^t$ represent ψ_x and $-j\psi_z$, respectively, in the element as follows:

$$\psi_x = \sum_{\ell=1}^{3} L_\ell \, u_\ell, \tag{6.164}$$

$$-j\psi_z = \sum_{\ell=1}^{3} L_\ell \, \mathbf{v}_\ell, \tag{6.165}$$

and $\{U\}$ and $\{\mathbf{V}\}$ are $N \times 1$ global column vectors representing ψ_x and $-j\psi_z$, respectively. Matrix elements of $\mathbf{G}_e$, $\mathbf{H}_e$, $\mathbf{R}_e$ and $\mathbf{T}_e$ are given by

$$\begin{cases} g_{11} = -\dfrac{1}{n_e^2} \iint_e \dfrac{\partial L_i}{\partial y} \cdot \dfrac{\partial L_i}{\partial y} dx\,dy + \left(k^2 - \dfrac{\beta^2}{n_e^2}\right) \iint_e L_i \cdot L_i \; dx\,dy \\ g_{12} = -\dfrac{1}{n_e^2} \iint_e \dfrac{\partial L_i}{\partial y} \cdot \dfrac{\partial L_j}{\partial y} dx\,dy + \left(k^2 - \dfrac{\beta^2}{n_e^2}\right) \iint_e L_i \cdot L_j \; dx\,dy = g_{21} \\ g_{13} = -\dfrac{1}{n_e^2} \iint_e \dfrac{\partial L_i}{\partial y} \cdot \dfrac{\partial L_k}{\partial y} dx\,dy + \left(k^2 - \dfrac{\beta^2}{n_e^2}\right) \iint_e L_i \cdot L_k \; dx\,dy = g_{31} \\ g_{22} = -\dfrac{1}{n_e^2} \iint_e \dfrac{\partial L_j}{\partial y} \cdot \dfrac{\partial L_j}{\partial y} dx\,dy + \left(k^2 - \dfrac{\beta^2}{n_e^2}\right) \iint_e L_j \cdot L_j \; dx\,dy \\ g_{23} = -\dfrac{1}{n_e^2} \iint_e \dfrac{\partial L_j}{\partial y} \cdot \dfrac{\partial L_k}{\partial y} dx\,dy + \left(k^2 - \dfrac{\beta^2}{n_e^2}\right) \iint_e L_j \cdot L_k \; dx\,dy = g_{32} \\ g_{33} = -\dfrac{1}{n_e^2} \iint_e \dfrac{\partial L_k}{\partial y} \cdot \dfrac{\partial L_k}{\partial y} dx\,dy + \left(k^2 - \dfrac{\beta^2}{n_e^2}\right) \iint_e L_k \cdot L_k \; dx\,dy \end{cases} \tag{6.166}$$

$$\begin{cases} h_{11} = -\dfrac{\beta}{n_e^2} \iint_e L_i \cdot \dfrac{\partial L_i}{\partial x} dx\,dy \\ h_{12} = -\dfrac{\beta}{n_e^2} \iint_e L_i \cdot \dfrac{\partial L_j}{\partial x} dx\,dy \\ h_{13} = -\dfrac{\beta}{n_e^2} \iint_e L_i \cdot \dfrac{\partial L_k}{\partial x} dx\,dy \\ h_{21} = -\dfrac{\beta}{n_e^2} \iint_e L_j \cdot \dfrac{\partial L_i}{\partial x} dx\,dy \\ h_{22} = -\dfrac{\beta}{n_e^2} \iint_e L_j \cdot \dfrac{\partial L_j}{\partial x} dx\,dy \\ h_{23} = -\dfrac{\beta}{n_e^2} \iint_e L_j \cdot \dfrac{\partial L_k}{\partial x} dx\,dy \\ h_{31} = -\dfrac{\beta}{n_e^2} \iint_e L_k \cdot \dfrac{\partial L_i}{\partial x} dx\,dy \\ h_{32} = -\dfrac{\beta}{n_e^2} \iint_e L_k \cdot \dfrac{\partial L_j}{\partial x} dx\,dy \\ h_{33} = -\dfrac{\beta}{n_e^2} \iint_e L_k \cdot \dfrac{\partial L_k}{\partial x} dx\,dy \end{cases} \tag{6.167}$$

$$\begin{cases} r_{11} = \iint\limits_e L_i \cdot \frac{\partial L_i}{\partial x} dx\,dy \\ r_{12} = \frac{1}{2}\iint\limits_e L_i \cdot \frac{\partial L_j}{\partial x} dx\,dy + \frac{1}{2}\iint\limits_e L_j \cdot \frac{\partial L_i}{\partial x} dx\,dy = r_{21} \\ r_{13} = \frac{1}{2}\iint\limits_e L_i \cdot \frac{\partial L_k}{\partial x} dx\,dy + \frac{1}{2}\iint\limits_e L_k \cdot \frac{\partial L_i}{\partial x} dx\,dy = r_{31} \\ r_{22} = \iint\limits_e L_j \cdot \frac{\partial L_j}{\partial x} dx\,dy \\ r_{23} = \frac{1}{2}\iint\limits_e L_j \cdot \frac{\partial L_k}{\partial x} dx\,dy + \frac{1}{2}\iint\limits_e L_k \cdot \frac{\partial L_j}{\partial x} dx\,dy = r_{32} \\ r_{33} = \iint\limits_e L_k \cdot \frac{\partial L_k}{\partial x} dx\,dy \end{cases} \tag{6.168}$$

$$\begin{cases} t_{11} = \beta \iint\limits_e L_i \cdot L_i dx\,dy \\ t_{12} = \beta \iint\limits_e L_i \cdot L_j dx\,dy = t_{21} \\ t_{13} = \beta \iint\limits_e L_i \cdot L_k dx\,dy = t_{31} \\ t_{22} = \beta \iint\limits_e L_j \cdot L_j dx\,dy \\ t_{23} = \beta \iint\limits_e L_j \cdot L_k dx\,dy = t_{32} \\ t_{33} = \beta \iint\limits_e L_k \cdot L_k dx\,dy. \end{cases} \tag{6.169}$$

Eliminating $\{\mathbf{V}\}$ from Eqs. (6.162) and (6.163), simultaneous equations for $\{\mathbf{U}\}$ is obtained as

$$[\mathbf{G} - \mathbf{H}\mathbf{T}^{-1}\mathbf{R}]\{U\} = \{0\}, \tag{6.170}$$

where $\mathbf{G}$, $\mathbf{H}$, $\mathbf{R}$ and $\mathbf{T}$ are $N \times N$ global matrices containing $\mathbf{G}_e$, $\mathbf{H}_e$, $\mathbf{R}_e$ and $\mathbf{T}_e$. For Eq. (6.170) to have a nontrivial solution other than $\{U\} = \{0\}$, the determinant of the matrix should be zero; that is,

$$\det[\mathbf{G} - \mathbf{H}\mathbf{T}^{-1}\mathbf{R}] = 0. \tag{6.171}$$

(6.171) is the dispersion (eigenvalue) equation for the Quasi-TM mode.

6A Derivation of Equation (6.59)

We assume that when the wave number k varies slightly, β and $E_t(r)$ become $\beta+\delta\beta$ and $E_t+\delta E_t$, respectively. In this case, Eq. (6.58) is expressed as

$$(\beta+\delta\beta)^2\int_0^\infty (E_t+\delta E_t)^2\ rdr+\int_0^\infty\left[\frac{d}{dr}(E_t+\delta E_t)\right]^2 rdr$$
$$-\int_0^\infty [kn+\delta(kn)]^2(E_t+\delta E_t)^2\ rdr=0. \qquad (6.172)$$

Neglecting the δ^2 term, we can rewrite this equation as

$$\left\{\beta^2\int_0^\infty E_t^2(r)\ rdr+\int_0^\infty\left(\frac{dE_t}{dr}\right)^2 rdr-\int_0^\infty k^2n^2(r)E_t^2(r)rdr\right\}$$
$$+\left\{\beta^2\int_0^\infty \delta E_t^2\ rdr+\int_0^\infty \delta\left(\frac{dE_t}{dr}\right)^2 rdr-\int_0^\infty k^2n^2(r)\delta E_t^2\ rdr\right\}$$
$$+2\{\beta\delta\beta\int_0^\infty E_t^2(r)\ rdr-\int_0^\infty kn\ \delta(kn)E_t^2(r)\ rdr\}=0. \qquad (6.173)$$

Substituting Eq. (6.58) in the first term of this equation, and also substituting the following relation obtained from the stationary condition $\delta\beta^2=0$,

$$\beta^2\int_0^\infty \delta E_t^2\ rdr+\int_0^\infty \delta\left(\frac{dE_t}{dr}\right)^2 rdr-\int_0^\infty k^2n^2(r)\delta E_t^2 rdr=0, \qquad (6.174)$$

in the second term of Eq. (6.174), we obtain

$$\beta\delta\beta\int_0^\infty E_t^2(r)rdr-\int_0^\infty kn\delta(kn)E_t^2(r)rdr=0. \qquad (6.175)$$

This can be rewritten as

$$\frac{\beta}{k}\frac{d\beta}{dk}=\frac{\int_0^\infty n(r)[d(kn)/dk]E_t^2(r)\ rdr}{\int_0^\infty E_t^2(r)\ rdr}. \qquad (6.176)$$

When we ignore the dispersion of refractive index, this is reduced to

$$\frac{\beta}{k}\frac{d\beta}{dk}=\frac{\int_0^\infty n^2(r)E_t^2(r)\ rdr}{\int_0^\infty E_t^2(r)\ rdr}. \qquad (6.177)$$

6B Proof of Equation (6.66)

We assume that $I[\phi]$ is stationary for $\phi(x, y)$ and consider the slightly deviated function

$$\phi_{\text{pert}}(x, y) = \phi(x, y) + \delta\eta(x, y), \tag{6.178}$$

where δ denotes a real small quantity and $\eta(x, y)$ is an arbitrary continuous function of x and y. Substituting $\phi_{\text{pert}}(x, y)$ in Eq. (6.66) and assuming that $I[\phi_{\text{pert}}]$ is stationary for $\delta = 0$, we obtain

$$\lim_{\partial \to 0}\left\{\frac{\partial}{\partial \delta} I[\phi_{\text{pert}}]\right\} = \int_{-\infty}^{\infty}\int_{-\infty}^{\infty}\left[\frac{\partial \phi}{\partial x}\frac{\partial \eta}{\partial x} + \frac{\partial \phi}{\partial y}\frac{\partial \eta}{\partial y} - (k^2n^2 - \beta^2)\phi\eta\right] dx\,dy = 0. \tag{6.179}$$

By partial integration, Eq. (6.179) is rewritten as

$$\int_{-\infty}^{\infty} dy\left[\eta\frac{\partial \phi}{\partial x}\right]_{x=-\infty}^{x=+\infty} + \int_{-\infty}^{\infty} dx\left[\eta\frac{\partial \phi}{\partial y}\right]_{y=-\infty}^{y=+\infty}$$
$$-\int_{-\infty}^{\infty}\int_{-\infty}^{\infty}\eta\left[\frac{\partial^2 \phi}{\partial x^2} + \frac{\partial^2 \phi}{\partial y^2} + (k^2n^2 - \beta^2)\phi\right] dx\,dy = 0. \tag{6.180}$$

Since $\eta(x, y)$ is an arbitrary function, the first, second, and the third terms of Eq. (6.180) shoud be zero independently. Then $\phi(x, y)$ satisfies the following wave equation and the boundary condition:

$$\frac{\partial^2 \phi}{\partial x^2} + \frac{\partial^2 \phi}{\partial y^2} + (k^2n^2 - \beta^2)\phi = 0, \tag{6.181}$$

$$\lim_{x \to \pm\infty}\frac{\partial \phi}{\partial x} = 0, \qquad \lim_{y \to \pm\infty}\frac{\partial \phi}{\partial y} = 0. \tag{6.182}$$

The second condition is a natural boundary condition that states that the field $\phi(x, y)$ decays to zero at infinity (the electromagnetic field is confined in the waveguide). It is then proved that the function $\phi(x, y)$ that makes the functional (6.66) to be stationary satisfies the wave equation (6.65) and the boundary condition (6.182) simultaneously.

REFERENCES

[1] Zienkiewicz, O. C. and Y. K. Cheung. 1971. *The Finite Element Method in Engineering Science*. New York: McGraw-Hill.

[2] Koshiba, M. 1992. *Optical Waveguide Theory by the Finite Element Method*. Tokyo: KTK Scientific.

[3] Itoh, T., G. Pelosi, and P. P. Silvester. 1996. *Finite Element Software for Microwave Engineering*. John Wiley & Sons, Inc., New York.

[4] Yamashita, E. 1990. *Analysis Methods for Electromagnetic Wave Problems*. Boston: Artech House.

[5] Okoshi, T. 1982. *Optical Fibers*. New York: Academic Press.

[6] Yeh, C., K. Ha, S. B. Dong, and W. P. Brown. 1979. Single-mode optical waveguide. *Appl. Opt.* 18:1490–1504.

[7] Hayata, K., M. Koshiba, M. Eguchi, and M. Suzuki. 1986. Vectorial finite-element method without any spurious solutions for dielectric waveguiding problem using transverse magnetic-field component. *IEEE Trans. Microwave Theory Tech.* MTT-34:1120–1124.

[8] Young, T. P. 1988. Design of integrated optical circuits using finite elements. *IEEE Proc., Part A* 135:135–144.

[9] Angkaew, T., M. Matsuhara, and N. Kumagai. 1987. Finite-element analysis of waveguide modes—A novel approach that eliminates spurious modes. *IEEE Trans. Microwave Theory Tech.* MTT-35:117–123.

[10] Golub, G. H. and C. F. van Loan. 1989. *Matrix Computations*. Baltimore: Johns-Hopkins University Press.

[11] Murata, H. 1987. *Handbook of Optical Fibers and Cables*. New York: Marcel Dekker.

[12] Turner, M. J., R. W. Clough, H. C. Martin, and L. J. Topp. 1956. Stiffness and deflection analysis of complex structures. *J. Aero. Sci.* 23:805–823.

[13] Timoshenko, S. and J. N. Goodier. 1951. *Theory of Elasticity*. New York: McGraw-Hill.

[14] Kressel, H. and J. K. Butler. 1977. *Semiconductor Lasers and Heterojunction LEDs*. New York: Academic Press.

[15] Dixon, R. W. 1967. Photoelastic properties of selected materials and their relevance for application to acoustic light modulators and scanners. *J. Appl. Phys.* 38:5149–5153.

[16] Lagakos, N., J. A. Bucaro, and R. Hughes. 1980. Acoustic sensitivity predictions of single-mode optical fibers using Brillouin scattering. *Appl. Opt.* 19:3668–3670.

[17] Manenkov, A. A. and A. I. Ritus. 1978. Determination of the elastic and elasto-optic constants and extinction coefficients of the laser glasses LGS-247-2, LGS-250-3, LGS-1, and KGSS-1621 by the Brillouin scattering technique. *Sov. J. Quantum Electron.* 8:78–80.

[18] Soref, R. A., J. Schmidtchen, and K. Petermann. 1991. Large single-mode rib waveguides in GeSi-Si and Si-on-SiO_2. *IEEE J. Quantum Electron.* 27:1971–1974.

[19] Jalali, B., S. Yegnanarayanan, T. Yoon, T. Yoshimoto, I. Rendina, and F. Coppinger. 1998. Advances in silicon-on-insulator optoelectronics. *IEEE J. Selected Topics in Quantum Electron.* 4:938–947.

[20] Little, B. E., S. T. Chu, P. P. Absil, J. V. Hryniewicz, F. G. Johnson, F. Seiferth, D. Gill, V. Van, O. King, and M. Trakalo. 2004. Very high-order microring resonator filters for WDM applications. *IEEE Photonics Tech. Lett.* 16:2263–2265.

[21] Tsuchizawa, T., K. Yamada, H. Fukuda, T. Watanabe, J. Takahashi, M. Takahashi, T. Shoji, E. Tamechika, S. Itabashi, and H. Morita. 2005. Microphotonics devices based on silicon microfabrication technology. *IEEE J. Selected Topics Quantum Electron.* 11:232–240.

[22] Bogaerts, W., R. Baets, P. Dumon, V. Wiaux, S. Beckx, D. Taillaert, B. Luyssaert, J. Campenhout, P. Bienstman, and D. Thourhout. 2005. Nanophotonic waveguides in silicon-on-insulator fabricated with CMOS technology. *IEEE J. Lightwave Tech.* 23:401–412.

[23] Huang, W. P. and C. L. Xu. 1993. Simulation of three-dimensional optical waveguides by a full-vector beam propagation method. *IEEE J. Quantum Electron.* 29:2639–2649.

[24] Jin, J. 2002. *The Finite Element Method in Electromagnetics*. John Wiley & Sons.

[25] Cucinotta, A., S. Selleri, and L. Vincetti. 1998. Finite-elements semivectorial beam propagation method for nonlinear integrated optical devices. *Integrated Photonic Research.* Victoria, British Columbia, Canada, IME3, pp. 62–64.

[26] Kawano, K., T. Kitoh, and M. Naganuma. 1999. Proposal of the accurate semi-vectorial finite element method for the 2-D cross-sectional optical waveguide analysis. *Transactions of The Institute of Electronics*, Information and Communication Engineers (Japanese Edition) C-II, J82-C-II:222–223.

Chapter 7

Beam Propagation Method

Curvilinear directional couplers, branching and combining waveguides, S-shaped bent waveguides and tapered waveguides are indispensable components in constructing integrated optical circuits. Mode-coupling phenomena in the parallel directional couplers have been investigated in Chapter 4. In practical directional couplers, however, light coupling in the S-shaped bent waveguide regions in the front and rear of parallel waveguides should be taken into account so as to evaluate the propagation characteristics precisely. For axially varying waveguides, the FEM stationary mode analysis described in Chapter 6 should be modified by using the paraxial wave approximation and Galerkin's method [1]. The Beam propagation method (BPM) is the most powerful technique to investigate linear and nonlinear lightwave propagation phenomena in axially varying waveguides such as curvilinear directional couplers, branching and combining waveguides, S-shaped bent waveguides, and tapered waveguides. BPM is also quite important for the analysis of ultrashort light pulse propagation in optical fibers. Two kinds of BPM procedures are described in this chapter: one based on the fast Fourier transform (FFT) and one based on the finite difference method (FDM).

7.1. BASIC EQUATIONS FOR BEAM PROPAGATION METHOD BASED ON THE FFT

7.1.1. Wave Propagation in Optical Waveguides

The three-dimensional scalar wave equation (Helmholtz equation), which is the basis of BPM, is expressed by

$$\frac{\partial^2 E}{\partial x^2}+\frac{\partial^2 E}{\partial y^2}+\frac{\partial^2 E}{\partial z^2}+k^2 n^2(x,y,z)E=0. \tag{7.1}$$

We separate electric field $E(x, y, z)$ into two parts: the axially slowly varying envelope term of $\phi(x, y, z)$ and the rapidly varying term of $\exp(-jk_{n_0}z)$. Here, n_0 is a refractive index in the cladding. Then, $E(x, y, z)$ is expressed by

$$E(x, y, z) = \phi(x, y, z) \exp(-jkn_0 z). \tag{7.2}$$

Substituting Eq. (7.2) in (7.1), we obtain

$$\nabla^2 \phi - j2kn_0 \frac{\partial \phi}{\partial z} + k^2(n^2 - n_0^2)\phi = 0, \tag{7.3}$$

where

$$\nabla^2 = \frac{\partial^2}{\partial x^2} + \frac{\partial^2}{\partial y^2}. \tag{7.4}$$

Assuming the weakly guiding condition, we can approximate $(n^2 - n_0^2) \cong 2_{n_0}(n - n_0)$ in Eq. (7.3). Then Eq. (7.3) can be rewritten as

$$\frac{\partial \phi}{\partial z} = -j\frac{1}{2kn_0}\nabla^2 \phi - jk(n - n_0)\phi. \tag{7.5}$$

When $n = n_0$, only the first term remains in the right-hand side of the above equation. Therefore, it is known that the first term of Eq. (7.5) represents free-space light propagation in the medium having refractive index n_0. The second term of Eq. (7.5) represents the guiding function or influence of the region having the refractive index $n(x, y, z)$. Both terms of Eq. (7.5) affect the light propagation simultaneously. However, in the BPM analysis, we assume that two terms can be separated and that each term affects the light propagation separately and alternately in the axially small distance h [2, 3]. This assumption is schematically illustrated for the tapered waveguide in Fig. 7.1. Figure 7.1(a) shows light propagation in the actual tapered waveguide over the small distance h, and Fig. 7.1(b) represents the separation of free-space propagation and the waveguide effect in BPM analysis. In BPM analysis, the electric field $\phi(x, z)$ is first propagated in the free space over a distance of $h/2$. Then phase retardation of the entire length h, which corresponds to the shaded area in Fig. 7.1(a), is taken into account at the center of propagation. This electric field is again propagated in the latter free space with distance $h/2$ to obtain $\phi(x, z + h)$. The Basic procedure of BPM is formulated over the small distance h so as to relate the transmitted field $\phi(x, z + h)$ to the initial field $\phi(x, z)$. Light propagation in various kinds of waveguides can be analyzed by repeating this same procedure many times.

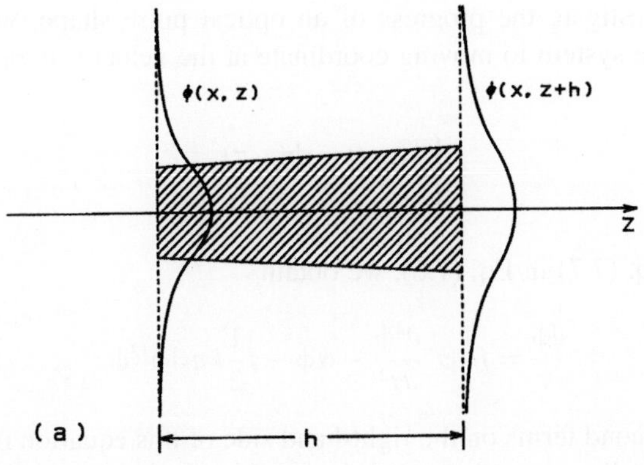

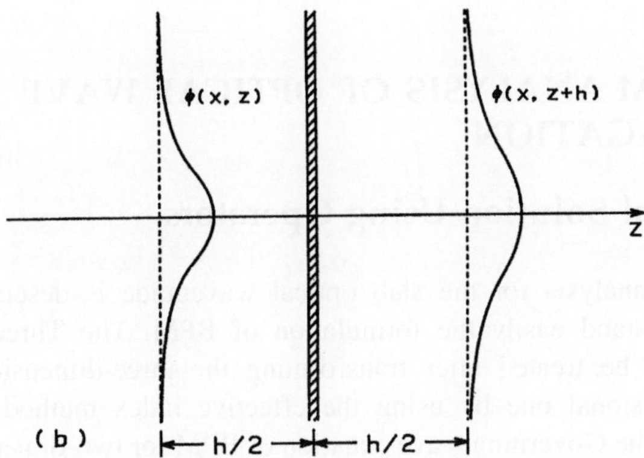

Figure 7.1 Schematic illustration of BPM analysis: (a) Light propagation in the taperd waveguide; (b) separation of free-space propagation and the waveguide effect in BPM.

7.1.2. Pulse Propagation in Optical Fibers

The nonlinear Schrödinger equation [Eq. (5.32)], which governs the envelope function of optical pulse $A(z, t)$ under the Kerr effect nonlinearity and loss (or gain) in the optical fibers, is expressed here again:

$$j\left(\frac{\partial A}{\partial z} + \beta' \frac{\partial A}{\partial t} + \alpha A\right) = -\frac{1}{2}\beta'' \frac{\partial^2 A}{\partial t^2} + \frac{1}{2} k n_2 |A|^2 A. \tag{7.6}$$

In order to investigate the progress of an optical pulse shape, we change the fixed coordinate system to moving coordinate at the velocity $\nu_g = 1/\beta'$:

$$\begin{cases} A(z,t) = \phi(z,\tau) & (7.7a) \\ \tau = t - \beta' z. & (7.7b) \end{cases}$$

Substituting Eq. (7.7) in Eq. (7.6), we obtain

$$\frac{\partial \phi}{\partial z} = j\frac{1}{2}\beta'' \frac{\partial^2 \phi}{\partial \tau^2} - \alpha\phi - j\frac{1}{2}kn_2|\phi|^2\phi. \tag{7.8}$$

The first and second terms on the right-hand side of this equation represent light propagation in a linear medium, and the third term represents the influence of Kerr-effect nonlinearity. Similar to BPM wave propagation analysis, we assume that light propagation in a linear medium and the influence of the nonlinear optical effect can be separated in the pulse propagation analysis by BPM.

7.2. FFTBPM ANALYSIS OF OPTICAL WAVE PROPAGATION

7.2.1. Formal Solution Using Operators

Here BPM analysis for the slab optical waveguide is described in order to move understand easily the formulation of BPM. The Three-dimensional waveguide can be treated after transforming the three-dimensional problem into two-dimensional one by using the effective index method described in Section 2.2.4. The Governing wave equation of BPM for two-dimensional waveguides is rewritten from Eq. (7.5) to

$$\frac{\partial \phi}{\partial z} = -j\frac{1}{2kn_0}\nabla^2\phi - \alpha\phi - jk[n(x,z) - n_0]\phi, \tag{7.9}$$

where the loss or gain term $-\alpha\phi$ is added and

$$\nabla^2 = \frac{\partial^2}{\partial x^2}. \tag{7.10}$$

Let us represent the free-space propagation effect [the first term in Eq. (7.9)] by operator **A** and the waveguiding effect [the second and third terms in Eq. (7.9)] by operator **B**. Using operator representation, Eq. (7.9) is formally expressed by

$$\frac{\partial \phi}{\partial z} = (\mathbf{A} + \mathbf{B})\phi, \tag{7.11}$$

$$\mathbf{A} = -j\frac{1}{2kn_0}\nabla^2, \tag{7.12a}$$

$$\mathbf{B} = -\alpha(x, z) - jk[n(x, z) - n_0]. \tag{7.12b}$$

If we assume that operator **B** has no z-dependence, Eq. (7.11) can be formally integrated as

$$\phi(x, z+h) = \exp[h(\mathbf{A}+\mathbf{B})]\phi(x, z). \tag{7.13}$$

Here we refer to Barker–Hausdorff theorem for noncommutative operators $\hat{\mathbf{a}}$ and $\hat{\mathbf{b}}$, which is expressed as [4]

$$\exp(\hat{\mathbf{a}})\exp(\hat{\mathbf{b}}) = \exp\left[\hat{\mathbf{a}} + \hat{\mathbf{b}} + \frac{1}{2}\left[\hat{\mathbf{a}}, \hat{\mathbf{b}}\right] + \frac{1}{12}\left[\hat{\mathbf{a}} - \hat{\mathbf{b}}, \left[\hat{\mathbf{a}}, \hat{\mathbf{b}}\right]\right] + \cdots\right], \tag{7.14}$$

where $[\hat{\mathbf{a}}, \hat{\mathbf{b}}] = \hat{\mathbf{a}}\hat{\mathbf{b}} - \hat{\mathbf{b}}\hat{\mathbf{a}}$. When we express $\hat{\mathbf{a}} = h\mathbf{A}$ and $\hat{\mathbf{b}} = h\mathbf{B}$ and assume that h is sufficiently small, we can ignore higher order term than $O(h^2)$. Therefore, we can approximate as

$$\exp(h\mathbf{A} + h\mathbf{B}) \cong \exp(h\mathbf{A})\exp(h\mathbf{B}). \tag{7.15}$$

Furthermore, it is known that accuracy of Eq. (7.15) can be improved to the order of $O(h^3)$ by modifying it into

$$\exp(h\mathbf{A} + h\mathbf{B}) = \exp\left(\frac{h\mathbf{A}}{2}\right)\exp(h\mathbf{B})\exp\left(\frac{h\mathbf{A}}{2}\right). \tag{7.16}$$

Substituting Eq. (7.16) in Eq. (7.13), we obtain formal solution of Eq. (7.11):

$$\phi(x, z+h) = \exp\left(\frac{h\mathbf{A}}{2}\right)\exp(h\mathbf{B})\exp\left(\frac{h\mathbf{A}}{2}\right)\phi(x, z). \tag{7.17}$$

This last equation says that the electric field $\phi(x, z)$ is first propagated in the free space (operator **A**) over a distance of $h/2$ and then the loss or gain and phase retardation of the entire length h is taken into account at the center of propagation (operator **B**). This electric field is again propagated in the latter free space (operator **A**) with distance $h/2$ to obtain $\phi(x, z+h)$.

However, Eq. (7.17) is merely a formal solution and even more z-dependence of **B** has been neglected. Therefore, we explain the physical meanings of operators **A, B** and Eq. (7.17) in the next section.

7.2.2. Concrete Numerical Procedures Using Split-step Fourier Algorithm

Let us first examine the meaning of operator **A** defined by Eq. (7.12a) and expressed in (7.17). By definition, operator **A** represents light propagation in free space having refractive index n_0. The wave equation describing free-space light propagation in the slab waveguide ($\partial/\partial y = 0$) is obtained from Eq. (7.1) as

$$\frac{\partial^2 \psi}{\partial x^2} + \frac{\partial^2 \psi}{\partial z^2} + k^2 n_0^2 \psi = 0, \tag{7.18}$$

where ψ denotes free space propagating electric field to discriminate it from E. We express the solution of the above wave equation in Fourier integral form as

$$\psi(x, z) = \int_{-\infty}^{\infty} \Psi(\rho, z) \exp(j2\pi\rho x) d\rho, \tag{7.19}$$

where $\Psi(\rho, z)$ is an amplitude of the plane wave having spatial frequency ρ. Substituting Eq. (7.19) in Eq. (7.18), we obtain the differential equation for $\Psi(\rho, z)$:

$$\frac{\partial^2 \Psi}{\partial z^2} + \beta^2 \Psi(\rho, z) = 0, \tag{7.20}$$

where β^2 is given by

$$\beta^2 = k^2 n_0^2 - (2\pi\rho)^2. \tag{7.21}$$

When the electric field at $z = z_0$ is known to be $\psi(x, z_0)$, its spatial frequency component $\Psi(\rho, z_0)$ is also given by

$$\Psi(\rho, z_0) = F[\psi(x, z_0)] = \int_{-\infty}^{\infty} \psi(x, z_0) \exp(-j2\pi\rho x) dx. \tag{7.22}$$

Here, the symbol $F[\ ]$ represents the Fourier transform. Using Eq. (7.22) as the initial condition, the solution of Eq. (7.20) is given by

$$\Psi(\rho, z) = \Psi(\rho, z_0) \exp[-j\beta(z - z_0)]. \tag{7.23}$$

Substituting Eq. (7.23) in Eq. (7.19), we obtain the solution for the slab wave equation (7.18):

$$\begin{aligned}\psi(x, z) &= F^{-1}[\Psi(\rho, z)] = F^{-1}[\Psi(\rho, z_0) \exp[-j\beta(z - z_0)]] \\ &= F^{-1}[F\{\psi(x, z_0)\} \exp[-j\beta(z - z_0)]].\end{aligned} \tag{7.24}$$

In this equation, $F^{-1}[]$ represents the inverse Fourier transform given by Eq. (7.19). Equation (7.24) represents the formulation that relates the free-space propagated light $\psi(x, z)$ over the distance of $(z - z_0)$ with the initial electric field $\psi(x, z_0)$ at $z = z_0$.

As shown in Eq. (7.2), the slowly varying envelope function $\phi(x, z)$ and the rapidly varying term $\exp(-jkn_0 z)$ in $\psi(x, z)$ are expressed separately as $\psi(x, z) = \phi(x, z)\exp(-jkn_0 z)$.

Substituting this in Eq. (7.24), we obtain the expression for the envelope function ϕ at $z = z_0 + h/2$:

$$\phi\left(x, z_0 + \frac{h}{2}\right)\exp\left(-\frac{jkn_0 h}{2}\right) = F^{-1}\left[F\{\phi(x, z_0)\}\exp\left(-\frac{j\beta h}{2}\right)\right]. \tag{7.25}$$

Introducing a new parameter, $\delta\beta$, which is defined by

$$\delta\beta = \beta - kn_0 = \left[k^2 n_0^2 - (2\pi\rho)^2\right]^{1/2} - kn_0 \tag{7.26}$$

and replacing z_0 with z, Eq. (7.25) can be rewritten as

$$\phi\left(x, z + \frac{h}{2}\right) = F^{-1}\left[\exp\left(-\frac{j\delta\beta h}{2}\right)F\{\phi(x, z)\}\right]. \tag{7.27}$$

When we compare Eq. (7.27) with Eq. (7.17), the physical meaning of operator $\mathbf{A}$ is described:

$$\phi\left(x, z + \frac{h}{2}\right) = \exp\left(\frac{h\mathbf{A}}{2}\right)\phi(x, z) = F^{-1}\left[\exp\left(-\frac{j\delta\beta h}{2}\right)F\{\phi(x, z)\}\right]. \tag{7.28}$$

Next we investigate the meaning of operator $\mathbf{B}$. If operator $\mathbf{A}$ is ignored in Eq. (7.11), the differential equation for operator $\mathbf{B}$ is expressed as

$$\frac{\partial\Theta}{\partial z} = \mathbf{B}\Theta. \tag{7.29}$$

Solution of this differential equation is given by

$$\Theta(x, z + h) = \Theta(x, z)\exp\left[\int_x^{z+h}\mathbf{B}d\zeta\right]. \tag{7.30}$$

If an integration step h is small, the integration term is approximated as

$$\int_z^{z+h}\mathbf{B}d\zeta \cong \frac{h}{2}[\mathbf{B}(z) + \mathbf{B}(z + h)]. \tag{7.31}$$

Therefore, operator $\mathbf{B}$ in (7.17) is expressed as

$$\exp(h\mathbf{B}) = \exp\left\{\frac{h}{2}[\mathbf{B}(z) + \mathbf{B}(z + h)]\right\}. \tag{7.32}$$

Since operator **B** is a scalar quantity, as shown in Eq. (7.12b), Eq. (7.32) means that the function of operator **B** is to add the loss (or gain) and phase retardation terms given by Eq. (7.12b) into the electric field ϕ.

When we recognize the meanings of operators **A** and **B**, the electric field $\phi(x, z+h)$ in Eq. (7.17) is obtained as follows:

1. Free-space propagation in the first half-step $h/2$:

$$\phi\left(x, z+\frac{h}{2}\right) = \exp\left(\frac{h\mathbf{A}}{2}\right)\phi(x, z)$$
$$= F^{-1}\left[\exp\left(-\frac{j\delta\beta h}{2}\right) F\{\phi(x, z)\}\right], \qquad (7.33a)$$

2. Loss (or gain) and phase retardation of the entire step h:

$$\phi^*\left(x, z+\frac{h}{2}\right) = \exp(h\mathbf{B})\phi\left(x, z+\frac{h}{2}\right)$$
$$= \exp\left\{\frac{h}{2}[\mathbf{B}(z)+\mathbf{B}(z+h)]\right\}\phi\left(x, z+\frac{h}{2}\right), \qquad (7.33b)$$

3. Free-space propagation in the second half-step $h/2$:

$$\phi(x, z+h) = \exp\left(\frac{h\mathbf{A}}{2}\right)\phi^*\left(x, z+\frac{h}{2}\right)$$
$$= F^{-1}\left[\exp\left(-\frac{j\delta\beta h}{2}\right) F\left\{\phi^*\left(x, z+\frac{h}{2}\right)\right\}\right]. \qquad (7.33c)$$

7.3. FFTBPM ANALYSIS OF OPTICAL PULSE PROPAGATION

When we represent the linear-space propagation effect [the first term in Eq. (7.8)] by operator **A** and the loss (or gain) and nonlinear effect [the second and third terms in Eq. (7.8)] by operator **B**, Eq. (7.8) is formally expressed as

$$\frac{\partial\phi}{\partial z} = (\mathbf{A}+\mathbf{B})\phi, \qquad (7.34)$$

$$\mathbf{A} = j\frac{1}{2}\beta''\frac{\partial^2}{\partial\tau^2}, \qquad (7.35a)$$

$$\mathbf{B} = -\alpha - j\frac{1}{2}kn_2|\phi|^2. \qquad (7.35b)$$

Similar to the waveguide analysis described in the previous section, the formal solution of Eq. (7.34) is obtained as

$$\phi(z+h,\tau)=\exp\left(\frac{h\mathbf{A}}{2}\right)\exp(h\mathbf{B})\exp\left(\frac{h\mathbf{A}}{2}\right)\phi(z,\tau). \tag{7.36}$$

By definition, operator **A** represents light propagation in linear space. The wave equation describing linear-space light propagation is obtained from Eq. (7.8):

$$\frac{\partial\psi}{\partial z}=j\frac{1}{2}\beta''\frac{\partial^2\psi}{\partial\tau^2}. \tag{7.37}$$

We express the solution of this wave equation in Fourier integral form:

$$\psi(z,\tau)=\int_{-\infty}^{\infty}\psi(z,f)\exp(j2\pi f\tau)df, \tag{7.38}$$

where $\psi(z,f)$ is a frequency spectral component. Substituting Eq. (7.38) in Eq. (7.37), we obtain the differential equation for $\psi(z,f)$:

$$\frac{\partial\psi}{\partial z}=-j\frac{\beta''}{2}(2\pi f)^2\psi(z,f). \tag{7.39}$$

When the pulse waveform at $z=z_0$ is known to be $\psi(z_0,\tau)$, its frequency spectrum component $\psi(z_0,f)$ is also given by

$$\psi(z_0,f)=F[\psi(z_0,\tau)]=\int_{-\infty}^{\infty}\psi(z_0,\tau)\exp(-j2\pi f\tau)d\tau. \tag{7.40}$$

Using Eq. (7.40) as the initial condition, the solution of Eq. (7.39) is given by

$$\psi(z,f)=\psi(z_0,f)\exp[-j\gamma(z-z_0)], \tag{7.41}$$

where γ is defined by

$$\gamma=\frac{\beta''}{2}(2\pi f)^2. \tag{7.42}$$

Substituting Eq. (7.42) in Eq. (7.38), we obtain the solution for Eq. (7.37):

$$\begin{aligned}\psi(z,\tau)&=F^{-1}[\psi(z,f)]=F^{-1}[\psi(z_0,f)\exp[-j\gamma(z-z_0)]]\\&=F^{-1}[F\{\psi(z_0,\tau)\}\exp[-j\gamma(z-z_0)]].\end{aligned} \tag{7.43}$$

Equation (7.43) represents the formulation that relates linear-space propagated light $\psi(z,\tau)$ over the distance of $(z-z_0)$ with the initial pulse waveform $\psi(z_0,\tau)$ at $z=z_0$.

When the propagation distance in linear space is $h/2$, Eq. (7.43) is rewritten as

$$\phi\left(z+\frac{h}{2},\tau\right)=F^{-1}\left[\exp\left(-\frac{j\gamma h}{2}\right)F\{\phi(z,\tau)\}\right], \qquad (7.44)$$

where ψ and z_0 are replaced with ϕ and z. Comparing Eq. (7.36) with Eq. (7.44), the physical meaning of operator **A** is described as

$$\phi\left(z+\frac{h}{2},\tau\right)=\exp\left(\frac{h\mathbf{A}}{2}\right)\phi(z,\tau)=F^{-1}\left[\exp\left(-\frac{j\gamma h}{2}\right)F\{\phi(z,\tau)\}\right]. \quad (7.45)$$

Following the similar procedure for operator **B** in waveguide analysis, we see that the physical meaning of operator **B** is expressed by

$$\exp(h\mathbf{B})=\exp\left\{\frac{h}{2}[\mathbf{B}(z)+\mathbf{B}(z+h)]\right\}, \qquad (7.46)$$

where **B** is given by Eq. (7.35b). However, the implementation of Eq. (7.46) is not simple since $\mathbf{B}(z+h)$ is unknown at the mid-segment located at $z+h/2$. It is necessary to follow an iterative procedure that is initiated by replacing $\mathbf{B}(z+h)$ by with $\mathbf{B}(z)$. Equation (7.46) is then used to estimate 0th-order approximation $\phi^{(0)}(z+h,\tau)$, which in turn is used to calculate the new value of $\mathbf{B}(z+h)$. Using this new value in Eq. (7.46), an improved approximation $\phi^{(1)}(z+h,\tau)$ is obtained. Although the iteration procedure is time-consuming, it can still reduce the overall computing time if the step size h can be increased because of the improved accuracy of the numerical algorithm. It is known that two iterations are generally enough in practice [5].

When we recognize the meanings of operators **A** and **B**, the pulse envelope $\phi(z+h,\tau)$ in Eq. (7.36) is obtained as follows:

1. Linear-space propagation in the first half step $h/2$:

$$\begin{aligned}\phi\left(z+\frac{h}{2},\tau\right)&=\exp\left(\frac{h\mathbf{A}}{2}\right)\phi(z,\tau)\\&=F^{-1}[\exp(-j\gamma h/2)F\{\phi(z,\tau)\}],\end{aligned} \qquad (7.47a)$$

2. Loss (or gain) and phase retardation of the entire step h:

$$\begin{aligned}\phi^*\left(z+\frac{h}{2},\tau\right)&=\exp(h\mathbf{B})\phi\left(z+\frac{h}{2},\tau\right)\\&=\exp\left\{\frac{h}{2}[\mathbf{B}(z)+\mathbf{B}(z+h)]\right\}\phi\left(z+\frac{h}{2},\tau\right),\end{aligned} \qquad (7.47b)$$

3. Linear-space propagation in the second half step $h/2$:

$$\begin{aligned}\phi(z+h,\tau) &= \exp\left(\frac{h\mathbf{A}}{2}\right)\phi^*\left(z+\frac{h}{2},\tau\right)\\ &= F^{-1}\left[\exp\left(-\frac{j\gamma h}{2}\right)F\left\{\phi^*\left(z+\frac{h}{2},\tau\right)\right\}\right].\end{aligned} \tag{7.47c}$$

7.4. DISCRETE FOURIER TRANSFORM

It is necessary to translate Fourier transforms in Eqs. (7.33) and (7.47) into discrete Fourier transforms [6] in order to calculate them numerically. Before describing the discrete Fourier transform (DFT), the sampling theorem [7] that is the basis of DFT will be explained.

Let us consider the electric field distribution $\psi(x)$ shown in Fig. 7.2(a). We assume that the spatial frequency spectrum $\Psi(\rho)$ is restricted inside of the spatial frequency range $-W \leqslant \rho \leqslant W$, as shown in Fig. 7.2(b); that is,

$$\Psi(\rho) = 0 \qquad (|\rho| > W). \tag{7.48}$$

Here W denotes the maximum spatial frequency. The Fourier integral to obtain $\psi(x)$ is then expressed by

$$\psi(x) = \int_{-\infty}^{\infty} \Psi(\rho)\exp(j2\pi\rho x)d\rho = \int_{-W}^{W} \Psi(\rho)\exp(j2\pi\rho x)d\rho. \tag{7.49}$$

Since spatial frequency components outside of $|\rho| > W$ are not necessary, we could freely assume the spatial frequency distributions in these regions. Here we

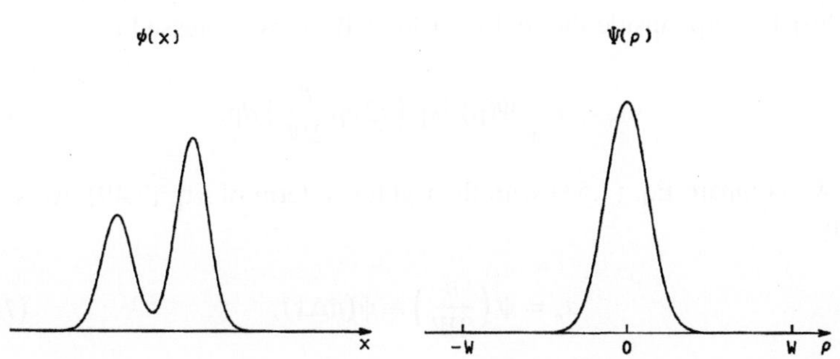

Figure 7.2 (a) Electric field distribution $\psi(x)$ and (b) its spatial frequency spectrum $\Psi(\rho)$.

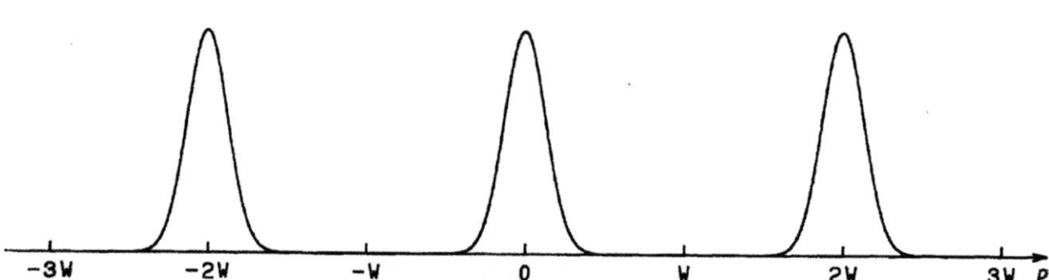

Figure 7.3 Spatial spectrum distribution $\tilde{\Psi}(\rho)$ in which $\Psi(\boldsymbol{\rho})$ inside of $|\boldsymbol{\rho}| \leqslant W$ is repeated periodically, with period of $2W$.

assume that the spatial spectrum distribution $\Psi(\rho)$ inside of $|\rho| \leqslant W$ is repeated periodically, with the period of $2W$ as shown in Fig. 7.3. This periodically repeated spectrum distribution is denoted by $\tilde{\Psi}(\rho)$. Equation (7.49) is then rewritten as

$$\psi(x) = \int_{-W}^{W} \tilde{\Psi}(\rho) \exp(j2\pi\rho x) d\rho. \tag{7.50}$$

The Periodical function $\tilde{\Psi}(\rho)$ is expressed by using the Fourier series:

$$\tilde{\Psi}(\rho) = \frac{1}{2W} \sum_{n=-\infty}^{\infty} a_n \exp\left(-j2\pi\rho \frac{n}{2W}\right), \tag{7.51}$$

where expansion coefficient a_n is given by

$$a_n = \int_{-W}^{W} \tilde{\Psi}(\rho) \exp\left(j2\pi\rho \frac{n}{2W}\right) d\rho. \tag{7.52}$$

Since $\tilde{\Psi}(\rho) = \Psi(\rho)$ inside the region of $|\rho| \leqslant W$, a_n is expressed as

$$a_n = \int_{-W}^{W} \Psi(\rho) \exp\left(j2\pi\rho \frac{n}{2W}\right) d\rho. \tag{7.53}$$

When we compare Eq. (7.53) with the rightmost term of Eq. (7.49), we see the equality

$$a_n = \psi\left(\frac{n}{2W}\right) \equiv \psi(n\Delta x), \tag{7.54a}$$

$$\Delta x = \frac{1}{2W}. \tag{7.54b}$$

Substituting Eq. (7.51) into Eq. (7.50) and denoting $a_n = \psi(n\Delta x) \equiv \psi_n$, $\psi(x)$ is given by

$$\psi(x) = \int_{-W}^{W} \tilde{\Psi}(\rho) \exp(j2\pi\rho x) d\rho = \frac{1}{2W} \sum_{n=-\infty}^{\infty} \psi_n \int_{-W}^{W} \exp\left[j\pi(2Wx - n)\frac{\rho}{W}\right] d\rho$$

$$= \sum_{n=-\infty}^{\infty} \psi_n \frac{\sin[\pi(2Wx - n)]}{\pi(2Wx - n)}. \tag{7.55}$$

The Function $\sin[\pi(2W\mathrm{x} - \mathrm{n})]/\pi(2W\mathrm{x} - \mathrm{n})$ is called *sampling function.* It is unity only at the sampling point $x = n/2W$ and becomes zero at other sampling points $x \neq n/2W$. It is therefore evident that $\psi(x)$, which is approximated by Eq. (7.55), passes through ψ_n at each sampling point. There seems to be plenty of curves that pass through ψ_n. However, the curve that is arbitrarily drawn to pass through ψ_n normally contains the higher-spatial-frequency component of $\rho > |W|$. Therefore, ψ_n is uniquely determined under the condition of $\rho \leqslant |W|$.

Equation (7.55) is an equation that gives continuous waveforms using discrete data on x-axis sampled at every $1/2W$ intervals. It is seen that when waveform $\psi(x)$, whose frequency spectrum is restricted below W, is sampled with the interval $\Delta x (\leqslant 1/2W)$, the series of sampled data $\{\psi(n\Delta x)\}$ (Figure 7.4) has sufficient information to reconstruct the original continuous waveform $\psi(x)$. This is called *sampling theorem.*

Based on the sampling theorem, the discrete Fourier transform is described. We assume that the electric field distribution $\psi(x)$ is confined inside of $0 \leqslant x \leqslant D$, as shown in Fig. 7.5, in addition and that its spatial frequency is restricted within $\rho \leqslant |W|$. Here, we consider the electric field profile $\tilde{\psi}(x)$, which is obtained by the repetition of $\psi(x)$, as shown in Fig. 7.6. Following procedures similar to Eqs. (7.49)–(7.53), we obtain

$$\tilde{\psi}(x) = \frac{1}{D} \sum_{\ell=-\infty}^{\infty} b_\ell \exp\left(j2\pi x \frac{\ell}{D}\right), \tag{7.56}$$

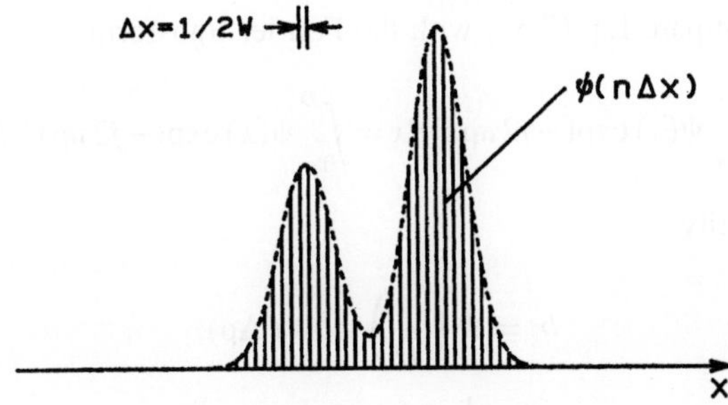

Figure 7.4 Series of sampled data $\{\psi(n\Delta x)\}$ that is sampled with the interval of $\Delta x = 1/2W$.

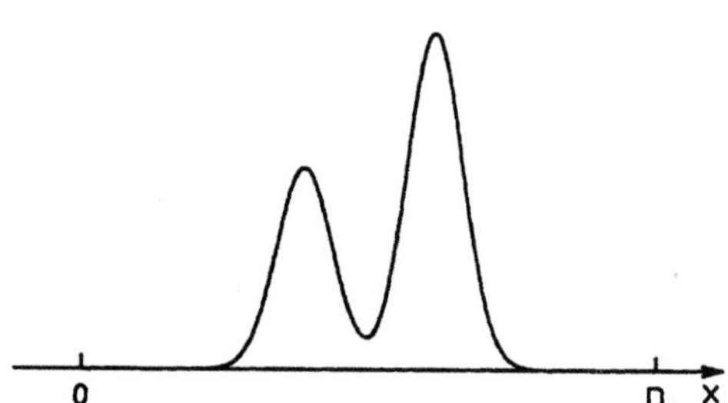

Figure 7.5 Electric field distribution $\psi(x)$ that is confined inside of $0 \leqslant x \leqslant D$.

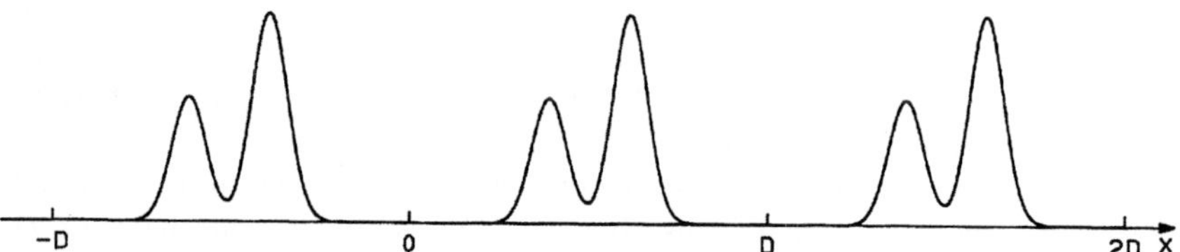

Figure 7.6 Electric field profile that is obtained by the repetition of $\psi(x)$ inside of $0 \leqslant x \leqslant D$.

$$
\begin{aligned}
b_\ell &= \int_0^D \tilde{\psi}(x) \exp\left(-j2\pi x \frac{\ell}{D}\right) dx \\
&= \int_0^D \psi(x) \exp\left(-j2\pi x \frac{\ell}{D}\right) dx.
\end{aligned} \tag{7.57}
$$

When we compare Eq. (7.57) with the Fourier transform

$$
\Psi(\rho) = \int_{-\infty}^{\infty} \psi(x) \exp(-j2\pi\rho x) dx = \int_0^D \psi(x) \exp(-j2\pi\rho x) dx, \tag{7.58}
$$

we see the equality

$$
b_\ell = \Psi\left(\frac{\ell}{D}\right) \equiv \Psi(\ell\,\Delta\rho), \tag{7.59a}
$$

$$
\Delta\rho = \frac{1}{D}. \tag{7.59b}
$$

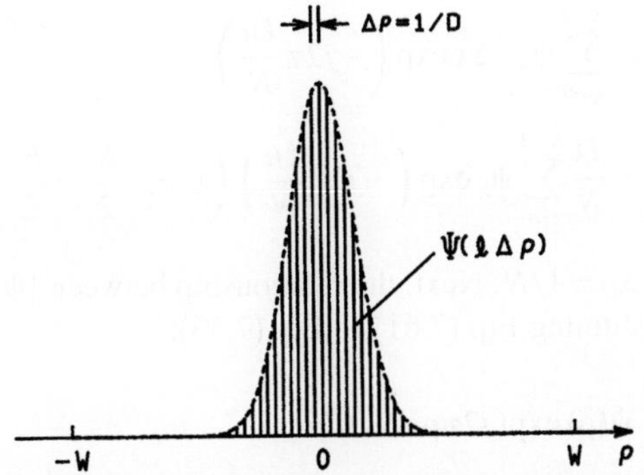

Figure 7.7 Series of sampled data $\{\psi(\ell\,\Delta\rho)\}$ that is sampled with the interval of $\Delta\rho = 1/D$.

Therefore, it is seen that when the spatial frequency distribution $\psi(\rho)$, whose corresponding electric field is restricted within $0 \leqslant x \leqslant D$, is sampled with the interval $\Delta\rho(\leqslant 1/D)$, the series of sampled data $\{\psi(\ell\,\Delta\rho)\}$ (Figure 7.7) has sufficient information to reconstruct the original continuous frequency distribution $\psi(\rho)$.

If the total number of sampling points is N for both the electric field distribution $\psi(x)$ and the spatial frequency spectra $\psi(\rho)$, they are approximated as

$$\psi(x) = \sum_{n=0}^{N-1} \psi_n \delta(x - n\Delta x) \cdot \Delta x, \tag{7.60}$$

$$\psi(\rho) = \sum_{\ell=-N/2}^{N/2-1} \psi(\ell\,\Delta\rho)\delta(\rho - \ell\,\Delta\rho) \cdot \Delta\rho, \tag{7.61}$$

where $\Delta x = D/N$ and $\Delta\rho = 2W/N$. Δx and $\Delta\rho$ are already given by Eqs. (7.54b) and (7.59b) as $\Delta x = 1/2W$ and $\Delta\rho = 1/D$. Therefore, it is known that total number of sampling points is related to W and D by

$$N = 2WD. \tag{7.62}$$

Substituting Eq. (7.60) in Eq. (7.58), we obtain the relationship between series of line spectra $\{\psi(\ell\,\Delta\rho)\}$ and the series of sampled electric field $\{\psi_n\}$:

$$\begin{aligned}\psi(\ell\,\Delta\rho) &= \int_0^D \psi(x)\exp(-j2\pi x\ell\,\Delta\rho)dx \\ &= \sum_{n=0}^{N-1} \psi_n \cdot \Delta x \int_0^D \delta(x - n\Delta x) \times \exp(-j2\pi x\ell\,\Delta\rho)dx\end{aligned}$$

$$= \sum_{n=0}^{N-1} \psi_n \cdot \Delta x \exp\left(-j2\pi \frac{\ell n}{N}\right)$$

$$= \frac{D}{N} \sum_{n=0}^{N-1} \psi_n \exp\left(-j2\pi \frac{\ell n}{N}\right) \left(\ell = -\frac{N}{2} - \frac{N}{2} - 1\right). \quad (7.63)$$

Here we used $\Delta x \cdot \Delta\rho = 1/N$. Next, the relationship between $\{\psi_n\}$ and $\{\psi(\ell\,\Delta\rho)\}$ is obtained by substituting Eq. (7.61) in Eq. (7.53):

$$\psi_n = \int_{-W}^{W} \psi(\rho) \exp(j2\pi\rho n \Delta x) d\rho$$

$$= \sum_{\ell=-N/2}^{N/2-1} \psi(\ell\,\Delta\rho) \cdot \Delta\rho \int_{-W}^{W} \delta(\rho - \ell\,\Delta\rho) \times \exp(j2\pi\rho n\,\Delta x) d\rho$$

$$= \sum_{\ell=-N/2}^{N/2-1} \psi(\ell\,\Delta\rho) \cdot \Delta\rho \exp\left(j2\pi \frac{\ell\, n}{N}\right)$$

$$= \frac{1}{D} \sum_{\ell=-N/2}^{N/2-1} \psi(\ell\,\Delta\rho) \exp\left(j2\pi \frac{\ell n}{N}\right) \quad (n = 0 - N - 1). \quad (7.64)$$

Equations (7.63) and (7.64) are equations of the forward and inverse Fourier transform. The range of parameter $\ell(= -N/2 - N/2 - 1)$ in Eq. (7.63) is different from that of $n(= 0 - N - 1)$ in Eq. (7.64). If the ranges of both ℓ and n are same, it is much more convenient for computer programming. Here, a new parameter, ℓ', is introduced for ℓ when it is in the range of $\ell = -N/2 \sim -1$; that is a

$$\ell' = \ell + N \qquad \left(\ell' = \frac{N}{2} - N - 1\right). \quad (7.65)$$

Equations (7.63) and (7.64) are then rewritten to

$$\begin{cases} \psi(\ell\,\Delta\rho) = \dfrac{D}{N} \displaystyle\sum_{n=0}^{N-1} \psi_n \exp\left(-j2\pi \frac{\ell n}{N}\right) & \left(\ell = 0 - \dfrac{N}{2} - 1\right) \quad (7.66a) \\ \psi[(\ell' - N)\Delta\rho] = \dfrac{D}{N} \displaystyle\sum_{n=0}^{N-1} \psi_n \exp\left(-j2\pi \frac{\ell' n}{N}\right) & \left(\ell' = \dfrac{N}{2} - N - 1\right) \quad (7.66b) \end{cases}$$

$$\psi_n = \frac{1}{D} \sum_{\ell=0}^{N/2-1} \psi(\ell\,\Delta\rho) \exp\left(j2\pi \frac{\ell n}{N}\right) + \frac{1}{D} \sum_{\ell'=N/2}^{N-1} \psi[(\ell' - N)\Delta\rho] \exp\left(j\,2\pi \frac{\ell' n}{N}\right). \quad (7.67)$$

When we replace ℓ' by ℓ in Eqs. (7.66b) and (7.67) and define ψ_ℓ as

$$\psi_\ell = \begin{cases} \dfrac{\sqrt{N}}{D}\psi(\ell\,\Delta\rho) & \left(\ell = 0 - \dfrac{N}{2} - 1\right) \quad (7.68a) \\ \dfrac{\sqrt{N}}{D}\psi[(\ell - N)\,\Delta\rho] & \left(\ell = \dfrac{N}{2} - N - 1\right), \quad (7.68b) \end{cases}$$

the forward and inverse discrete Fourier transforms (IDFT) are expressed by

$$\psi_\ell = \mathrm{DFT}(\psi_n) = \frac{1}{\sqrt{N}} \sum_{n=0}^{N-1} \psi_n \exp\left(-j2\pi \tfrac{\ell n}{N}\right) \; (\ell = 0 - N - 1) \qquad (7.69)$$

$$\psi_n = \mathrm{IDFT}(\psi_\ell) = \frac{1}{\sqrt{N}} \sum_{\ell=0}^{N-1} \psi_\ell \exp\left(j2\pi \tfrac{\ell n}{N}\right) \; (n = 0 - N - 1). \qquad (7.70)$$

We should note here that the negative spectral component in Fig. 7.7 is transposed into spectral region higher than W, as shown in Fig. 7.8, since we introduced a parameter transformation in Eq. (7.68b). Equations (7.69) and (7.70) are counterparts of the continuous forward and inverse Fourier transforms

$$\psi(\rho) = F(\psi) = \int_{-\infty}^{\infty} \psi(x) \exp(-j2\pi\rho x)\, dx, \qquad (7.71)$$

$$\psi(x) = F^{-1}(\psi) = \int_{-\infty}^{\infty} \psi(\rho) \exp(j2\pi\rho x)\, d\rho. \qquad (7.72)$$

Figures 7.9 and 7.10 show the relationships between the electric field distribution and its spatial frequency spectra for continuous and discrete Fourier transforms, respectively.

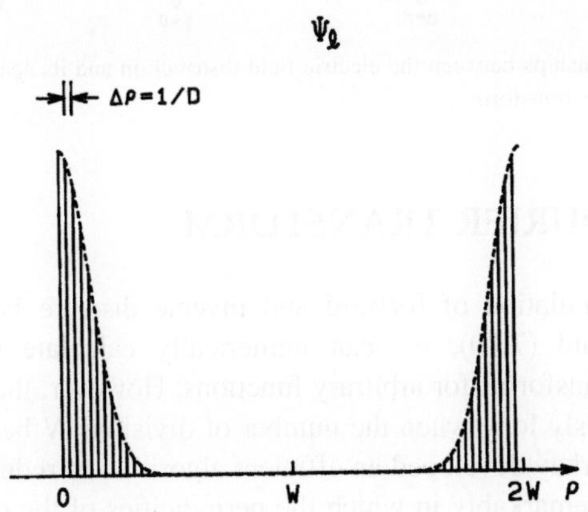

Figure 7.8 New line spectrum series $\{\Psi_\ell\}$ defined by Eq. (7.68).

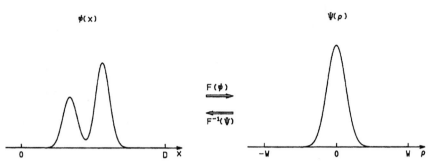

Figure 7.9 Relationships between the electric field distribution and its spatial frequency spectra for the continuous Fourier transform.

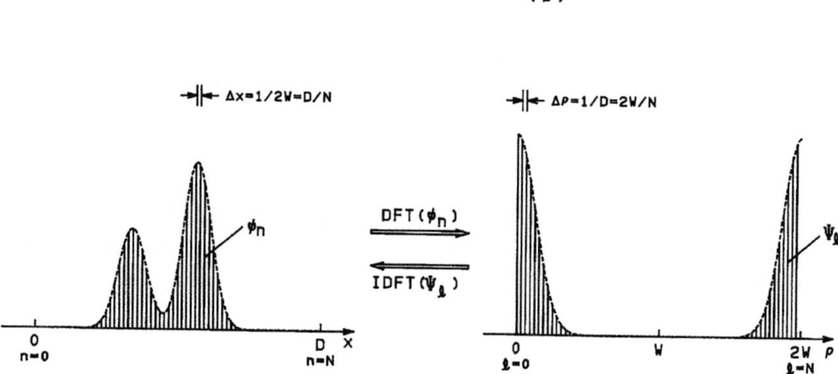

Figure 7.10 Relationships between the electric field distribution and its spatial frequency spectra for the discrete Fourier transform.

7.5. FAST FOURIER TRANSFORM

Using the formulation of forward and inverse discrete Fourier transforms of Eqs. (7.69) and (7.70), we can numerically calculate the forward and inverse Fourier transforms for arbitrary functions. However, the calculation time becomes enormously long when the number of divisions N becomes large.

Cooley and Turkey developed an efficient algorithm to reduce computational time of the DFT remarkably in which the periodicities of the exponential terms are ingeniously utilized [8]. This is called the *fast Fourier transform (FFT)* [6, 8].

The forward and inverse DFTs in Eqs. (7.69) and (7.70) are mathematically identical, since the difference is only in the sign of the exponential terms. Therefore, we describe the formulation of the FFT by using forward DFT. To begin with, Eq. (7.69) is rewritten as

$$F_\ell = \sum_{n=0}^{N-1} f_n G^{\ell n} \qquad (\ell = 0 - N-1), \tag{7.73}$$

where $f_n = \psi_n/\sqrt{N}$, $F_\ell = \Psi_\ell$, and G is defined by

$$G = \exp\left(-\frac{j2\pi}{N}\right). \tag{7.74}$$

The matrix representation of Eq. (7.73) for $N = 2^3 = 8$ becomes

$$\begin{bmatrix} F_0 \\ F_1 \\ F_2 \\ F_3 \\ F_4 \\ F_5 \\ F_6 \\ F_7 \end{bmatrix} = \begin{bmatrix} 1 & 1 & 1 & 1 & 1 & 1 & 1 & 1 \\ 1 & G & G^2 & G^3 & G^4 & G^5 & G^6 & G^7 \\ 1 & G^2 & G^4 & G^6 & G^8 & G^{10} & G^{12} & G^{14} \\ 1 & G^3 & G^6 & G^9 & G^{12} & G^{15} & G^{18} & G^{21} \\ 1 & G^4 & G^8 & G^{12} & G^{16} & G^{20} & G^{24} & G^{28} \\ 1 & G^5 & G^{10} & G^{15} & G^{20} & G^{25} & G^{30} & G^{35} \\ 1 & G^6 & G^{12} & G^{18} & G^{24} & G^{30} & G^{36} & G^{42} \\ 1 & G^7 & G^{14} & G^{21} & G^{28} & G^{35} & G^{42} & G^{49} \end{bmatrix} \begin{bmatrix} f_0 \\ f_1 \\ f_2 \\ f_3 \\ f_4 \\ f_5 \\ f_6 \\ f_7 \end{bmatrix} \tag{7.75}$$

$G^{\ell n}$ ranges from G^0 to G^{49} in this equation. However, if we notice the periodicity of $G^{\ell n}$, Eq. (7.73) or (7.75) can be simplified. We separate N sampled values from f_0 to f_{N-1} into two groups, with $n = 0 - (N/2 - 1)$ and $n = N/2 - (N-1)$. Then Eq. (7.73) is expressed by

$$F_\ell = \sum_{n=0}^{N/2-1} f_n G^{\ell n} + \sum_{n=N/2}^{N-1} f_n G^{\ell n}. \tag{7.76}$$

The second term of this equation can be rewritten as

$$\sum_{n=N/2}^{N-1} f_n G^{\ell n} = \sum_{n=0}^{N/2-1} f_{n+N/2} G^{\ell(n+N/2)} = \sum_{n=0}^{N/2-1} f_{n+N/2} G^{\ell n} G^{\ell N/2}. \tag{7.77}$$

From Eq. (7.74), $G^{\ell N/2}$ is obtained by

$$G^{\ell N/2} = \exp\left(-j\frac{2\pi\ell}{N}\frac{N}{2}\right) = \exp(-j\pi\ell) = (-1)^\ell. \tag{7.78}$$

Then Eq. (7.76) is expressed by

$$F_\ell = \sum_{n=0}^{N/2-1} [f_n + (-1)^\ell f_{n+N/2}] G^{\ell n}. \tag{7.79}$$

The matrix representation of Eq. (7.79) for $N = 8$ is:

$$\begin{bmatrix} F_0 \\ F_2 \\ F_4 \\ F_6 \\ F_1 \\ F_3 \\ F_5 \\ F_7 \end{bmatrix} = \begin{bmatrix} 1 & 1 & 1 & 1 & 0 & 0 & 0 & 0 \\ 1 & G^2 & G^4 & G^6 & 0 & 0 & 0 & 0 \\ 1 & G^4 & G^8 & G^{12} & 0 & 0 & 0 & 0 \\ 1 & G^6 & G^{12} & G^{18} & 0 & 0 & 0 & 0 \\ 0 & 0 & 0 & 0 & 1 & G & G^2 & G^3 \\ 0 & 0 & 0 & 0 & 1 & G^3 & G^6 & G^9 \\ 0 & 0 & 0 & 0 & 1 & G^5 & G^{10} & G^{15} \\ 0 & 0 & 0 & 0 & 1 & G^7 & G^{14} & G^{21} \end{bmatrix} \begin{bmatrix} f_0 + f_4 \\ f_1 + f_5 \\ f_2 + f_6 \\ f_3 + f_7 \\ f_0 - f_4 \\ f_1 - f_5 \\ f_2 - f_6 \\ f_3 - f_7 \end{bmatrix} \tag{7.80}$$

Equation (7.80) shows that the 8×8 matrix operation is reduced into two sets of 4×4 matrix operations. The matrix operation of Eq. (7.80) can be further reduced into 2×2 matrix operations in the same way as can Eq. (7.79). Such reductions of matrix operations are systematically formulated in the FFT algorithm [6, 9].

7.6. FORMULATION OF NUMERICAL PROCEDURES USING DISCRETE FOURIER TRANSFORM

Here we rewrite BPM formulations for waveguide analysis [Eq. (7.33)] and pulse propagation analysis [Eq. (7.47)] into those that use the discrete Fourier transform in order to utilize FFT subroutine. We should note here that the negative spectral component in the frequency domain is transposed into the spectral region higher than half of the spectral window, as shown in Fig. 7.10(b).

BPM procedures for the waveguide analysis described in Eq. (7.33) are rewritten in the discretized form as:

1. Free space propagation in the first half-step $h/2$:

$$\begin{aligned} \phi(m\,\Delta x, z + h/2) &= \exp(h\mathbf{A}/2)\phi(m\,\Delta x, z) \\ &= \mathrm{IDFT}[\exp(-j\delta\beta_\ell h/2)\mathrm{DFT}\{\phi(m\Delta x, z)\}] \\ &\quad \times (m = 0 - N - 1) \end{aligned} \tag{7.81a}$$

2. Loss (or gain) and phase retardation of entire step h:

$$\begin{aligned} \phi^*(m\Delta x, z + h/2) &= \exp(h\mathbf{B})\phi(m\Delta x, z + h/2) \\ &= \exp\left\{\frac{h}{2}[\mathbf{B}(z) + \mathbf{B}(z+h)]\right\}\phi(m\Delta x, z + h/2) \\ &\quad \times (m = 0 - N - 1) \end{aligned} \tag{7.81b}$$

3. Free-space propagation in the second half-step $h/2$:

$$\begin{aligned}\phi(m\Delta x, z+h) &= \exp(h\mathbf{A}/2)\phi^*(m\Delta x, z+h/2)\\ &= \mathrm{IDFT}[\exp(-j\delta\beta_\ell h/2)\mathrm{DFT}\{\phi^*(m\Delta x, z+h/2)\}]\\ &\qquad (m=0-N-1)\end{aligned} \tag{7.81c}$$

Here, $\delta\beta_\ell$ and $\mathbf{B}$ are given by

$$\delta\beta_\ell = \begin{cases}\left[k^2n_0^2-(2\pi\ell\Delta\rho)^2\right]^{1/2}-kn_0 & (\ell=0-N/2-1)\\ \left\{k^2n_0^2-[2\pi(\ell-N)\Delta\rho]^2\right\}^{1/2}-kn_0 & (\ell=N/2-N-1)\end{cases} \tag{7.82}$$

$$\mathbf{B} = -\alpha(m\Delta x, z) - jk[n(m\Delta x, z)-n_0] \qquad (m=0-N-1) \tag{7.83}$$

BPM procedures for the pulse propagation analysis described in Eq. (7.47) are rewritten in the discretized form as:

1. Linear-space propagation in the first half-step $h/2$:

$$\begin{aligned}\phi(z+h/2, m\Delta\tau) &= \exp(h\mathbf{A}/2)\phi(z, m\Delta\tau)\\ &= \mathrm{IDFT}[\exp(-j\gamma_\ell h/2)\mathrm{DFT}\{\phi(z, m\Delta\tau)\}]\\ &\qquad (m=0-N-1)\end{aligned} \tag{7.84a}$$

2. Loss (or gain) and phase retardation of entire step h:

$$\begin{aligned}\phi^*(z+h/2, m\Delta\tau) &= \exp(h\mathbf{B})\phi(z+h/2, m\Delta\tau)\\ &= \exp\left\{\frac{h}{2}[\mathbf{B}(z)+\mathbf{B}(z+h)]\right\}\phi(z+h/z, m\Delta\tau)\\ &\qquad (m=0-N-1)\end{aligned} \tag{7.84b}$$

3. Linear-space propagation in the second half-step $h/2$:

$$\begin{aligned}\phi(z+h, m\Delta\tau) &= \exp(h\mathbf{A}/2)\phi^*(z+h/2, m\Delta\tau)\\ &= \mathrm{IDFT}[\exp(-j\gamma_\ell h/2)\mathrm{DFT}\{\phi^*(z+h/2, m\Delta\tau)\}]\\ &\qquad (m=0-N-1).\end{aligned} \tag{7.84c}$$

Here, $\Delta\tau = T/N = 1/2W$, where T and W denote time window and the maximum frequency of temporal pulse, respectively. When we denote the frequency step $\Delta f = 2W/N = 1/T$, γ_ℓ and $\mathbf{B}$ are given by

$$\gamma_\ell = \begin{cases} \dfrac{\beta''}{2}(2\pi\ell\,\Delta f)^2 & (\ell = 0 - N/2 - 1) \\ \dfrac{\beta''}{2}[2\pi(\ell - N)\Delta f]^2 & (\ell = N/2 - N - 1) \end{cases} \tag{7.85}$$

$$\mathbf{B} = -\alpha(z, m\Delta\tau) - j\frac{1}{2}kn_2|\phi(z, m\Delta\tau)|^2 \qquad (m = 0 - N - 1). \tag{7.86}$$

Since terms inside of square root in Eq. (7.82) should be positive, we have the following relations for integer variable ℓ:

$$kn_0 \geqslant 2\pi\frac{\ell}{D} \qquad (\ell = 0 - N/2 - 1)$$

and

$$kn_0 \geqslant 2\pi\frac{(N - \ell)}{D} \qquad (\ell = N/2 - N - 1).$$

The range of variable ℓ is then determined from the above equations as

$$\ell \leqslant \left[\frac{n_0 D}{\lambda}\right] \equiv \ell_{\max} \qquad (\ell = 0 - N/2 - 1) \tag{7.87a}$$

$$N - \ell \leqslant \left[\frac{n_0 D}{\lambda}\right] \qquad (\ell = N/2 - N - 1), \tag{7.87b}$$

where [ ] denotes Gauss' sign. If $\ell_{\max}$ is smaller than $N/2$, allowable range for ℓ is given by

$$\ell = 0 - \ell_{\max} \tag{7.88a}$$

and

$$\ell = N - \ell_{\max} - N - 1. \tag{7.88b}$$

Frequency spectrum component in the parameter range of $\ell = \ell_{\max} + 1 - N - \ell_{\max} - 1$ should be set to $\Psi_\ell = 0$.

7.7. APPLICATIONS OF FFTBPM

Applications of BPM based on FFT to optical pulse propagation have been shown in Figs. 5.6, 5.7 and 5.9 in Section 5.3. Therefore, we will explain here applications of BPM to optical waveguide problems.

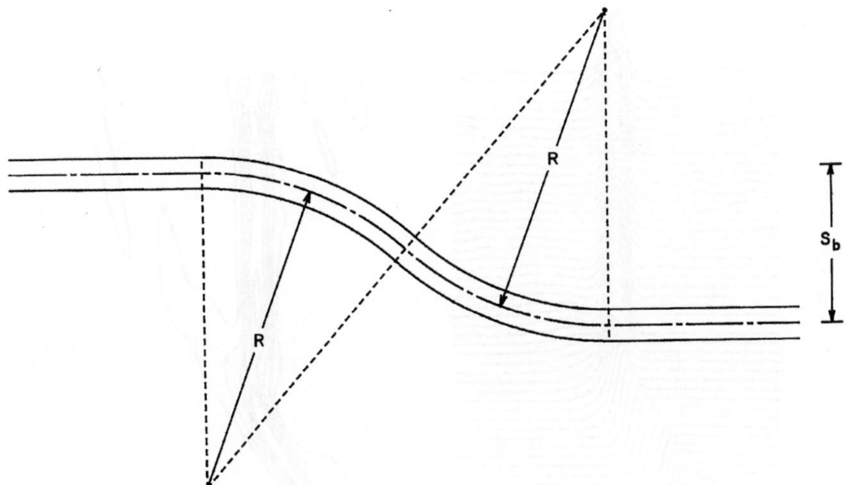

Figure 7.11 S-shaped bent waveguide without offset.

First of all, we explain the BPM investigation to reduce propagation loss in S-shaped bent (S-bend) waveguides [10]. The S-shaped bent waveguide connects two parallel waveguides separated by the distance S_b, as shown in Fig. 7.11. S-bend waveguides are important as input/output waveguides for directional couplers and as waveguide path transformers in various circuits. There are basically two kinds of S-bend waveguides: the S-bend waveguide consisting of a fixed radius of curvature R, as shown in Fig. 7.11, and S-bend waveguide with the functional shape of $y = az + b\sin(cz)$ in which radius of curvature varies continuously. Here we treat the former fixed-R S-bends.

Figure 7.12 shows BPM simulation of the light propagation at $\lambda = 1.55\,\mu\text{m}$ in S-bend waveguide shown in Fig. 7.11. The parameters of the S-bend waveguide are as follows: core width $2a = 8\,\mu\text{m}$, core thickness $2d = 8\,\mu\text{m}$, refractive-index difference $\Delta = 0.3\%$, radius of curvature $R = 10\,\text{mm}$, and waveguide separation $S_b = 25\,\mu\text{m}$, respectively. Here, three-dimensional waveguide problem is transformed into two-dimensional one by using an effective-index method. Lefthand-side figure of Fig. 7.12 shows light intensity waveforms and righthand-side figure shows contour plots of intensity.

In Fig. 7.12 and figures of the following BPM analyses, we should note that the propagation length along z-axis direction is much longer than the horizontal x-axis window size. The width of the BPM analysis in the x-axis direction in Fig. 7.12 is $D = 102.4\mu\text{m}$ and number of division is $N = 512(\Delta x = D/N = 0.2\,\mu\text{m})$. The calculation step along the z-axis direction is $h = 0.5\,\mu\text{m}$. Figure 7.12 shows that light cannot negotiate the curved waveguide and is radiated into cladding when bend is steep. The bend-induced radiation loss in Fig. 7.12 is about 1.45 dB. The straightforward method to reduce bend-induced loss is to

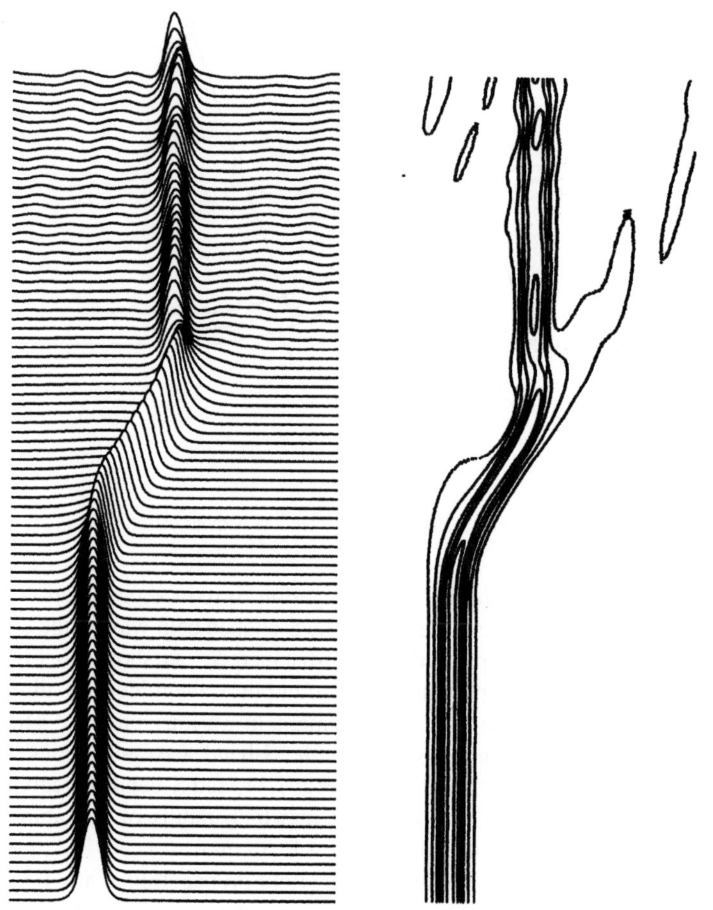

Figure 7.12 BPM simulation of the light propagation in an S-bend waveguide consisting of a fixed radius of curvature without offset.

increase the refractive-index difference Δ of the waveguide and to confine the optical field tightly inside the core.

However, there is another possible way to reduce bending loss without increasing Δ, that is, to introduce waveguide offset, as shown in Fig. 7.13 [11]. The waveguide offset is introduced at the interface between the straight and bent waveguides or at interface between the two oppositely bent waveguides (Fig. 7.13). In the bent waveguide, the light field is pressed slightly to the outer core–cladding interface and is somewhat deformed from its original profile. The waveguide is usually shifted to the inward direction by the offset. Then the waveguide offset compensates for the field deformation and thus alleviates the bend-induced radiation loss. Figure 7.14 shows a BPM simulation of the light propagation

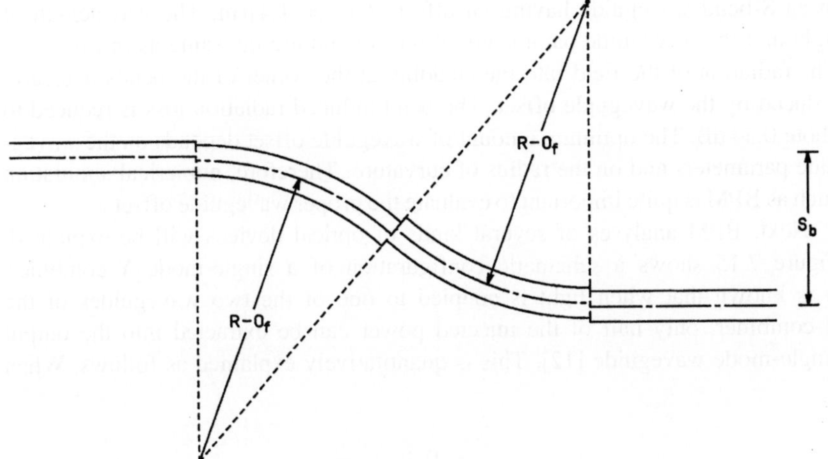

Figure 7.13 S-shaped bent waveguide with a waveguide offset.

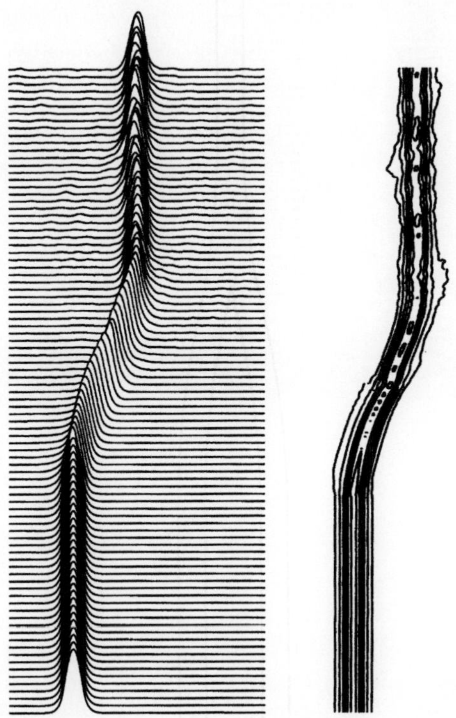

Figure 7.14 BPM simulation of the light propagation in an S-bend waveguide having an offset of $O_f = 1.4\,\mu\text{m}$.

in an S-bend waveguide having an offset of $O_f = 1.4\,\mu\text{m}$. The wavelength of light and the waveguide parameters of the S-bend are the same as in Fig. 7.12. The radiation of the field into the cladding at the corner of the bends is clearly reduced by the waveguide offset. The bend-induced radiation loss is reduced to about 0.44 dB. The optimum amount of waveguide offset depends on the waveguide parameters and on the radius of curvature. Therefore, numerical simulation such as BPM is quite important to evaluate the proper waveguide offset.

Next, BPM analyses of several kinds of optical devices will be explained. Figure 7.15 shows a schematic configuration of a single-mode Y-combiner. It is known that when light is coupled to one of the two waveguides of the Y-combiner, only half of the injected power can be extracted into the output single-mode waveguide [12]. This is quantitatively explained as follows. When

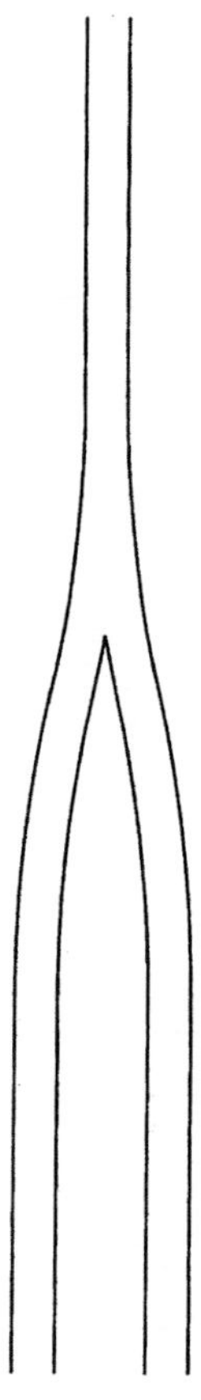

Figure 7.15 Schematic configuration of a Y-combiner consisting of single-mode waveguides.

light is coupled into one of the waveguides, even and odd modes are generated at the combining region, where the waveguide is wider than the single-mode waveguide (refer to Fig. 4.12). The electric field amplitude of each mode is about $1/\sqrt{2}$. Beyond the combining region, the waveguide width gradually decreases to that of the single-mode waveguide. Then, higher-order odd mode becomes cut off and radiated into the cladding. Thus the transmitted light is only an even mode, and about 3 dB light power is lost.

Figure 7.16 shows BPM analysis of single-mode Y-combiner when light is coupled into one of the two waveguides. The parameters of the Y-combiner are as follows: core width $2a = 8\,\mu\text{m}$, core thickness $2d = 8\,\mu\text{m}$, refractive-index

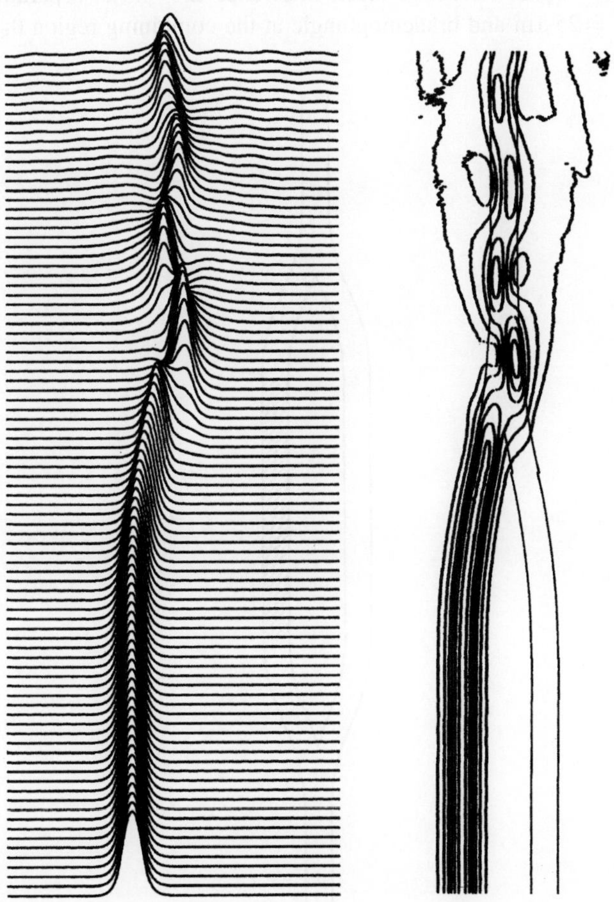

Figure 7.16 BPM analysis of single-mode Y-combiner when light is coupled into one of the two waveguides.

difference $\Delta = 0.3\%$, separation of the two waveguides 25 μm, branching angle at the combining region $\theta_B = 1.2°$, and output waveguide length = 1 mm. The light beam undulation in the combining region of Fig. 7.16 is considered to be due to the interference effect between even, odd and radiation modes. The transmitted eigen-mode light power in the output waveguide of Fig. 7.16 is 0.488367 (3.1 dB loss). It is confirmed by the BPM numerical simulation that there is about 3-dB excess loss in the single-mode Y-combiners.

Figure 7.17 shows a Y-branch type optical intensity modulator [13]. The hatched region in Fig. 7.17 is a switching part in which the phase retardation of the light (actually a refractive index of the waveguide) is varied. The parameters of Y-branch type of modulator are as follows: core width $2a = 8$ μm, core thickness $2d = 8$ μm, refractive-index difference $\Delta = 0.3\%$, separation of two waveguides = 25 μm and branching angle at the combining region $\theta_B = 1.2°$.

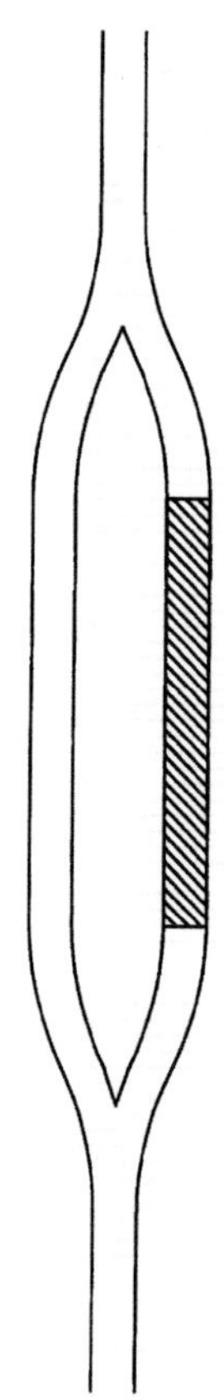

Figure 7.17 Y-branch type of optical intensity modulator.

When the refractive index of the switching region is not varied, the two light beams are combined with the same phase retardation (in phase) at Y-combiner. Therefore, almost 100% light transmission is achieved in the output waveguide, as shown in Fig. 7.18. In contrast, when refractive index of the switching region is varied by δn, the relative phase retardation between the two arms becomes $\phi = \delta\beta \cdot L$, where L denotes the length of switching region. If relative phase retardation satisfies

$$\delta\beta \cdot L = \frac{2\pi}{\lambda}\delta n_{\mathrm{eff}} \cdot L = \pi, \tag{7.89}$$

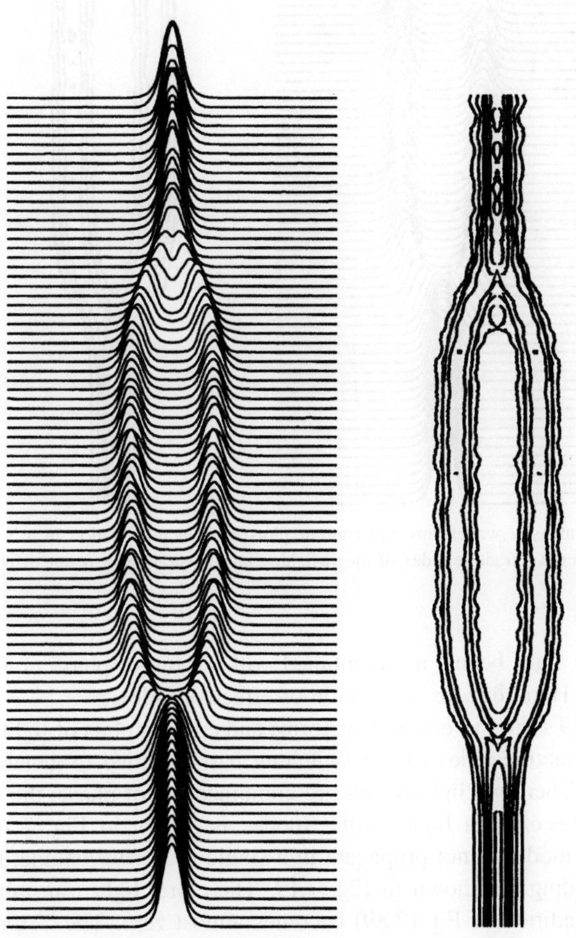

Figure 7.18 Intensity waveforms and contour plots of light propagation in a Y-branch type of modulator when the refractive index of the switching part is not varied.

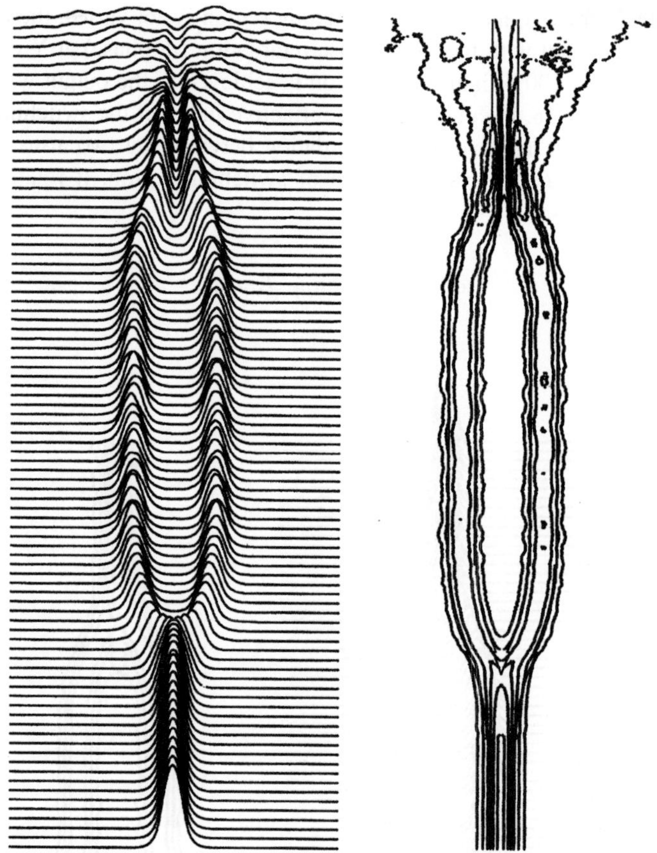

Figure 7.19 Intensity waveforms and contour plots of light propagation in a Y-branch type of modulator when the refractive index of the switching part is varied to generate π·phase shift.

then the two light beams are combined with an out-of-phase condition at the Y-combiner. Here, δn_{eff} is a variation of effective index.

Figure 7.19 shows intensity waveforms and contour plots of light propagation when the refractive index of the switching part is varied to generate $\pi \cdot$ phase phase shift. When two light beams are combined out of phase, the electric field distribution becomes a higher-order mode, as shown in Fig. 2.7(b). Since a higher-order mode cannot propagate in a single-mode waveguide, it is radiated into the cladding, as shown in Fig. 7.19. Therefore, light transmittance at the switching condition of Eq. (7.89) becomes almost zero. The Y-branch type of modulator acts as an on–off type of optical switch or as an optical intensity modulator.

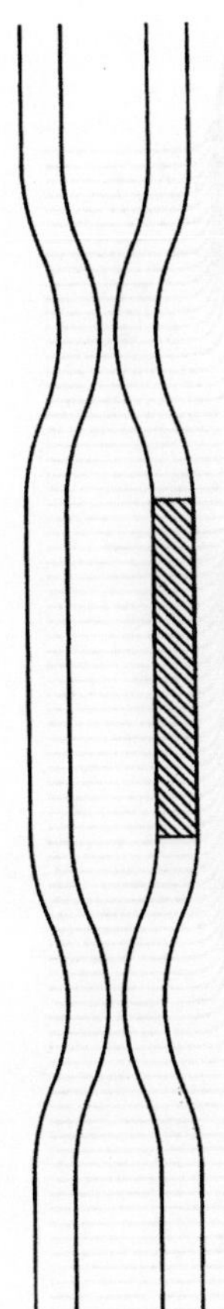

Figure 7.20 Mach–Zehnder type of optical switch. The hatched region is the switching region.

Figure 7.20 shows a schematic configuration of the Mach–Zehnder (MZ) type of optical switch [14]. The operational principle of Mach–Zehnder switch has been explained analytically in Section 4.5.1. Here, the transmission characteristics of the MZ switch will be analyzed numerically by BPM. The parameters of the MZ switch are as follows: core width $2a = 8\,\mu\text{m}$, core thickness $2d = 8\,\mu\text{m}$, refractive-index difference $\Delta = 0.3\%$, and separation of the two waveguides $= 25\,\mu\text{m}$. The two directional couplers are 3-dB couplers. When the refractive index of the switching region is not varied, the light beam exits from the cross-port, as shown in Fig. 7.21. This corresponds to the condition of $\phi = \delta\beta \cdot L = 0$ in Eq. (4.150). In contrast, if the refractive index of the switching region is varied such that Eq. (7.89) is satisfied, the light beam is switched into the through-port as shown in Fig. 7.22. This corresponds to the condition of $\phi = \delta\beta \cdot L = \pi$ in Eq. (4.150).

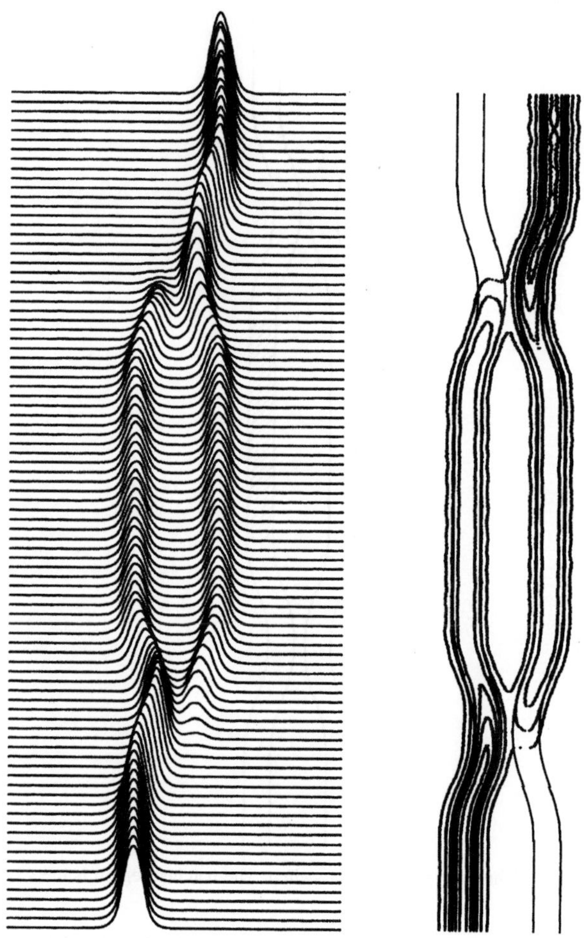

Figure 7.21 Intensity waveforms and contour plots of light propagation in the MZ switch when the refractive index of the switching region is not varied.

Finally, BPM analysis of an all-optical switch [15] will be described. In this all-optical switch, the directional coupler consists of a Kerr medium whose refractive index changes in proportion to the light intensity. A Schematic configuration of an all-optical switch is shown in Fig. 7.23. The hatched region indicates the Kerr medium; and the other region is a linear medium. The parameters of the all-optical switch are as follows: core width $2a = 8\,\mu\text{m}$, core thickness $2d = 8\,\mu\text{m}$, refractive-index difference $\Delta = 0.3\%$, and separation of the two waveguides $= 50\,\mu\text{m}$. The gap of the waveguide edges in a 3-dB directional

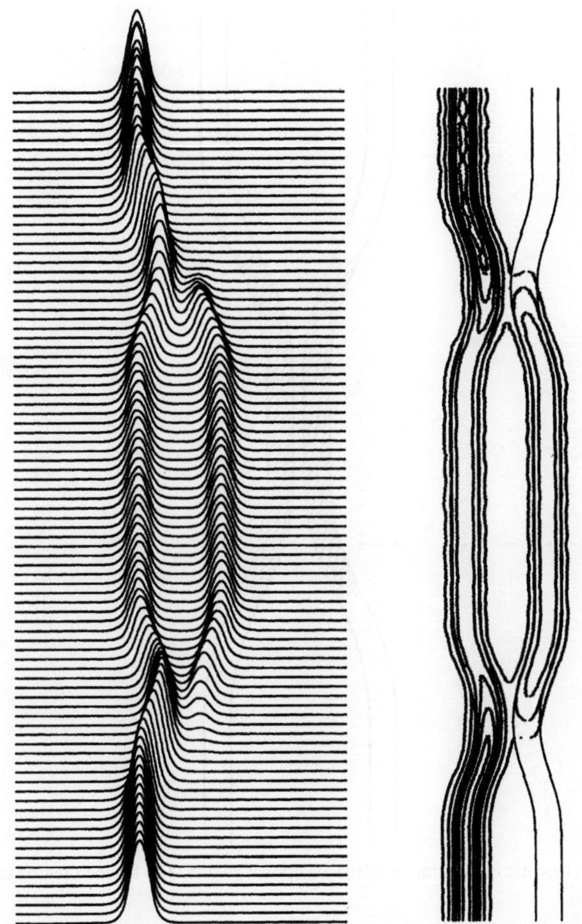

Figure 7.22 Intensity waveforms and contour plots of light propagation in the MZ switch when the refractive index of the switching region is varied.

coupler is 3 μm and the straight waveguide length of the coupler is 800 μm. We assume here semiconductor-doped glass as the Kerr medium [16]. The Kerr coefficient is $n_2 = 2 \times 10^{-14}\, \mathrm{m^2/W}$.

Figure 7.24 shows the light propagation characteristics for 1 mW of input power (light intensity of $I = 1.9 \times 10^7\, \mathrm{W/m^2}$). In this case, since the light intensity is low, a nonlinear optical effect is not observed. Then, the directional-coupler type of switch acts as a linear switch, and the light beam exits from the cross-port as designed. In contrast, when the light intensity is increased,

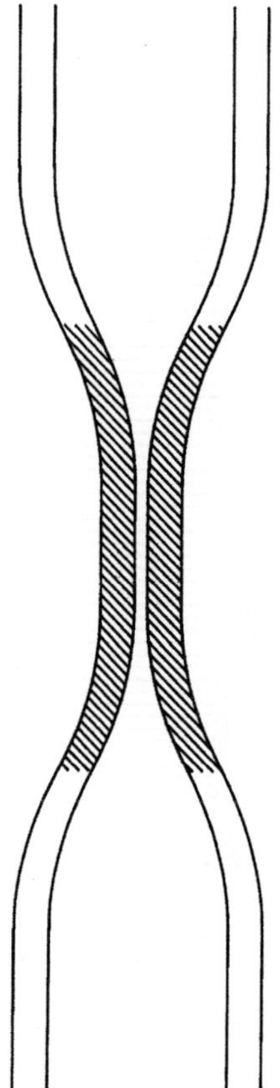

Figure 7.23 Schematic configuration of the all-optical switch. The hatched region consists of Kerr medium.

the directional coupler becomes unbalanced, since the refractive index of the waveguide into which the light is coupled increases. As shown in Eqs. (4.40)–(4.41) and Fig. 4.4(b), the coupling efficiency to the cross-port decreases when the refractive-index asymmetry between the two waveguides (refer to Eq. (4.20)) becomes large. Figure 7.25 shows the light propagation characteristics for 2.2 W of input power (light intensity of $I = 4.1 \times 10^{10}\,\mathrm{W/m^2}$). Since the directional coupler becomes unbalanced, most of the light beam exits from the through-port.

In a directional coupler consisting of a Kerr medium, the light path is automatically switched, depending on the light intensity itself, as shown in Figs. 7.24 and 7.25. This all-optical switch is expected to be applied as an optical limiter and bistable optical switch [17, 18]. Waveguide material with a large Kerr

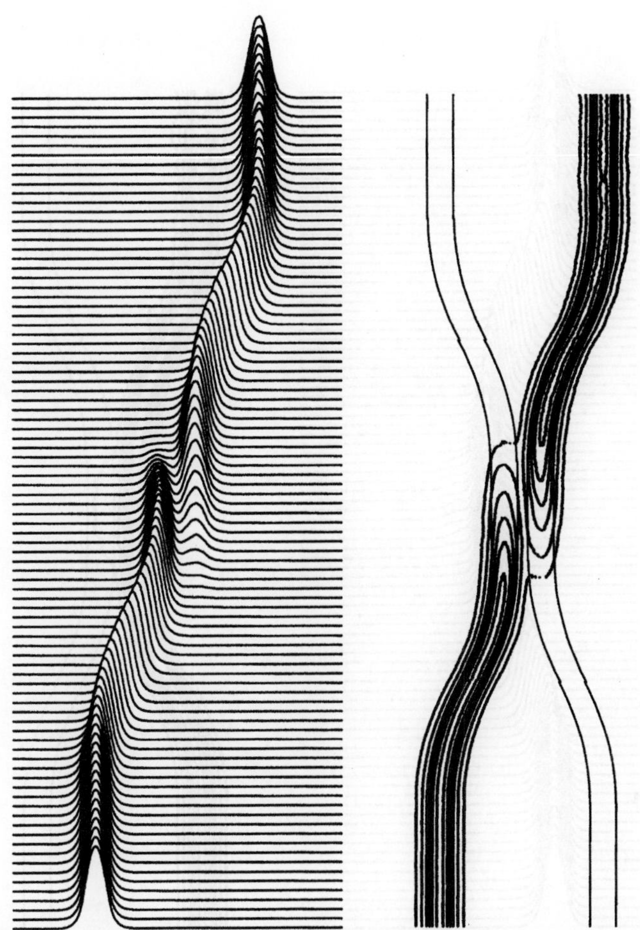

Figure 7.24 Light propagation characteristics for **1 mW** of input power. Since the light intensity is low, a nonlinear optical effect is not observed.

coefficient is required to reduce the self-switching power of the all-optical switch. We should note here that Figs. 7.24 and 7.25 are transmission characteristics for cw (continuous wave) light. When a temporal optical pulse is injected into an all-optical switch, the switch behaves as a linear directional coupler for the weak-intensity part of the pulse. Therefore, the weak part of the pulse couples to the cross-port of the coupler even when high-intensity light is injected to the all-optical coupler. This causes crosstalk degradation of the device. Several methods are proposed to solve such problems [19, 20].

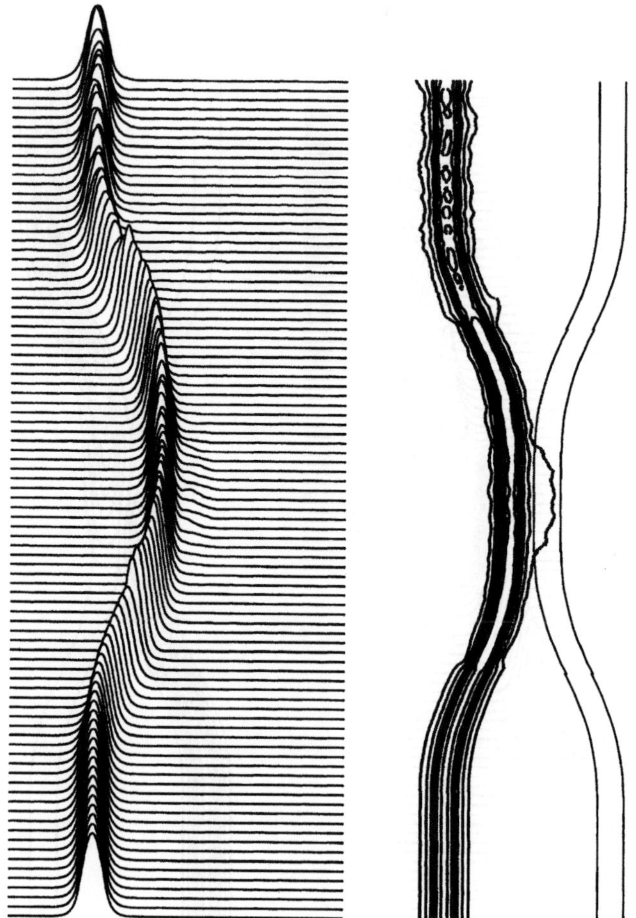

Figure 7.25 Light propagation characteristics for **2.2 W** of input power.

7.8. FINITE DIFFERENCE METHOD ANALYSIS OF PLANAR OPTICAL WAVEGUIDES

7.8.1. Derivation of Basic Equations

BPM analyses described in the previous sections are based on FFT and are therefore called FFTBPM. Here we describe another BPM based on the finite difference method (FDMBPM). Since FDMBPM does not rely on the sampling theorem, it has a great advantage over FFTBPM which will be shown later in comparing the two BPMs. First, we consider lightwave propagation in slab waveguides. The two-dimensional scalar wave equation is given, from Eq. (7.5), by

$$\frac{\partial \phi}{\partial z} = -j\frac{1}{2kn_0}\frac{\partial^2 \phi}{dx^2} - \alpha(x, z)\phi - j\frac{k}{2n_0}[n^2(x, z) - n_0^2]\phi. \tag{7.90}$$

Here, $\partial^2\phi/\partial z^2$ has been neglected by assuming $|\partial^2\phi/\partial z^2| \ll 2kn_0|\partial\phi/\partial z|$. This approximation is called a *paraxial approximation* or *Fresnel approximation*. In Eq. (7.90), we do not approximate as $(n^2 - n_0^2) \cong 2n_0(n - n_0)$, which was adopted in Eqs. (7.5) and (7.9). Generally, a differential equation of the form

$$\frac{\partial \phi}{\partial z} = \mathbf{A}(x, z)\frac{\partial^2 \phi}{\partial x^2} + \mathbf{B}(x, z)\phi \tag{7.91}$$

can be approximated by the finite difference method as

$$\frac{\partial \phi}{\partial z} \to \frac{\phi_i^{m+1} - \phi_i^m}{\Delta z}, \tag{7.92}$$

$$\mathbf{A}(x, z)\frac{\partial^2 \phi}{\partial x^2} \to \frac{1}{2}\mathbf{A}_i^{m+1/2}\left\{\frac{\phi_{i-1}^m - 2\phi_i^m + \phi_{i+1}^m}{(\Delta x)^2} + \frac{\phi_{i-1}^{m+1} - 2\phi_i^{m+1} + \phi_{i+1}^{m+1}}{(\Delta x)^2}\right\}, \tag{7.93}$$

$$\mathbf{B}(x, z)\phi \to \frac{1}{2}\mathbf{B}_i^{m+1/2}\left(\phi_i^{m+1} + \phi_i^m\right), \tag{7.94}$$

where Δx and Δz denote the calculation step in the x- and z-axis directions and subscript i and superscript m are sampling points along x- and z-axis directions, respectively. The numbers of divisions along the x- and z-axis directions are $N(i = 0 - N)$ and $M(m = 0 - M)$, respectively. Therefore, ϕ_i^m represents the electric field amplitude at $x = x_i = i\Delta x$ and $z = z_m = m\Delta z$. Comparing Eqs. (7.90) and (7.91), we see that

$$A = -j\frac{1}{2kn_0}, \tag{7.95}$$

$$B = -\alpha(x, z) - j\frac{k}{2n_0}[n^2(x, z) - n_0^2]. \tag{7.96}$$

Substituting Eqs. (7.92) – (7.96) in Eq. (7.90), we obtain the following simultaneous equation:

$$-\phi_{i-1}^{m+1} + s_i^m\phi_i^{m+1} - \phi_{i+1}^{m+1} = \phi_{i-1}^m + q_i^m\phi_i^m + \phi_{i+1}^m \equiv d_i^m \quad (i = 1 - N - 1), \tag{7.97}$$

where

$$s_i^m = 2 - k^2(\Delta x)^2\left[(n_i^{m+1/2})^2 - n_0^2\right] + j\frac{4kn_0(\Delta x)^2}{\Delta z} + j2kn_0(\Delta x)^2\alpha_i^{m+1/2}, \quad (7.98)$$

$$q_i^m = -2 + k^2(\Delta x)^2\left[(n_i^{m+1/2})^2 - n_0^2\right] + j\frac{4kn_0(\Delta x)^2}{\Delta z} - j2kn_0(\Delta x)^2\alpha_i^{m+1/2}. \quad (7.99)$$

When the initial electric field distribution $\phi_i^{m=0}(i=0-N)$ at the input position $(m=0)$ is given, electric field profile ϕ_i^m at $z=z_m=m\Delta z$ $(m=1\text{–}M)$ is successively calculated by using Eq. (7.97). It should be noted here that there are only $(N-1)$ equations in Eq. (7.97) for $(N+1)$ unknown variables. Two boundary equations are lacking, at $x=0$ and $x=N\Delta x\equiv D$. In stationary electric field problems, the Dirichlet condition $(\phi=0)$ or the Neumann condition $(\partial\phi/\partial x=0)$ at the boundary is given. However, such boundary conditions are not sufficient in lightwave propagation analyses, since we should treat the radiation fields that penetrate away from the calculation window.

7.8.2. Transparent Boundary Conditions

In order to solve the preceding difficulty, the transparent boundary condition (TBC) has been introduced to FDMBPM [21]. This treatment of the boundary condition is described at the right-hand boundary, $x=D$. In the TBC method, the electric field at the boundary is assumed to be expressed by the plane wave:

$$\phi = C\exp(-j\kappa x). \quad (7.100)$$

Here κ and C are generally complex number. When we know the electric field distribution ϕ_i^m at mth axial step, we assume that wavenumber κ at the $(m+1)$th axial step is given by

$$\frac{\phi_N^m}{\phi_{N-1}^m} = \exp(-j\kappa\Delta x). \quad (7.101)$$

If the real part of κ is positive, then the plane wave expressed by Eq. (7.100) propagates toward the outside of the boundary. Then the right-hand boundary value at the $(m+1)$th axial step is given by

$$\phi_N^{m+1} = \phi_{N-1}^{m+1}\exp(-j\kappa\Delta x). \quad (7.102)$$

However, if the real part of κ is negative, the plane wave of Eq. (7.100) propagates toward the inside of the boundary. When we are dealing with a waveguiding structure that has no reflecting element, an inward-propagating wave should not exist. Therefore, in such a case κ_r (real part of κ) must be made positive:

$$\kappa_r \geqslant 0. \tag{7.103}$$

The imaginary part of κ, which is denoted by κ_i, is used as in any case. When we define the κ that is obtained by the foregoing procedures as

$$\kappa_{\text{right}} = \kappa_r + j\kappa_i, \tag{7.104}$$

the boundary condition at the righthand-side boundary is given by

$$\phi_N^{m+1} = \phi_{N-1}^{m+1} \exp(-j\kappa_{\text{right}}\Delta x). \tag{7.105}$$

The wavenumber of the outgoing plane wave at the left-hand boundary κ_{left} is obtained in the similar manner. The boundary condition at the left-hand boundary is then given by

$$\phi_0^{m+1} = \phi_1^{m+1} \exp(-j\kappa_{\text{left}}\Delta x). \tag{7.106}$$

Substituting Eqs. (7.105) and (7.106) into Eq. (7.97), we obtain $(N-1)$ simultaneous equations for $(N-1)$ unknown variables $(\phi_1^{m+1} - \phi_{N-1}^{m+1})$ as

$$-a_i\phi_{i-1}^{m+1} + b_i\phi_i^{m+1} - c_i\phi_{i+1}^{m+1} = d_i^m \qquad (i = 1 - N - 1), \tag{7.107}$$

where

$$a_1 = 0, \quad b_1 = s_1^m - \exp(-j\kappa_{left}\Delta x), \quad c_1 = 1 \tag{7.108a}$$

$$a_i = 1, \quad b_i = s_i^m, \quad c_i = 1 \qquad (i = 2 - N - 2) \tag{7.108b}$$

$$a_{N-1} = 1, \quad b_{N-1} = s_{N-1}^m - \exp(-j\kappa_{\text{right}}\Delta x), \quad c_{N-1} = 0 \tag{7.108c}$$

Equation (7.107) is expressed in the matrix form by

$$\mathbf{A}\Phi = \mathbf{D}, \tag{7.109}$$

where $\mathbf{A}$ is an $(N-1) \times (N-1)$ matrix whose elements are given by Eqs. (7.108), Φ is a column vector of electric field ϕ_i^{m+1}, and $\mathbf{D}$ is a column vector of d_i^m. The solution of Eq. (7.109) is generally given by $\Phi = \mathbf{A}^{-1}\mathbf{D}$. However, since Eq. (7.109) is a tridiagonal matrix, solution Φ can be obtained via the recurrence formula without calculating the inverse matrix $\mathbf{A}^{-1}$.

7.8.3. Solution of Tri-diagonal Equations

We first express the electric field ϕ_i^{m+1} in the recurrence form:

$$\phi_i^{m+1} = \alpha_i \phi_{i+1}^{m+1} + \beta_i. \tag{7.110}$$

When we set $i \to i-1$ in this relation, we have $\phi_{i-1}^{m+1} = \alpha_{i-1}\phi_i^{m+1} + \beta_{i-1}$. Substituting this ϕ_{i-1}^{m+1} into Eq. (7.107), we obtain

$$-a_i(\alpha_{i-1}\phi_i^{m+1} + \beta_{i-1}) + b_i\phi_i^{m+1} - c_i\phi_{i+1}^{m+1} = d_i^m.$$

ϕ_i^{m+1} is then expressed as

$$\phi_i^{m+1} = \frac{c_i}{b_i - a_i\alpha_{i-1}}\phi_{i+1}^{m+1} + \frac{d_i^m + a_i\beta_{i-1}}{b_i - a_i\alpha_{i-1}}. \tag{7.111}$$

Comparing Eqs. (7.110) and (7.111), we obtain the recurrence equations for α_i and β_i:

$$\alpha_i = \frac{c_i}{b_i - a_i\alpha_{i-1}} \qquad (i = 1 - N - 1) \tag{7.112a}$$

$$\beta_i = \frac{d_i^m + a_i\beta_{i-1}}{b_i - a_i\alpha_{i-1}} \qquad (i = 1 - N - 1). \tag{7.112b}$$

Since we know $a_1 = 0$ and $c_1 = 1$ for $i = 1$ from Eq. (7.108a), α_1 and β_1 are given by

$$\alpha_1 = \frac{c_1}{b_1 - a_1\alpha_0} = \frac{1}{b_1}, \tag{7.113a}$$

$$\beta_1 = \frac{d_1^m + a_1\beta_0}{b_1 - a_1\alpha_0} = \frac{d_1^m}{b_1}. \tag{7.113b}$$

$\alpha_2 - \alpha_{N-1}$ and $\beta_2 - \beta_{N-1}$ are then calculated successively from Eqs. (7.112) and (7.113). Since we know $c_{N-1} = 0$ for $i = N-1$ from Eq. (7.108c), α_{N-1} is given by

$$\alpha_{N-1} = \frac{c_{N-1}}{b_{N-1} - a_{N-1}\alpha_{N-2}} = 0. \tag{7.114}$$

Therefore, ϕ_{N-1}^{m+1} is obtained from Eq. (7.110) as

$$\phi_{N-1}^{m+1} = \beta_{N-1}. \tag{7.115}$$

Electric field $\phi_{N-2}^{m+1} - \phi_1^{m+1}$ are then calculated by using the recurrence relation of Eq. (7.110). The boundary values ϕ_0^{m+1} and ϕ_N^{m+1} at $x = 0$ and $x = D$ are already given by Eqs. (7.105) and (7.106).

Figure 7.26(a) shows intensity waveforms and contour plots of Gaussian beam propagation in the free space using FDMBPM. The analysis window and the number of divisions are $D = 260\,\mu\text{m}$ and $N = 1024(\Delta x = 0.25\,\mu\text{m})$ respectively. The calculation step along the axial direction is $\Delta z = 2\,\mu\text{m}$. It is confirmed in Fig. 7.26(a) that light beam propagation is correctly analyzed even when it coincides with the analysis window. In contrast, Fig. 7.26(b) shows intensity waveforms and contour plots of Gaussian beam propagation in the free space under the same condition as Fig. 7.26(a) by using FFTBPM. In FFTBPM, it is

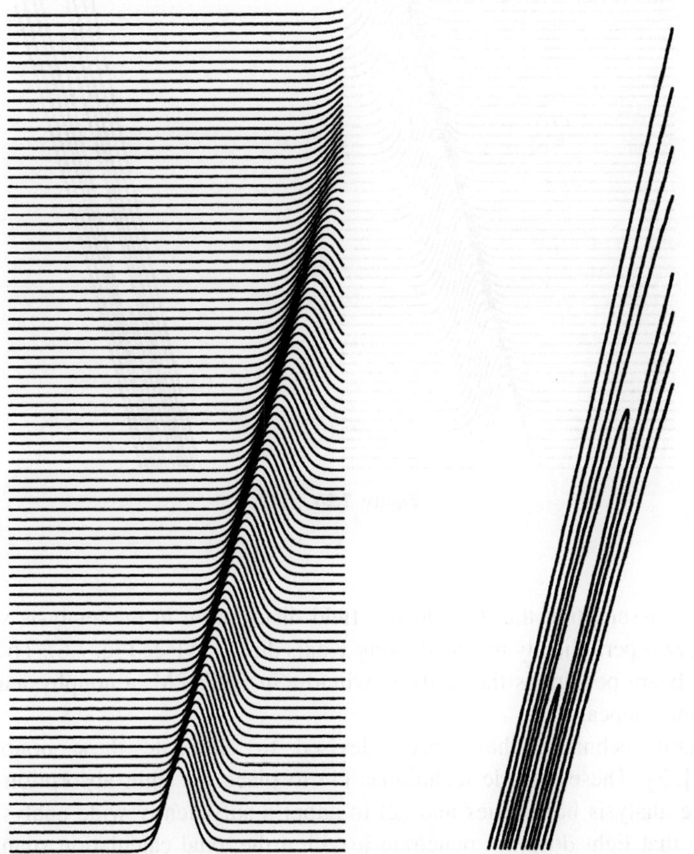

Figure 7.26 Intensity waveforms and contour plots of Gaussian beam propagation in the free space using (a) FDMBPM and (b) FFTBPM.

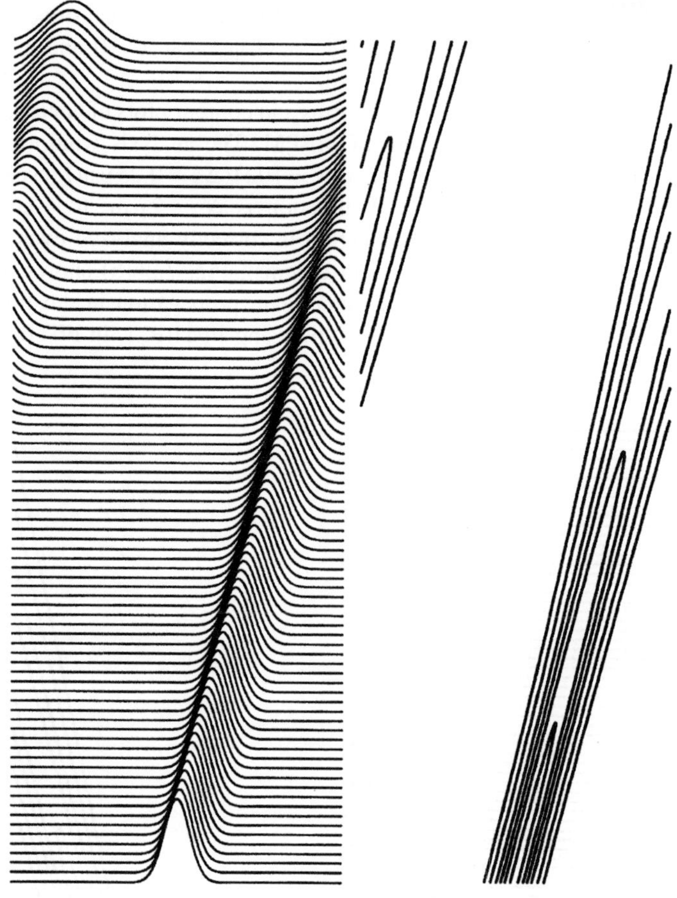

Figure 7.26 (b)

the basic assumption that the electric field distribution in the analysis window $0 \leqslant x \leqslant D$ is periodically repeated along x-axis direction (see Fig. 7.6). Therefore, if light beam penetrates the analysis window in FFTBPM, a nonphysical wave sometimes appears.

Several techniques have been devised to eliminate these nonphysical waves [22]. These include techniques (1) to place the light absorption region near the analysis boundaries and (2) to adopt a sufficiently wide analysis window so that light does not penetrate it within the axial calculation span. Since the optimum shape and width of the absorption window are different for each problem, the first technique is rather cumbersome and inefficient. In the second technique, a large number of divisions along the x-axis direction is required. Therefore, computation time increases substantially.

In the FDMBPM method utilizing TBC, since analysis window can be placed in the vicinitiy of the optical device under investigation, the number of divisions N can be reduced.

7.9. FDMBPM ANALYSIS OF RECTANGULAR WAVEGUIDES

In three-dimensional wave equation corresponding to Eq. (7.3) is given by

$$\frac{\partial \phi}{\partial z} = -j\frac{1}{2kn_0}\nabla^2\phi - \alpha(x, y, z)\phi - j\frac{k}{2n_0}[n^2(x, y, z) - n_0^2]\phi. \tag{7.116}$$

As shown in the previous section, electric field at the grid point of $x = i\Delta x$, $y = \ell\ \Delta y$ and $z = m\Delta z$ is expressed by

$$\phi(i\Delta x, \ell\Delta y, m\Delta z) = \phi_{i,\ell}^m. \tag{7.117}$$

Using the above notation of the field, Eq. (7.116) is approximated by the finite difference form as

$$\begin{aligned} A(\phi_{i,\ell}^{m+1} - \phi_{i,\ell}^m) = & \frac{\phi_{i-1,\ell}^m - 2\phi_{i,\ell}^m + \phi_{i+1,\ell}^m + \phi_{i-1,\ell}^{m+1} - 2\phi_{i,\ell}^{m+1} + \phi_{i+1,\ell}^{m+1}}{2(\Delta x)^2} \\ & + \frac{\phi_{i,\ell-1}^m - 2\phi_{i,\ell}^m + \phi_{i,\ell+1}^m + \phi_{i,\ell-1}^{m+1} - 2\phi_{i,\ell}^{m+1} + \phi_{i,\ell+1}^{m+1}}{2(\Delta y)^2} \\ & + B\left(\phi_{i,\ell}^{m+1} + \phi_{i,\ell}^m\right), \end{aligned} \tag{7.118}$$

where

$$A = \frac{j2kn_0}{\Delta z}, \tag{7.119}$$

$$B = -jkn_0\alpha(i, \ell, m + 1/2) + \frac{k^2}{2}\left[n^2(i, \ell, m + 1/2) - n_0^2\right]. \tag{7.120}$$

Notice here that the definitions of A and B are different from those in Eqs. (7.95) and (7.96). This finite difference equation (7.118) for the three-dimensional problem is not a tri-diagonal equation as in the two-dimensional problems. Therefore, generally an inverse matrix operation is required. However, the following approximate solution method which is called *alternating-direction implicit finite difference method* (ADIFDM) [23] can greatly simplify the calculation procedures of Eq. (7.118).

In ADIFDM, the calculation step Δz along the z-direction is split into two steps of $\Delta z/2$. The intermediate electric field $\phi_{j,\ell}^{m+1/2}$ $(j = i-1, i, \text{and } i+1)$ is approximated as the average of $\phi_{j,\ell}^{m}$ and $\phi_{j,\ell}^{m+1}$ by

$$\phi_{j,\ell}^{m+1/2} = \frac{\phi_{j,\ell}^{m+1} + \phi_{j,\ell}^{m}}{2} \qquad (j = i-1, i, \text{and } i+1). \tag{7.121}$$

By using this equation, Eq. (7.118) can be separated into two finite difference equations:

$$A\left(\phi_{i,\ell}^{m+1/2} - \phi_{i,\ell}^{m}\right) = \frac{\phi_{i-1,\ell}^{m+1/2} - 2\phi_{i,\ell}^{m+1/2} + \phi_{i+1,\ell}^{m+1/2}}{2(\Delta x)^2} + \frac{\phi_{i,\ell-1}^{m} - 2\phi_{i,\ell}^{m} + \phi_{i,\ell+1}^{m}}{2(\Delta y)^2} + \frac{B}{2}\left(\phi_{i,\ell}^{m+1/2} + \phi_{i,\ell}^{m}\right). \tag{7.122}$$

$$A\left(\phi_{i,\ell}^{m+1} - \phi_{i,\ell}^{m+1/2}\right) = \frac{\phi_{i-1,\ell}^{m+1/2} - 2\phi_{i,\ell}^{m+1/2} + \phi_{i+1,\ell}^{m+1/2}}{2(\Delta x)^2} + \frac{\phi_{i,\ell-1,}^{m+1} - 2\phi_{i,\ell}^{m+1} + \phi_{i,\ell+1}^{m+1}}{2(\Delta y)^2} + \frac{B}{2}\left(\phi_{i,\ell}^{m+1} + \phi_{i,\ell}^{m+1/2}\right). \tag{7.123}$$

Equations (7.122) and (7.123) are further rewritten to

$$-\phi_{i-1,\ell}^{m+1/2} + s_{i,\ell}^{m}\phi_{i,\ell}^{m+1/2} - \phi_{i+1,\ell}^{m+1/2} = \frac{(\Delta x)^2}{(\Delta y)^2}\left(\phi_{i,\ell-1}^{m} + Q_{i,\ell}^{m}\phi_{i,\ell}^{m} + \phi_{i,\ell+1}^{m}\right) \equiv d_{i,\ell}^{m} \tag{7.124}$$

$$-\phi_{i,\ell-1}^{m+1} + S_{i,\ell}^{m}\phi_{i,\ell}^{m+1} - \phi_{i,\ell+1}^{m+1} = \frac{(\Delta y)^2}{(\Delta x)^2}\left(\phi_{i-1,\ell}^{m+1/2} + q_{i,\ell}^{m}\phi_{i,\ell}^{m+1/2} + \phi_{i+1,\ell}^{m+1/2}\right) \equiv h_{i,\ell}^{m+1/2}, \tag{7.125}$$

where

$$s_{i,\ell}^{m} = \left\{2 - \frac{k^2(\Delta x)^2}{2}\left[n^2(i, \ell, m+1/2) - n_0^2\right]\right\} + j\left\{\frac{4kn_0(\Delta x)^2}{\Delta z} + kn_0(\Delta x)^2\alpha(i, \ell, m+1/2)\right\} \tag{7.126}$$

$$S_{i,\ell}^{m} = \left\{2 - \frac{k^2(\Delta y)^2}{2}\left[n^2(i, \ell, m+1/2) - n_0^2\right]\right\} + j\left\{\frac{4kn_0(\Delta y)^2}{\Delta z} + kn_0(\Delta y)^2\alpha(i, \ell, m+1/2)\right\} \tag{7.127}$$

$$q_{i,\ell}^{m} = \left\{-2 + \frac{k^2(\Delta x)^2}{2}\left[n^2(i,\ell,m+1/2) - n_0^2\right]\right\} + j\left\{\frac{4kn_0(\Delta x)^2}{\Delta z} - kn_0(\Delta x)^2\alpha(i,\ell,m+1/2)\right\} \tag{7.128}$$

$$Q_{i,\ell}^{m} = \left\{-2 + \frac{k^2(\Delta y)^2}{2}\left[n^2(i,\ell,m+1/2) - n_0^2\right]\right\} + j\left\{\frac{4kn_0(\Delta y)^2}{\Delta z} - kn_0(\Delta y)^2\alpha(i,\ell,m+1/2)\right\}. \tag{7.129}$$

The electric field distribution at the intermediate step $z = (m + 1/2)\Delta z$ is first calculated by using Eq. (7.124). Substitution of the field at $z = (m + 1/2)\Delta z$ into Eq. (7.125) then gives the field distribution at $z = (m + 1)\Delta z$. Since Eqs. (7.124) and (7.125) are tri-diagonal equations, the solutions of the problems are efficiently obtained as shown in the previous section. Moreover, since the transparent boundary condition is also applicable in ADIFDM, the analysis window can be placed at the vicinity of the optical device under investigation, and thus computational time can be reduced.

Figure 7.27 shows contour plots of Gaussian beam propagation in the free space calculated by ADIFDM. The analysis windows and the number of divisions along x- and y-axis directions are $D_x = D_y = 100\,\mu$m and $N_x = N_y = 256(\Delta x = \Delta y = 0.39\,\mu\text{m})$, respectively. The calculation step along the z-axis direction is $\Delta z = 2\,\mu$m. It is confirmed that nonphysical reflection of the field by the analysis window is eliminated by TBC. Figures 7.28(a) and (b) show contour plots of beam propagation in a Mach–Zehnder optical switch for (a) the "off" and (b) the "on" state having similar configuration as in Fig. 7.20. In two-dimensional BPM calculation of Fig. 7.20, we used the effective index method to transform the three-dimensional refractive-index structure into a two-dimensional one. However, three-dimensional BPM analysis can be efficiently performed by using ADIFDM.

In FDMBPM analysis, the paraxial approximation (or the Fresnel approximation) has been adopted, as shown in Eq. (7.90) or (7.116). Therefore, when we analyze light beam propagation in a highly tilted waveguide from the z-axis direction, calculation error becomes large. On the other hand, since paraxial approximation has not been used in FFTBPM, as shown in Eq. (7.18), FFTBPM can be applied to the beam propagation calculation in a highly-tilted waveguide from z-axis direction. Several techniques to improve the accuracy of FDMBPM have been proposed [24, 25], which make the mathematical formulation of FDMBPM rather cumbersome. Both FFTBPM and FDMBPM have their own merits and demerits. Therefore, it is necessary to consider which technique is suitable for the waveguide analysis under investigation.

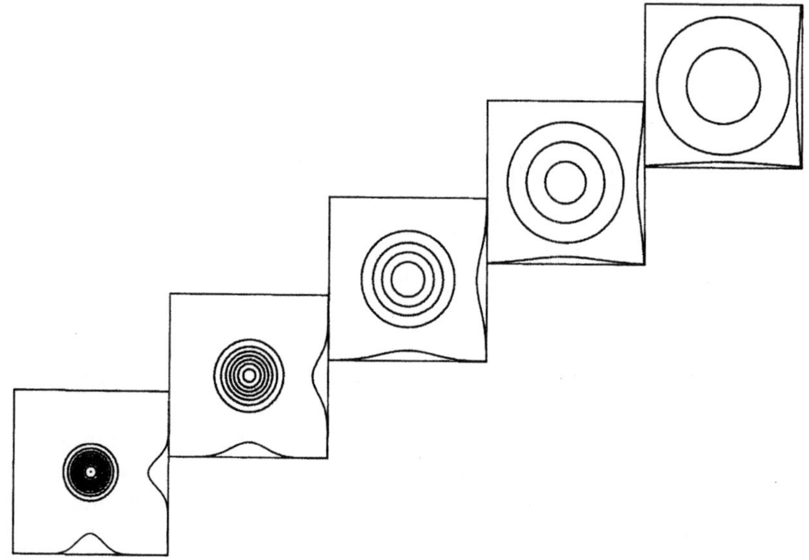

Figure 7.27 Contour plots of Gaussian beam propagation in the free space calculated by ADIFDM.

7.10. FDMBPM ANALYSIS OF OPTICAL PULSE PROPAGATION

Nonlinear Schrödinger equation [Eq. (7.8)] which governs the envelope function of optical pulse $\phi(z, \tau)$ under Kerr effect nonlinearity and loss (or gain) in the optical fibers is given here again:

$$\frac{\partial \phi}{\partial z} = j\frac{1}{2}\beta'' \frac{\partial^2 \phi}{\partial \tau^2} - \alpha\phi - j\frac{1}{2}kn_2|\phi|^2\phi. \tag{7.130}$$

Generally, differential equation of the form

$$\frac{\partial \phi}{\partial z} = A(z)\frac{\partial^2 \phi}{\partial \tau^2} + B(z, \tau)\phi \tag{7.131}$$

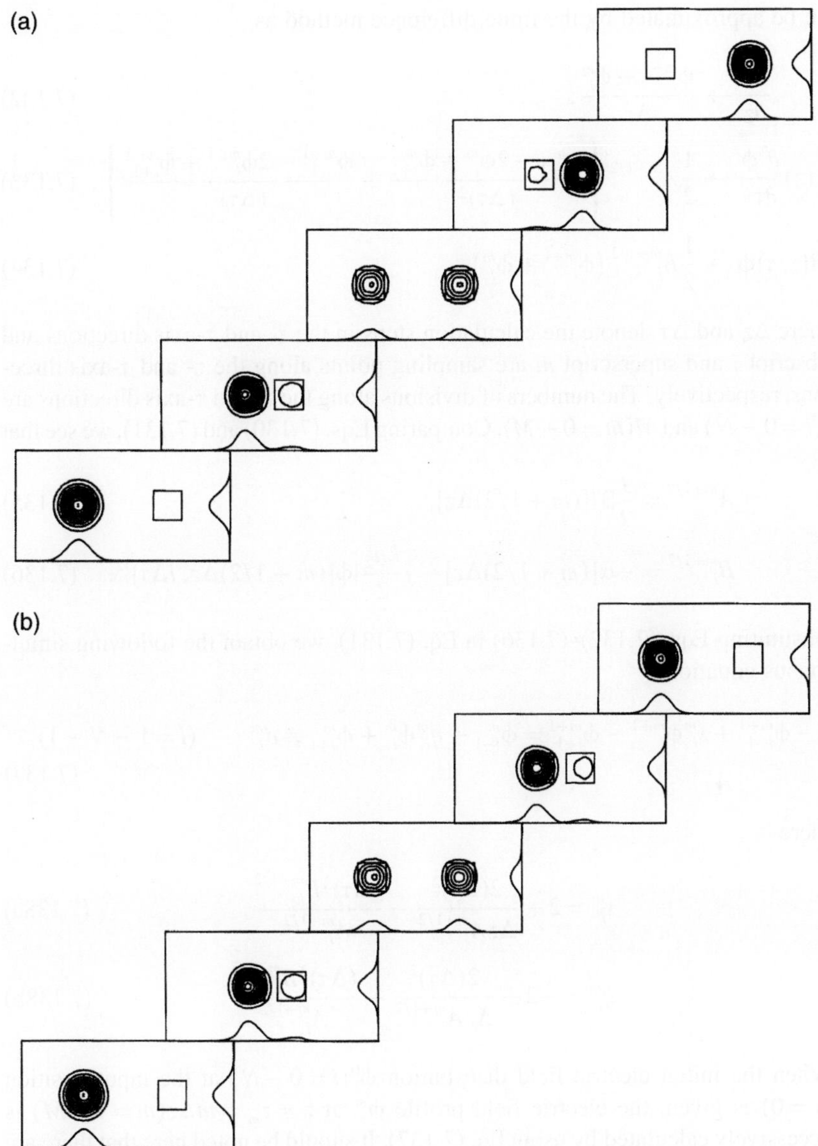

Figure 7.28 Contour plots of beam propagation in a Mach–Zehnder optical switch having a similar configuration to that in Fig. 7.20. The switch is "off" in (a) and "on" in (b).

can be approximated by the finite difference method as

$$\frac{\partial \phi}{\partial z} \rightarrow \frac{\phi_i^{m+1} - \phi_i^m}{\Delta z}, \tag{7.132}$$

$$A(z)\frac{\partial^2 \phi}{\partial \tau^2} \rightarrow \frac{1}{2} A_i^{m+1/2} \left\{ \frac{\phi_{i-1}^m - 2\phi_i^m + \phi_{i+1}^m}{(\Delta\tau)^2} + \frac{\phi_{i-1}^{m+1} - 2\phi_i^{m+1} + \phi_{i+1}^{m+1}}{(\Delta\tau)^2} \right\}, \tag{7.133}$$

$$B(z,\tau)\phi \rightarrow \frac{1}{2} B_i^{m+1/2} \left(\phi_i^{m+1} + \phi_i^m\right), \tag{7.134}$$

where Δz and $\Delta\tau$ denote the calculation steps in the z- and τ-axis directions and subscript i and superscript m are sampling points along the z- and τ-axis directions, respectively. The numbers of divisions along the z- and τ-axis directions are $N(i=0-N)$ and $M(m=0-M)$. Comparing Eqs. (7.130) and (7.131), we see that

$$A_i^{m+1/2} = \frac{j}{2}\beta''[(m+1/2)\Delta z], \tag{7.135}$$

$$B_i^{m+1/2} = -\alpha[(m+1/2)\Delta z] - j\frac{kn_2}{2}|\phi[(m+1/2)\Delta z, i\Delta\tau]|^2. \tag{7.136}$$

Substituting Eqs. (7.132)–(7.136) in Eq. (7.131), we obtain the following simultaneous equation:

$$-\phi_{i-1}^{m+1} + s_i^m \phi_i^{m+1} - \phi_{i+1}^{m+1} = \phi_{i-1}^m + q_i^m \phi_i^m + \phi_{i+1}^m \equiv d_i^m \qquad (i=1-N-1), \tag{7.137}$$

where

$$s_i^m = 2 + \frac{2(\Delta\tau)^2}{\Delta z A_i^{m+1/2}} - \frac{(\Delta\tau)^2 B_i^{m+1/2}}{A_i^{m+1/2}}, \tag{7.138a}$$

$$q_i^m = -2 + \frac{2(\Delta\tau)^2}{\Delta z A_i^{m+1/2}} + \frac{(\Delta\tau)^2 B_i^{m+1/2}}{A_i^{m+1/2}}. \tag{7.138b}$$

When the initial electric field distribution $\phi_i^0(i=0-N)$ at the input position $(m=0)$ is given, the electric field profile ϕ_i^m at $z=z_m=m\Delta z(m=1-M)$ is successively calculated by using Eq. (7.137). It should be noted here that there are only $(N-1)$ equations in (7.137) for $(N+1)$ unknown variables. Two boundary equations are lacking at $\tau=0$ and $\tau=N\Delta\tau(=T)$. In stationary electric field problems, the Dirichlet condition $(\phi=0)$ or the Neumann condition $(\partial\phi/\partial\tau=0)$ at the boundary is given. However, such boundary conditions are not sufficient in temporal pulse propagation analyses, since we should treat the radiation fields that penetrate away from the calculation window. In order to solve this difficulty, the transparent boundary condition (TBC) is adopted in the FDMBPM analysis of optical pulse propagation. The TBC procedure in temporal pulse analysis is the same as described in Section 7.8.2. After some calculation, we obtain $(N-1)$ simultaneous equations for $(N-1)$ unknown variables $(\phi_1^{m+1} - \phi_{N-1}^{m+1})$ as

$$-a_i\phi_{i-1}^{m+1} + b_i\phi_i^{m+1} - c_i\phi_{i+1}^{m+1} = d_i^m \qquad (i=1-N-1), \tag{7.139}$$

where

$$a_1 = 0, \quad b_1 = s_1^m - \exp(-j\kappa_{\text{left}}\Delta\tau), \quad c_1 = 1 \tag{7.140a}$$

$$a_i = 1, \quad b_i = s_i^m, \quad c_i = 1 \qquad (i=2-N-2) \tag{7.140b}$$

$$a_{N-1} = 1, \quad b_{N-1} = s_{N-1}^m - \exp(-j\kappa_{\text{right}}\Delta\tau), \quad c_{N-1} = 0. \tag{7.140c}$$

Equation (7.139) is expressed in the matrix form by

$$\mathbf{A}^{m+1/2}\Phi^{m+1} = \mathbf{D}^m, \tag{7.141}$$

where $\mathbf{A}^{m+1/2}$ is an $(N-1)\times(N-1)$ matrix whose elements are given by Eqs. (7.140), Φ^{m+1} is a column vector of electric field ϕ_i^{m+1} and $\mathbf{D}^m$ is a column vector of d_i^m. The solution of (7.141) is generally given by $\Phi^{m+1} = [\mathbf{A}^{m+1/2}]^{-1}\mathbf{D}^m$. However, since Eq. (7.141) is a tri-diagonal matrix, solution Φ^{m+1} can be obtained via the recurrence formula without calculating the inverse matrix $[\mathbf{A}^{m+1/2}]^{-1}$ as described in Section 7.8.3.

Some of the matrix elements of $\mathbf{A}^{m+1/2}$ contains s_i^m's as shown in Eqs. (7.139) and (7.140). In order to calculate s_i^m's, $\phi_i^{m+1/2}$'s should be known in advance as defined by Eqs. (7.136) and (7.138a). Of course, it is generally impossible since we only know up to ϕ_i^m's and $\phi_i^{m+1/2}$'s are unknown values to be determined. In such a case, leapfrog (LF) method is quite useful. When values of ϕ are known up to step m, these values are used to calculate the auxiliary values $\phi_i^{m+1/2}$ by shifting a step in Eq. (7.137) with a half step as

$$\begin{aligned} -\phi_{i-1}^{m+1/2} + s_i^{m-1/2}\phi_i^{m+1/2} - \phi_{i+1}^{m+1/2} &= \phi_{i-1}^{m-1/2} + q_i^{m-1/2}\phi_i^{m-1/2} + \phi_{i+1}^{m-1/2} \\ &\equiv d_i^{m-1/2}(i=1-N-1), \end{aligned} \tag{7.142}$$

where

$$s_i^{m-1/2} = 2 + \frac{2(\Delta\tau)^2}{\Delta z A_i^m} - \frac{(\Delta\tau)^2 B_i^m}{A_i^m}, \tag{7.143a}$$

$$q_i^{m-1/2} = -2 + \frac{2(\Delta\tau)^2}{\Delta z A_i^m} + \frac{(\Delta\tau)^2 B_i^m}{A_i^m}. \tag{7.143b}$$

Then the values $\phi_i^{m+1/2}$ are utilized to calculate the nonlinear term in Eq. (7.138), to perform the effective propagation step. In the first auxiliary step with $m=0$, the righthand term of Eq. (7.142) is replaced by ϕ_i^0, since leapfrog method cannot be used.

7.11. SEMI-VECTOR FDMBPM ANALYSIS OF HIGH-INDEX CONTRAST WAVEGUIDES

Semi-vector wave equations for the extremely high-index contrast (EH-Δ) waveguides [26–30] have been obtained in Section 6.6. Semi-vector wave equations based on the E-field formulation are expressed by

$$\frac{\partial}{\partial x}\left[\frac{1}{n^2}\frac{\partial(n^2E_x)}{\partial x}\right]+\frac{\partial^2 E_x}{\partial y^2}+\frac{\partial^2 E_x}{\partial z^2}+k^2n^2E_x=0,\quad \text{Quasi-TE Mode} \tag{7.144}$$

$$\frac{\partial^2 E_y}{\partial x^2}+\frac{\partial}{\partial y}\left[\frac{1}{n^2}\frac{\partial(n^2E_y)}{\partial y}\right]+\frac{\partial^2 E_y}{\partial z^2}+k^2n^2E_y=0,\quad \text{Quasi-TE Mode} \tag{7.145}$$

and wave equations based on the H-field formulation are given as

$$n^2\frac{\partial}{\partial x}\left(\frac{1}{n^2}\frac{\partial H_y}{\partial x}\right)+\frac{\partial^2 H_y}{\partial y^2}+\frac{\partial^2 H_y}{\partial z^2}+n^2\frac{\partial(1/n^2)}{\partial z}\frac{\partial H_y}{\partial z}+k^2n^2H_y=0,\quad \text{Quasi-TE Mode} \tag{7.146}$$

$$\frac{\partial^2 H_x}{\partial x^2}+n^2\frac{\partial}{\partial y}\left(\frac{1}{n^2}\frac{\partial H_x}{\partial y}\right)+\frac{\partial^2 H_x}{\partial z^2}+n^2\frac{\partial(1/n^2)}{\partial z}\frac{\partial H_x}{\partial z}+k^2n^2H_x=0.\quad \text{Quasi-TE Mode} \tag{7.147}$$

We assume that $E_t=\phi_t(x,y,z)\exp(-jkn_{\text{ref}}z)$ and $H_t=\psi_t(x,y,z)\exp(-jkn_{\text{ref}}z)$ where n_{ref} denotes a reference refractive index and the subscript t represents x or y. Substitute these equations into Eqs. (7.144)–(7.147) and by making use of the slowly varying envelope approximation, i.e.,

$$\left|\frac{\partial^2\phi_t}{\partial z^2}\right|\ll 2kn_{\text{ref}}\left|\frac{\partial\phi_t}{\partial z}\right|, \tag{7.148}$$

$$\left|\frac{\partial^2\psi_t}{\partial z^2}\right|\ll 2kn_{\text{ref}}\left|\frac{\partial\psi_t}{\partial z}\right|, \tag{7.149}$$

we obtain the paraxial semi-vector BPM equations

$$j2kn_{\text{ref}}\frac{\partial\phi_x}{\partial z}=\frac{\partial}{\partial x}\left[\frac{1}{n^2}\frac{\partial(n^2\phi_x)}{\partial x}\right]+\frac{\partial^2\phi_x}{\partial y^2}+(k^2n^2-k^2n_{\text{ref}}^2)\phi_x,\quad \text{Quasi-TE Mode} \tag{7.150}$$

$$j2kn_{\text{ref}}\frac{\partial\phi_y}{\partial z}=\frac{\partial^2\phi_y}{\partial x^2}+\frac{\partial}{\partial y}\left[\frac{1}{n^2}\frac{\partial(n^2\phi_y)}{\partial y}\right]+(k^2n^2-k^2n_{\text{ref}}^2)\phi_y,\quad \text{Quasi-TE Mode} \tag{7.151}$$

and

$$j2kn_{\text{ref}}\frac{\partial\psi_y}{\partial z} = n^2\frac{\partial}{\partial x}\left(\frac{1}{n^2}\frac{\partial\psi_y}{\partial x}\right) + \frac{\partial^2\psi_y}{\partial y^2} + \left[k^2n^2 - k^2n_{\text{ref}}^2 - jkn_{\text{ref}}n^2\frac{\partial(1/n^2)}{\partial z}\right]\psi_y,$$

Quasi-TE Mode (7.152)

$$j2kn_{\text{ref}}\frac{\partial\psi_x}{\partial z} = \frac{\partial^2\psi_x}{\partial x^2} + n^2\frac{\partial}{\partial y}\left(\frac{1}{n^2}\frac{\partial\psi_x}{\partial y}\right) + \left[k^2n^2 - k^2n_{\text{ref}}^2 - jkn_{\text{ref}}n^2\frac{\partial(1/n^2)}{\partial z}\right]\psi_x.$$

Quasi-TE Mode (7.153)

The terms $kn_{\text{ref}}n^2\partial(1/n^2)/\partial z$ in Eqs. (7.152) and (7.153) have been retained in order to keep the power conservation properties [31].

Equations (7.150)–(7.153) can be solved by using a finite difference method. In the finite difference solutions, the continuous space is replaced by a discrete lattice structure defined in the computational region. The fields at the lattice point of $x = i\Delta x$, $y = \ell\Delta y$, and $z = m\Delta z$ are represented by their discrete expressions. The differential operators in the E- and H-field formulations are also approximated by the finite difference. The discrete form of the differential operators in the governing Eqs. (7.150)–(7.153) may be found in a straightforward way. At the index discontinuities, although the normal electric fields are not continuous, the displacement vectors $n^2\phi_x$ and $n^2\phi_y$ are continuous across the index interfaces along the x- and y-axes, respectively. Therefore the central difference scheme can be applied directly. In the following sections, Eqs. (7.150) and (7.153) will be used in the derivation of the semi-vector FDMBPM equations for Quasi-TE and Quasi-TM nodes, respectively.

7.11.1. Quasi-TE Modes

Rewriting ϕ_x to ϕ in Eq. (7.150), semi-vector FDMBPM equation for Quasi-TE mode is expressed by

$$j2kn_{\text{ref}}\frac{\partial\phi}{\partial z} = \frac{\partial}{\partial x}\left[\frac{1}{n^2}\frac{\partial(n^2\phi)}{\partial x}\right] + \frac{\partial^2\phi}{\partial y^2}$$
$$+\left\{-j2kn_{\text{ref}}\alpha(x,y,z) + k^2\left[n^2(x,y,z) - n_{\text{ref}}^2\right]\right\}\phi, \quad (7.154)$$

where the loss or gain term $-j2kn_{\text{ref}}\alpha(x,y,z)\phi$ is added for the generality. Finite difference expressions for the operators in the above equation are found to be as follows [32]:

$$\frac{\partial\phi}{\partial z} \to \frac{(\phi_{i,\ell}^{m+1} - \phi_{i,\ell}^{m})}{\Delta z}, \quad (7.155)$$

$$\phi \to \frac{(\phi_{i,\ell}^{m+1} + \phi_{i,\ell}^{m})}{2}, \quad (7.156)$$

$$\frac{\partial}{\partial x}\left[\frac{1}{n^2}\frac{\partial(n^2\phi)}{\partial x}\right] \to \frac{1}{2}\cdot\left\{\frac{\xi^m_{i,\ell}\phi^m_{i-1,\ell} - 2\eta^m_{i,\ell}\phi^m_{i,\ell} + \zeta^m_{i,\ell}\phi^m_{i+1,\ell}}{(\Delta x)^2} + \frac{\xi^m_{i,\ell}\phi^{m+1}_{i-1,\ell} - 2\eta^m_{i,\ell}\phi^{m+1}_{i,\ell} + \zeta^m_{i,\ell}\phi^{m+1}_{i+1,\ell}}{(\Delta x)^2}\right\}, \tag{7.157}$$

$$\frac{\partial^2\phi}{\partial y^2} \to \frac{1}{2}\cdot\left\{\frac{\phi^m_{i,\ell-1} - 2\phi^m_{i,\ell} + \phi^m_{i,\ell+1}}{(\Delta y)^2} + \frac{\phi^{m+1}_{i,\ell-1} - 2\phi^{m+1}_{i,\ell} + \phi^{m+1}_{i,\ell+1}}{(\Delta y)^2}\right\}, \tag{7.158}$$

where

$$\xi^m_{i,\ell} = \frac{2n^2(i-1,\ell,m)}{n^2(i-1,\ell,m)+n^2(i,\ell,m)}, \tag{7.159a}$$

$$\eta^m_{i,\ell} = \frac{n^2(i,\ell,m)}{n^2(i-1,\ell,m)+n^2(i,\ell,m)} + \frac{n^2(i,\ell,m)}{n^2(i,\ell,m)+n^2(i+1,\ell,m)}, \tag{7.159b}$$

$$\zeta^m_{i,\ell} = \frac{2n^2(i+1,\ell,m)}{n^2(i,\ell,m)+n^2(i+1,\ell,m)}. \tag{7.159c}$$

By substituting Eqs. (7.155)–(7.159) in Eq. (7.154), it is expressed by the finite difference form as

$$\begin{aligned} A(\phi^{m+1}_{i,\ell} - \phi^m_{i,\ell}) = {} & \frac{\xi^m_{i,\ell}\phi^m_{i-1,\ell} - 2\eta^m_{i,\ell}\phi^m_{i,\ell} + \zeta^m_{i,\ell}\phi^m_{i+1,\ell}}{2(\Delta x)^2} \\ & + \frac{\xi^m_{i,\ell}\phi^{m+1}_{i-1,\ell} - 2\eta^m_{i,\ell}\phi^{m+1}_{i,\ell} + \zeta^m_{i,\ell}\phi^{m+1}_{i+1,\ell}}{2(\Delta x)^2} + \frac{\phi^m_{i,\ell-1} - 2\phi^m_{i,\ell} + \phi^m_{i,\ell+1}}{2(\Delta y)^2} \\ & + \frac{\phi^{m+1}_{i,\ell-1} - 2\phi^{m+1}_{i,\ell} + \phi^{m+1}_{i,\ell+1}}{2(\Delta y)^2} + B(\phi^{m+1}_{i,\ell} + \phi^m_{i,\ell}), \end{aligned} \tag{7.160}$$

where

$$A = \frac{j2kn_{\text{ref}}}{\Delta z}, \tag{7.161}$$

$$B = -jkn_{\text{eff}}\alpha(i,\ell,m+1/2) + \frac{k^2}{2}\left[n^2(i,\ell,m+1/2) - n^2_{\text{ref}}\right]. \tag{7.162}$$

Equation (7.160) is solved by using the *alternating-direction implicit finite difference method* (ADIFDM) which was described in Section 7.9.

7.11.2. Quasi-TM Modes

Similar to the previous Quasi-TE mode treatment, we rewrite ψ_x to ψ in Eq. (7.153), and semi-vector FDMBPM equation for Quasi-TM mode is expressed by

$$j2kn_{\text{ref}}\frac{\partial\psi}{\partial z} = \frac{\partial^2\psi}{\partial x^2} + n^2\frac{\partial}{\partial y}\left(\frac{1}{n^2}\frac{\partial\psi}{\partial y}\right) + \left[-j2kn_{\text{ref}}\alpha + k^2n^2 - k^2n_{\text{ref}}^2 - jkn_{\text{ref}}n^2\frac{\partial(1/n^2)}{\partial z}\right]\psi. \quad (7.163)$$

Finite difference expressions for the operators in the above equation are found to be as follows:

$$\frac{\partial\psi}{\partial z} \to \frac{(\psi_{i,\ell}^{m+1} - \psi_{i,\ell}^m)}{\Delta z}, \quad (7.164)$$

$$\psi \to \frac{(\psi_{i,\ell}^{m+1} + \psi_{i,\ell}^m)}{2}, \quad (7.165)$$

$$\frac{\partial^2\psi}{\partial x^2} \to \frac{1}{2}\cdot\left\{\frac{\psi_{i-1,\ell}^m - 2\psi_{i,\ell}^m + \psi_{i+1,\ell}^m}{(\Delta x)^2} + \frac{\psi_{i-1,\ell}^{m+1} - 2\psi_{i,\ell}^{m+1} + \psi_{i+1,\ell}^{m+1}}{(\Delta x)^2}\right\}, \quad (7.166)$$

$$n^2\frac{\partial}{\partial y}\left(\frac{1}{n^2}\frac{\partial\psi}{\partial y}\right) \to \frac{1}{2}\cdot\left\{\frac{\xi_{i,\ell}^m\psi_{i,\ell-1}^m - 2\eta_{i,\ell}^m\psi_{i,\ell}^m + \zeta_{i,\ell}^m\psi_{i,\ell+1}^m}{(\Delta y)^2} + \frac{\xi_{i,\ell}^m\psi_{i,\ell-1}^{m+1} - 2\eta_{i,\ell}^m\psi_{i,\ell}^{m+1} + \zeta_{i,\ell}^m\psi_{i,\ell+1}^{m+1}}{(\Delta y)^2}\right\}, \quad (7.167)$$

where

$$\xi_{i,\ell}^m = \frac{2n^2(i,\ell,m)}{n^2(i,\ell-1,m) + n^2(i,\ell,m)}, \quad (7.168a)$$

$$\eta_{i,\ell}^m = \frac{n^2(i,\ell,m)}{n^2(i,\ell-1,m) + n^2(i,\ell,m)} + \frac{n^2(i,\ell,m)}{n^2(i,\ell,m) + n^2(i,\ell+1,m)}, \quad (7.168b)$$

$$\zeta_{i,\ell}^m = \frac{2n^2(i,\ell,m)}{n^2(i,\ell,m) + n^2(i,\ell+1,m)}. \quad (7.168c)$$

The term $n^2\partial(1/n^2)/\partial z$ in Eq. (7.163) is approximated by [31]

$$n^2\frac{\partial(1/n^2)}{\partial z} \to \frac{(u_{i,\ell}^{m+1} - u_{i,\ell}^{m-1})}{\Delta z}, \quad (7.169)$$

where

$$u_{i,\ell}^{m-1} = \frac{2n^2(i,\ell,m)}{n^2(i,\ell,m-1)+n^2(i,\ell,m)}, \tag{7.170a}$$

$$u_{i,\ell}^{m+1} = \frac{2n^2(i,\ell,m)}{n^2(i,\ell,m)+n^2(i,\ell,m+1)}. \tag{7.170b}$$

By substituting Eqs. (7.164)–(7.170) in Eq. (7.163), it is expressed by the finite difference form as

$$\begin{aligned} A(\psi_{i,\ell}^{m+1}-\psi_{i,\ell}^{m}) = {} & \frac{\psi_{i-1,\ell}^{m}-2\psi_{i,\ell}^{m}+\psi_{i+1,\ell}^{m}}{2(\Delta x)^2} + \frac{\psi_{i-1,\ell}^{m+1}-2\psi_{i,\ell}^{m+1}+\psi_{i+1,\ell}^{m+1}}{2(\Delta x)^2} \\ & + \frac{\xi_{i,\ell}^{m}\psi_{i,\ell-1}^{m}-2\eta_{i,\ell}^{m}\psi_{i,\ell}^{m}+\zeta_{i,\ell}^{m}\psi_{i,\ell+1}^{m}}{2(\Delta y)^2} \\ & + \frac{\xi_{i,\ell}^{m}\psi_{i,\ell-1}^{m+1}-2\eta_{i,\ell}^{m}\psi_{i,\ell}^{m+1}+\zeta_{i,\ell}^{m}\psi_{i,\ell+1}^{m+1}}{2(\Delta y)^2} + B(\psi_{i,\ell}^{m+1}+\psi_{i,\ell}^{m}), \end{aligned} \tag{7.171}$$

where

$$A = \frac{j2kn_{\mathrm{ref}}}{\Delta z}, \tag{7.172}$$

$$\begin{aligned} B = {} & -jkn_{\mathrm{ref}}\left[\alpha(i,\ell,m+1/2)+\frac{(u_{i,\ell}^{m+1}-u_{i,\ell}^{m-1})}{2\Delta z}\right] \\ & +\frac{k^2}{2}[n^2(i,\ell,m+1/2)-n_{\mathrm{ref}}^2]. \end{aligned} \tag{7.173}$$

Equation (7.171) is solved by using the *alternating-direction implicit finite difference method* (ADIFDM) which was described in Section 7.9.

7.11.3. Polarization Splitter Using Silicon-on-Insulator (SOI) Waveguide

The polarization dependent behavior of optical waveguides has two main sources as described in Section 3.9; they are, geometrical birefringence and stress-induced birefringence. It was shown that the geometrical birefringence increases substantially in proportion to the refractive-index difference Δ (refer to Fig. 3.33). In silicon-on-insulator (SOI) waveguides, the refractive-index difference becomes of the order of $\Delta=\left[1-(n_0/n_1)^2\right]/2=0.41$, where $n_1(=3.48)$ and $n_0(=1.444)$ are refractive indices of silicon and silica glass at $\lambda=1.55\,\mu\mathrm{m}$

region, respectively. Then the polarization dependence becomes conspicuous in SOI waveguides.

Semi-vector BPM analysis of the polarization splitter using SOI rib waveguide is described in the following section. Figure 7.29 shows a cross-sectional geometry of the SOI rib directional coupler. Core width W and height H are both chosen to be 1 μm, while the slab height $h = 0.45$ μm. After several runs of semi-vector BPM simulations, it was confirmed that the almost perfect polarization splitting is obtainable with a gap value of $g = 0.7$ μm. Since the refractive-index difference between the core and cladding is very large, the calculation step Δz was chosen to be 0.001 μm. Figure 7.30 is a schematic configuration of the polarization splitter, where L_{st} is the length of the single waveguide and L_{cpl} is the coupler length,

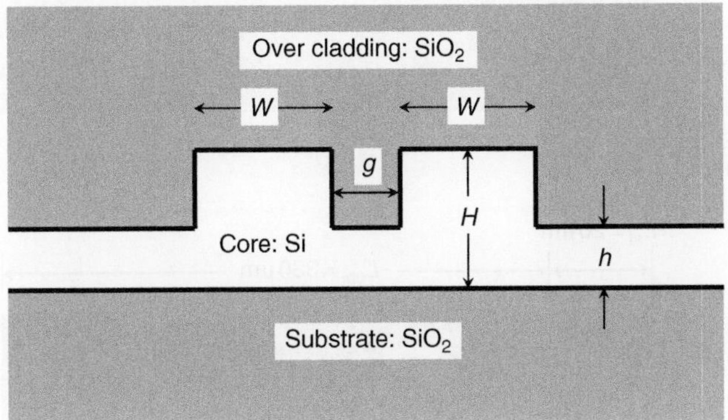

Figure 7.29 Cross-sectional geometry of the SOI rib directional coupler.

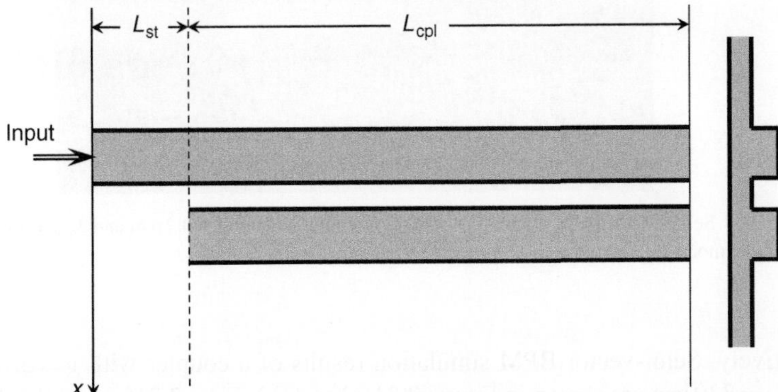

Figure 7.30 Schematic configuration of the polarization splitter. L_{st}: length of the single waveguide, L_{cpl}: coupler length.

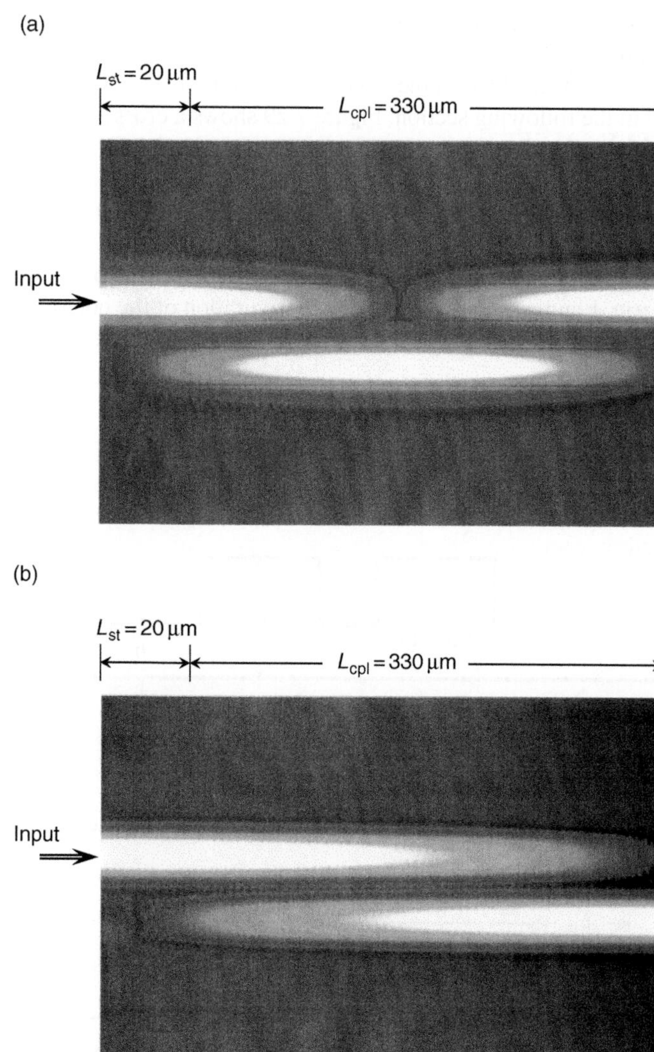

Figure 7.31 Semi-vector BPM simulation results of a coupler with $g = 0.7\,\mu m$ and $L_{cpl} = 330\,\mu m$. (a) Quasi-TE mode (E_x). (b) Quasi-TM mode (H_x).

respectively. Semi-vector BPM simulation results of a coupler with $g = 0.7\,\mu m$ and $L_{cpl} = 330\,\mu m$ are shown in Figure 7.31(a) and (b). Figs. 7.31(a) and (b) show waveform transients of Quasi-TE mode (E_x) and Quasi-TM mode (H_x), respectively. Quasi-TE mode couples back and forth and exits at the original upper port. On the other hand, Quasi-TM mode couples only once and exits at the lower port, thus enabling polarization beam splitting operation [33].

7.12. FINITE DIFFERENCE TIME DOMAIN (FDTD) METHOD

The FDTD method is an approach that directly solves Maxwell's equations by a proper discretization of both time and space domains [34]. Maxwell's equations in a homogeneous and non-dispersive medium are written as

$$\nabla \times \mathbf{E} = -\frac{\partial \mathbf{B}}{\partial t}, \tag{7.174}$$

$$\nabla \times \mathbf{H} = -\frac{\partial \mathbf{D}}{\partial t} + \mathbf{J}. \tag{7.175}$$

Substituting the relation for the electric field $\mathbf{E}$, magnetic field $\mathbf{H}$, electric flux density $\mathbf{D}$, and magnetic flux density $\mathbf{B}$ as

$$\mathbf{B} = \mu \mathbf{H}, \tag{7.176a}$$

$$\mathbf{D} = \varepsilon \mathbf{E}, \tag{7.176b}$$

$$\mathbf{J} = \sigma \mathbf{E}, \tag{7.176c}$$

into Eqs. (7.174) and (7.175), we obtain

$$\frac{\partial \mathbf{E}}{\partial t} = -\frac{\sigma}{\varepsilon}\mathbf{E} + \frac{1}{\varepsilon}\nabla \times \mathbf{H}, \tag{7.177}$$

$$\frac{\partial \mathbf{H}}{\partial t} = -\frac{1}{\mu}\nabla \times \mathbf{E}. \tag{7.178}$$

The above equations are expressed in the centered difference forms as

$$\frac{\mathbf{E}^{n} - \mathbf{E}^{n-1}}{\Delta t} = -\frac{\sigma}{\varepsilon}\mathbf{E}^{n-\frac{1}{2}} + \frac{1}{\varepsilon}\nabla \times \mathbf{H}^{n-\frac{1}{2}}, \tag{7.179}$$

$$\frac{\mathbf{H}^{n+\frac{1}{2}} - \mathbf{H}^{n-\frac{1}{2}}}{\Delta t} = -\frac{1}{\mu}\nabla \times \mathbf{E}^{n}, \tag{7.180}$$

where $t = (n-1)\Delta t$ with Δt representing the increment in time. Since the centered difference points for the electric field $\mathbf{E}$ are taken at $n-1$ and n, $\mathbf{E}^{n-1/2}$ in (7.179) is approximated by

$$\sigma \mathbf{E}^{n-\frac{1}{2}} \cong \sigma \cdot \frac{\mathbf{E}^{n} + \mathbf{E}^{n-1}}{2}. \tag{7.181}$$

Then (7.179) is reduced to

$$\frac{\mathbf{E}^n - \mathbf{E}^{n-1}}{\Delta t} = -\frac{\sigma}{\varepsilon} \cdot \frac{\mathbf{E}^n + \mathbf{E}^{n-1}}{2} + \frac{1}{\varepsilon} \nabla \times \mathbf{H}^{n-\frac{1}{2}}. \tag{7.182}$$

Solving Eqs. (7.180) and (7.182), we obtain expressions for $\mathbf{E}^n$ and $\mathbf{H}^{n+1/2}$ as

$$\mathbf{E}^n = \frac{1 - \dfrac{\sigma\Delta t}{2\varepsilon}}{1 + \dfrac{\sigma\Delta t}{2\varepsilon}} \mathbf{E}^{n-1} + \frac{\Delta t/\varepsilon}{1 + \dfrac{\sigma\Delta t}{2\varepsilon}} \nabla \times \mathbf{H}^{n-\frac{1}{2}}, \tag{7.183}$$

$$\mathbf{H}^{n+\frac{1}{2}} = \mathbf{H}^{n-\frac{1}{2}} - \frac{\Delta t}{\mu} \nabla \times \mathbf{E}^n. \tag{7.184}$$

In order to solve the set of Eqs. (7.183) and (7.184), Yee introduced the leap-frog schemes using the cubic cell as shown in Fig. 7.32. Δx, Δy and Δz are the discretization increments along the x, y and z axis directions. The electric and magnetic field components are located at the edges and on the surface of the cell, respectively, and are half-step offset in both space and time domain. The flow chart of FDTD analysis is shown in Fig. 7.33. Absorbing boundary condition [35] will be described later in this section.

Derivation of the finite difference equation for E_x^n using Eq. (7.183) is first described in detail. Applying Eq. (10.44) to Eq. (7.183), E_x^n is expressed by

$$\mathbf{E}_x^n = \frac{1 - \dfrac{\sigma\Delta t}{2\varepsilon}}{1 + \dfrac{\sigma\Delta t}{2\varepsilon}} E_x^{n-1} + \frac{\Delta t/\varepsilon}{1 + \dfrac{\sigma\Delta t}{2\varepsilon}} \left(\frac{\partial H_z^{n-1/2}}{\partial y} - \frac{\partial H_y^{n-1/2}}{\partial z} \right). \tag{7.185}$$

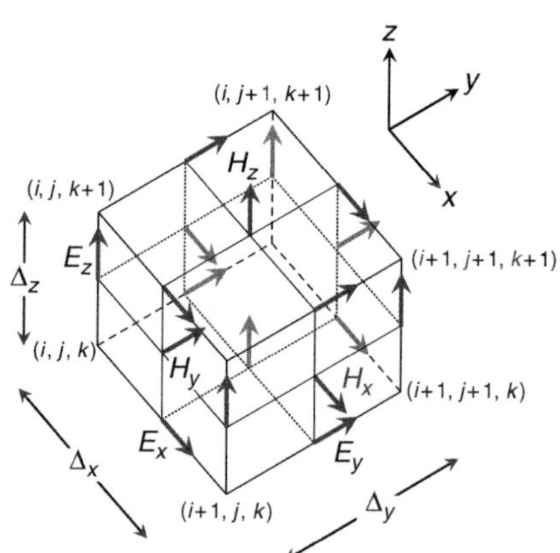

Figure 7.32 Yee's unit cell.

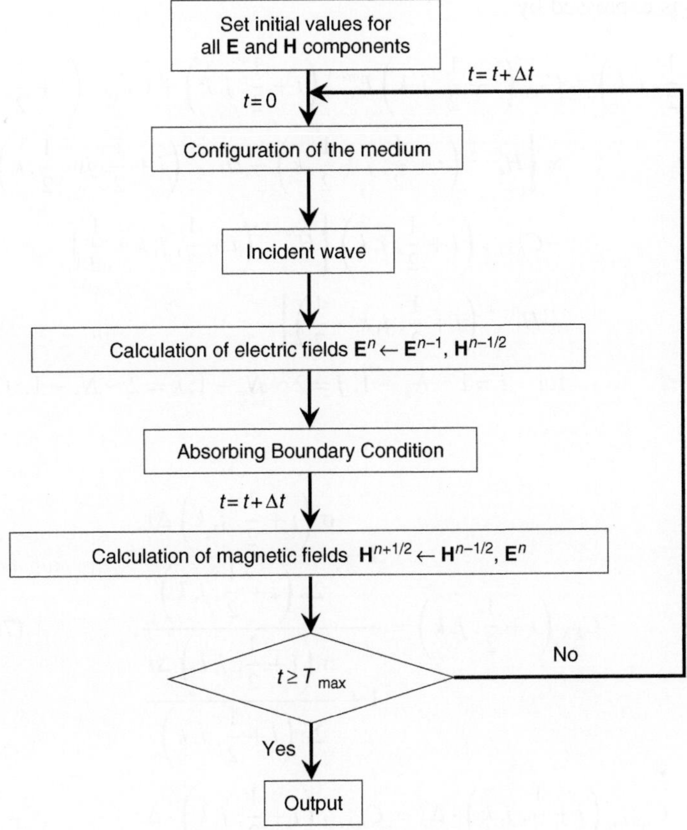

Figure 7.33 Flow chart of FDTD analysis.

Since E_x is located at $(i+1/2, j, k)$ as shown in Fig. 7.32, $\partial H_z^{n-1/2}/\partial y$ and $\partial H_y^{n-1/2}/\partial z$ are evaluated at $(i+1/2, j, k)$ as follows:

$$\left.\frac{\partial H_z^{n-1/2}}{\partial y}\right|_{\left(i+\frac{1}{2},j,k\right)} = \frac{H_z^{n-\frac{1}{2}}\left(i+\frac{1}{2}, j+\frac{1}{2}, k\right) - H_z^{n-\frac{1}{2}}\left(i+\frac{1}{2}, j-\frac{1}{2}, k\right)}{\Delta y} \quad (7.186a)$$

$$\left.\frac{\partial H_y^{n-1/2}}{\partial z}\right|_{\left(i+\frac{1}{2},j,k\right)} = \frac{H_y^{n-\frac{1}{2}}\left(i+\frac{1}{2}, j, k+\frac{1}{2}\right) - H_y^{n-\frac{1}{2}}\left(i+\frac{1}{2}, j, k-\frac{1}{2}\right)}{\Delta z}. \quad (7.186b)$$

Then E_x is expressed by

$$E_x^n\left(i+\frac{1}{2},j,k\right)=C_{EX}\left(i+\frac{1}{2},j,k\right)E_x^{n-1}\left(i+\frac{1}{2},j,k\right)+C_{EXLY}\left(i+\frac{1}{2},j,k\right)$$
$$\times\left\{H_z^{n-\frac{1}{2}}\left(i+\frac{1}{2},j+\frac{1}{2},k\right)-H_z^{n-\frac{1}{2}}\left(i+\frac{1}{2},j-\frac{1}{2},k\right)\right\}$$
$$-C_{EXLZ}\left(i+\frac{1}{2},j,k\right)\left\{H_y^{n-\frac{1}{2}}\left(i+\frac{1}{2},j,k+\frac{1}{2}\right)\right.$$
$$\left.-H_y^{n-\frac{1}{2}}\left(i+\frac{1}{2},j,k-\frac{1}{2}\right)\right\}$$
$$\text{for}\quad i=1\sim N_x-1,\,j=2\sim N_y-1,\,k=2\sim N_z-1,\tag{7.187}$$

where

$$C_{EX}\left(i+\frac{1}{2},j,k\right)=\frac{1-\dfrac{\sigma\left(i+\frac{1}{2},j,k\right)\Delta t}{2\varepsilon\left(i+\frac{1}{2},j,k\right)}}{1+\dfrac{\sigma\left(i+\frac{1}{2},j,k\right)\Delta t}{2\varepsilon\left(i+\frac{1}{2},j,k\right)}},\tag{7.188a}$$

$$C_{EXLY}\left(i+\frac{1}{2},j,k\right)\cdot\Delta y=C_{EXLZ}\left(i+\frac{1}{2},j,k\right)\cdot\Delta z$$
$$=\frac{\Delta t/\varepsilon\left(i+\frac{1}{2},j,k\right)}{1+\dfrac{\sigma\left(i+\frac{1}{2},j,k\right)\Delta t}{2\varepsilon\left(i+\frac{1}{2},j,k\right)}}.\tag{7.188b}$$

In the similar manner, finite difference equations for E_y and E_z are obtained as

$$E_y^n\left(i,j+\frac{1}{2},k\right)=C_{EY}\left(i,j+\frac{1}{2},k\right)E_y^{n-1}\left(i,j+\frac{1}{2},k\right)+C_{EYLZ}\left(i,j+\frac{1}{2},k\right)$$
$$\times\left\{H_x^{n-\frac{1}{2}}\left(i,j+\frac{1}{2},k+\frac{1}{2}\right)-H_x^{n-\frac{1}{2}}\left(i,j+\frac{1}{2},k-\frac{1}{2}\right)\right\}$$

$$-C_{EYLX}\left(i,j+\frac{1}{2},k\right)\left\{H_z^{n-\frac{1}{2}}\left(i+\frac{1}{2},j+\frac{1}{2},k\right)\right.$$
$$\left.-H_z^{n-\frac{1}{2}}\left(i-\frac{1}{2},j+\frac{1}{2},k\right)\right\}$$
$$\text{for}\quad i=2\sim N_x-1,\, j=1\sim N_y-1,\, k=2\sim N_z-1, \tag{7.189}$$

where

$$C_{EY}\left(i,j+\frac{1}{2},k\right)=\frac{1-\dfrac{\sigma\left(i,j+\frac{1}{2},k\right)\Delta t}{2\varepsilon\left(i,j+\frac{1}{2},k\right)}}{1+\dfrac{\sigma\left(i,j+\frac{1}{2},k\right)\Delta t}{2\varepsilon\left(i,j+\frac{1}{2},k\right)}}, \tag{7.190a}$$

$$C_{EYLZ}\left(i,j+\frac{1}{2},k\right)\cdot\Delta z=C_{EYLX}\left(i,j+\frac{1}{2},k\right)\cdot\Delta x$$
$$=\frac{\Delta t/\varepsilon\left(i,j+\frac{1}{2},k\right)}{1+\dfrac{\sigma\left(i,j+\frac{1}{2},k\right)\Delta t}{2\varepsilon\left(i,j+\frac{1}{2},k\right)}}, \tag{7.190b}$$

$$E_z^n\left(i,j,k+\frac{1}{2}\right)=C_{EZ}\left(i,j,k+\frac{1}{2}\right)E_z^{n-1}\left(i,j,k+\frac{1}{2}\right)+C_{EZLX}\left(i,j,k+\frac{1}{2}\right)$$
$$\times\left\{H_y^{n-\frac{1}{2}}\left(i+\frac{1}{2},j,k+\frac{1}{2}\right)-H_y^{n-\frac{1}{2}}\left(i-\frac{1}{2},j,k+\frac{1}{2}\right)\right\}$$
$$-C_{EZLY}\left(i,j,k+\frac{1}{2}\right)\left\{H_x^{n-\frac{1}{2}}\left(i,j+\frac{1}{2},k+\frac{1}{2}\right)\right.$$
$$\left.-H_x^{n-\frac{1}{2}}\left(i,j-\frac{1}{2},k+\frac{1}{2}\right)\right\}$$
$$\text{for}\quad i=2\sim N_x-1,$$
$$j=2\sim N_y-1,\, k=1\sim N_z-1 \tag{7.191}$$

where

$$C_{EZ}\left(i,j,k+\frac{1}{2}\right)=\frac{1-\dfrac{\sigma\left(i,j,k+\frac{1}{2}\right)\Delta t}{2\varepsilon\left(i,j,k+\frac{1}{2}\right)}}{1+\dfrac{\sigma\left(i,j,k+\frac{1}{2}\right)\Delta t}{2\varepsilon\left(i,j,k+\frac{1}{2}\right)}}, \tag{7.192a}$$

$$\begin{aligned} C_{EZLX}\left(i,j,k+\frac{1}{2}\right)\cdot\Delta x &= C_{EZLY}\left(i,j,k+\frac{1}{2}\right)\cdot\Delta y \\ &= \frac{\Delta t/\varepsilon\left(i,j,k+\frac{1}{2}\right)}{1+\dfrac{\sigma\left(i,j,k+\frac{1}{2}\right)\Delta t}{2\varepsilon\left(i,j,k+\frac{1}{2}\right)}}. \end{aligned} \tag{7.192b}$$

Next, derivation of the finite difference equation for $H_x^{n+1/2}$ using (7.184) is described in detail. Applying Eq. (10.44) to Eq. (7.184), $H_x^{n+1/2}$ is expressed by

$$H_x^{n+\frac{1}{2}}=H_x^{n-\frac{1}{2}}-\frac{\Delta t}{\mu}\left(\frac{\partial E_z^n}{\partial y}-\frac{\partial E_y^n}{\partial z}\right). \tag{7.193}$$

Since $H_x^{n+1/2}$ is located at $(i, j+1/2, k+1/2)$ as shown in Fig. 7.32, $\partial E_z^n/\partial y$ and $\partial E_y^n/\partial z$ are evaluated at $(i, j+1/2, k+1/2)$ as follows:

$$\left.\frac{\partial E_z^n}{\partial y}\right|_{\left(i,j+\frac{1}{2},k+\frac{1}{2}\right)}=\frac{E_z^n\left(i,j+1,k+\frac{1}{2}\right)-E_z^n\left(i,j,k+\frac{1}{2}\right)}{\Delta y}, \tag{7.194a}$$

$$\left.\frac{\partial E_y^n}{\partial z}\right|_{\left(i,j+\frac{1}{2},k+\frac{1}{2}\right)}=\frac{E_y^n\left(i,j+\frac{1}{2},k+1\right)-E_y^n\left(i,j+\frac{1}{2},k\right)}{\Delta z}. \tag{7.194b}$$

Then $H_x^{n+1/2}$ is expressed by

$$H_x^{n+\frac{1}{2}}\left(i, j+\frac{1}{2}, k+\frac{1}{2}\right) = H_x^{n-\frac{1}{2}}\left(i, j+\frac{1}{2}, k+\frac{1}{2}\right) - C_{HXLY}\left(i, j+\frac{1}{2}, k+\frac{1}{2}\right)$$
$$\times\left\{E_z^n\left(i, j+1, k+\frac{1}{2}\right) - E_z^n\left(i, j, k+\frac{1}{2}\right)\right\}$$
$$+C_{HXLZ}\left(i, j+\frac{1}{2}, k+\frac{1}{2}\right)$$
$$\times\left\{E_y^n\left(i, j+\frac{1}{2}, k+1\right) - E_y^n\left(i, j+\frac{1}{2}, k\right)\right\}$$
$$\text{for}\quad i=2\sim N_x-1, j=1\sim N_y-1, k=1\sim N_z-1, \tag{7.195}$$

where

$$C_{HXLY}\left(i, j+\frac{1}{2}, k+\frac{1}{2}\right) = \frac{\Delta t}{\mu\left(i, j+\frac{1}{2}, k+\frac{1}{2}\right)}\cdot\frac{1}{\Delta y}, \tag{7.196a}$$

$$C_{HXLZ}\left(i, j+\frac{1}{2}, k+\frac{1}{2}\right) = \frac{\Delta t}{\mu\left(i, j+\frac{1}{2}, k+\frac{1}{2}\right)}\cdot\frac{1}{\Delta z}. \tag{7.196b}$$

In the similar manner, finite difference equations for $H_y^{n+1/2}$ and $H_z^{n+1/2}$ are obtained as

$$H_y^{n+\frac{1}{2}}\left(i+\frac{1}{2}, j, k+\frac{1}{2}\right) = H_y^{n-\frac{1}{2}}\left(i+\frac{1}{2}, j, k+\frac{1}{2}\right) - C_{HYLZ}\left(i+\frac{1}{2}, j, k+\frac{1}{2}\right)$$
$$\times\left\{E_x^n\left(i+\frac{1}{2}, j, k+1\right) - E_x^n\left(i+\frac{1}{2}, j, k\right)\right\}$$
$$+C_{HYLX}\left(i+\frac{1}{2}, j, k+\frac{1}{2}\right)$$
$$\times\left\{E_z^n\left(i+1, j, k+\frac{1}{2}\right) - E_z^n\left(i, j, k+\frac{1}{2}\right)\right\}$$
$$\text{for}\quad i=1\sim N_x-1, j=2\sim N_y-1, k=1\sim N_z-1, \tag{7.197}$$

where

$$C_{HYLZ}\left(i+\frac{1}{2}, j, k+\frac{1}{2}\right) = \frac{\Delta t}{\mu\left(i+\frac{1}{2}, j, k+\frac{1}{2}\right)}\cdot\frac{1}{\Delta z}, \tag{7.198a}$$

$$C_{HYLX}\left(i+\frac{1}{2}, j, k+\frac{1}{2}\right)=\frac{\Delta t}{\mu\left(i+\frac{1}{2}, j, k+\frac{1}{2}\right)}\cdot\frac{1}{\Delta x}, \tag{7.198b}$$

$$\begin{aligned} H_z^{n+\frac{1}{2}}\left(i+\frac{1}{2}, j+\frac{1}{2}, k\right) = {} & H_z^{n-\frac{1}{2}}\left(i+\frac{1}{2}, j+\frac{1}{2}, k\right) - C_{HZLX}\left(i+\frac{1}{2}, j+\frac{1}{2}, k\right) \\ & \times\left\{E_y^n\left(i+1, j+\frac{1}{2}, k\right) - E_y^n\left(i, j+\frac{1}{2}, k\right)\right\} \\ & + C_{HZLY}\left(i+\frac{1}{2}, j+\frac{1}{2}, k\right) \\ & \times\left\{E_x^n\left(i+\frac{1}{2}, j+1, k\right) - E_x^n\left(i+\frac{1}{2}, j, k\right)\right\} \\ \text{for}\quad & i=1\sim N_x-1, j=1\sim N_y-1, k=2\sim N_z-1, \end{aligned} \tag{7.199}$$

where

$$C_{HZLX}\left(i+\frac{1}{2}, j+\frac{1}{2}, k\right)=\frac{\Delta t}{\mu\left(i+\frac{1}{2}, j+\frac{1}{2}, k\right)}\cdot\frac{1}{\Delta x}, \tag{7.200a}$$

$$C_{HZLY}\left(i+\frac{1}{2}, j+\frac{1}{2}, k\right)=\frac{\Delta t}{\mu\left(i+\frac{1}{2}, j+\frac{1}{2}, k\right)}\cdot\frac{1}{\Delta y}. \tag{7.200b}$$

The time step size Δt should satisfy the following Courant condition in order to guarantee the numerical stability:

$$c\Delta t \leqslant \frac{1}{\sqrt{\left(\frac{1}{\Delta x}\right)^2+\left(\frac{1}{\Delta y}\right)^2+\left(\frac{1}{\Delta z}\right)^2}}, \tag{7.201}$$

where c is the speed of light.

At the edge of the calculation region, a proper absorbing boundary condition (ABC) should be imposed to avoid undesirable (non-physical) reflections. The most popular ABC in the FDTD analysis is the one developed by Mur [35].

Mur's ABC will be described using one-way wave equation for E_y, which travels in the $-x$ direction as shown in Fig. 7.34. Absorbing boundary is placed

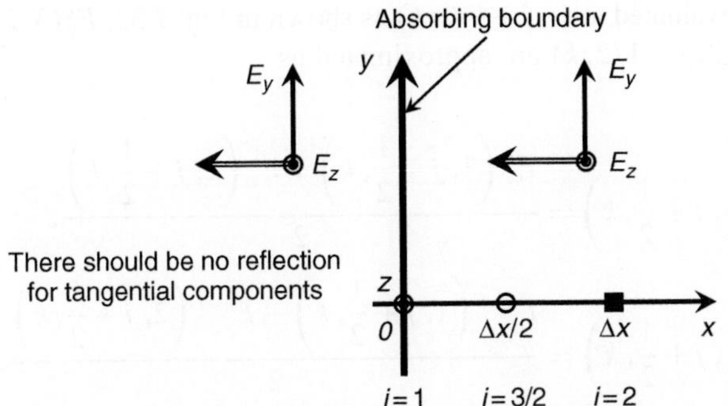

Figure 7.34 Geometry to explain Mur's absorbing boundary condition (ABC).

at $x=0$. Electric field E_y, which is traveling in the negative x direction with the velocity V_x, is expressed by

$$E_y = E_y(x + V_x t), \tag{7.202a}$$

$$V_x = \frac{\omega}{\beta_x}, \tag{7.202b}$$

where β_x is the propagation constant along x direction. E_y satisfies the following relation

$$\frac{\partial E_y}{\partial t} = V_x \cdot \frac{\partial E_y}{\partial x}. \tag{7.203}$$

This is an expression of the one-way wave equation. Since there is no physical boundary at $x=0$ (although there exists a boundary of computational region), Eq. (7.203) should be satisfied at $x=0$. When we discretize Eq. (7.203) with respect to time, we obtain

$$\left.\frac{\partial E_y}{\partial t}\right|_{t=\left(n-\frac{1}{2}\right)\Delta t} = \left.\frac{\left(E_y^n - E_y^{n-1}\right)}{\Delta t}\right|_{x=\Delta x/2} = \mathrm{V}_x \cdot \left.\frac{\partial E_y^{n-\frac{1}{2}}}{\partial x}\right|_{x=\Delta x/2}. \tag{7.204}$$

Equation (7.204) is expressed more precisely by

$$\frac{E_y^n\left(\frac{3}{2}, j+\frac{1}{2}, k\right) - E_y^{n-1}\left(\frac{3}{2}, j+\frac{1}{2}, k\right)}{\Delta t} = V_x \cdot \frac{E_y^{n-\frac{1}{2}}\left(2, j+\frac{1}{2}, k\right) - E_y^{n-\frac{1}{2}}\left(1, j+\frac{1}{2}, k\right)}{\Delta x}. \tag{7.205}$$

Since E_y is evaluated at $(i, j+1/2, k)$ as shown in Fig. 7.32, $E_y^n(3/2, j+1/2, k)$ and $E_y^{n-1}(3/2, j+1/2, k)$ are approximated as

$$E_y^n\left(\frac{3}{2}, j+\frac{1}{2}, k\right) = \frac{E_y^n\left(1, j+\frac{1}{2}, k\right) + E_y^n\left(2, j+\frac{1}{2}, k\right)}{2}, \tag{7.206a}$$

$$E_y^{n-1}\left(\frac{3}{2}, j+\frac{1}{2}, k\right) = \frac{E_y^{n-1}\left(1, j+\frac{1}{2}, k\right) + E_y^{n-1}\left(2, j+\frac{1}{2}, k\right)}{2}. \tag{7.206b}$$

Similarly, because the centered difference point for the electric field **E** is taken at $n-1$ and n, $E_y^{n-1/2}$ in (7.205) is approximated as

$$E_y^{n-\frac{1}{2}}\left(1, j+\frac{1}{2}, k\right) = \frac{E_y^n\left(1, j+\frac{1}{2}, k\right) + E_y^{n-1}\left(1, j+\frac{1}{2}, k\right)}{2}, \tag{7.207a}$$

$$E_y^{n-\frac{1}{2}}\left(2, j+\frac{1}{2}, k\right) = \frac{E_y^n\left(2, j+\frac{1}{2}, k\right) + E_y^{n-1}\left(2, j+\frac{1}{2}, k\right)}{2}. \tag{7.207b}$$

Substituting Eqs. (7.206)–(7.207) to (7.205), we obtain

$$\begin{aligned} E_y^n\left(1, j+\frac{1}{2}, k\right) &= E_y^{n-1}\left(2, j+\frac{1}{2}, k\right) + \frac{(V_x\Delta t - \Delta x)}{(V_x\Delta t + \Delta x)} \\ &\quad \times \left\{E_y^n\left(2, j+\frac{1}{2}, k\right) - E_y^{n-1}\left(1, j+\frac{1}{2}, k\right)\right\} \\ &\quad \text{for} \quad j=2 \sim N_y-2,\ k=2 \sim N_z-1. \end{aligned} \tag{7.208}$$

The above equation is the Mur's ABC for E_y at $x=0$. ABC for E_z at $x=0$ is given by

$$\begin{aligned} E_z^n\left(1, j, k+\frac{1}{2}\right) &= E_z^{n-1}\left(2, j, k+\frac{1}{2}\right) + \frac{(V_x\Delta t - \Delta x)}{(V_x\Delta t + \Delta x)} \\ &\quad \times \left\{E_z^n\left(2, j, k+\frac{1}{2}\right) - E_z^{n-1}\left(1, j, k+\frac{1}{2}\right)\right\} \\ &\quad \text{for} \quad j=2 \sim N_y-1,\ k=2 \sim N_z-2. \end{aligned} \tag{7.209}$$

ABCs for E_y and E_z at $x = D_x = (N_x - 1)\Delta x$ are obtained in the similar manner as

$$E_y^n\left(N_x, j+\frac{1}{2}, k\right) = E_y^{n-1}\left(N_x - 1, j+\frac{1}{2}, k\right) + \frac{(V_x\Delta t - \Delta x)}{(V_x\Delta t + \Delta x)}$$
$$\times\left\{E_y^n\left(N_x - 1, j+\frac{1}{2}, k\right) - E_y^{n-1}\left(N_x, j+\frac{1}{2}, k\right)\right\}$$
$$\text{for} \quad j = 2 \sim N_y - 2, k = 2 \sim N_z - 1 \qquad (7.210)$$

and

$$E_z^n\left(N_x, j, k+\frac{1}{2}\right) = E_z^{n-1}\left(N_x - 1, j, k+\frac{1}{2}\right) + \frac{(V_x\Delta t - \Delta x)}{(V_x\Delta t + \Delta x)}$$
$$\times\left\{E_z^n\left(N_x - 1, j, k+\frac{1}{2}\right) - E_z^{n-1}\left(N_x, j, k+\frac{1}{2}\right)\right\}$$
$$\text{for} \quad j = 2 \sim N_y - 1, k = 2 \sim N_z - 2. \qquad (7.211)$$

The Mur's ABC annihilates a normally incident wave with high accuracy. However, for obliquely incident waves, large reflections can occur. Other boundary operators have been introduced to annihilate waves at multiple angles [36, 37].

REFERENCES

[1] Koch, T. B., J. B. Davies, and D. Wickramasinghe. 1989. Finite element/finite difference propagation algorithm for integrated optical device. *Electron. Lett.* 25:514–516.

[2] Fleck, J. A., J. R. Morris, and M. D. Feit. 1976. Time-dependent propagation of high energy laser beams through the atmosphere. *Appl. Phys.* 10:129–160.

[3] Feit, M. D., and J. A. Fleck. 1978. Light propagation in graded-index optical fibers. *Appl. Opt.* 17:3990–3998.

[4] Lax, M., J. H. Batteh, and G. P. Agrawal. 1981. Channeling of intense electromagnetic beams. *J. Appl. Phys.* 52:109–125.

[5] Agrawal, G. P., and M. J. Potasek. 1986. Nonlinear pulse distortion in single-mode optical fibers at the zero-dispersion wavelength. *Phys. Rev. A* 33:1765–1776.

[6] Bringham, E. O. 1974. *The Fast Fourier Transform.* Euglewood Cliffs, NJ: Prentice-Hall.

[7] Oliver, B. M., J. R. Pierce, and C. E. Shannon. 1948. The philosophy of PCM. *Proc.* of the IRE. 36:1324–1331.

[8] Cooley, J. W., and J. W. Turkey. 1965. An algorithm for the machine calculation of complex Fourier series. *Math. Comp.* 19:297–301.

[9] Golub, G. H., and C. F. van Loan. 1989. *Matrix Computations*. Baltimore: Johns Hopkins University Press.

[10] Hutcheson, L. D., I. A. White, and J. J. Burke. 1980. Comparison of bending losses in integrated optical circuits. *Opt. Lett.* 5:276–278.

[11] Neumann, E. G., and R. Nat. 1982. Curved dielectric optical waveguides with reduced transition loss. *IEE Proc., Pt. H* 129:278–280.

[12] Izutsu, M., Y. Nakai, and T. Sueta. 1982. Operation mechanism of the single-mode optical waveguide Y-junction. *Opt. Lett.* 7:136–138.

[13] Ranganath, T. R., and S. Wang. 1977. Ti-diffuse $LiNbO_3$ branched-waveguide modulators-performance and design. *IEEE J. of Quantum Electron.* QE-13:290–295.

[14] Schmidt, R. V., and L. L. Buhl. 1976. Experimental 4×4 optical switching network. *Electron. Lett.* 12:575–577.

[15] Jensen, S. M. 1982. The nonlinear coherent coupler. *IEEE Trans. on Microwave Theory and Tech.* MTT-30:1568–1571.

[16] Ironside, C. N., J. F. Duffy, R. Hutchins, W. C. Bany, C. T. Seaton, and G. I. Stegeman. 1985. Waveguide fabrication in nonlinear semiconductor-doped glasses. *Proc. 11th European Conf. Opt. Commun.*, Venetia, Italy, pp.237–240.

[17] Stegeman, G. I., E. M. Wright, N. Finlayson, R. C. Zanoni and C. T. Seaton. 1988. Third order nonlinear integrated optics. *IEEE J. of Lightwave Tech.* LT-6:953–970.

[18] Aitchison, J. S., A. H. Kean, C. N. Ironside, A. Villeneuve, and G. I. Stegeman. 1991. Ultrafast all-optical switching in $Al_{0.18}Ga_{0.82}$ As directional coupler in 1.55 μm spectral region. *Electron. Lett.* 27:1709–1710.

[19] Doran, N. J., and D. Wood. 1988. Nonlinear-optical loop mirror. *Opt. Lett.* 13:56–58.

[20] Nelson, B. P., K. J. Blow, P. D. Constantine, N. J. Doran, J. K. Lucek, I. W. Marshall, and K. Smith. 1991. All-optical Gbit/s switching using nonlinear optical loop mirror. *Electron. Lett.* 27:704–705.

[21] Hadley, G. R. 1992. Transparent boundary condition for beam propagation method. *IEEE J. of Quantum Electron.* QE-28:363–370.

[22] Yevick, D., and B. Hermansson. 1989. New formulations of the matrix beam propagation method: Application to rib waveguides. *IEEE J. of Quantum Electron.* QE-25:221–229.

[23] Press, W. H., B. P. Flannery, S. A. Teukolsky, and W. T. Vettering. 1986. *Numerical Recipes: The Art of Scientific Computing.* New York: Cambridge University Press.

[24] Ratowsky, R. P., and J. A. Fleck Jr. 1991. Accurate numerical solution of the Helmholz equation by iterative Lanczos reduction. *Opt. Lett.* 16:787–789.

[25] Hadley, G. R. 1992. Wide-angle beam propagation using Pade approximant operators. *Opt. Lett.* 17:1426–1428.

[26] Soref, R. A., J. Schmidtchen, and K. Petermann. 1991. Large single-mode rib waveguides in GeSi-Si and Si-on-SiO_2. *IEEE J. Quantum Electron.* 27:1971–1974.

[27] Jalali, B., S. Yegnanarayanan, T. Yoon, T. Yoshimoto, I. Rendina, and F. Coppinger. 1998. Advances in silicon-on-insulator optoelectronics. *IEEE J. Selected Topics in Quantum Electron.* 4:938–947.

[28] Little, B. E., S. T. Chu, P. P. Absil, J. V. Hryniewicz, F. G. Johnson, F. Seiferth, D. Gill, V. Van, O. King, and M. Trakalo. 2004. Very high-order microring resonator filters for WDM applications. *IEEE Photonics Tech. Lett.* 16:2263–2265.

[29] Yamada, K., T. Tsuchizawa, T. Watanabe, J. Takahashi, E. Tamechika, M. Takahashi, S. Uchiyama, H. Fukuda, T. Shoji, S. Itabashi, and H. Morita. 2004. Microphotonics devices based on silicon wire waveguiding system. *IEICE Trans. Electron.* E87-C:351–358.

[30] Bogaerts, W., R. Baets, P. Dumon, V. Wiaux, S. Beckx, D. Taillaert, B. Luyssaert, J. Campenhout, P. Bienstman, and D. Thourhout. 2005. Nanophotonic waveguides in silicon-on-insulator fabricated with CMOS technology. *IEEE J. Lightwave Tech.* 23:401–412.

[31] Yamauchi, J. 2003. Propagating beam analysis of optical waveguides, Chapter 8. Research Studies Press Ltd., England.

[32] Huang W. P., and C. L. Xu. 1993. Simulation of three-dimensional optical waveguides by a full-vector beam propagation method. *IEEE J. Quantum Electron.* 29:2639–2649.

[33] Kiyat, I., A. Aydinli, and N. Dagli. 2005. A compact silicon-on-insulator polarization splitter. *IEEE Photon. Tech. Lett.* 17:100–102.

[34] Yee, K. S. 1966. Numerical solution of initial boundary value problems involving Maxwell's equations in isotropic media. *IEEE Trans. Antennas Propag.* AP-14:302–307.

[35] Mur, G. 1981. Absorbing boundary conditions for the finite-difference approximation of the time-domain electromagnetic field equations. *IEEE Trans. Electromagnetic Compat.* EMC-23(4):377–382.

[36] Higdon, R. L. 1986. Absorbing boundary conditions for difference approximations to the multi-dimensional wave equation. *Math. Comp.* 47:437–459.

[37] Berenger, J.-P. 1994. A perfectly matched layer for the absorption of electromagnetic waves. *Jour. Comput. Phys.* 114:185–200.

Chapter 8

Staircase Concatenation Method

For axially varying waveguides, the beam propagation method described in the preceding chapter is the most powerful technique for investigating linear and nonlinear lightwave propagation phenomena. In comparison with BPM, the staircase concatenation method is a classical technique that has been utilized for the analysis of axially varying waveguides. As explained in Chapter 7, the step size of numerical analysis in BPM is something between a fraction of the wavelength and several times the wavelength. Therefore calculation time and rounding errors will increase in the analysis of optical devices of several centimeters length. The staircase concatenation method is suitable for the analysis of such long devices. In this chapter, the basic concepts and procedures of the staircase concatenation method are explained via the example of fused-taper fiber couplers.

8.1. STAIRCASE APPROXIMATION OF WAVEGUIDE BOUNDARY

We will investigate here the transmission characteristics of the fused-taper (fused and elongated) coupler [1, 2] shown in Fig. 8.1. The fused-taper coupler is fabricated by first fusing the two parallel fibers with a burner or heater and then elongating it. The total diameter of the minimum waist region reaches about 20–30 μm from the original diameter of the two fibers. In this case, the core diameter of each fiber becomes about 1 μm (one-tenth of the original core diameter). Therefore, most of the light is not confined in the core region, and it spreads to the entire cladding. Light confinement is then provided by the air

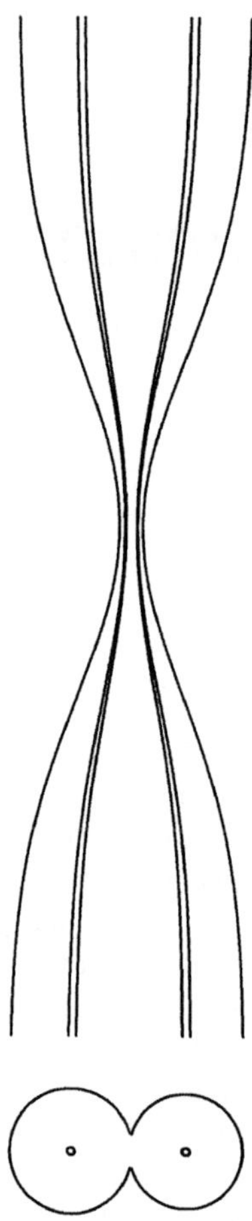

Figure 8.1 Schematic configuration of a fused and elongated fiber coupler.

cladding. Since the refractive-index difference between the glass core and the air cladding is about 25%, theoretically many modes can exist. However, if the taper inclination is sufficiently low, higher-order modes can seldom be generated by mode conversion. It has been confirmed that the insertion loss of the fabricated fusion-type fiber coupler is of the order of 0.1 dB [3].

The first step of the analysis of the fused-taper coupler is the staircase approximation of the smooth coupling region, as shown in Fig. 8.2. In each staircase-approximated region, the cross-sectional geometrical structure is assumed to be constant. Light coupling phenomena and propagation characteristics can be analyzed by an analysis based on the interaction between even and odd modes, as described in Section 4.4.3. The transmission function from a particular stair-

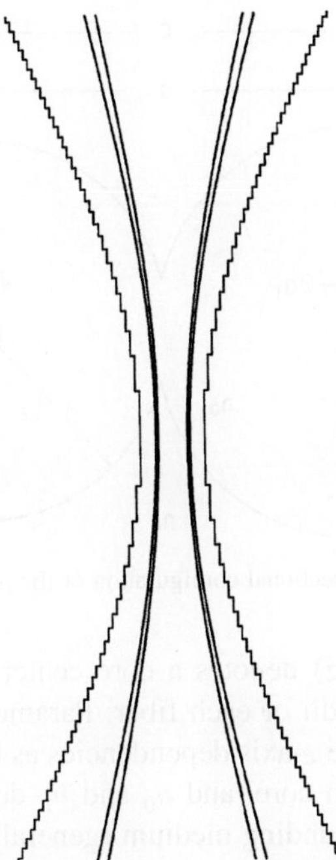

Figure 8.2 Staircase approximation of the light coupling region (staircase approximation of cores are not shown because they are too small).

case region to the consecutive one is given by the analytical formulation, which will be shown next. Then, if we specify the initial condition of the electric field distribution at a position relatively far from the coupling region, we can calculate the light propagation phenomena in the entire coupler [4]. In each staircase region, the electric field distributions of even and odd modes are obtained as follows: (1) the three-dimensional refractive-index profile of the coupler is transformed into a two-dimensional one based on the effective index method and (2) then it is analyzed by using the finite element method for slab waveguides with arbitrary index profiles, as shown in Section 6.2. Numerical calculation for two-dimensional analysis is much faster and more efficient than that for three-dimensional analysis in terms of CPU time and memory size.

The taper shape of the fused-taper coupler shown in Fig. 8.1 is known to be approximated by [5]

$$c(z) = c_0 - (c_0 - c_{\min}) \exp\left[-\left(\frac{z}{z_0}\right)^2\right], \tag{8.1}$$

where $c(z)$ is the outer diameter of the coupler defined in Fig. 8.3, z_0 represents a taper length, and c_0 and $c_{\min}$ denote the initial and the minimum diameters,

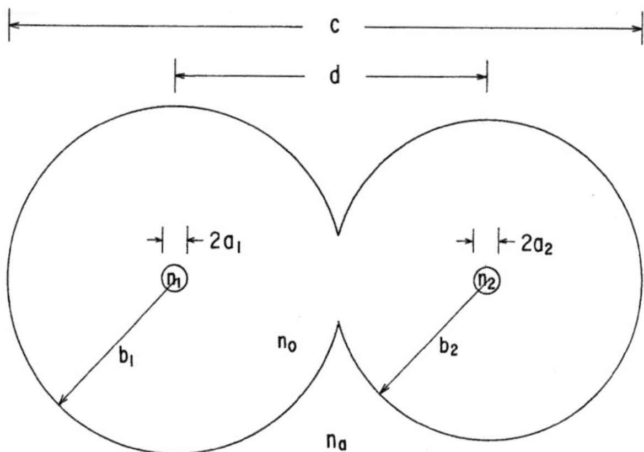

Figure 8.3 Cross-sectional configuration of the fused-taper coupler.

respectively. In Fig. 8.3, $d(z)$ denotes a core center separation, and $b_1(z)$ and $b_2(z)$ denote the cladding radii of each fiber. Parameters $d(z), b_1(z)$, and $b_2(z)$ are assumed to have the same z-axis dependencies as those of $c(z)$. n_1 and n_2 are the refractive indices of each core, and n_0 and n_a denote the refractive indices of the cladding and the surrounding medium (generally air). $2a_1$ and $2a_2$ are the diameters of each core. In the present analysis, we assume the following typical waveguide parameters:

$$2a_1 = 2a_2 = 8\,\mu\text{m},$$
$$\Delta_1 = \Delta_2 = 0.3\%,$$
$$n_0 = 1.45, \qquad n_a = 1.0,$$
$$2b_1 = 125\,\mu\text{m}.$$

Calculation of the mode coupling phenomena using the staircase approximation method starts at the position $z = -z_{\text{in}}$, where coupling between the two cores is negligible. Similarly, calculation is carried out up to the position $z = z_{\text{out}}$, where mutual coupling becomes negligible. In the following analysis, $-z_{\text{in}}$ and z_{out} are determined to be the position at which the mode coupling coefficient κ becomes

$$\frac{\kappa}{k} \approx 10^{-8}. \tag{8.2}$$

The interval between $z = -z_{\text{in}}$ and z_{out} is approximated by the staircase function with N steps. Typically N is about 40–50. Here, we introduce two important parameters:

$$\eta = \frac{d}{b_1 + b_2}, \tag{8.3}$$

$$\tau = \frac{c_{\min}}{c_0}, \tag{8.4}$$

where η represents a degree of fusion between the two fibers and τ expresses the elongation ratio. Since d, b_1, and b_2 are assumed to have the same z-dependencies, η is constant at any axial position. The two fibers are in point contact for $\eta = 1$, and η becomes smaller as the two fibers are fused tightly.

8.2. AMPLITUDES AND PHASES BETWEEN THE CONNECTING INTERFACES

Figure 8.4 shows a cross-sectional view of the fused-taper coupler at axial position z and its effective index distribution $n_{\text{eff}}(x)$. Even and odd modes in the slab waveguide having the effective index profile $n_{\text{eff}}(x)$ can be obtained by the FEM analysis described in Section 6.2. The total electric field distribution at the mth $(m = 0 - N)$ staircase region is expressed by

$$E_m(x, z) = A_{e,m}\phi_{e,m}(x)\exp[-j\beta_{e,m}(z + z_{\text{in}})] + A_{o,m}\phi_{o,m}(x)\exp[-j\beta_{o,m}(z + z_{\text{in}})] \quad (m = 0 - N). \tag{8.5}$$

Here, $A_{e,m}$, $\phi_{e,m}$, and $\beta_{e,m}$ are the amplitude, the eigen mode, and the propagation constant of the even mode and $A_{o,m}$, $\phi_{o,m}$, and $\beta_{o,m}$ are the amplitude, the eigen mode, and the propagation constant of the odd mode, respectively.

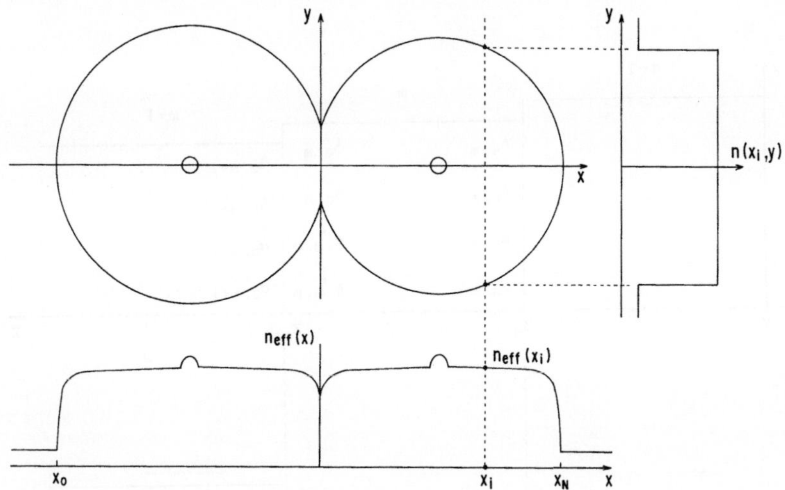

Figure 8.4 Cross-sectional view of the fused coupler and its effective index profile.

Generally speaking, higher-order modes and radiation modes should be taken into account in Eq. (8.5). However, since the insertion loss of the practical fused-taper fiber coupler is very small, we can assume that mode coupling occurs predominantly only between even and odd modes. $\phi_{e,m}$, $\phi_{o,m}$, $\beta_{e,m}$, and $\beta_{o,m}$ are obtained by FEM for the refractive-index profile $n_{\text{eff}}(x)$ at every step of the staircase-approximated region. Therefore, if we determine the amplitudes $A_{e,m}$ and $A_{o,m}$ for the even and odd modes in each step, we can evaluate the light coupling phenomena in the entire coupling region.

Basically, the amplitude and phase-transmission coefficients from the initial position of the mth step ($z = z_m$) to that of the $(m+1)$th step ($z = z_{m+1}$), as shown in Fig. 8.5, should be calculated. The continuity conditions at $z = z_{m+1}$ for the electromagnetic fields give the following relations:

$$\begin{aligned} &A_{e,m}\phi_{e,m}(x)\exp(-j\alpha'_{e,m}) + A_{o,m}\phi_{o,m}(x)\exp(-j\alpha'_{o,m}) \\ &\quad + B_{e,m}\phi_{e,m}(x)\exp(j\gamma_{e,m}) + B_{o,m}\phi_{o,m}(x)\exp(j\gamma_{o,m}) \\ &= A_{e,m+1}\phi_{e,m+1}(x)\exp(-j\alpha_{e,m+1}) + A_{o,m+1}\phi_{o,m+1}(x)\exp(-j\alpha_{o,m+1}) \end{aligned} \tag{8.6}$$

$$\begin{aligned} &\beta_{e,m}A_{e,m}\phi_{e,m}(x)\exp(-j\alpha'_{e,m}) + \beta_{o,m}A_{o,m}\phi_{o,m}(x)\exp(-j\alpha'_{o,m}) \\ &\quad - \beta_{e,m}B_{e,m}\phi_{e,m}(x)\exp(j\gamma_{e,m}) - \beta_{o,m}B_{o,m}\phi_{o,m}(x)\exp(j\gamma_{o,m}) \\ &= \beta_{e,m+1}A_{e,m+1}\phi_{e,m+1}(x)\exp(-j\alpha_{e,m+1}) \\ &\quad + \beta_{o,m+1}A_{o,m+1}\phi_{o,m+1}(x)\exp(-j\alpha_{o,m+1}), \end{aligned} \tag{8.7}$$

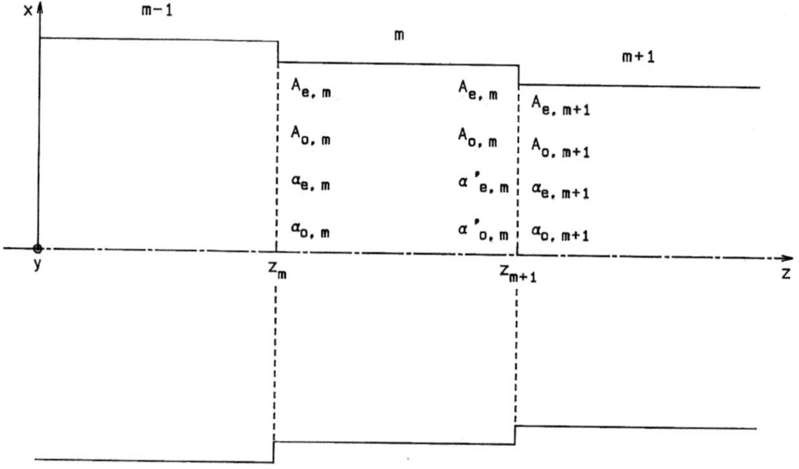

Figure 8.5 Amplitudes and phases between the two staircase-approximated regions.

where

$$\alpha_{e,m} = \beta_{e,m}(z_m + z_{\text{in}}) \tag{8.8a}$$

$$\alpha_{o,m} = \beta_{o,m}(z_m + z_{\text{in}}) \tag{8.8b}$$

$$\alpha'_{e,m} = \beta_{e,m}(z_{m+1} + z_{\text{in}}) = \alpha_{e,m} + \beta_{e,m}(z_{m+1} - z_m) \tag{8.8c}$$

$$\alpha'_{o,m} = \beta_{o,m}(z_{m+1} + z_{\text{in}}) = \alpha_{o,m} + \beta_{o,m}(z_{m+1} - z_m), \tag{8.8d}$$

$B_{\ell,m}$ and $\gamma_{\ell,m}(\ell = e$ or $o)$ are the amplitude and the phase of the reflected wave, respectively. When we calculate the following integral:

$$\int_{-\infty}^{\infty} [8.6 \times \beta_{e,m+1} - 8.7]\phi^*_{e,m+1}(x)dx,$$

we obtain

$$B_{e,m}\exp(j\gamma_{e,m}) \cong \frac{\beta_{e,m} - \beta_{e,m+1}}{\beta_{e,m} + \beta_{e,m+1}} A_{e,m}\exp(-j\alpha'_{e,m}). \tag{8.9}$$

Here we used the following orthogonality and normalization relations:

$$\frac{\beta_{p,m}}{2\omega\mu_0}\int_{-\infty}^{\infty} \phi_{p,m}(x)\phi^*_{q,m}(x)dx = \delta_{pq} \quad (p, q = e \text{ or } o) \tag{8.10a}$$

$$\int_{-\infty}^{\infty} \phi_{p,m}(x)\phi^*_{q,m+1}(x)dx \cong 0 \quad (p \neq q). \tag{8.10b}$$

Equation (8.10b) is a good approximation as long as the change between the two coupler diameters at $z = z_{m+1}$ is sufficiently small. Similarly, the integral of the form

$$\int_{-\infty}^{\infty} [8.6 \times \beta_{o,m+1} - 8.7]\phi^*_{o,m+1}(x)dx$$

gives

$$B_{o,m}\exp(j\gamma_{o,m}) \cong \frac{\beta_{o,m} - \beta_{o,m+1}}{\beta_{o,m} + \beta_{o,m+1}} A_{o,m}\exp(-j\alpha'_{o,m}), \tag{8.11}$$

where we used Eq. (8.10). Substituting Eqs. (8.9) and (8.11) into Eqs. (8.6) and (8.7), we obtain

$$\frac{2\beta_{e,m}}{\beta_{e,m} + \beta_{e,m+1}} A_{e,m}\phi_{e,m}(x)\exp(-j\alpha'_{e,m}) + \frac{2\beta_{o,m}}{\beta_{o,m} + \beta_{o,m+1}} A_{o,m}\phi_{o,m}(x)\exp(-j\alpha'_{o,m})$$
$$= A_{e,m+1}\phi_{e,m+1}(x)\exp(-j\alpha_{e,m+1}) + A_{o,m+1}\phi_{o,m+1}(x)\exp(-j\alpha_{o,m+1}) \tag{8.12}$$

$$\frac{2\beta_{e,m}\beta_{e,m+1}}{\beta_{e,m}+\beta_{e,m+1}} A_{e,m}\phi_{e,m}(x)\exp(-j\alpha'_{e,m})$$
$$+\frac{2\beta_{o,m}\beta_{o,m+1}}{\beta_{o,m}+\beta_{o,m+1}} A_{o,m}\phi_{o,m}(x)\exp(-j\alpha'_{o,m})$$
$$=\beta_{e,m+1}A_{e,m+1}\phi_{e,m+1}(x)\exp(-j\alpha_{e,m+1})$$
$$+\beta_{o,m+1}A_{o,m+1}\phi_{o,m+1}(x)\exp(-j\alpha_{o,m+1}). \tag{8.13}$$

When we further calculate the integral of the form

$$\int_{-\infty}^{\infty}[8.12\times\beta_{e,m}+8.13]\phi^*_{e,m+1}(x)dx,$$

we obtain

$$A_{e,m+1}\exp(-j\alpha_{e,m+1}) = \frac{2\beta_{e,m}}{\beta_{e,m}+\beta_{e,m+1}}A_{e,m}\exp(-j\alpha'_{e,m})\frac{\int_{-\infty}^{\infty}\phi_{e,m}\phi^*_{e,m+1}dx}{\int_{-\infty}^{\infty}|\phi_{e,m+1}|^2dx}$$
$$+\frac{2\beta_{o,m}}{\beta_{e,m}+\beta_{e,m+1}}\frac{\beta_{e,m}+\beta_{o,m+1}}{\beta_{o,m}+\beta_{o,m+1}}A_{o,m}\exp(-j\alpha'_{o,m})$$
$$\times\frac{\int_{-\infty}^{\infty}\phi_{o,m}\phi^*_{e,m+1}dx}{\int_{-\infty}^{\infty}|\phi_{e,m+1}|^2dx}. \tag{8.14}$$

In Eq. (8.14), the overlap integral between even and odd modes is rigorously calculated without approximating it to be zero as is done in Eq. (8.10b). Similarly, the integral of the form

$$\int_{-\infty}^{\infty}[8.12\times\beta_{o,m}+8.13]\phi^*_{o,m+1}(x)dx$$

gives

$$A_{o,m+1}\exp(-j\alpha_{o,m+1}) = \frac{2\beta_{e,m}}{\beta_{e,m}+\beta_{e,m+1}}\frac{\beta_{o,m}+\beta_{e,m+1}}{\beta_{o,m}+\beta_{o,m+1}}A_{e,m}\exp(-j\alpha'_{e,m})$$
$$\times\frac{\int_{-\infty}^{\infty}\phi_{e,m}\phi^*_{o,m+1}dx}{\int_{-\infty}^{\infty}|\phi_{o,m+1}|^2dx}+\frac{2\beta_{o,m}}{\beta_{o,m}+\beta_{o,m+1}}A_{o,m}\exp(-j\alpha'_{o,m})$$
$$\times\frac{\int_{-\infty}^{\infty}\phi_{o,m}\phi^*_{o,m+1}dx}{\int_{-\infty}^{\infty}|\phi_{o,m+1}|^2dx}. \tag{8.15}$$

Here we introduce a new parameter, $c^{(m)}_{p,q}$, which is defined by

$$c^{(m)}_{p,q} = \frac{2\sqrt{\beta_{p,m}\beta_{q,m+1}}}{\beta_{p,m}+\beta_{p,m+1}}\frac{\beta_{q,m}+\beta_{p,m+1}}{\beta_{q,m}+\beta_{q,m+1}}$$
$$\times\frac{\int_{-\infty}^{\infty}\phi_{p,m}\phi^*_{q,m+1}dx}{[\int_{-\infty}^{\infty}|\phi_{p,m}|^2dx\int_{-\infty}^{\infty}|\phi_{q,m+1}|^2dx]^{1/2}} \quad (p,q=e \text{ or } o). \tag{8.16}$$

Then Eqs. (8.14) and (8.15) are expressed by

$$A_{e,m+1}\exp(-j\alpha_{e,m+1}) = c^{(m)}_{e,e} A_{e,m}\exp(-j\alpha'_{e,m}) + c^{(m)}_{o,e} A_{o,m}\exp(-j\alpha'_{o,m}), \quad (8.17)$$

$$A_{o,m+1}\exp(-j\alpha_{o,m+1}) = c^{(m)}_{e,o} A_{e,m}\exp(-j\alpha'_{e,m}) + c^{(m)}_{o,o} A_{o,m}\exp(-j\alpha'_{o,m}). \quad (8.18)$$

Since $A_{p,m}$ and $c^{(m)}_{p,q}$ in the last two equations are real number, the phase values $\alpha_{e,m+1}$ and $\alpha_{o,m+1}$ in the $(m+1)$th step are given by

$$\alpha_{e,m+1} = \tan^{-1}\left[\frac{c^{(m)}_{e,e} A_{e,m}\sin(\alpha'_{e,m}) + c^{(m)}_{o,e} A_{o,m}\sin(\alpha'_{o,m})}{c^{(m)}_{e,e} A_{e,m}\cos(\alpha'_{e,m}) + c^{(m)}_{o,e} A_{o,m}\cos(\alpha'_{o,m})}\right], \quad (8.19)$$

$$\alpha_{o,m+1} = \tan^{-1}\left[\frac{c^{(m)}_{e,o} A_{e,m}\sin(\alpha'_{e,m}) + c^{(m)}_{o,o} A_{o,m}\sin(\alpha'_{o,m})}{c^{(m)}_{e,o} A_{e,m}\cos(\alpha'_{e,m}) + c^{(m)}_{o,o} A_{o,m}\cos(\alpha'_{o,m})}\right]. \quad (8.20)$$

Amplitudes in the $(m+1)$th step are then expressed by

$$A_{e,m+1} = c^{(m)}_{e,e} A_{e,m}\cos(\alpha'_{e,m} - \alpha_{e,m+1}) + c^{(m)}_{o,e} A_{o,m}\cos(\alpha'_{o,m} - \alpha_{e,m+1}), \quad (8.21)$$

$$A_{o,m+1} = c^{(m)}_{e,o} A_{e,m}\cos(\alpha'_{e,m} - \alpha_{o,m+1}) + c^{(m)}_{o,o} A_{o,m}\cos(\alpha'_{o,m} - \alpha_{o,m+1}). \quad (8.22)$$

Equations (8.19)–(8.22) give the relations of amplitudes and phases between the two positions of $z = z_m$ and $z = z_{m+1}$ in the staircase approximation method. By successively repeating the calculation, we can investigate the light coupling phenomena in the entire coupling region.

The initial amplitude and phase at $z = z_{m=0} = -z_{\text{in}}$ are expressed by

$$E_{\text{in}}(x) \equiv E_0(x, -z_{\text{in}}) = A_{e,0}\phi_{e,0}(x) + A_{o,0}\phi_{o,0}(x), \quad (8.23)$$

$$\alpha_{e,0} = \alpha_{o,0} = 0, \quad (8.24)$$

where $E_{\text{in}}(x)$ denotes the electric field profile at $z = -z_{\text{in}}$. By applying the orthogonality relation of Eq. (8.10) into the last two equations, $A_{e,0}$ and $A_{o,0}$ are given by

$$A_{e,0} = \int_{-\infty}^{\infty} E_{\text{in}}(x)\phi^*_{e,0}(x)dx, \quad (8.25a)$$

$$A_{o,0} = \int_{-\infty}^{\infty} E_{\text{in}}(x)\phi^*_{o,0}(x)dx. \quad (8.25b)$$

The electric field distribution in the mth staircase region $(z_m \leq z \leq z_{m+1})$ is then expressed, by using Eqs. (8.5), (8.8), and (8.25), as

$$E_m(x, z) = A_{e,m}\phi_{e,m}(x)\exp\{-j[\beta_{e,m}(z - z_m) + \alpha_{e,m}]\}$$
$$+ A_{o,m}\phi_{o,m}(x)\exp\{-j[\beta_{o,m}(z - z_m) + \alpha_{o,m}]\}. \quad (8.26)$$

In the following sections, light propagation phenomena in (a) the wavelength division multiplexing (WDM) coupler and (b) the wavelength-flattened coupler (WFC) will be described using the staircase approximation method.

8.3. WAVELENGTH DIVISION MULTIPLEXING COUPLERS

In the symmetrical coupler that consists of two identical fibers, 100% light transfer from the excited core to the other one is possible (refer to Section 4.2). Here, we define the cumulative phase difference between even and odd modes as

$$\Theta = \int_{-z_{in}}^{z} [\beta_e(\zeta) - \beta_o(\zeta)]d\zeta. \tag{8.27}$$

When we have a coupler structure that satisfies $\Theta(z_{out}) = \pi$ for light with $\lambda = 1.3\,\mu m$ and $\Theta(z_{out}) = 2\pi$ for light with $\lambda = 1.55\,\mu m$ simultaneously, it functions as the WDM coupler [6]. Figure 8.6 shows the progress of electric field profiles of even and odd modes when light is coupled into the left-hand core of a WDM coupler with the parameters of $\eta = 0.6$, $\tau = 0.34$, and $z_0 = 22.25\,mm$. As shown in Section 4.4.3, when light is coupled into only one of the two cores, we have the relations as

$$E_{in}(x) = C \cdot [\phi_{e,0}(x) + \phi_{o,0}(x)], \tag{8.28}$$

$$A_{e,0} = A_{o,0} = C. \tag{8.29}$$

It is confirmed that the even and odd modes are equally excited at the input position. Since even and odd modes are always orthogonal to each other in the symmetrical coupler, mode coupling does not take place and power transfer between the two waveguides is brought about by the interference effect among the even and odd modes. The cumulative phase difference in a WDM coupler with $\eta = 0.6$, $\tau = 0.34$, and $z_0 = 22.25\,mm$ is shown in Fig. 8.7. It is confirmed that the WDM condition is satisfied for both the $\lambda = 1.3\,\mu m$ and the $\lambda = 1.55\,\mu m$ wavelengths simultaneously. Light intensity waveforms and the wavelength-dependent coupling ratio are shown in Figs. 8.8 and 8.9, respectively.

8.4. WAVELENGTH-FLATTENED COUPLERS

Figure 8.10 shows variations of even and odd modes in the asymmetrical coupler consisting of $2b_1 = 125\,\mu m$, $2b_2 = 115\,\mu m (b_2/b_1 = 0.92)$, $\eta = 0.962$, $\tau = 0.1$, and $z_0 = 2.89\,mm$. It should be noted that the even and odd modes are localized

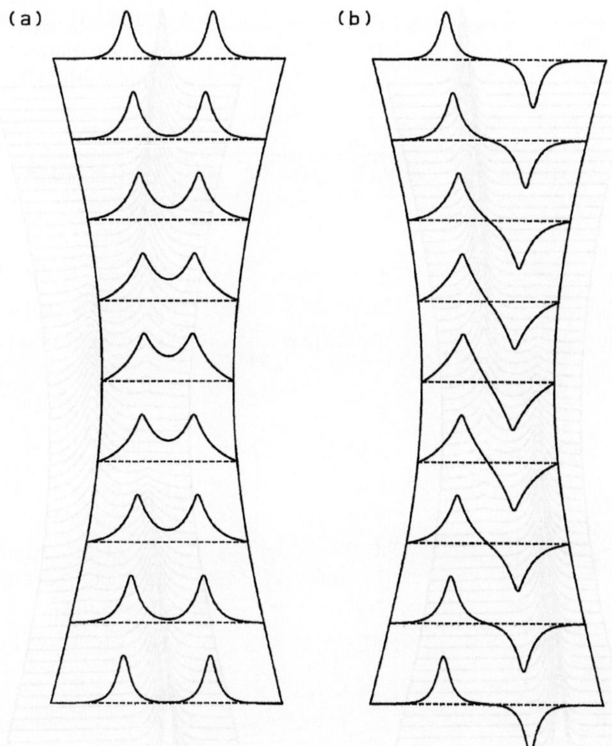

Figure 8.6 Progress of electric field profiles of (a) even modes and (b) odd modes in the WDM coupler.

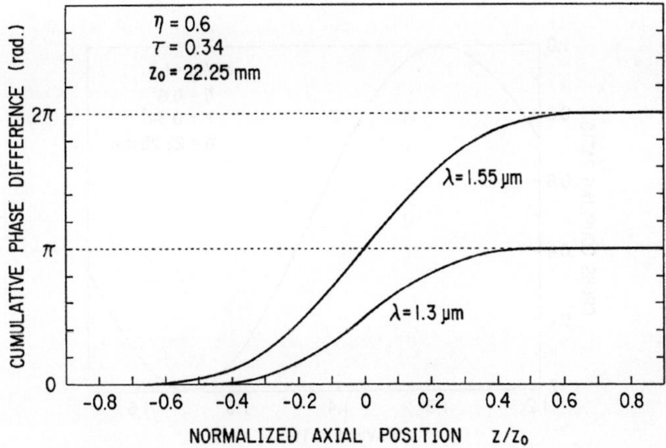

Figure 8.7 Cumulative phase difference in the WDM coupler.

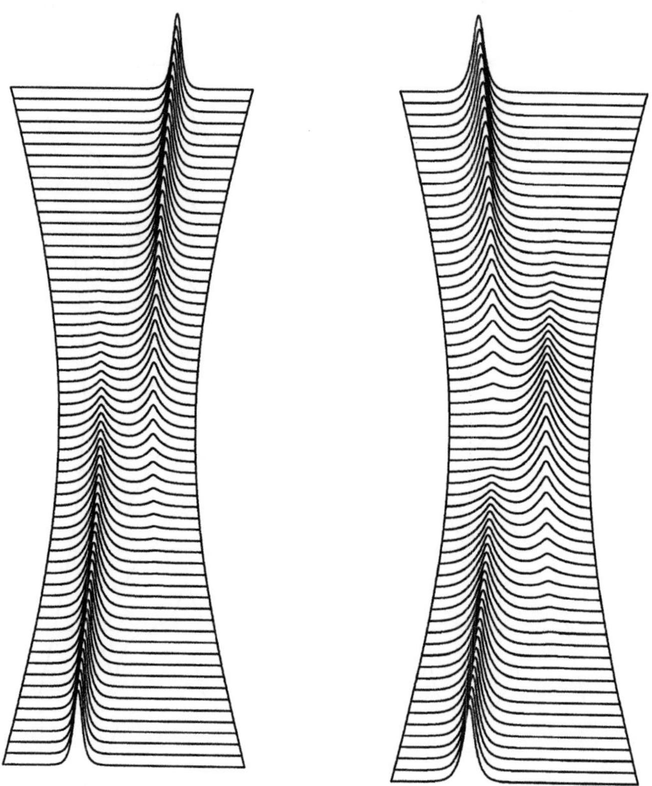

Figure 8.8 Light intensity waveforms in the WDM coupler for (a) $\lambda = 1.3\,\mu m$ and (b) $\lambda = 1.55\,\mu m$.

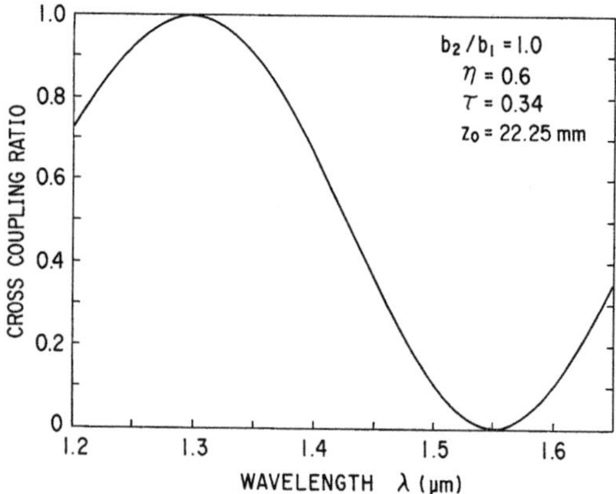

Figure 8.9 Wavelength dependency of the coupling ratio in the WDM coupler.

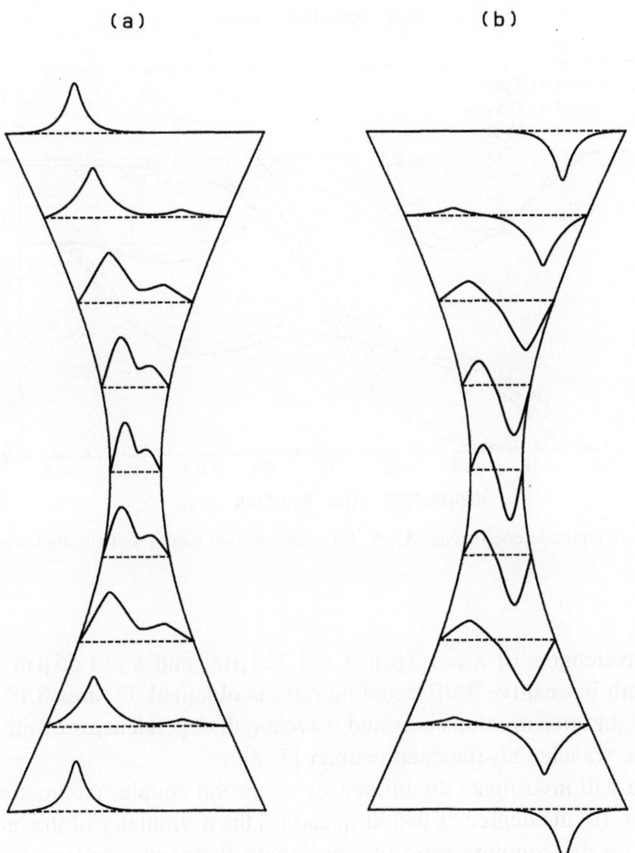

Figure 8.10 (a) Even and (b) odd modes in the asymmetrical coupler.

in either one of the two cores in the asymmetrical coupler when two cores are sufficiently apart from each other. Therefore, when light is coupled into the left-hand core, only the even mode is excited. In order to obtain a 3-dB coupling ratio in the asymmetrical coupler, proper mode coupling should take place from the excited (even) mode to the other (odd) mode. Amplitude coefficients A_e, A_o for even and odd modes and cumulative phase difference Θ in the asymmetrical coupler consisting of $b_2/b_1 = 0.92$, $\eta = 0.962$, $\tau = 0.1$, and $z_0 = 2.89\,\text{mm}$ are shown in Fig. 8.11. It is confirmed that the amplitude coefficients at the output end are

$$A_e \cong A_o \cong \frac{1}{\sqrt{2}} \tag{8.30}$$

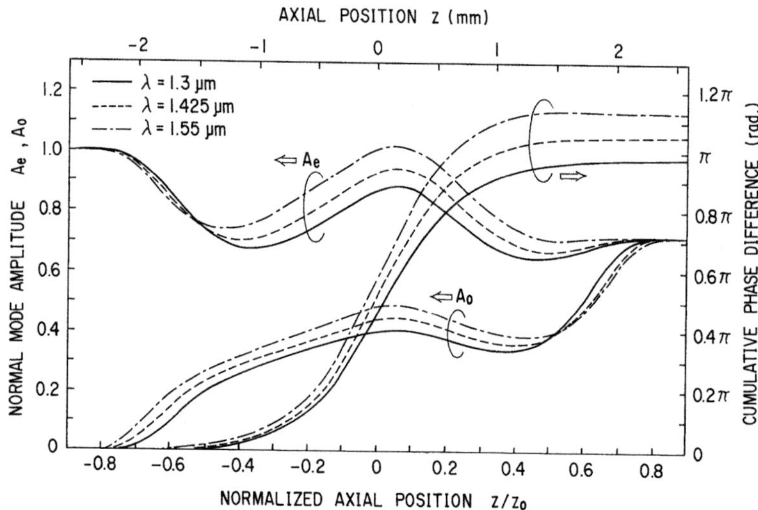

Figure 8.11 Amplitude coefficients A_e, A_o for even and odd modes and cummulative phase difference Θ.

for any wavelengths of $\lambda = 1.3\,\mu\text{m}$, $\lambda = 1.425\,\mu\text{m}$, and $\lambda = 1.55\,\mu\text{m}$, and thus a wavelength-insensitive 3-dB coupling ratio is obtained. Figures 8.12 and 8.13 show the light intensity transients and wavelength dependencies of the coupling ratios in the wavelength-flattened coupler [7, 8].

Next we will investigate the influences of several coupler parameters: (a) the taper ratio τ, (b) the degree of fusion η, and (c) the asymmetry of the outer diameter b_2/b_1 on the coupling ratio of wavelength-flattened couplers. Figure 8.14 shows the influences of (a) the taper ratio τ, (b) the degree of fusion η, and (c) the asymmetry of the outer diameter b_2/b_1 on the coupling ratio of wavelength-flattened couplers. In Fig. 8.14(a), taper length z_0 is optimized for each τ when b_2/b_1 and η are fixed at $b_2/b_1 = 0.92$ and $\eta = 0.962$. Similarly, τ and b_2/b_1 are fixed in Fig. 8.14(b) and τ and η are fixed in Fig. 8.14(c). It is seen from Fig. 8.14(a) that taper length z_0 becomes very short (long) when taper ratio τ is smaller (larger) than 0.1. When taper length is very short, the insertion loss increases, since the width of the coupling region varies quite rapidly. In contrast, if taper length is very long, the coupler becomes rather impractical because of the long device length. It is therefore known that a taper ratio of about $\tau = 0.1$ is the preferable value. From Fig. 8.14(b), it is seen that the coupling ratio becomes large for small η (tightly fused coupler). In contrast, the coupling ratio becomes small for large η (lightly fused coupler). From Fig. 8.14(c), it is seen that the coupling ratio becomes smaller (larger) when b_2/b_1 is small (large). Taking the results of Figs. 8.14(a), (b), and (c) into account, it is seen that there are

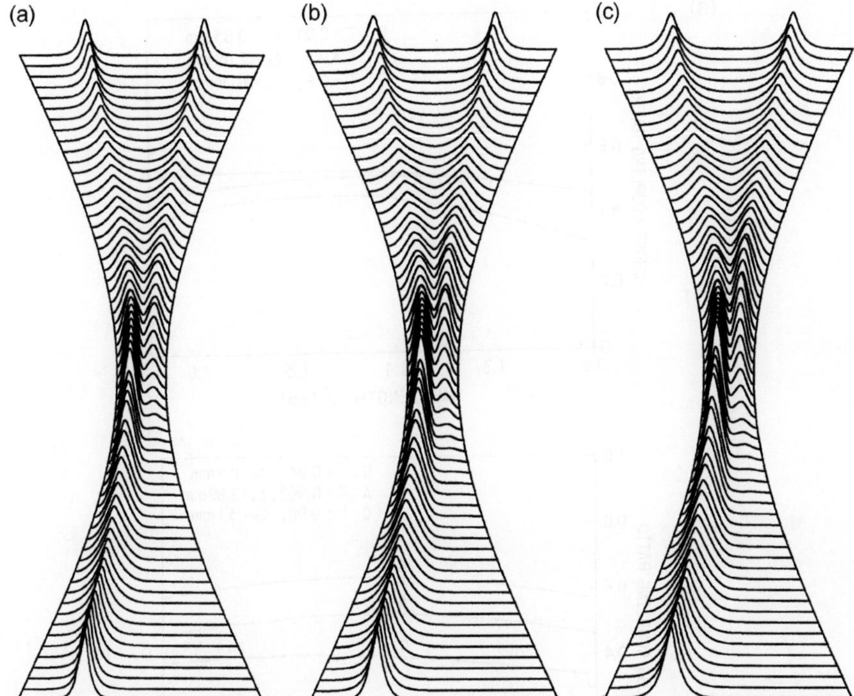

Figure 8.12 Light intensity transients at (a) $\lambda = 1.3\,\mu m$, (b) $\lambda = 1.425\,\mu m$, and (c) $\lambda = 1.55\,\mu m$ in the wavelength-flattened coupler.

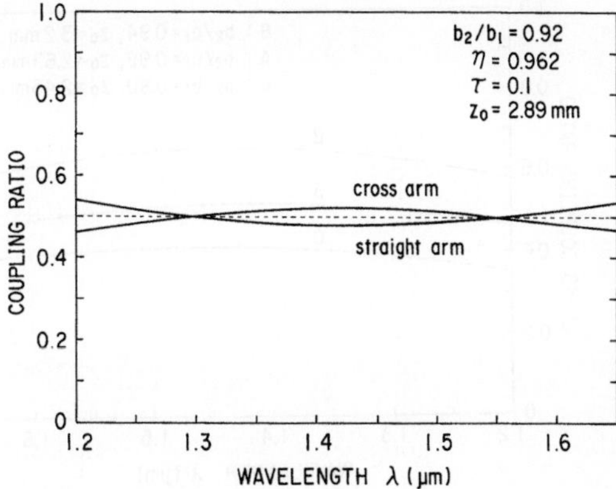

Figure 8.13 Wavelength dependencies of the coupling ratios in the wavelength-flattened coupler.

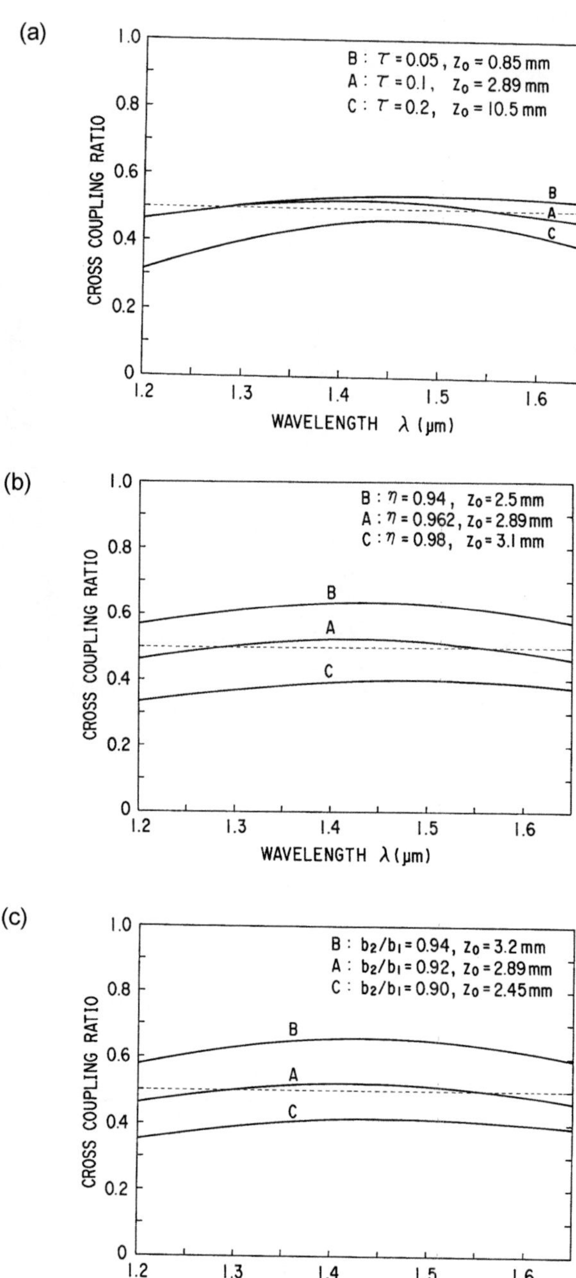

Figure 8.14 Influences of (a) taper ratio τ, (b) degree of fusion η, and (c) asymmetry of the outer diameter b_2/b_1 on the coupling ratio of wavelength-flattened couplers.

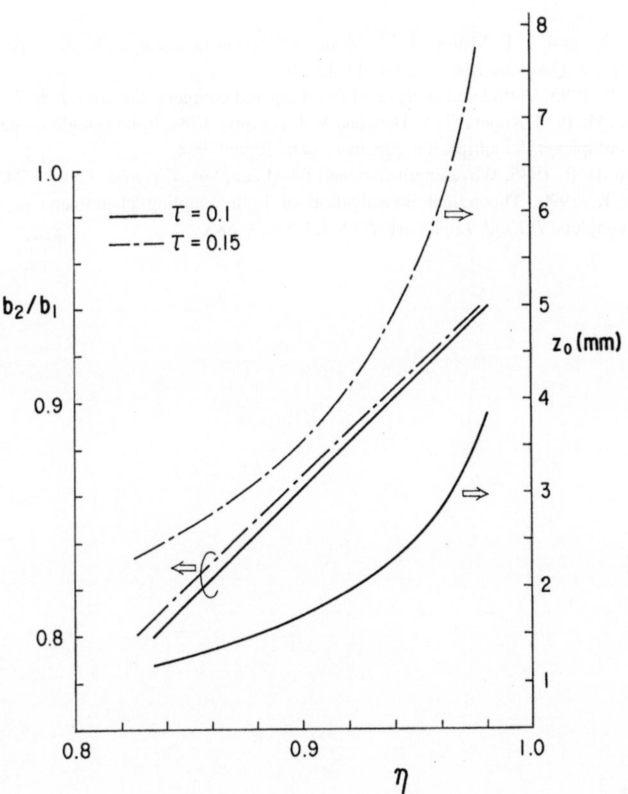

Figure 8.15 Optimum relationships among η, b_2/b_1, and z_0 when taper ratio τ is fixed at $\tau = 0.1$ and $\tau = 0.15$.

several possible choices of coupler parameters for wavelength-flattened couplers. Figure 8.15 shows the optimum relationships among η, b_2/b_1, and z_0 when taper ratio τ is fixed at $\tau = 0.1$ and $\tau = 0.15$ [8]. Similar wavelength-flattened characteristics to that of Fig. 8.13 are obtainable with any parameter combinations of τ, η, b_2/b_1, and z_0.

REFERENCES

[1] Kawasaki, B. S., K. O. Hill, and R. G. Lamont. 1981. Biconical-taper single-mode fiber coupler. *Opt. Lett.* 6:327–328.

[2] Yokohama, I., K. Okamoto, M. Kawachi, and J. Noda. 1984. Polarizing fiber coupler with high extinction ratio. *Electron. Lett.* 20:1004–1005.

[3] Yokohama, I., J. Noda, and K. Okamoto. 1987. Fiber-coupler fabrication with automatic fusion-elongation process for low excess loss and high coupling-ratio accuracy. *IEEE J. Lightwave Tech.* LT-5:910–915.

[4] Burns, W. K., and A. F. Milton. 1975. Mode conversion in planar-dielectric separating waveguides. *IEEE J. Quantum Electron.* QE-11:32–39.
[5] Wright, J. V. 1985. Variational analysis of fused tapered couplers. *Electron. Lett.* 21:1064–1065.
[6] Lawson, C. M., P. M. Kopera, T. Y. Hsu, and V. J. Tekippe. 1984. In-line single-mode wavelength division multiplexer/demultiplexer. *Electron. Lett.* 20:963–964.
[7] Mortimore, D. B. 1985. Wavelength-flattened fused couplers. *Electron. Lett.* 21:742–743.
[8] Okamoto, K. 1990. Theoretical investigation of light coupling phenomena in wavelength-flattened couplers. *IEEE J. Lightwave Tech.* LT-8:678–683.

Chapter 9

Planar Lightwave Circuits

Upgrading telecommunication networks to increase their capacity is becoming increasingly important due to the rapid increase in network traffic caused by multimedia communications. Although optical technologies are replacing most transmission lines, the nodes of the networks, such as switching and cross-connect nodes, are still depend on relatively slow electrical technologies. This will be a serious problem because nodes in the networks will limit the throughput all over the networks, due to the limitations of the electrical circuits. Making the nodes optical, therefore, is important for solving these issues. It requires multiplexing and demultiplexing (mux/demux) via optical technologies. The time-division multiplexing, or TDM, systems that are widely used in existing optical communications systems, are inherently depend on electrical circuits for multiplexing and demultiplexing. The nodes in TDM systems use optical–electrical conversion, electrical demulti- and multiplexing, and electrical–optical conversion. This means the throughput of the node is limited by the processing speed in the electrical circuits. Wavelength division multiplexing, or WDM, technologies, on the other hand, enable optical multi- and demultiplexing because individual signals have different light wavelengths and can be separated easily by wavelength-selective optical elements. This may enable us to construct WDM networks in which node functionality is supported by optical technologies without electrical mux/demux.

The most prominent feature of the silica waveguides is their simple and well-defined waveguide structures [1]. This allows us to fabricate multibeam or multi-stage interference devices, such as arrayed-waveguide gratings and lattice-form programmable dispersion equalizers. A variety of passive PLCs, such as $N \times N$ star couplers, $N \times N$ arrayed-waveguide grating multiplexers, and thermo-optic matrix switches have been developed [2, 3]. Hybrid optoelectronics integration based on the terraced-silicon platform technologies are also important, both to the fiber-to-the-home (FTTH) applications and high-speed signal processing devices [4, 5]. Synthesis theory of the lattice-form programmable optical filters has been developed [6] and implemented to the fabrication of variable group-delay dispersion equalizers [7].

In this chapter, various kinds of planar lightwave circuit (PLC) devices for optical WDM systems and subscriber networks are described.

9.1. WAVEGUIDE FABRICATION

Planar lightwave circuits using silica-based optical waveguides are fabricated on silicon or silica substrate by a combination of flame hydrolysis deposition (FHD) and reactive ion etching (RIE). Figure 9.1 shows a planar waveguide fabrication technique. Fine glass particles are produced in the oxy-hydrogen flame and deposited on the substrates. After depositing undercladding and core glass layers, the wafer is heated to high temperature for consolidation. The circuit pattern is fabricated by photolithography and reactive ion etching. Then core ridge structures are covered with an overcladding layer and consolidated again.

Since the typical bending radius R of silica waveguide is around 2–25 mm, the chip size of the large-scale integrated circuit becomes several centimeters square. Therefore, reduction of propagation loss and the uniformity of refractive indices and core geometries throughout the wafer are strongly required. A Propagation loss of 0.1 dB/cm was obtained in a 2-m-long waveguide with $\Delta = 2\%$ index difference ($R = 2$ mm) [8], and loss of 0.035 dB/cm was obtained in a 1.6-m-long waveguide with $\Delta = 0.75\%$ index difference ($R = 5$ mm) [9]. Further loss reduction down to 0.017 dB/cm has been achieved (Fig. 9.2) in a 10-m long

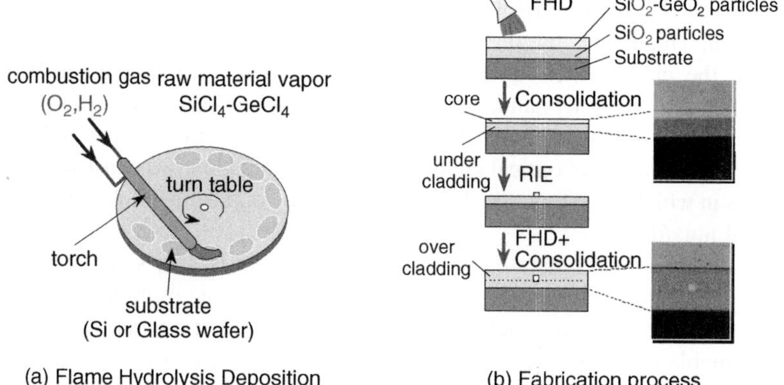

(a) Flame Hydrolysis Deposition (b) Fabrication process

Figure 9.1 Planar waveguide fabrication technique.

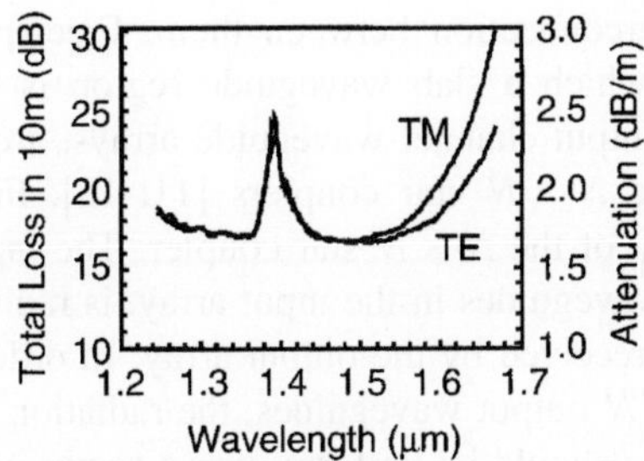

Figure 9.2 Loss spectra of 10-m-long waveguide.

Table 9.1
Waveguide parameters and propagation characteristics of four kinds of waveguides.

	Low-Δ	Medium-Δ	High-Δ	Superhigh-Δ
Index difference(%)	0.3	0.45	0.75	1.5–2.0
Core size(μm)	8 × 8	7 × 7	6 × 6	4.5 × 4.5 − 3 × 3
Loss (dB/cm)	<0.01	0.02	0.04	0.07
Coupling loss (dB/point)	<0.1	0.1	0.4	2.0
Bending radius (mm)	25	15	5	2

waveguide with $\Delta = 0.45\%$ index difference ($R = 15$ mm) [10]. The higher loss for TM mode (electric field vector is perpendicular to the waveguide plane) may be due to the roughness of waveguide wall caused by RIE etching process. However the mode conversion from TE to TM mode or vice versa was less than the 20 dB in 10-m-long waveguides.

Various kinds of waveguides are utilized depending on the circuit configurations. Table 9.1 summarizes the waveguide parameters and propagation characteristics of four kinds of waveguides. The propagation losses of low-Δ and medium-Δ waveguides are about 0.01 dB/cm and those of high-Δ and super high-Δ waveguides are about 0.04–0.07 dB/cm. The low-Δ waveguides are superior to the high-Δ waveguides in terms of fiber coupling losses with the standard single-mode fibers. On the other hand, the minimum bending radii for high-Δ waveguides are much smaller than those of low-Δ waveguides. Therefore, high-Δ waveguides are indispensable to construction highly integrated and large-scale optical circuits such as $N \times N$ star couplers, arrayed-waveguide grating multiplexers, and dispersion equalizers.

9.2. $N \times N$ STAR COUPLER

$N \times N$ star couplers are quite useful in high-speed, multiple-access optical networks, since they distribute the input signal evenly among many receivers and make possible the interconnection between them. Free-space-type integrated-optic star coupler, in which a slab waveguide region is located between the fan-shaped input and output channel waveguide arrays, are quite advantageous constructing large-scale $N \times N$ star couplers [11, 12]. Figure 9.3 shows the schematic configuration of the $N \times N$ star coupler. The input power, from any one of the N channel waveguides in the input array, is radiated to the slab (free space) region and it is received by the output array. In order to get the uniform power distribution into N output waveguides, the radiation pattern at the output side slab–array interface should be uniform over a sector of N waveguides.

Since the radiation pattern is the Fraunhofer pattern (Fourier transform) of the field profile at the input side slab–array interface, proper sidelobes must be produced by the mode coupling from the excited input waveguide to neighboring guides so as to make rectangular field pattern. Therefore, the dummy waveguides are necessary for the marginal guides to guarantee the same coupling condition as the central guides. Figure 9.4 shows an enlarged view of the central coupling region. The core width W near the slab region is tapered so as to control the mode coupling precisely. The star coupler parameters, such as the aperture angle θ, radius of slab region f, taper length L_t, recess distance L_f, and taper ratio α, were optimized by using beam propagation method [13] so as to get the maximum output and good splitting uniformity.

Figure 9.5 shows the waveform transients of the optical intensity at the $\lambda = 1.55\,\mu m$ wavelength in the optimized 144×144 star coupler when light is coupled into the leftmost waveguide. It is clearly shown that multiple mode coupling takes place in the input array and uniform radiation pattern is generated

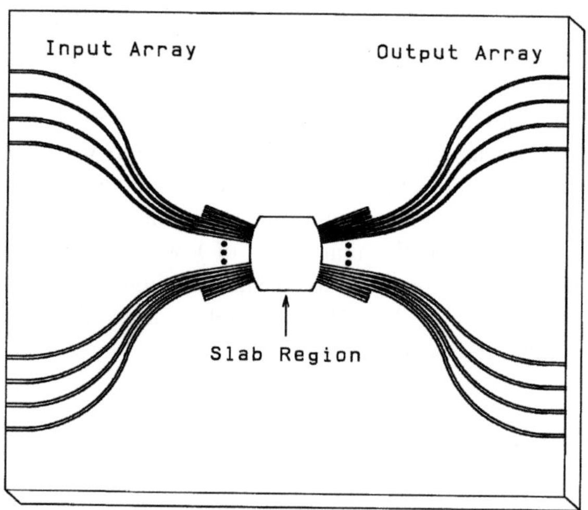

Figure 9.3 Schematic configuration of $N \times N$ star coupler.

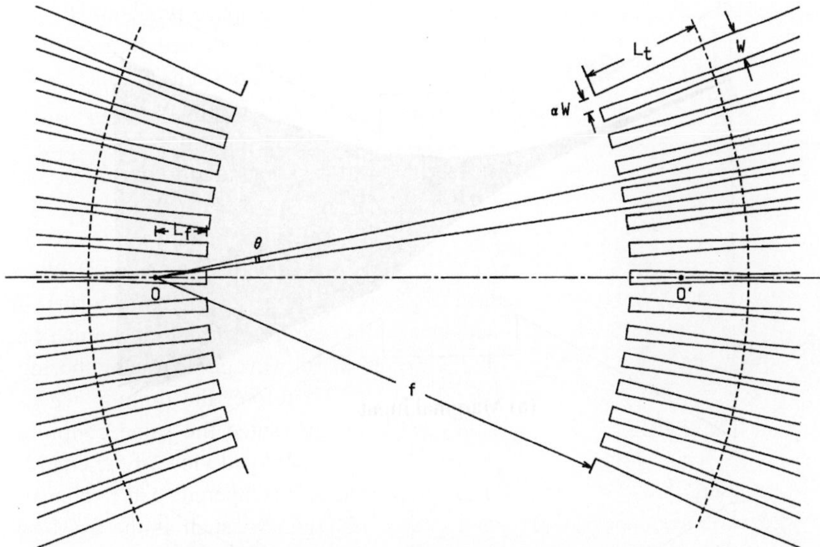

Figure 9.4 Enlarged view of the central coupling region.

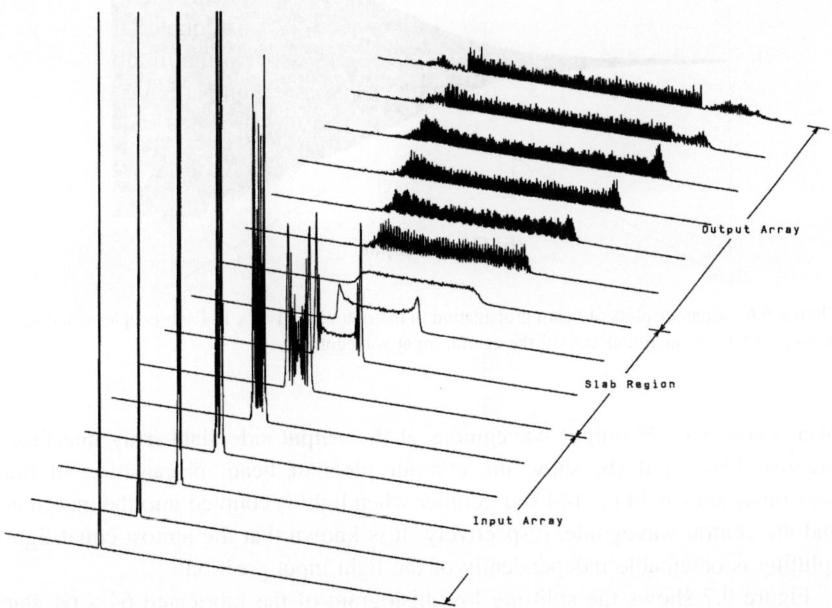

Figure 9.5 Waveform transients of the optical intensity at $\lambda = 1.55\,\mu m$ wavelength in the optimized 144×144 star coupler when light is coupled into the leftmost waveguide.

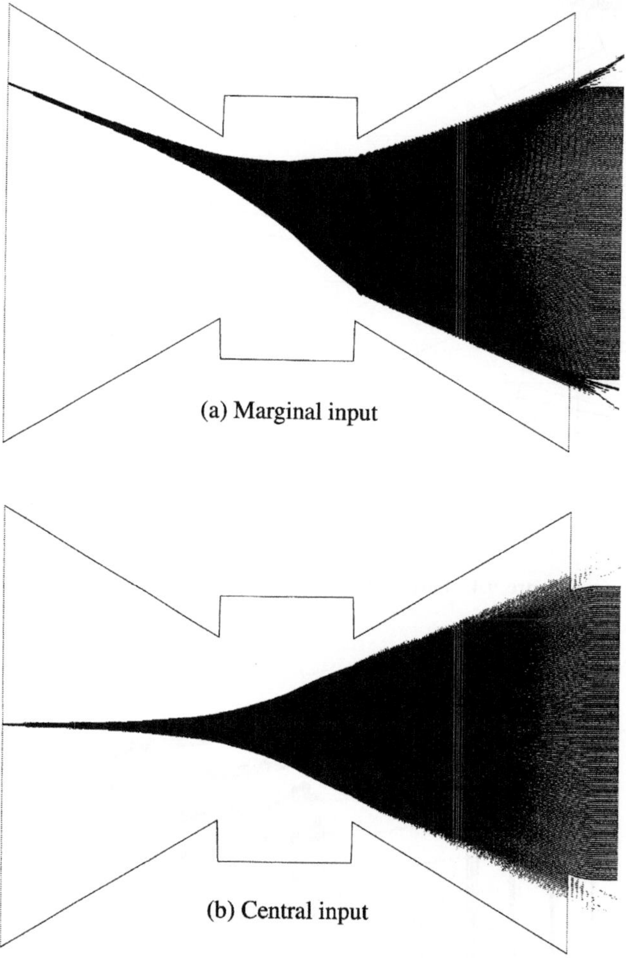

Figure 9.6 Contour plots of beam propagation in the optimized 144 × 144 star coupler when light is coupled into (a) marginal and (b) the central input waveguides.

over a sector of N output waveguides at the output side slab–array interface. Figures 9.6(a) and (b) show the contour plots of beam propagation in the previously shown 144 × 144 star coupler when light is coupled into the marginal and the central waveguide, respectively. It is known that the almost-equal light splitting is obtainable independently of the light input position.

Figure 9.7 shows the splitting loss histogram of the fabricated 64 × 64 star coupler measured at $\lambda = 1.55\,\mu m$ [14]. The essential splitting loss when light is evenly distributed into 64 output waveguides is 18.1 dB. Therefore, the average

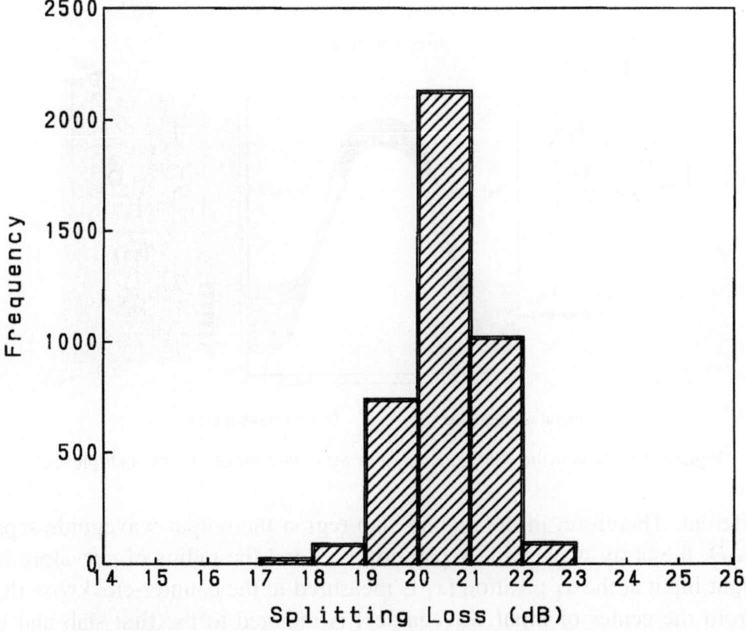

Figure 9.7 Splitting loss histogram of the 64 × 64 star coupler.

of the excess losses is 2.5 dB, and the standard deviation of the splitting losses is 0.8 dB. Within the 2.5-dB additional loss, the inevitable imperfection (theoretical) loss is about 1.5 dB, the propagation loss is about 0.6 dB, and coupling loss with single-mode fiber is 0.2 dB/facet. Various kinds of star couplers, ranging from 8 × 8 to 256 × 256, have been fabricated.

9.3. ARRAYED-WAVEGUIDE GRATING

9.3.1. Principle of Operation and Fundamental Characteristics

An $N \times N$ arrayed-waveguide grating (AWG) multiplexer is very attractive in optical WDM networks since it is capable of increasing the aggregate transmission capacity of single-strand optical fiber [15, 16]. The AWG consists of input/output waveguides, two focusing slab regions and a phase array of multiple channel waveguides with the constant path-length difference ΔL between neighboring waveguides (Fig. 9.8). In the first slab region, input waveguide separation is D_1, the array waveguide separation is d_1 and the radius of curvature is f_1. Generally the waveguide parameters in the first and the second slab regions may

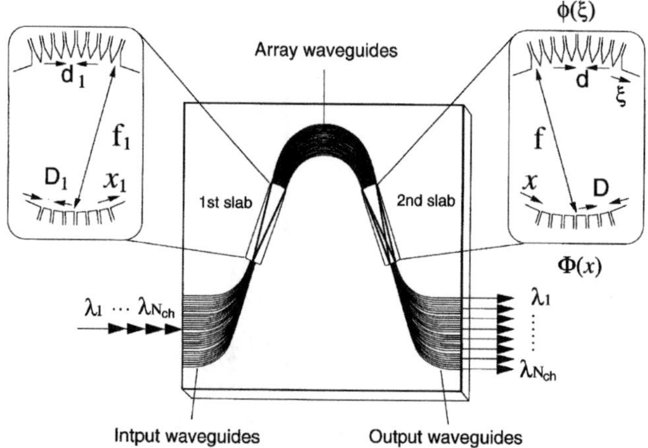

Figure 9.8 Schematic configuration of arrayed-waveguide grating multiplexer.

be different. Therefore, in the second slab region the output waveguide separation is D, the array waveguide separation is d and the radius of curvature is f. The light input at the x_1 position (x_1 is measured in the counter-clockwise direction from the center of input waveguides) is radiated to the first slab and then excites the arrayed waveguides. The excited electric field amplitude in each array waveguide is $a_i(i = 1\text{–}N)$ where N is the total number of array waveguides. The amplitude profile a_i is usually a Gaussian distribution. After traveling through the arrayed waveguides, the light beams constructively interfere into one focal point x(x is measured in the counter -clockwise direction from the center of output waveguides) in the second slab. The location of this focal point depends on the signal wavelength since the relative phase delay in each waveguide is given by $\Delta L/\lambda$.

Figure 9.9 shows an enlarged view of the second slab region. Let us consider the phase retardations for two light beams passing through the $(i-1)$-th and i-th array waveguides. The geometrical distances between two beams in the second slab region are approximated as shown in Fig. 9.9. We have similar configurations in the first slab region as those in Fig. 9.9. The difference between the total phase retardations for the two light beams passing through the $(i-1)$-th and i-th array waveguides must be an integer multiple of 2π in order for the two beams constructively interfere at the focal point x. Therefore we have the interference condition expressed by

$$\beta_s(\lambda_0)\left(f_1 - \frac{d_1 x_1}{2f_1}\right) + \beta_c(\lambda_0)[L_c + (i-1)\Delta L] + \beta_s(\lambda_0)\left(f + \frac{dx}{2f}\right)$$
$$= \beta_s(\lambda_0)\left(f_1 + \frac{d_1 x_1}{2f_1}\right) + \beta_c(\lambda_0)[L_c + i\Delta L] + \beta_s(\lambda_0)\left(f - \frac{dx}{2f}\right) - 2m\pi, \tag{9.1}$$

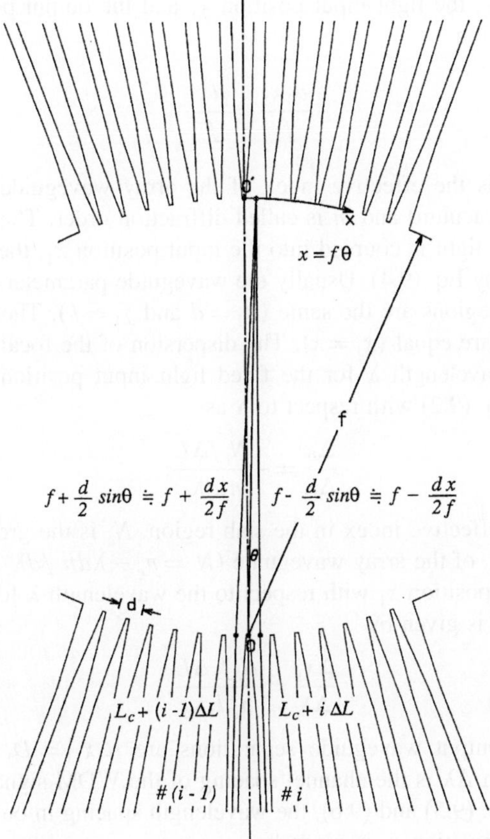

Figure 9.9 Enlarged view of the second slab region.

where β_s and β_c denote the propagation constants in the slab region and array waveguide, m is an integer, λ_0 is the center wavelength of WDM system and L_c is the minimum array waveguide length. Subtracting common terms from Eq. (9.1), we obtain

$$\beta_s(\lambda_0)\frac{d_1x_1}{f_1}-\beta_s(\lambda_0)\frac{dx}{f}+\beta_c(\lambda_0)\Delta L=2m\pi. \tag{9.2}$$

When the condition $\beta_c(\lambda_0)\Delta L=2m\pi$ or

$$\lambda_0=\frac{n_c\Delta L}{m} \tag{9.3}$$

is satisfied for λ_0, the light input position x_1 and the output position x should satisfy the condition

$$\frac{d_1 x_1}{f_1} = \frac{dx}{f}. \tag{9.4}$$

In Eq. (9.3) n_c is the effective index of the array waveguide ($n_c = \beta_c/k$, k: wavenumber in vacuum) and m is called diffraction order. The above equation means that when light is coupled into the input position x_1, the output position x is determined by Eq. (9.4). Usually the waveguide parameters in the first and the second slab regions are the same ($d_1 = d$ and $f_1 = f$). Therefore input and output distances are equal ($x_1 = x$). The dispersion of the focal position x with respect to the wavelength λ for the fixed light input position x_1 is given by differentiating Eq. (9.2) with respect to λ as

$$\frac{\Delta x}{\Delta\lambda} = -\frac{N_c f \Delta L}{n_s d \lambda_0}, \tag{9.5}$$

where n_s is the effective index in the slab region, N_c is the group index of the effective index n_c of the array waveguide ($N_c = n_c - \lambda dn_c/d\lambda$). The dispersion of the input-side position x_1 with respect to the wavelength λ for the fixed light output position x is given by

$$\frac{\Delta x_1}{\Delta\lambda} = \frac{N_c f_1 \Delta L}{n_s d_1 \lambda_0}. \tag{9.6}$$

The input and output waveguide separations are $|\Delta x_1| = D_1$ and $|\Delta x| = D$, respectively when $\Delta\lambda$ is the channel spacing of the WDM signal. Putting these relations into Eqs. (9.5) and (9.6), the wavelength spacing in output side for the fixed light input position x_1 is given by

$$\Delta\lambda_{\text{out}} = \frac{n_s d D \lambda_0}{N_c f \Delta L} \tag{9.7}$$

and the wavelength spacing in input side for the fixed light output position x is given by

$$\Delta\lambda_{\text{in}} = \frac{n_s d_1 D_1 \lambda_0}{N_c f_1 \Delta L}. \tag{9.8}$$

Generally the waveguide parameters in the first and the second slab regions are the same; they are, $D_1 = D$, $d_1 = d$ and $f_1 = f$. Then the channel spacings are the same as $\Delta\lambda_{\text{in}} = \Delta\lambda_{\text{out}} \equiv \Delta\lambda$. The path length difference ΔL is obtained from Eq. (9.7) or (9.8) as

$$\Delta L = \frac{n_s d D \lambda_0}{N_c f \Delta\lambda}. \tag{9.9}$$

The spatial separation of the m-th and $(m+1)$-th focused beams for the same wavelength is given from Eq. (9.2) as

$$X_{\mathrm{FSR}} = x_m - x_{m+1} = \frac{\lambda_0 f}{n_s d}. \tag{9.10}$$

X_{FSR} represents the free spatial range of AWG. Number of available wavelength channels N_{ch} is given by dividing X_{FSR} by the output waveguide separation D as

$$N_{\mathrm{ch}} = \frac{X_{\mathrm{FSR}}}{D} = \frac{\lambda_0 f}{n_s d D}. \tag{9.11}$$

Figures 9.10(a) and (b) show BPM simulation of the light focusing property in the second slab region for the (a) central wavelength λ_0 and (b) the shorter wavelength component $\lambda < \lambda_0$. For the signal component which converges into the off-center output port as in Fig. 9.10(b), higher or lower order diffraction beams appear. Since one of the two diffraction beams in Fig. 9.10(b) is usually thrown away, the insertion loss for the peripheral output port becomes 2–3 dB higher than that for the central output port.

The electric field profile $\Phi(x)$ at the output plane of AWG (Fig. 9.8) is the summation of the farfield patterns of ϕ_i's from each array waveguide. Therefore,

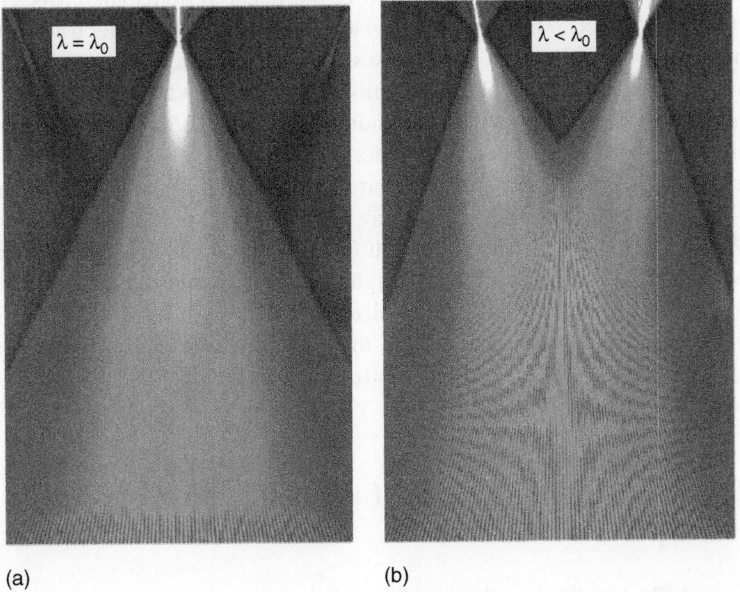

Figure 9.10 BPM simulation of the light focusing property in the second slab region for the (a) central wavelength λ_0 and (b) shorter wavelength component $\lambda < \lambda_0$.

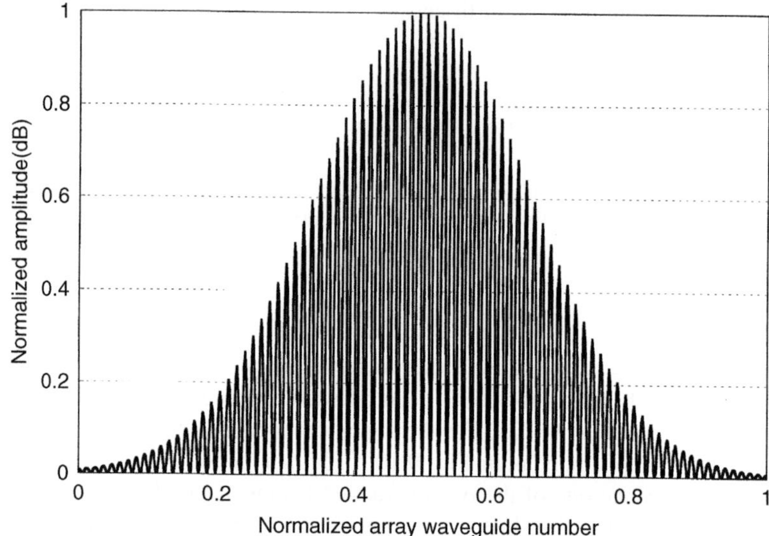

Figure 9.11 Schematic electric field distribution in the array waveguide.

$\Phi(x)$ is the summation of the spatial Fourier transforms of ϕ_i's. Summation and Fourier transformation can be exchanged in the linear system. Then it is shown that the focused electric field profile $\Phi(x)$ at the output is the Fourier transform of the entire electric field profile $\phi(\xi)$ at the slab–array interface. Figure 9.11 shows schematically the electric field distribution in the array waveguide. Horizontal axis is a normalized array waveguide number $i/N(i = 1\text{–}N)$, where N denotes total number of array waveguides. In order to minimize the light capture loss into the array waveguides, the number of array waveguides should be sufficiently large. Since the electric field in the array waveguide is segmented as shown in Fig. 9.11, that is, the field is not smooth Gaussian, Fourier-transformed field at the focal position has certain level of higher spatial components or sidelobes as shown in Fig. 9.12, which shows normalized frequency response of AWG. Such sidelobes cause theoretical crosstalk in the AWG. Theoretical crosstalk power level in the typical AWG is about −60 dB. It depends on the AWG channel numbers and also waveguide design.

9.3.2. Analytical Treatment of AWG Demultiplexing Properties

Focused electric field at the interface of the second slab and output waveguide can be almost completely expressed by the analytical form. Position of the

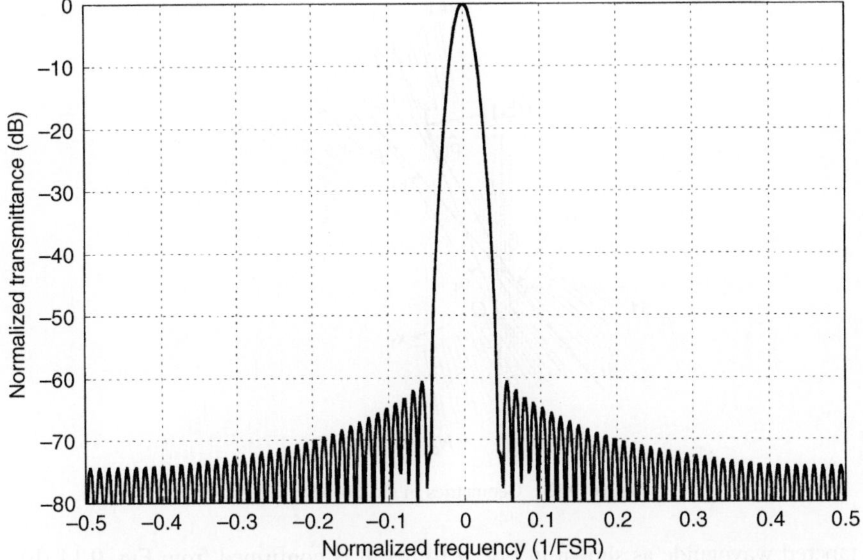

Figure 9.12 Normalized frequency response of arrayed-waveguide grating.

focused electric field moves in proportion to the wavelength shift $\Delta\lambda$ as shown in Eq. (9.5). Demultiplexing property of AWG is then given by the overlap integral of the focused electric field with the eigen mode of the output waveguide.

In this section, analytical treatment of AWG demultiplexing property is described in detail. Figure 9.13 shows waveguide geometries in the first slab region. $e(x_1)$ is an electric field distribution at the interface between the input waveguide and the first slab, where x_1 denotes the geometrical position on the interface. $f(\xi_1)$ is an electric field distribution at the interface between the first slab and the array waveguides, where ξ_1 denotes the geometrical position on the interface. $\hat{\sigma}_\ell$ and $\hat{\rho}_i$ are angles of the center of i-th input WG and ℓ-th array WG, respectively. $\hat{L}_{i,\ell}$ is the distance from the i-th input waveguide to the ℓ-th array waveguide.

Similar to the reciprocity of directivity in the transmission and receiving antennas, acceptability of waveguide is expected to be the same as the farfield pattern (FFP) from the waveguide. Figure 9.14 (a) shows the geometry to calculate FFP from waveguide. FFP $g(\rho)$ from the waveguide is obtained by the Fourier transform of the electric field at the endface of the waveguide as described in Section 2.3. Here waveguide geometries are $2a = 6\,\mu\text{m}$, $2d = 6\,\mu\text{m}$, refractive-index difference $\Delta = 0.75\%$, and tapered waveguide width and length are $18\,\mu\text{m}$ and 1.8 mm, respectively. Circles in Fig. 9.14 (b) show FFP from the waveguide with respect to the radiation angle ρ. Acceptability of the waveguide is calculated in the BPM numerical simulation by coupling plane wave to the

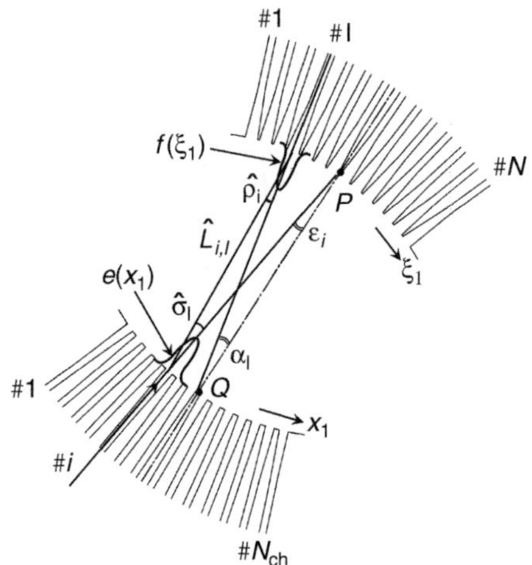

Figure 9.13 Geometries in the first slab region.

tapered waveguide as shown in Fig. 9.14 (c). It is confirmed from Fig. 9.14 (b) that the acceptability of waveguide $\Gamma(\rho)$ exactly matches with the FFP from the waveguide $g(\rho)$.

Next, we calculate how much electric field amplitude is coupled from the input waveguide to each array waveguide in Fig. 9.13. We define here the FFP

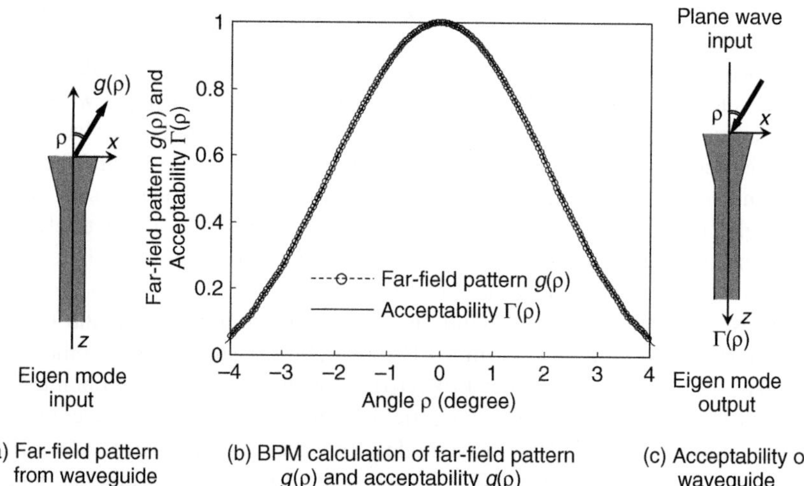

Figure 9.14 (a) Geometry to calculate FFP from the waveguide $g(\rho)$. (b) FFP from the waveguide $g(\rho)$ and acceptability of the waveguide $\Gamma(\rho)$ with respect to the radiation angle ρ. (c) Geometry to calculate acceptability of the waveguide $\Gamma(\rho)$.

of the electric field $e(x_1)$ as $h(\hat{\sigma}_\ell)$ and that of the electric field $f(\xi_1)$ as $g(\hat{\rho}_i)$. As described in Fig. 9.14 (b), FFP $g(\hat{\rho}_i)$ represents amplitude acceptability to the incoming field with angle $\hat{\rho}_i$. Since the radiation amplitude from the input waveguide #i to the array waveguide #ℓ is given by $h(\hat{\sigma}_\ell)$, electric field amplitude that is coupled from the input waveguide to the array waveguide is expressed by

$$b(\ell) = h(\hat{\sigma}_\ell) g(\hat{\rho}_i) \exp\left(-j\beta_s \hat{L}_{i,\ell}\right). \tag{9.12}$$

Figure 9.15 shows waveguide geometries in the second slab region. $f(\xi)$ is an electric field distribution at the interface between the array waveguide and the second slab, where ξ denotes the geometrical position on the interface. $e(x)$ is an electric field distribution at the interface between the second slab and the output waveguide, where x denotes the geometrical position on the interface. ρ_k and σ_ℓ are angles of the center of ℓ-th array WG and k-th output WG, respectively. $L_{\ell,k}$ is the distance from the ℓ-th array WG to k-th output WG.

Electric field amplitude in the ℓ-th array waveguide is expressed by

$$\begin{aligned} s(\ell) &= b(\ell) \exp[-j(N-\ell)\beta_c \Delta L] \\ &= h(\hat{\sigma}\ell) g(\hat{\rho}_i) \exp\left\{-j\left[\beta_s \hat{L}_{i,\ell} + (N-\ell)\beta_c \Delta L\right]\right\}, \end{aligned} \tag{9.13}$$

where N-th (the shortest) array waveguide length is assumed to be zero for simplicity.

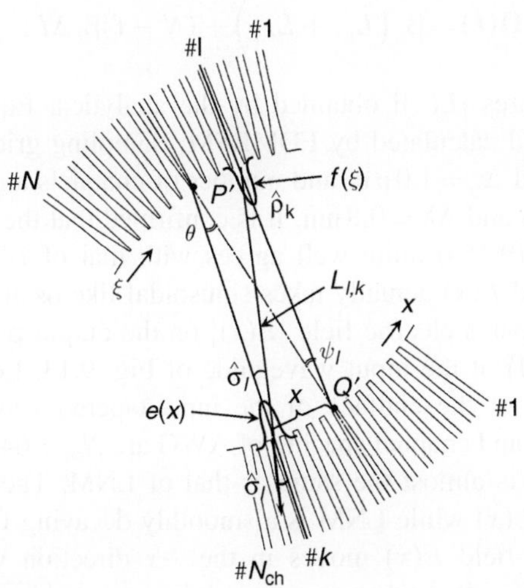

Figure 9.15 Geometries in the second slab region.

We define the FFP of the electric field $f(\xi)$ as $g(\rho_k)$ and that of the electric field $e(x)$ as $h(\sigma_\ell)$. In a similar manner to the first slab region, we intend to calculate how much electric field amplitude is coupled from the array waveguide to the output waveguide by using FFPs $g(\rho_k)$ and $h(\sigma_\ell)$. However, since multiple radiation fields interfere on the interface of the second slab and output waveguides, we can not simply use light acceptability $h(\sigma_\ell)$ because it does not take into account the phase of the radiation field. Therefore, we first obtain focused electric field at the interface of the second slab and output waveguides, and coupling efficiency is then calculated by numerically coupling the focused electric field to the output waveguide.

Since the radiation amplitude from the j-th array waveguide to the k-th output WG is given by $g(\rho_k)$, radiation field at x on the interface of the second slab and output waveguide is given by

$$s(\ell)g(\rho_k)\cos(\sigma_\ell)\exp(-j\beta_s L_{\ell,k}), \tag{9.14}$$

where $\cos(\sigma_\ell)$ is multiplied to take into account the component that is normal to the propagation axis of the k-th output waveguide.

Then, focused electric field at position x is obtained by using Eqs. (9.12)–(9.14) as

$$E(x) = \sum_{\ell=1}^{N} c(\ell)\exp[-j\Omega(\ell)], \tag{9.15a}$$

$$c(\ell) = h(\hat{\sigma}_\ell)g(\hat{\rho}_i)g(\rho_k)\cos(\sigma_\ell), \tag{9.15b}$$

$$\Omega(\ell) = \beta_s\left(\hat{L}_{i,\ell} + L_{\ell,k}\right) + (N-\ell)\beta_c\Delta L. \tag{9.15c}$$

Figure 9.16 compares $|E(x)|$ obtained by the analytical Eq. (9.15a) with the focused electric field calculated by FDMBPM. Sampling grid spacing in BPM is $\Delta x = 0.05\,\mu\text{m}$ and $\Delta z = 1.0\,\mu\text{m}$ and number of channels and channel spacing of AWG are $N_{\text{ch}} = 4$ and $\Delta\lambda = 0.8\,\text{nm}$. It is confirmed that the analytical electric field given by Eq. (9.15a) quite well agrees with that of BPM. Ripple in the focused electric field $E(x)$ actually takes sinusoidal-like oscillation.

Figure 9.17 compares electric field $|E(x)|$ on the output plane with the local normal mode (LNM) of the input waveguide of Fig. 9.13. Local normal mode is the electric field at the endface of the input-tapered waveguide. Here the number of channels and channel spacing of AWG are $N_{\text{ch}} = 64$ and $\Delta\lambda = 0.8\,\text{nm}$, respectively. $|E(x)|$ is almost the same as that of LNM. The difference is that there is a ripple in $E(x)$ while LNM is a smoothly decaying function.

Focused electric field $E(x)$ moves in the $-x$ direction with the speed of $\Delta x/\Delta\lambda = -N_c f\Delta L/(n_s d\lambda_0)$ when wavelength is increased by $\Delta\lambda$. Then, demultiplexing property at the output port #k is obtained by the overlap integral of

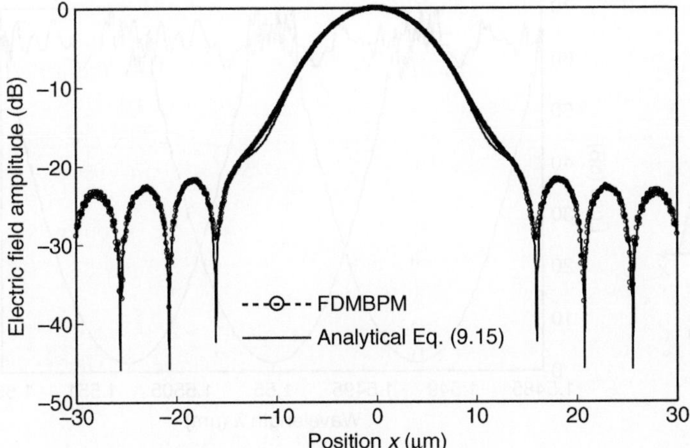

Figure 9.16 Electric field $|E(x)|$ obtained by the analytical equation (9.15) and the field calculated by FDMBPM. Sampling grid spacing in BPM is $\Delta x = 0.05\,\mu\text{m}$ and $\Delta z = 1.0\,\mu\text{m}$, respectively.

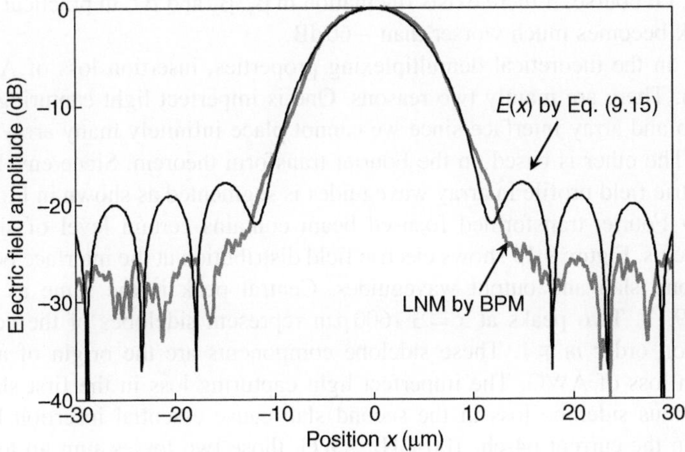

Figure 9.17 Comparison of focused electric field $|E(x)|$ on the output plane with the local normal mode (LNM) in the input waveguide.

$E(x)$ with the LNM of k-th output waveguide. Overlap integral is carried out by BPM, where initial field $E(x)$ is coupled into the taper waveguide of BPM simulation. In the numerical calculation, the entire input field $E(x)$ should be shifted by the amount of $\Delta x = -[N_c f \Delta L/(n_s d \lambda_0)]\Delta\lambda$ for the wavelength component $\lambda = \lambda_0 + \Delta\lambda$.

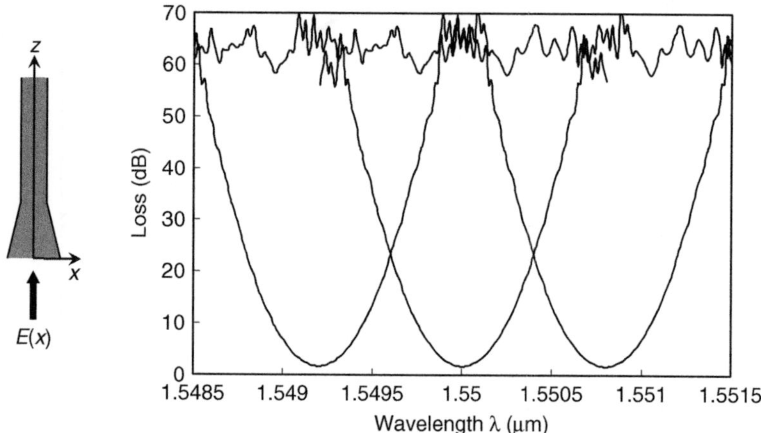

Figure 9.18 Theoretical demultiplexing properties of 64-ch, 100-GHz AWG.

Figure 9.18 shows the theoretical demultiplexing properties of 64-ch, 100-GHz AWG. Theoretical crosstalk of the current model of AWG is about $-60\,\text{dB}$. Of course, if there exists fluctuation in β_s, β_c and ΔL in practical AWG, crosstalk becomes much worser than $-60\,\text{dB}$.

Even in the theoretical demultiplexing properties, insertion loss of AWG is not zero. There are mainly two reasons. One is imperfect light capturing at the first slab and array interface since we cannot place infinitely many array waveguides. The other is based on the Fourier transform theorem. Since envelope of the electric field profile in array waveguides is segmented as shown in Fig. 9.11, spatially Fourier-transformed focused beam contains certain level of sidelobe components. Figure 9.19 shows electric field distribution at the interface between the second slab and output waveguides. Central peak is the same as $|E(x)|$ in Fig. 9.17. Two peaks at $x \cong \pm 1600\,\mu\text{m}$ represent sidelobes of the adjacent diffraction order $m \mp 1$. These sidelobe components are the origin of another insertion loss of AWG. The imperfect light capturing loss in the first slab and the spurious sidelobe loss in the second slab cause essential insertion loss of AWG. In the current 64-ch, 100-GHz AWG, those two losses sum up to about 1.7 dB as shown in Fig. 9.18.

9.3.3. Waveguide Layout of AWG

Figure 9.20 shows the schematic waveguide layout for AWG design. Each arm in the waveguide array consists of two straight waveguides of variable length on both sides and they are smoothly connected to a nonconcentric waveguide bend. The parameters to be determined are angle of slab $\alpha(=\angle PQQ')$ and the

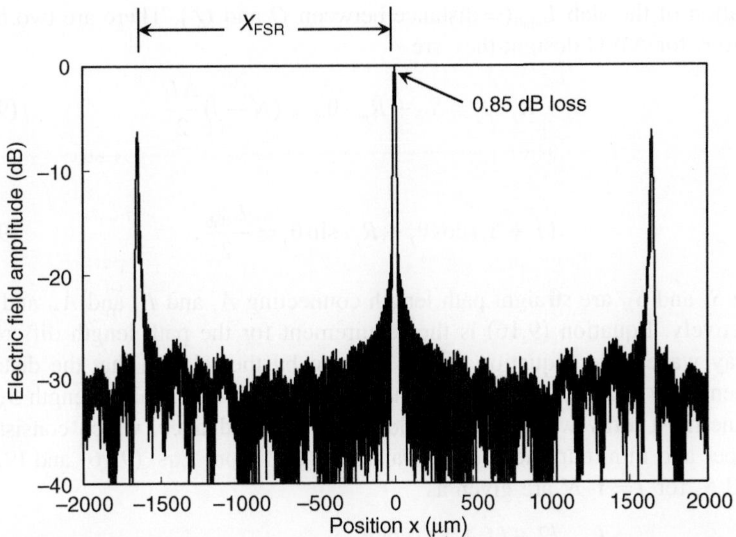

Figure 9.19 Electric field distribution at the interface between the second slab and output waveguides.

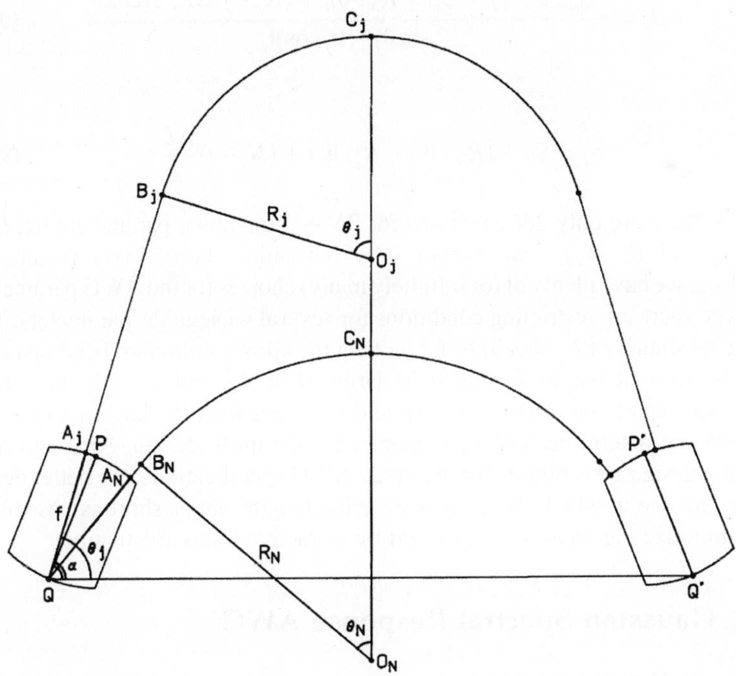

Figure 9.20 Schematic waveguide layout for AWG design.

separation of the slab L_{slab}(= distance between Q and Q'). There are two basic equations for AWG design; they are

$$S_j + R_j \cdot \theta_j = S_N + R_N \cdot \theta_N + (N - j)\frac{\Delta L}{2} \quad (9.16)$$

and

$$(f + S_j)\cos\theta_j + R_j \cdot \sin\theta_j = \frac{L_{slab}}{2}, \quad (9.17)$$

where S_j and S_N are straight path length connecting A_j and B_j and A_N and B_N, respectively. Equation (9.16) is the requirement for the path length difference of array waveguide. Equation (9.17) is given by the relation that the distance between point Q and the center line should be $L_{slab}/2$. The straight length S_N for the innermost array waveguide should be given in advance, which consists of the taper and minimum necessary straight length. From Eqs. (9.16) and (9.17), R_j and S_j for $j = 1$–N are given as

$$R_N = \frac{L_{slab}/2 - (f + S_N)\cos\theta_N}{\sin\theta_N}, \quad (9.18)$$

$$R_j = \frac{L_{slab}/2 - [f + S_N + R_N \cdot \theta_N + (N - j)\Delta L/2]\cos\theta_j}{\sin\theta_j - \theta_j\cos\theta_j} \quad (9.19)$$

and

$$S_j = S_N + (R_N \cdot \theta_N - R_j \cdot \theta_j) + (N - j)\frac{\Delta L}{2}. \quad (9.20)$$

Since there are only $2N$ equations for $2N + 1$ unknown parameters (α, L_{slab}, S_1–S_{N-1} and R_1–R_N), we cannot fully determine these AWG parameters. Therefore, we have plenty of (or infinitely many) choices for the AWG parameters. However, there are restricting conditions for several waveguide parameters; they are, the minimum of R_j should be larger than the known minimum bending radius R_{min}, the straight length S_j should be larger than S_N, and the minimum array waveguide separation at the center should be larger than the known value S_{min}. Then we can determine AWG parameters for the mask design. Although there are many design possibilities for the given AWG specifications, the better design may be the one in which the array waveguide lengths are as short as possible so as to minimize the phase errors caused by refractive-index fluctuations.

9.3.4. Gaussian Spectral Response AWG

Gaussian AWG denotes that the frequency response is Gaussian shape and not flat response. Figure 9.21 shows the waveguide layout of 32-ch, 100-GHz-

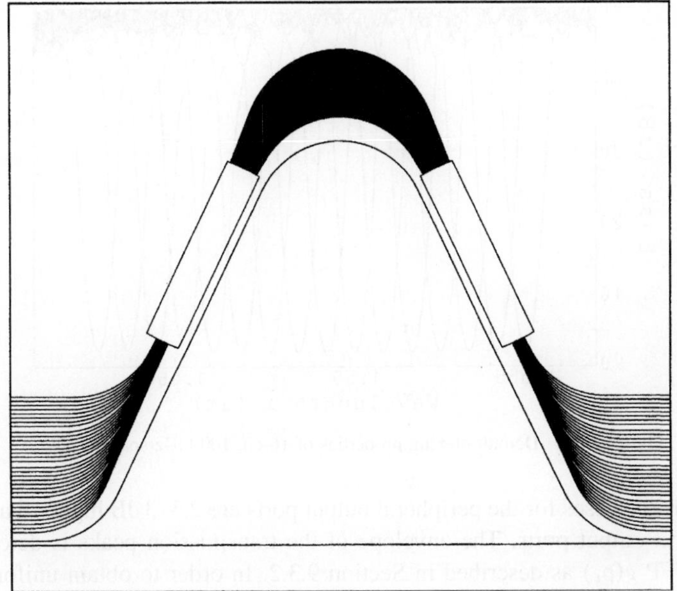

Figure 9.21 waveguide layout of 32-ch, 100-GHz-spacing AWG.

spacing AWG. It consists of 32 input/output waveguides, slab regions with arc length of 11.35 mm and waveguide array of 100-ch waveguides with the constant path length difference ΔL between neighboring waveguides. The path length difference ΔL is 63 μm; the corresponding grating order at $\lambda_0 = 1.55$ μm is $m = 59$, which gives a free spectral range of 25.6 nm (3.2 THz) and a channel spacing of 0.8 nm (100 GHz). Each arm in waveguide array consists of two straight waveguides of variable length on both sides and they are smoothly connected to a non-concentric waveguide bend. The core size and refractive-index difference between the channel waveguides are 7 μm × 7 μm and 0.75%, respectively. The bending radius in the array varies from 5 mm to 6.3 mm and the minimum waveguide separation is 30 μm. The total device size is 30 μm × 26 μm. Various kinds of multiplexers ranging from 50-nm spacing 8-channel AWG to 25-GHz spacing AWG have been fabricated [17–19]. Figure 9.22 shows the measured loss spectra of 16-ch, 100-GHz $(N_{\text{system}} = 16)$ AWG when light from tunable laser is coupled into central input port. Here N_{system} is the channel number which is required from a WDM system. On the other hand, the total number of channels N_{ch} of AWG itself is 32 $(N_{\text{system}} = 0.5 \times N_{\text{ch}})$. The relation of N_{system} to N_{ch} will be described in the following discussion. Crosstalks of AWG, which is defined by the light leakage at the center of the neighboring channel, are about −40 dB. Figure 9.23 shows the measured transmission spectra of 32-ch, 50-GHz-spacing AWG over four diffraction orders. As explained by the BPM simulations in Figs. 9.10(a) and

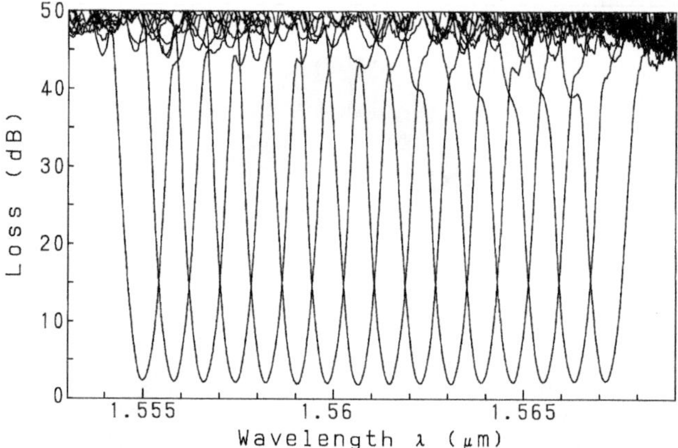

Figure 9.22 Demultiplexing properties of 16-ch, 100-GHz-spacing AWG.

(b), insertion losses for the peripheral output ports are 2.5–3 dB higher than those for central output ports. The envelope of the transmission peaks is determined by the FFP $g(\rho_k)$ as described in Section 9.3.2. In order to obtain uniform loss characteristics in WDM system applications, the total number of channels N_{ch} of AWG should be larger than the channel number N_{system} of the system. Number of output ports N_{system} is usually about $(0.5 \sim 0.6) \times N_{ch}$ to guarantee loss variation of less than 1 dB.

Figure 9.24 shows the demultiplexing properties of 64-ch, 50-GHz-spacing AWG. Crosstalks of about −40 dB have been achieved in 64-ch, 50-GHz spacing

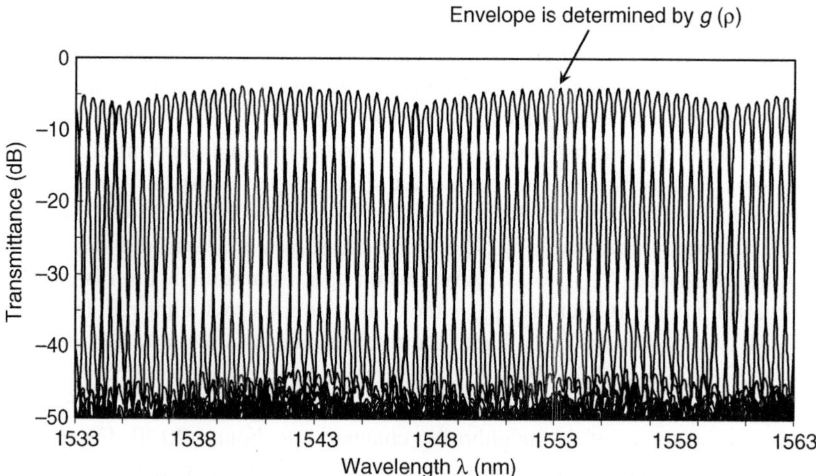

Figure 9.23 Demultiplexing properties of 32-ch, 50-GHz-spacing AWG over four diffraction orders.

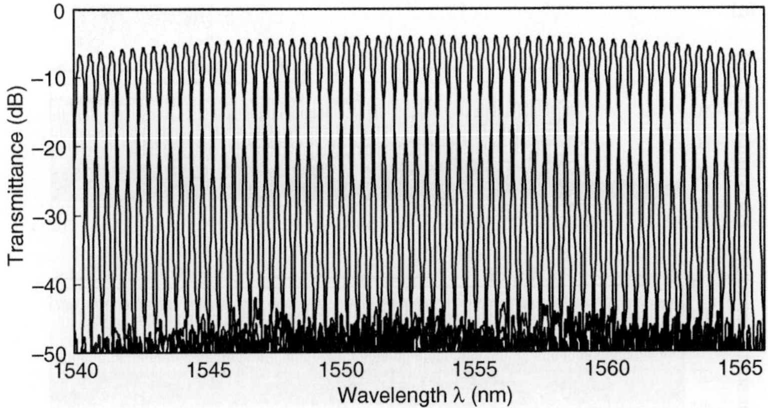

Figure 9.24 Demultiplexing properties of 64-ch-50-GHz-spacing AWG.

AWG. By the improvement of the fabrication technology and the optimization of the waveguide configurations, good crosstalk characteristics have been achieved even in 10–25 GHz spacing AWGs, as shown in Figs. 9.25 and 9.26. Superhigh-Δ waveguide with refractive-index difference of 1.5% was used in 400-ch, 25-GHz AWG so as to minimize the area of array waveguide region. The adjacent channel crosstalk and background crosstalk were less than −20 dB and −30 dB, respectively. Figure 9.25(b) shows a single channel demultiplexing property at the central output port. The inset of the figure shows close-up demultiplexing properties for the three output ports. Figure 9.26 shows the demultiplexing properties of 32-ch, 10-GHz-spacing AWG without using a post process for the phase-error (non-uniformity in the optical path length difference $n_c\Delta L$) compensation. Here the high-Δ waveguide with refractive-index difference of 0.75% was used. Adjacent channel crosstalk of about −30 dB has been achieved even in the 10-GHz spacing AWG. Phase-error compensation technique can further improve the crosstalk of AWGs. It will be described in Section 9.5.8.

9.3.5. Polarization Dependence of Pass Wavelength

Polarization dependence of pass wavelength in AWG is mainly determined by the birefringence of the waveguide. Center wavelength of the passband is expressed by Eq. (9.2) as $\lambda_0 = n_c\Delta L/m$. When effective indices for TE and TM modes are different, it causes polarization-dependent pass wavelength difference, which is given by

$$\delta\lambda = \lambda_{\rm TE} - \lambda_{\rm TM} = \frac{[n_c({\rm TE}) - n_c({\rm TM})]}{m}\Delta L. \tag{9.21}$$

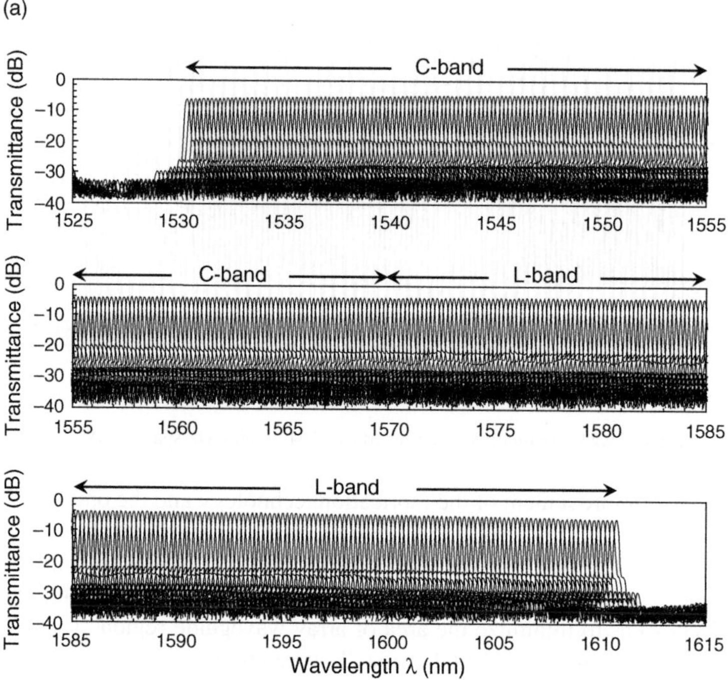

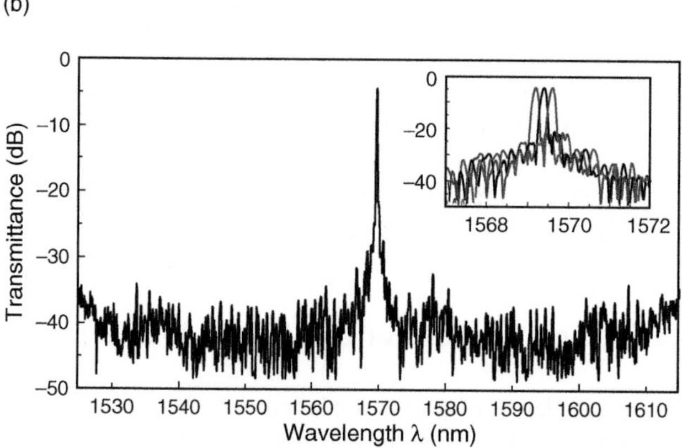

Figure 9.25 (a) Demultiplexing properties of 400-ch-25-GHz-spacing AWG. (b) Single channel demultiplexing property at the central output port. The inset of the figure shows a close-up of demultiplexing properties for the three output ports.

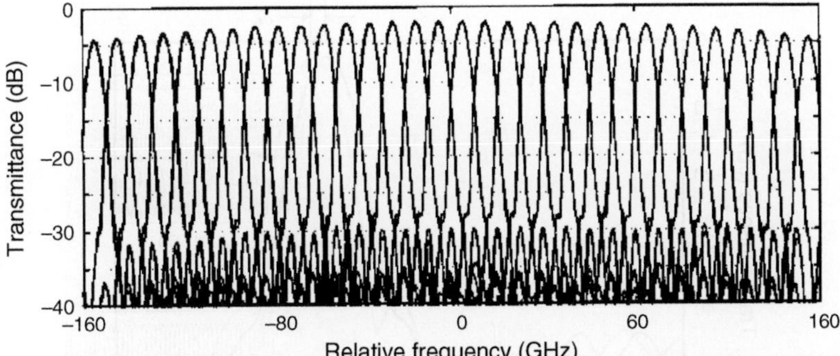

Figure 9.26 Demultiplexing properties of 32-ch, 10-GHz-spacing AWG without using a post process for the phase-error compensation.

Here $\delta\lambda$ is called PDλ (polarization dependent λ). Birefringence of the waveguide in silica PLC is mainly caused by the stress anisotropy along x and y directions. Then, PDλ is expressed by using Eqs. (9.21) and (3.240) as

$$\delta\lambda = C \cdot (\sigma_x - \sigma_y) \cdot \frac{\Delta L}{m}, \tag{9.22}$$

where $C = 3.36 \times 10^{-5}\left(\text{mm}^2/\text{kg wt}\right)$, σ_x and σ_y are stress in the core center along x and y directions, respectively. In the normal silica on silicon waveguide, both σ_x and σ_y are negative and $|\sigma_x| > |\sigma_y|$. Then, $\delta\lambda$ is negative ($\lambda_{\text{TE}} < \lambda_{\text{TM}}$) in the normal AWG. Figure 9.27 shows the polarization-dependent pass wavelength difference in AWG using silica core and silicon substrate. PDλ is normally of the order of 0.1–0.2 nm.

Figure 9.28(a) shows an under-cladding ridge structure to eliminate the PDλ of AWG [20]. When we etch the core ridge structure excessively down into the under-cladding region, we can change the magnitude of σ_x and σ_y in and around the core region. At the proper excess-etching depth d, we can eliminate the stress difference between σ_x and σ_y. Since the origin of σ_x is the contraction of the silicon substrate, which acts through the under-cladding layer, σ_x will decrease with an increase in the ridge height. On the other hand, since the origin of σ_y is the contraction of the over-cladding, σ_y will increase with an increase in the ridge height. Figure 9.28(b) shows the transmission spectra of an AWG with $d = 3\,\mu\text{m}$. Here, we used high-Δ waveguide with $6 \times 6\,\mu\text{m}^2$ core and $\Delta = 0.75\%$. The transmission spectra for both polarizations overlap almost completely. PDλ of less than 0.01 nm is successfully obtained at $d = 3\,\mu\text{m}$. The insertion loss is about 2.5 dB, and the background crosstalk is less than −40 dB. These results mean that there is no degradation in the optical characteristics when we incorporate the under-cladding ridge structure in the AWGs.

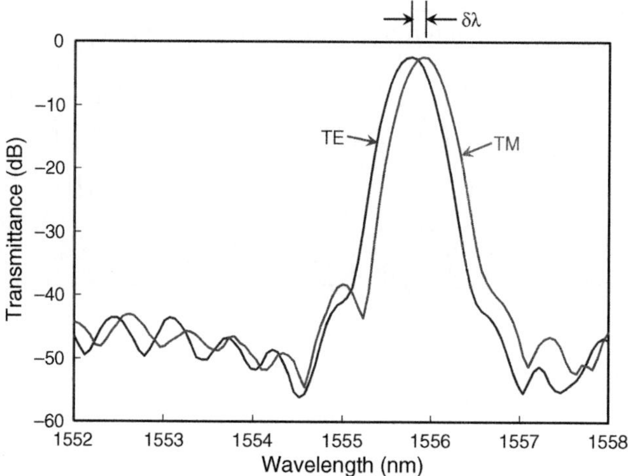

Figure 9.27 Polarization dependent pass wavelength difference in the normal AWG using silica core and silicon substrate.

9.3.6. Vernier Technique for the Center Wavelength Adjustment

When some of the waveguide parameters in the first slab (D_1, d_1 and f_1) and those in the second slab region (D, d and f) are different, the channel spacing $\Delta\lambda_{out}$ becomes different from $\Delta\lambda_{in}$ as shown in Eqs. (9.7) and (9.8). Putting

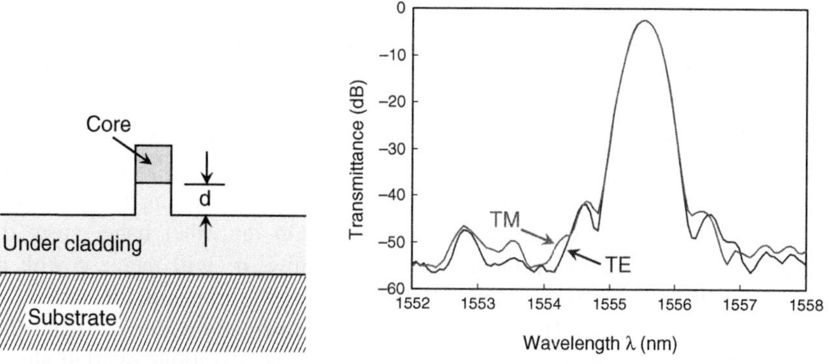

Figure 9.28 (a) Under-cladding ridge structure in the polarization-insensitive AWG. (b) Demultiplexing properties of the AWG using under-cladding ridge structure. (After Ref. [20]).

$x_1 = jD_1$ and $x = jD(j = \pm 1, \pm 2, \pm 3, \ldots)$ in Eq. (9.2), it can be rewritten as

$$n_s(\lambda) j \left(\frac{d_1 D_1}{f_1} - \frac{dD}{f} \right) + n_c(\lambda) \Delta L = m\lambda. \tag{9.23}$$

The above equation is satisfied with the following center wavelength

$$\lambda = \lambda_0 + j \frac{N_c}{n_c} \left(\frac{d_1 D_1 f}{dD f_1} - 1 \right) \Delta\lambda_{\text{out}}, \tag{9.24}$$

where we used Eq. (9.9). Equation (9.24) indicates that the center pass wavelength of AWG can be tuned up or down by choosing the proper j-th input–output pair. Such vernier design was demonstrated [21] in those cases where input and output waveguide separations D_1 and D were different while $d_1 = d$, and $f_1 = f$. Vernier AWG can compensate for the possible center wavelength shift due to the slight fabrication error in waveguide parameters n_c and ΔL. Vernier AWG can also be realized by changing at least one of the waveguide parameters in the first slab (D_1, d_1 and f_1) and those in the second slab region (D, d, and f). Figure 9.29 shows the measured center wavelengths in 32-ch, 100-GHz AWG having array-side vernier. The input and output waveguide separations in array-side vernier AWG was $d_1 = 18\,\mu\text{m}$ and $d = 20\,\mu\text{m}$ while $D_1 = D = 25\,\mu\text{m}$ and $f_1 = f = 13.7\,\text{mm}$. The straight line in Fig. 9.29 indicates the vernier line for the center path wavelengths. For the $1 \times N$ wavelength filter applications, the vernier technique is quite effective in compensating the possible fabrication errors in center wavelength of AWG.

9.4. CROSSTALK AND DISPERSION CHARACTERISTICS OF AWGs

9.4.1. Crosstalk of AWGs

Crosstalk of AWG is attributed to the phase and amplitude fluctuations in the entire electric field profile at the output side array–slab interface since the focused beam profile at the output plane is the spatial Fourier transform of the electric field in the array waveguides. Amplitude and/or phase fluctuations in the entire electric field profile cause imperfect focused beam profile in which sidelobe level becomes higher than that of Fig. 9.16. Then, the crosstalk level becomes much worse than $-60\,\text{dB}$ as shown in Fig. 9.18. The amplitude fluctuation is caused by non-uniformity in the array waveguides. The phase fluctuation is actually an optical path length fluctuation in each array waveguide. It is caused by the non-uniformity in refractive indices and core geometries in the array waveguide region.

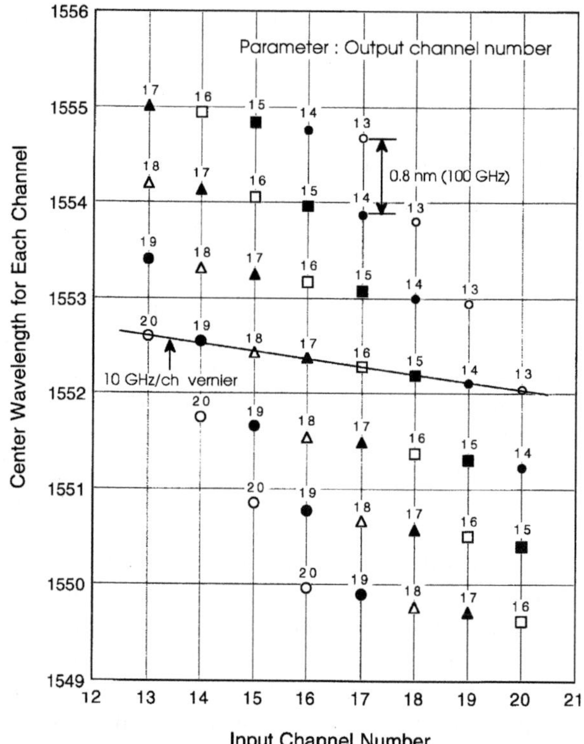

Figure 9.29 Center wavelengths in array-side vernier AWG.

First, the influence of amplitude fluctuation will be investigated. For simplicity, the sinusoidal amplitude fluctuation with the amplitude δc and the half period of fluctuation Λ is assumed. The actual fluctuation may be expressed by the summation of series of sinusoidal fluctuations with different period Λ. The focused electric field under a single sinusoidal amplitude fluctuation is given from Eq. (9.15) as

$$E(x) = \sum_{\ell=1}^{N} \left[c(\ell) + \delta c \cdot \sin\left(\ell \frac{\pi}{\Lambda}\right) \right] \exp[-j\Omega(\ell)]. \tag{9.25}$$

Figure 9.30 shows the envelope of the entire electric field profile at the output side array–slab interface with a sinusoidal amplitude fluctuation of $\delta_c = 0.095$ and $\Lambda = N/5$. Demultiplexing properties of AWG having fluctuation can be obtained in a similar manner to those described in Section 9.3.2.

Figures 9.31(a) and (b) show the demultiplexing properties of AWGs having sinusoidal amplitude fluctuations of $\delta_c = 0.0095$, 0.03 and 0.095 with $\Lambda = N/5$ for

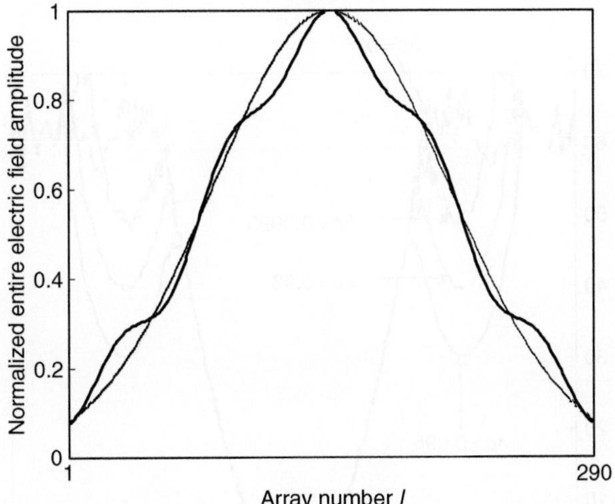

Figure 9.30 Envelope of the entire electric field profile at the output side array–slab interface with a sinusoidal amplitude fluctuation of $\delta c = 0.095$ and $\Lambda = N/5$.

two kinds of AWGs with 100-GHz and 25-GHz channel spacing. Location of the crosstalk degradation depends on the spatial frequency $2\pi/\Lambda$ of the fluctuation. Sidelobe peak goes far from the passband center when spatial frequency $2\pi/\Lambda$ increases. It is known that crosstalk degrades by about 10 dB when δc becomes 3.2 ($\sqrt{10}$) times larger. Also, it is known from these figures that the sidelobe level does not depend on the channel spacing.

Next, the influence of phase fluctuation will be investigated. Here, the sinusoidal effective-index fluctuation with the amplitude δn and the half period of fluctuation Λ is assumed. Actual fluctuation may be expressed by the summation of series of sinusoidal fluctuations with different half period Λ. The focused electric field under a single sinusoidal effective-index fluctuation is given from Eqs. (9.15) as

$$E(x) = \sum_{\ell=1}^{N} c(\ell) \exp[-j\Omega(\ell)], \tag{9.26a}$$

$$\begin{aligned}\Omega(\ell) &= \beta_s \left(\hat{L}_{i,\ell} + L_{\ell,k}\right) + (N-\ell)\beta_c \Delta L = \beta_s \left(\hat{L}_{i,\ell} + L_{\ell,k}\right) \\ &\quad + (N-\ell)\frac{2\pi}{\lambda}\left[n_c(\ell) + \delta n \cdot \sin\left(\ell \frac{\pi}{\Lambda}\right)\right]\Delta L.\end{aligned} \tag{9.26b}$$

Figures 9.32 (a) and (b) show the focused electric field profile at the output plane and the demultiplexing properties in the 100-GHz spacing AWG having sinusoidal phase fluctuation of $\delta n = 5 \times 10^{-5}$ and $\Lambda = N/2$. When spatial frequency

(a)

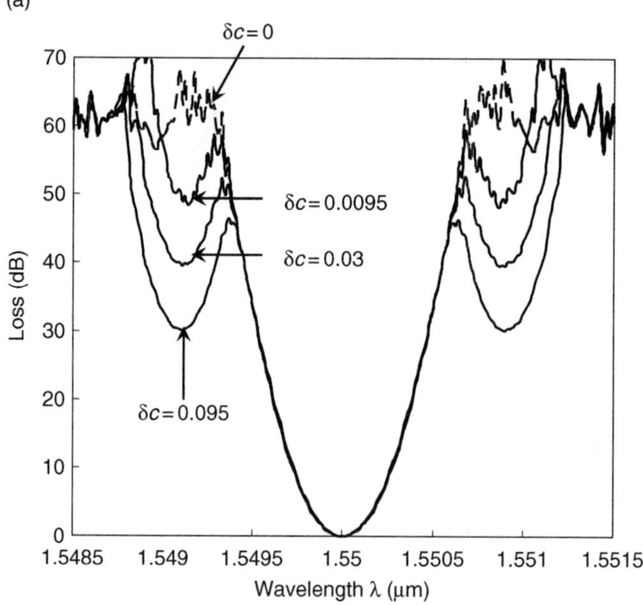

(b)

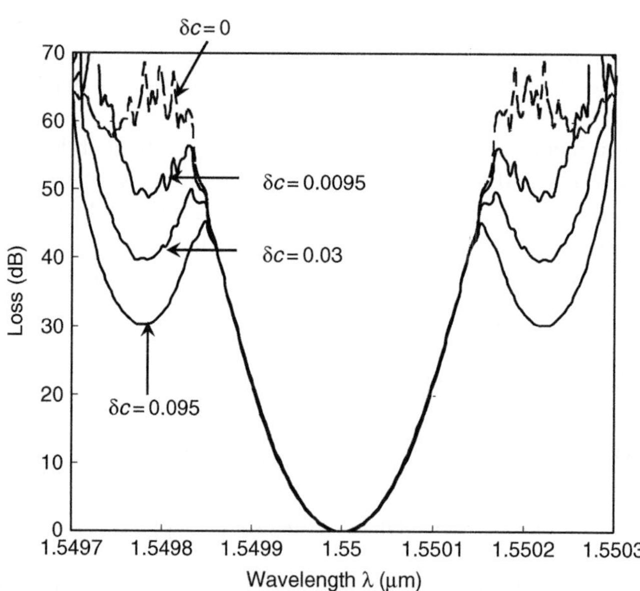

Figure 9.31 Demultiplexing properties of AWGs having sinusoidal amplitude fluctuations of $\delta c = 0.0095, 0.03$ and 0.095 with $\Lambda = N/5$ for two kinds of AWGs with (a) 100-GHz and (b) 25-GHz channel spacings.

(a)

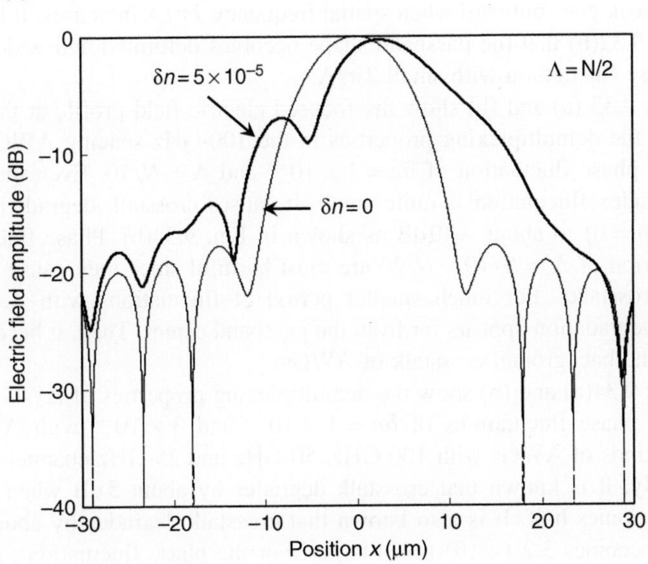

(b)

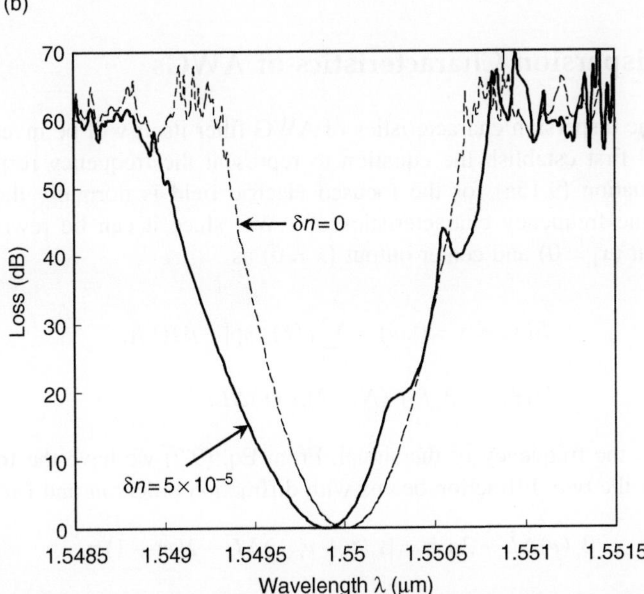

Figure 9.32 (a) The focused electric field profile at the output plane and (b) the demultiplexing properties in the 100-GHz-spacing AWG having sinusoidal phase fluctuation of $\delta n = 5 \times 10^{-5}$ and $\Lambda = N/2$.

of the fluctuation $2\pi/\Lambda$ is small, influence appears near the passband center. Sidelobe peak goes outward when spatial frequency $2\pi/\Lambda$ increases. It is known from Fig. 9.32(b) that the passband shape becomes deformed and widened due to the phase fluctuation with small $2\pi/\Lambda$.

Figures 9.33 (a) and (b) show the focused electric field profile at the output plane and the demultiplexing properties in the 100-GHz spacing AWG having sinusoidal phase fluctuation of $\delta n = 1 \times 10^{-6}$ and $\Lambda = N/10$. Even though the effective-index fluctuation is quite small, it causes crosstalk degradation from -60 dB($\delta n = 0$) to about -40 dB as shown in Fig. 9.33(b). Phase fluctuations having period of $\Lambda \approx N/10 \sim N/20$ are most harmful since they cause adjacent channel crosstalks. For much smaller period of fluctuations with $\Lambda < N/20$, crosstalk degradation appears far from the passband center. Then, it becomes the origin of the background crosstalk of AWGs.

Figures 9.34(a) and (b) show the demultiplexing properties of AWGs having sinusoidal phase fluctuations of $\delta n = 1 \times 10^{-6}$ and 3×10^{-7} with $\Lambda = N/10$ for three kinds of AWGs with 100-GHz, 50-GHz and 25-GHz channel spacing, respectively. It is known that crosstalk degrades by about 5 dB when channel spacing becomes half. It is also known that crosstalk degrades by about 10 dB when δn becomes 3.2 ($\sqrt{10}$) times larger. For the phase fluctuations, sidelobe level strongly depends on the channel spacing.

9.4.2. Dispersion Characteristics of AWGs

Next, the dispersion characteristics of AWG filter itself will be investigated. We should first establish the equation to represent the frequency response of AWG. Equation (9.15a) for the focused electric field is normally thought to represent the frequency characteristics of AWG since it can be rewritten for center input ($x_1 = 0$) and center output ($x = 0$) as

$$E(x_1 = x = 0, \nu) = \sum_{\ell=1}^{N} c(\ell) \exp[-j\Omega(\ell)], \tag{9.27a}$$

$$\Omega(\ell) = 2\beta_s f + (N - \ell)\beta_c(\nu)\Delta L, \tag{9.27b}$$

where ν is the frequency of the signal. From Eq. (9.2) we have the following relation for the two diffraction beams with diffraction orders m and $(m+1)$ as

$$\beta_c(\nu)\Delta L - 2m\pi = \beta_c(\nu + \nu_{FSR})\Delta L - 2(m+1)\pi, \tag{9.28}$$

where ν_{FSR} is a free spectral range (FSR). ν_{FSR} is obtained from Eq. (9.28) as

$$\nu_{FSR} = \frac{n_c}{N_c} \cdot \frac{\nu_0}{m}, \tag{9.29}$$

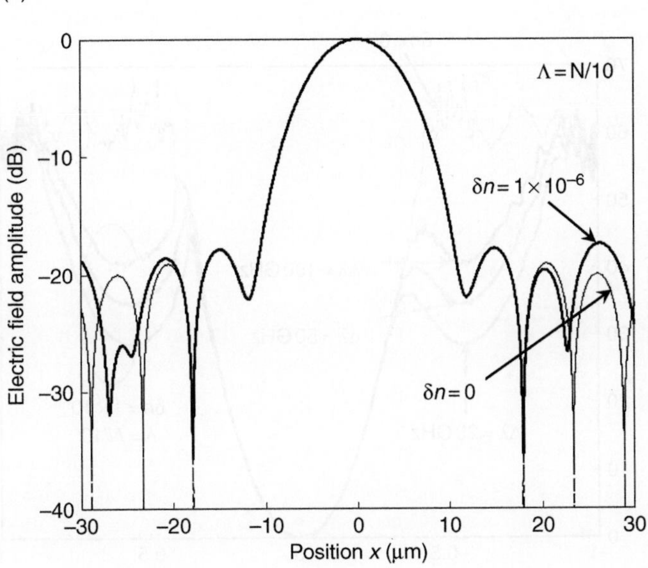

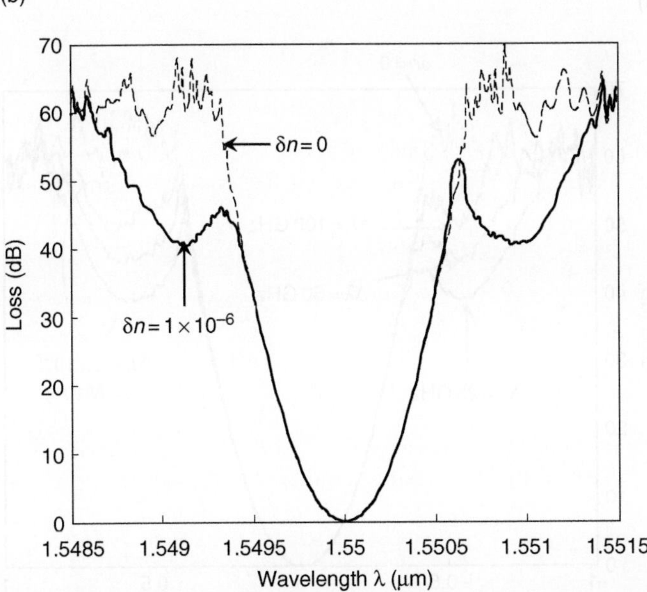

Figure 9.33 (a) The focused electric field profile at the output plane and (b) the demultiplexing properties in the 100-GHz spacing AWG having sinusoidal phase fluctuation of $\delta n = 1 \times 10^{-6}$ and $\Lambda = N/10$.

(a)

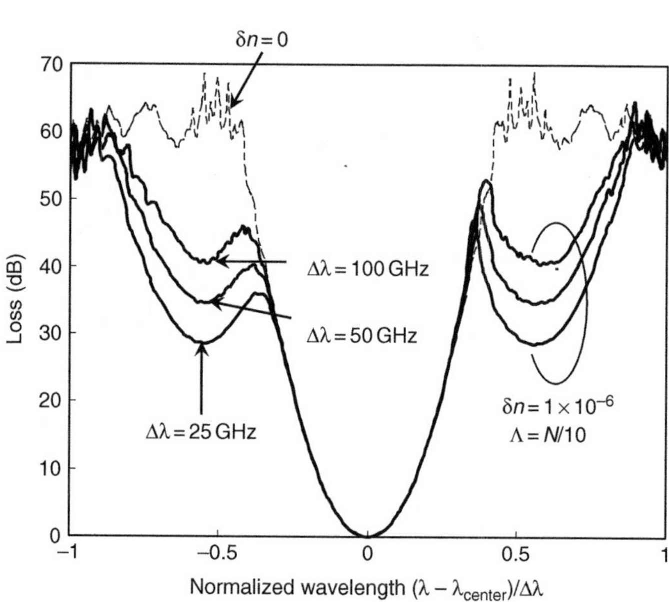

(b)

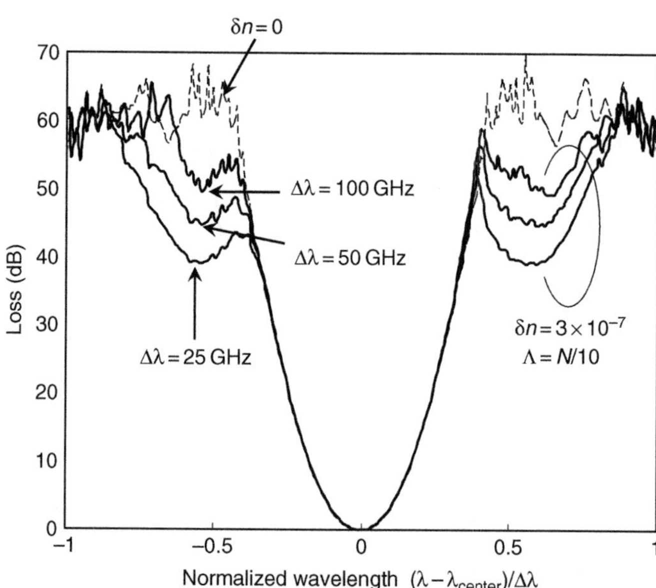

Figure 9.34 Demultiplexing properties of AWGs having sinusoidal phase fluctuations of (a) $\delta n = 1 \times 10^{-6}$ (b) $\delta n = 3 \times 10^{-7}$ with $\Lambda = N/10$ for three kinds of AWGs with 100-GHz, 50-GHz and 25-GHz channel spacings.

where ν_0 is the center frequency $(= c/\lambda_0)$. ν_{FSR} is also expressed by using Eqs. (9.3) and (9.29) as

$$\nu_{\mathrm{FSR}} = \frac{c}{N_c \Delta L}. \tag{9.30}$$

The above equation is a universal expression of FSR in the PLC interference device which has a path length difference of ΔL (see Eq. (4.166a)). $\beta_c(\nu)\Delta L$ in Eq. (9.27b) can be rewritten by using the above equation as

$$\beta_c(\nu)\Delta L = \frac{2\pi\nu n_c}{c}\Delta L = 2\pi \frac{n_c}{N_c}\frac{\nu}{\nu_{\mathrm{FSR}}} \cong 2\pi \frac{\nu}{\nu_{\mathrm{FSR}}}. \tag{9.31}$$

Here we assumed $n_c/N_c \cong 1$ since $N_c =_{n_c} -\lambda_{n_c}/d\lambda \cong 1.016 n_c$ in silica PLC at 1.55-μm wavelength region. Then, Eq. (9.27a) reduces to

$$E(x_1 = x = 0, \nu) = e^{-j2\beta_s f} \sum_{\ell=1}^{N} c(\ell) \exp\left[-j(N-\ell)2\pi \frac{\nu}{\nu_{\mathrm{FSR}}}\right]. \tag{9.32}$$

Since frequency dependence of the term $\exp[-j2\beta_s(\nu)f]$ in the above equation can be neglected when compared to that of the second term, the frequency characteristics of AWG can be expressed by

$$E(\nu) = \sum_{\ell=1}^{N} c(\ell) \exp\left[-j(N-\ell)2\pi \frac{\nu}{\nu_{\mathrm{FSR}}}\right]. \tag{9.33}$$

Validity of the above equation should be first examined by comparing its frequency response with that of the numerical overlap integral described in Section 9.3.2. Figure 9.35 compares the frequency responses of Gaussian AWG calculated by the numerical overlap integral with the analytical frequency response by using Eq. (9.33). It is known that the analytical frequency response well approximates the Gaussian AWG response around the passband center. Since we are interested in the frequency characteristics of AWG around the passband center, it is confirmed that Eq. (9.33) can be used to investigate the frequency response and dispersion characteristics of Gaussian AWGs.

Next, validity of Eq. (9.33) to the flat spectral response AWG will be examined. Principle of operation in the flat spectral response AWG will be described in Section 9.5.1. We can apply numerical overlap integral described in Section 9.3.2 to the flat AWG. Figure 9.36 compares the frequency responses of sinc-type flat AWG [22] calculated by the numerical overlap integral with the analytical frequency response by using Eq. (9.33). Though agreement is not so well as that for the Gaussian AWG, we can utilize Eq. (9.33) to investigate the frequency response and dispersion characteristics of flat AWG. We should bear in mind

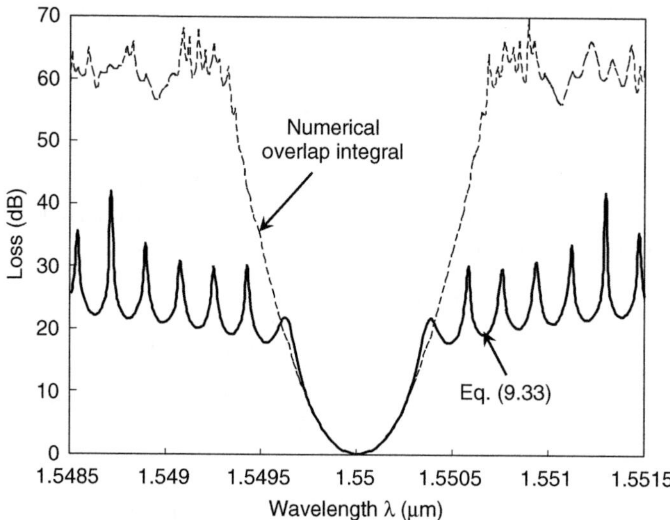

Figure 9.35 Comparison of the frequency response of Gaussian AWG calculated by the numerical overlap integral with the response by using Eq. (9.33).

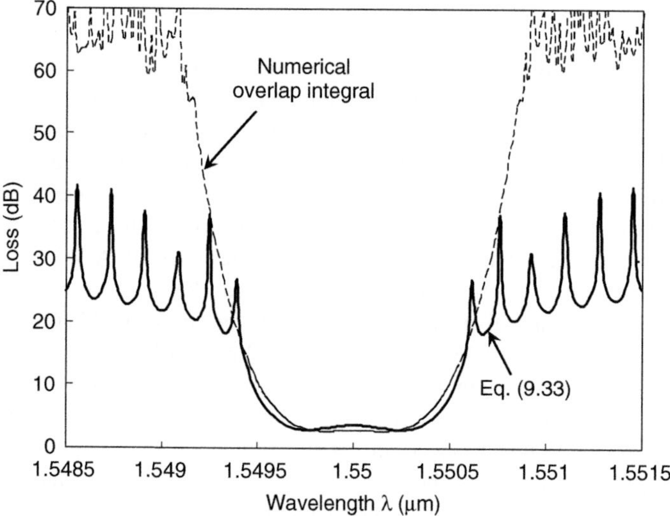

Figure 9.36 Comparison of the frequency responses of sinc-type flat AWG calculated by the numerical overlap integral with the analytical frequency response by using Eq. (9.33).

that the frequency response obtained by Eq. (9.33) has slight error when we apply it to the flat AWGs.

Generally, delay time τ of the transmission medium is given by

$$\tau = -\frac{1}{2\pi}\frac{d}{d\nu}[\arg(E)] = -\frac{1}{2\pi}\text{Im}\left[\frac{E'(\nu)}{E(\nu)}\right], \tag{9.34}$$

where $E(\nu)$ is a frequency response of the medium and Im[ ] denotes the imaginary part of the argument. Chromatic dispersion σ is obtained by differentiating τ with respect to the wavelength λ (refer to Eqs. (3.118) and (3.143)) as

$$\sigma = \frac{d\tau}{d\lambda}. \tag{9.35}$$

Dispersion of AWG is then obtained by putting the frequency response $E(\nu)$ (Eq. (9.33)) into Eqs. (9.34) and (9.35).

First, dispersion of AWG without any amplitude or phase fluctuations is investigated. Figure 9.37 shows the chromatic dispersion characteristics of 64-ch, 100-GHz Gaussian AWG without having any amplitude or phase fluctuations. It is known that there is no (within the accuracy of the numerical analysis) dispersion in Gaussian AWG. Contrary to Gaussian AWGs, some types of flat response AWGs have intrinsic dispersions based on the mechanism of passband broadening. Dispersions in flat AWGs will be described in Section 9.5.1.

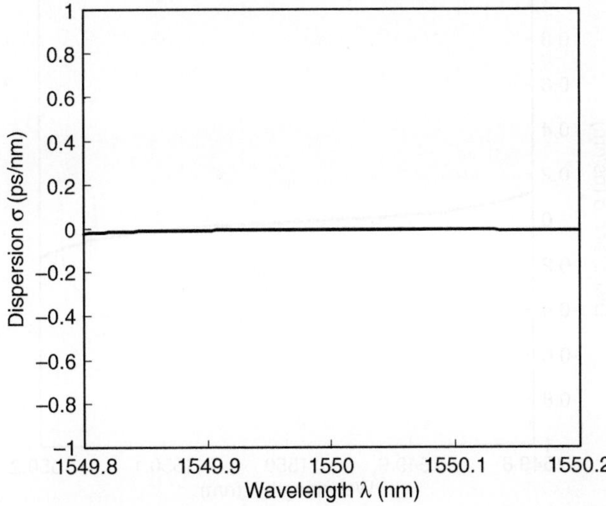

Figure 9.37 Chromatic dispersion characteristics of 64-ch, 100-GHz Gaussian AWG without having any amplitude or phase fluctuations.

Next, dispersion caused by the amplitude fluctuations in array waveguides will be investigated. Similar to the analysis in Section 9.4.1, the frequency response of AWG having sinusoidal amplitude fluctuation with the amplitude δc and half period Λ is expressed by using Eq. (9.33) as

$$E(\nu)=\sum_{\ell=1}^{N}\left[c(\ell)+\delta c\cdot\sin\left(\ell\frac{\pi}{\Lambda}\right)\right]\exp\left[-j(N-\ell)2\pi\frac{\nu}{\nu_{\mathrm{FSR}}}\right]. \tag{9.36}$$

Chromatic dispersion characteristics of 64-ch, 100-GHz Gaussian AWG having sinusoidal amplitude fluctuation with the amplitude $\delta c=0.03$ and half period $\Lambda=N/5$ are shown in Fig. 9.38. It is known that the amplitude fluctuation in the array waveguides does not cause any substantial dispersion in AWGs.

Next, dispersion caused by the phase fluctuations in array waveguides will be investigated. Frequency response of AWG having sinusoidal phase fluctuation with the amplitude δn and half period Λ is expressed by using Eqs. (9.26) and (9.33) by

$$E(\nu)=\sum_{\ell=1}^{N}c(\ell)\exp\left[-j(N-\ell)\left(2\pi\frac{\nu}{\nu_{\mathrm{FSR}}}+\phi_{\ell}\right)\right], \tag{9.37a}$$

$$\phi_{\ell}=2\pi\frac{\nu}{\nu_{\mathrm{FSR}}}\frac{\delta n}{n_c}\sin\left(\ell\frac{\pi}{\Lambda}\right). \tag{9.37b}$$

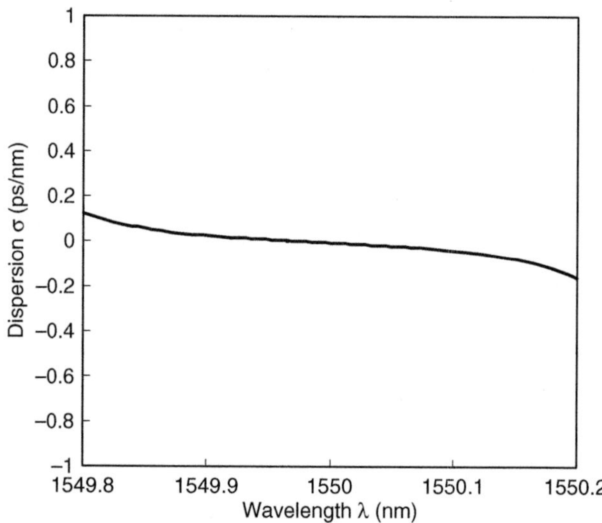

Figure 9.38 Chromatic dispersion characteristics of 64-ch, 100-GHz Gaussian AWG having sinusoidal amplitude fluctuation with the amplitude $\delta c=0.03$ and half period $\Lambda=N/5$.

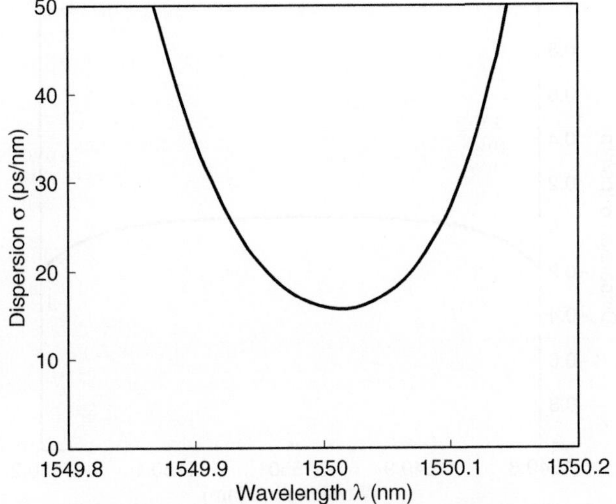

Figure 9.39 Chromatic dispersion characteristics of 64-ch, 100-GHz Gaussian AWG having phase fluctuation with the amplitude $\delta n = 2 \times 10^{-5}$ and half period of $\Lambda = N/3$.

Putting Eq. (9.37) into (9.35) gives us dispersion characteristics of AWG having phase fluctuations. Figure 9.39 shows the chromatic dispersion characteristics of 64-ch, 100-GHz Gaussian AWG having phase fluctuation with the amplitude $\delta n = 2 \times 10^{-5}$ and half period of $\Lambda = N/3$. Chromatic dispersion caused by the phase fluctuation depends on the type of fluctuations. Though, phase fluctuation with $\delta n = 2 \times 10^{-5}$ and $\Lambda = N/3$ brings dispersion $\sigma \sim 16\,\text{ps/nm}$, fluctuation with $\delta n = 5 \times 10^{-5}$ and $\Lambda = N$ causes dispersion $\sigma \sim -16\,\text{ps/nm}$. Since the influence of fluctuation goes far from the central passband for the higher spatial frequency component (smaller period Λ), dispersion becomes negligible as shown in Fig. 9.40. Figure 9.40 shows the dispersion characteristics of AWG having phase fluctuation with the amplitude $\delta n = 1 \times 10^{-6}$ and half period $\Lambda = N/10$.

Finally, dependence of the dispersion σ on the channel spacing of AWG will be investigated. Dispersion characteristics of AWGs having phase fluctuations of $\delta n = 2.5 \times 10^{-6}$ with $\Lambda = N/3$ for three kinds of AWGs with 100-GHz, 50-GHz and 25-GHz channel spacing are shown in Figs. 9.41(a), (b) and (c), respectively. Dispersions at the passband center are 1.9 ps/nm, 16.1 ps/nm and 129.5 ps/nm for 100-GHz, 50-GHz and 25-GHz channel spacing, respectively. It is known from these results that dispersion becomes about 8 times larger when channel spacing becomes half. In other words, dispersion is proportional to $1/(\text{channel spacing})^3$. Therefore, quite strict effective-index control is required to keep dispersion small, especially in the narrow-spacing AWGs.

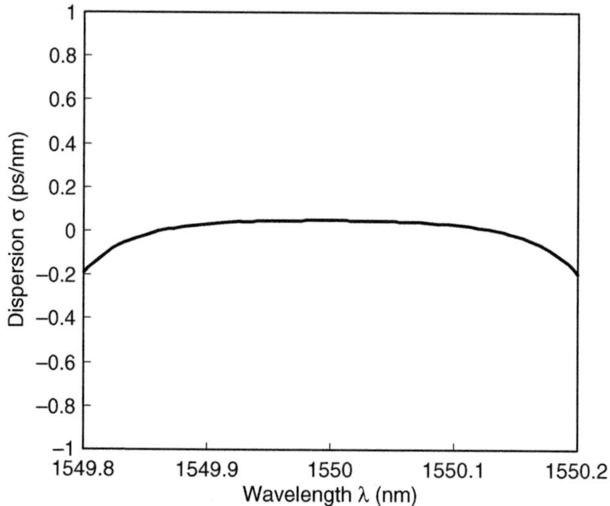

Figure 9.40 Chromatic dispersion characteristics of AWG having phase fluctuation with the amplitude $\delta n = 1 \times 10^{-6}$ and half period of $\Lambda = N/10$.

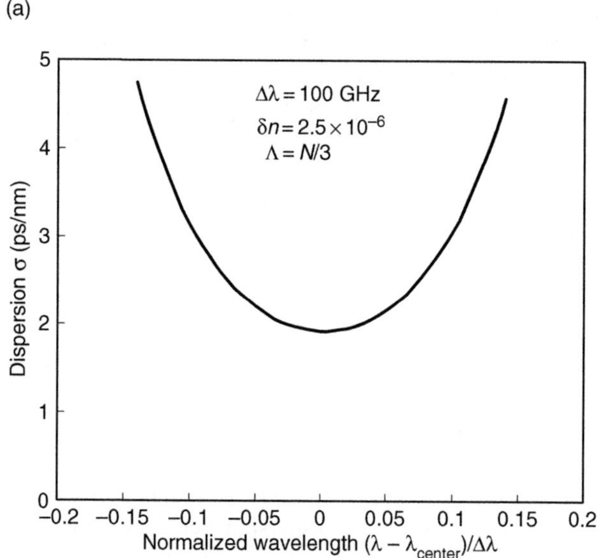

Figure 9.41 Chromatic dispersion characteristics of AWGs having phase fluctuations of $\delta n = 2.5 \times 10^{-6}$ with $\Lambda = N/3$ for three kinds of AWGs with (a) 100-GHz.

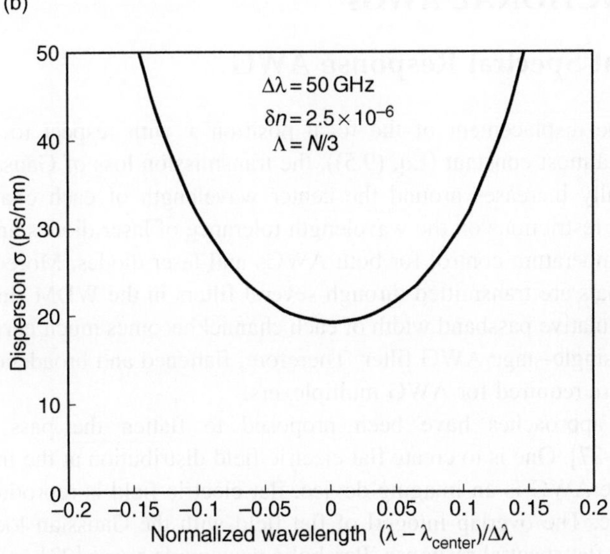

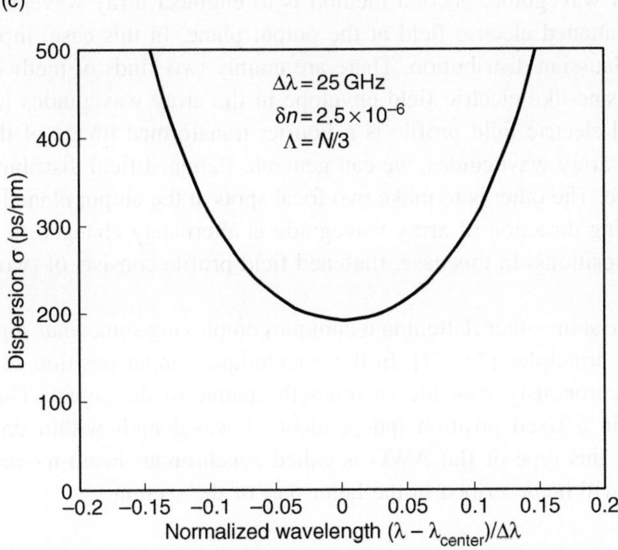

Figure 9.41 (*Continued*) (b) 50-GHz and (c) 25-GHz channel spacing.

9.5. FUNCTIONAL AWGs

9.5.1. Flat Spectral Response AWG

Since the displacement of the focal position x with respect to the wavelength λ is almost constant (Eq. (9.5)), the transmission loss of Gaussian AWG monotonically increases around the center wavelength of each channel. This places tight restrictions on the wavelength tolerance of laser diodes and requires accurate temperature control for both AWGs and laser diodes. Moreover, since optical signals are transmitted through several filters in the WDM ring/bus networks, cumulative passband width of each channel becomes much narrower than that of the single-stage AWG filter. Therefore, flattened and broadened spectral responses are required for AWG multiplexers.

Several approaches have been proposed to flatten the pass bands of AWGs [22–27]. One is to create flat electric field distribution at the input waveguide. Since AWG is an imaging device, flat electric field is reproduced at the output plane. The overlap integral of flat field with the Gaussian local normal mode gives flat spectral response. Parabolic waveguide horns [23] or 1×2 multimode interference couplers [24] are used to create flat electric field distribution at the input waveguide. Second method is to engineer array waveguide design to create flattened electric field at the output plane. In this case, input field is a normal Gaussian distribution. There are mainly two kinds of methods. One is to make a sinc-like electric field envelope in the array waveguides [22]. Since the focused electric field profile is a Fourier-transformed image of the electric field in the array waveguides, we can generate flattened field distribution at the output plane. The other is to make two focal spots at the output plane [25]. Here, light focusing direction of array waveguide is alternately changed to two separate focal positions. In this case, flattened field profile consists of two Gaussian beams.

There are some other flattening techniques employing somewhat sophisticated operational principles [26, 27]. In these techniques, input position of the beam moves synchronously with the wavelength change of the signal. Then, output beam lies in a fixed position independent of wavelength within one channel span. Here, this type of flat AWG is called synchronous-beam-movement-type AWG and will be described in the latter part of the section.

9.5.1.1. Parabola-type AWG

Figure 9.42 shows the enlarged view of the interface between (a) parabola-shaped input waveguides and first slab and (b) second slab and normal output

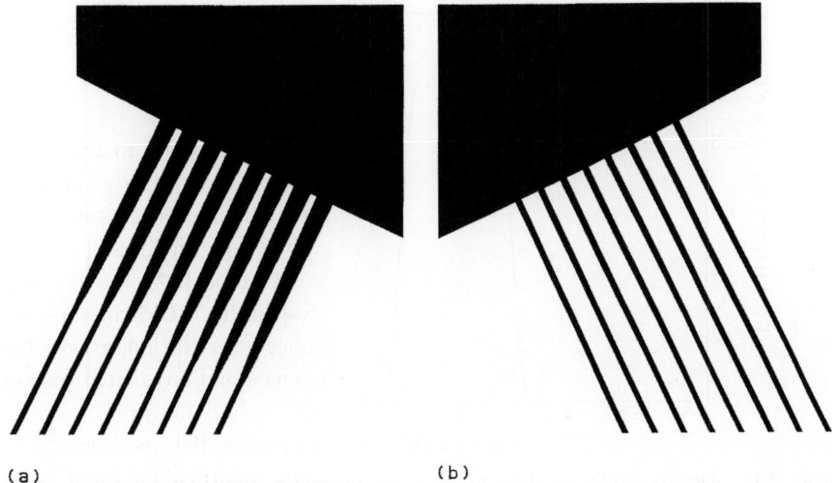

Figure 9.42 Enlarged view of the interface between (a) input waveguides and first slab and (b) second slab and normal output waveguides.

waveguides, respectively. The width of the parabolic horn along the propagation direction z is given by [28]

$$W(z) = \sqrt{2\alpha\lambda_g z + (2a)^2}, \tag{9.38}$$

where α is a constant less than unity, λ_g is the wavelength in the guide ($\lambda_g = \lambda/n_c$) and $2a$ is the core width of the channel waveguide (see inset of Fig. 9.43). At the proper horn length ($z = \ell$) less than the collimator length, a slightly double-peaked intensity distribution can be obtained as shown in Fig. 9.43. A broadened and sharp falling optical intensity profile is obtainable by the parabolic waveguide horn, which is quite advantageous for achieving wide passband without deteriorating the nearest neighbor crosstalk characteristics. The broadened and double-peaked field is imaged onto the entrance of an output waveguide having normal core width. The overlap integral of the focused field with the local normal mode of the output waveguide gives the flattened spectral response of AWG. Figure 9.44 shows the demultiplexing properties of 16-ch, 100-GHz spacing AWG having parabolic horns with $W = 40\,\mu\text{m}$ and $\ell = 800\,\mu\text{m}$. The crosstalks to the neighboring channels are less than -35 dB and the on-chip loss is about 7.0 dB. The average 1-dB, 3-dB and 20-dB bandwidths are 86.4 GHz, 100.6 GHz and 143.3 GHz, respectively.

In parabola-type flat AWG, double-peaked electric field distribution is created by the interference of the fundamental mode and 2nd-order mode as shown in Fig. 9.45. Generally, phase retardations of the fundamental mode and 2nd-order

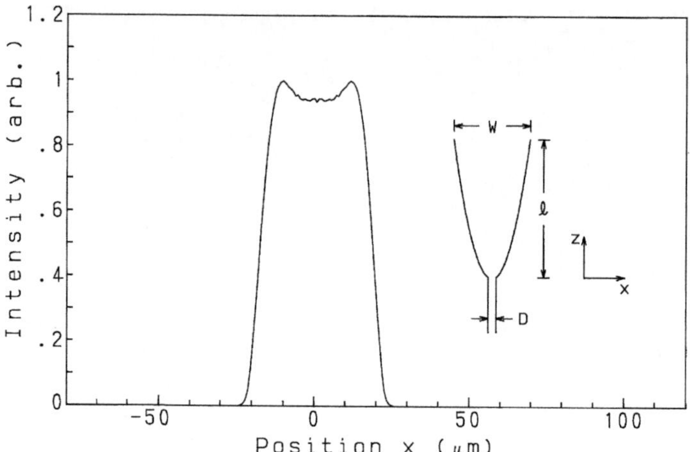

Figure 9.43 Intensity profile calculated by the beam propagation method for the parabolic horn with $W = 40\,\mu\text{m}$ and $\ell = 800\,\mu\text{m}$. Inset shows the schematic configuration of parabolic waveguide horn.

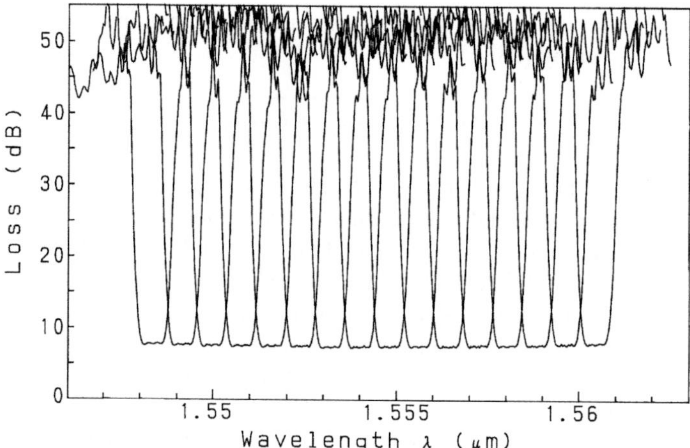

Figure 9.44 Demultiplexing properties of 16-ch, 100-GHz-spacing AWG having parabolic horns with $W = 40\,\mu\text{m}$ and $\ell = 800\,\mu\text{m}$.

mode are different. Therefore, the total phase at the end of the parabolic waveguide horn is not a uniform phase as shown in Fig. 9.46. Here geometries of parabolic horn are $W = 26.1\,\mu\text{m}$ and $\ell = 270\,\mu\text{m}$. Non-uniform phase distribution in the parabola input waveguide causes non-uniformity of phase in the array waveguides. Frequency response of AWG having non-uniform phase distribution

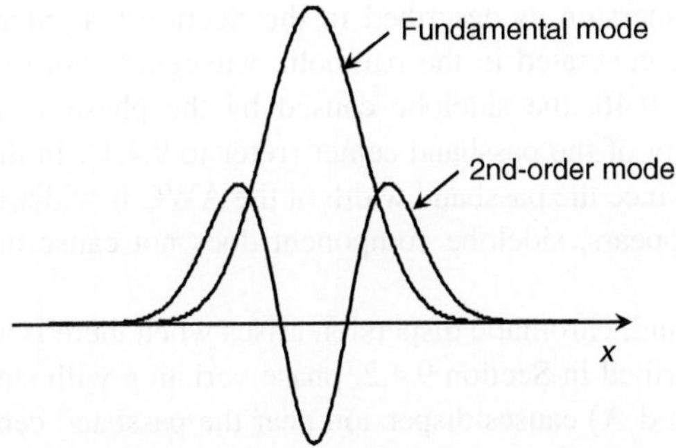

Figure 9.45 Fundamental mode and 2nd-order mode in a parabolic waveguide horn.

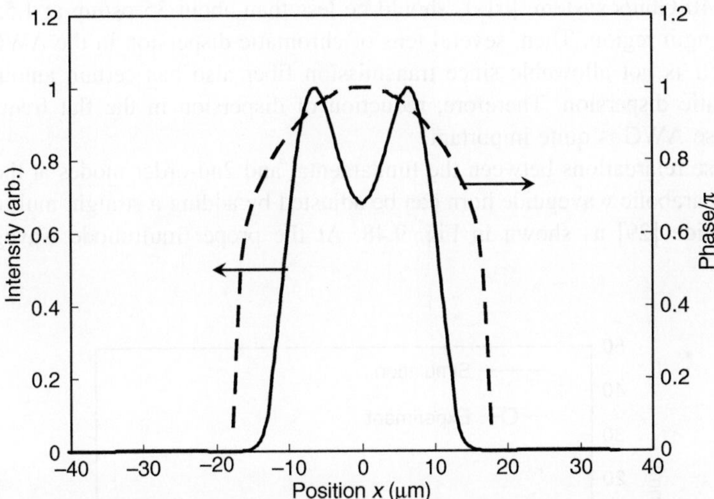

Figure 9.46 Intensity and phase distribution at the end of the parabolic waveguide horn with $W = 26.1\,\mu\text{m}$ and $\ell = 270\,\mu\text{m}$.

is expressed as

$$E(\nu) = \sum_{\ell=1}^{N} c(\ell) \exp\left[-j(N-\ell)2\pi\frac{\nu}{\nu_{\text{FSR}}} - j\theta_\ell\right], \tag{9.39}$$

where θ_ℓ denotes the non-uniform phase in the ℓ-th array waveguide. When we compare the above equation with Eq. (9.37), it is known that the non-uniform phase is similar to the effective-index fluctuations in the array waveguides. Then, the non-uniform phase θ_ℓ is estimated to cause crosstalk degradation and chromatic dispersion as described in the Section 9.4. Since the period of phase variation Λ generated in the parabolic waveguide horn is large ($\Lambda \approx N$) as shown in Fig. 9.46, the sidelobe caused by the phase variation manifests itself in the vicinity of the passband center (refer to 9.4.1). In the flat frequency response AWGs, since the passband width of the AWG is wider than the location where sidelobe appears, sidelobe component does not cause harmful crosstalk degradations.

On the other hand, chromatic dispersion arises when there is a phase variation in AWG. As described in Section 9.4.2, phase variation with small spatial component (large period Λ) causes dispersion near the passband center. Figure 9.47 shows theoretical and experimental dispersion characteristics of 32-ch, 100-GHz parabola-type flat AWG. Moreover, Eq. (3.213) gives the maximum limit of the dispersion $\cdot$ length product $|\sigma| \cdot L$ for the transmission system with B Gbit/s. In the 40-Gbit/s system, $|\sigma| \cdot L$ should be less than about 35 ps/nm at 1.55-μm wavelength region. Then, several tens of chromatic dispersion in the AWG filter itself is not allowable since transmission fiber also has certain amount of chromatic dispersion. Therefore, reduction of dispersion in the flat frequency response AWG is quite important.

Phase retardations between the fundamental and 2nd-order modes at the end of the parabolic waveguide horn can be adjusted by adding a straight multimode waveguide [29] as shown in Fig. 9.48. At the proper multimode waveguide

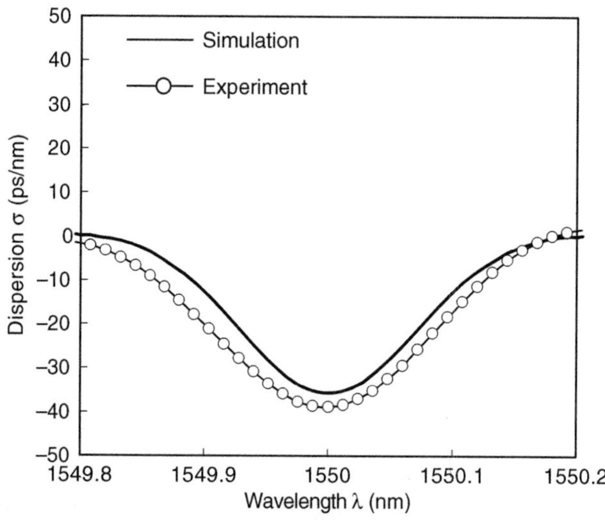

Figure 9.47 (a) Theoretical and (b) experimental dispersion characteristics of 32-ch, 100-GHz parabola-type flat AWG.

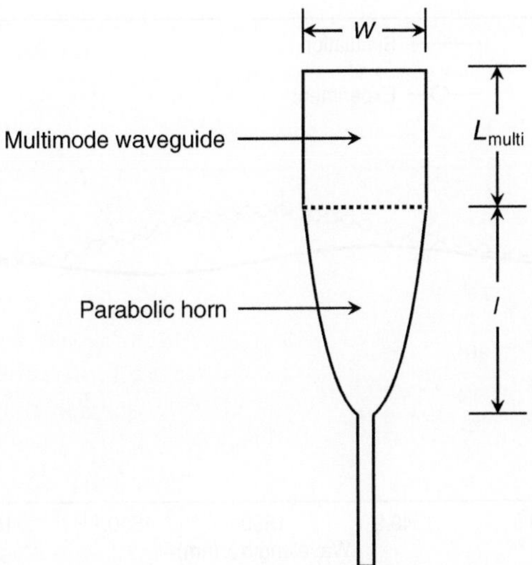

Figure 9.48 Parabolic waveguide horn having a straight multimode waveguide.

length, phase retardations of the fundamental and 2nd-order modes are almost equalized. Figure 9.49 shows the optical intensity and phase distribution at the end of the straight multimode waveguide with $L_{multi} = 85\,\mu m$. Total phase distribution becomes uniform while double-peaked electric field distribution is

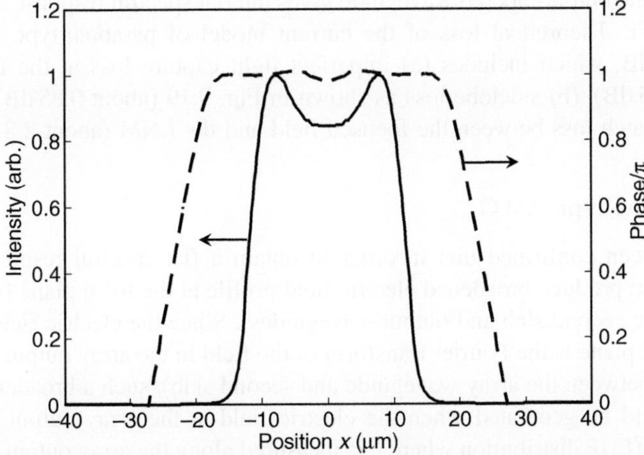

Figure 9.49 Intensity and phase distribution at the end of the straight multimode waveguide with $L_{multi} = 85\,\mu m$.

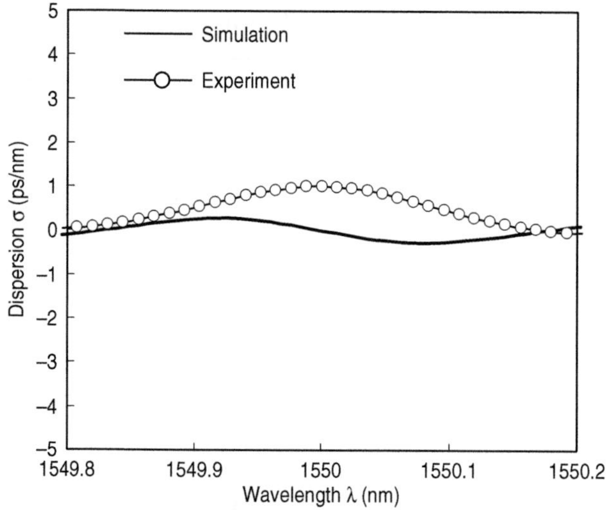

Figure 9.50 Theoretical and experimental dispersion characteristics of 32-ch, 100-GHz parabola-type flat AWG with $W = 26.1\,\mu\text{m}$, $\ell = 270\,\mu\text{m}$ and $L_{\text{multi}} = 85\,\mu\text{m}$, respectively.

maintained. Theoretical and experimental dispersion characteristics of 32-ch, 100-GHz parabola-type flat AWG with $W = 26.1\,\mu\text{m}$, $\ell = 270\,\mu\text{m}$ and $L_{\text{multi}} = 85\,\mu\text{m}$ are shown in Fig. 9.50.

Chromatic dispersion has been reduced to negligible value. Overlap integral of the broadened and slightly double-peaked field with the local normal mode (LNM) in the output-tapered waveguide gives the flat spectral response as shown in Fig. 9.51. Theoretical loss of the current model of parabola-type AWG is about 4.5 dB, which includes (a) imperfect light capture loss at the first slab (about 0.85 dB), (b) sidelobe loss as shown in Fig. 9.19 (about 0.85 dB) and (c) field mismatch loss between the focused field and the LNM (about 2.8 dB).

9.5.1.2. Sinc-type AWG

It has been confirmed that in order to obtain a flat spectral response, it is necessary to produce broadened electric field profile at the focal plane (interface between the second slab and output waveguides). Since the electric field profile in the focal plane is the Fourier transform of the field in the array output aperture (interface between the array waveguide and second slab), such a broadened field profile could be generated when the electric field at the array output aperture obeys a $\sin(\xi)/\xi$ distribution where ξ is measured along the array output aperture (see Fig. 9.8) [22]. Normal tapered waveguide is used in the input waveguide. Then, Gaussian envelope distribution is excited at the interface between the first

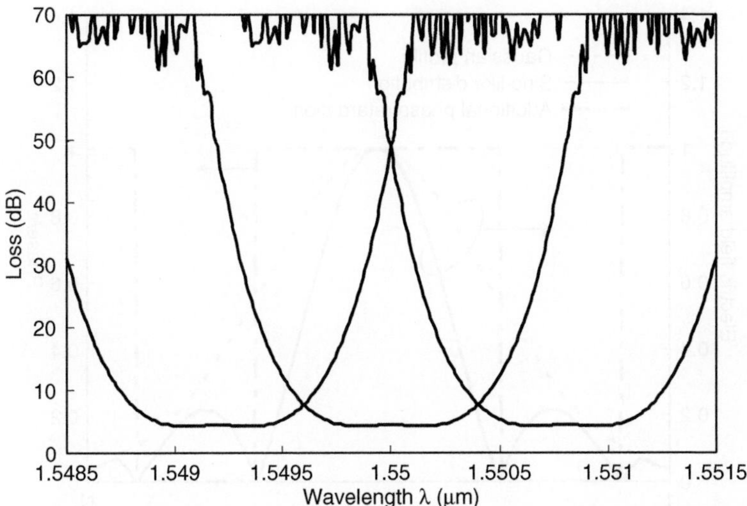

Figure 9.51 Theoretical flat spectral response of the parabola-type 32-ch, 100-GHz AWG.

slab and array waveguides. In order to create sinc-like envelope electric field distribution, proper loss and phase retardation are added to the corresponding waveguides. Figure 9.52 shows Gaussian envelope distribution (dotted line), sinc-like envelope electric field distribution (solid line) and additional phase retardation (dot and broken line) in 64-ch, 100-GHz AWG. Additional loss is realized by providing a waveguide gap or waveguide offset in the array waveguide. Plus or minus π phase shift is realized by making the array waveguide longer or shorter with the amount of $\lambda/(2n_c)$.

Generated sinc-like electric field distribution is shown in Fig. 9.53. Electric field profiles in the peripheral array waveguides are truncated since the sinc-like distribution is determined by the original Gaussian profile. Focused electric field distribution is obtained by using Eq. (9.15) as

$$E(x) = \sum_{\ell=1}^{N} c(\ell) \exp[-j\Omega(\ell)], \tag{9.40a}$$

$$c(\ell) = s(\ell) g(\hat{\rho}_k) \cos(\sigma_\ell), \tag{9.40b}$$

$$\Omega(\ell) = \beta_s \left(\hat{L}_{i,\ell} + L_{\ell,k}\right) + (N - \ell)\beta_c \Delta L, \tag{9.40c}$$

where $s(\ell)$ is a sinc-like field distribution given by Fig. 9.53. Figure 9.54 shows the electric field distribution at the interface between the second slab and output waveguides. Overlap integral of the broadened and slightly double-peaked field

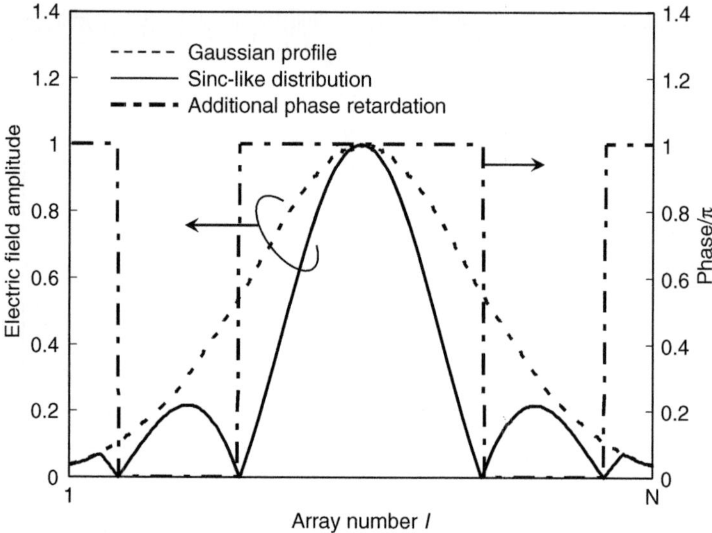

Figure 9.52 Gaussian envelope distribution (dotted line), sinc-like envelope electric field distribution (solid line) and excess phase retardation (dot and broken line), respectively.

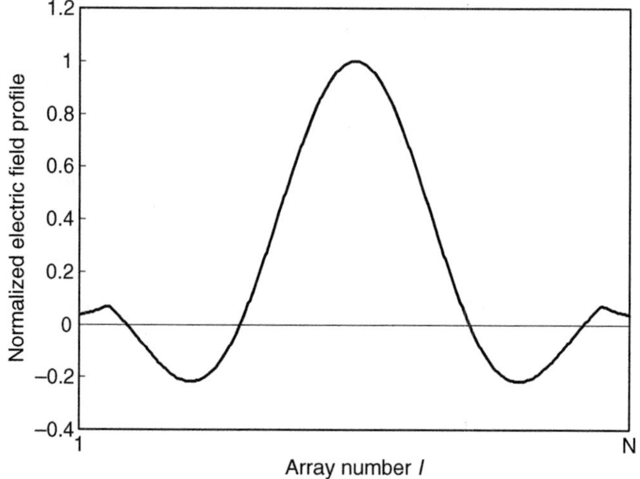

Figure 9.53 Generated sinc-like electric field distribution.

with the LNM in the output-tapered waveguide gives the flat spectral response as shown in Fig. 9.55. Theoretical loss of the current model of sinc-type AWG is about 6.8 dB, which includes (a) imperfect light capture loss at the first slab (about 0.85 dB), (b) additional loss in array waveguide to form sinc-like profile

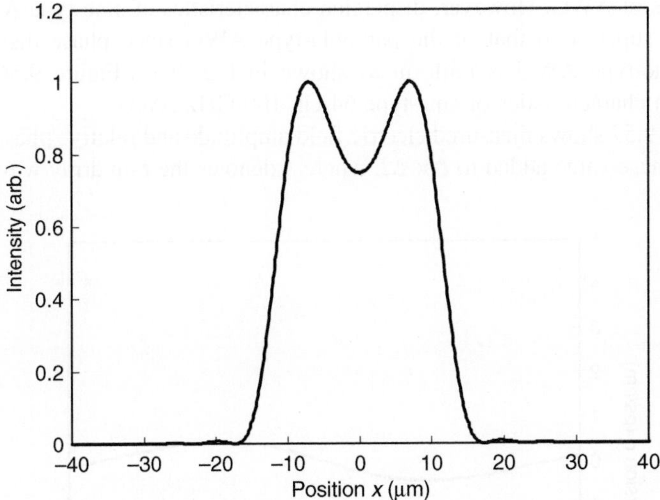

Figure 9.54 Electric field distribution at the interface between the second slab and output waveguides.

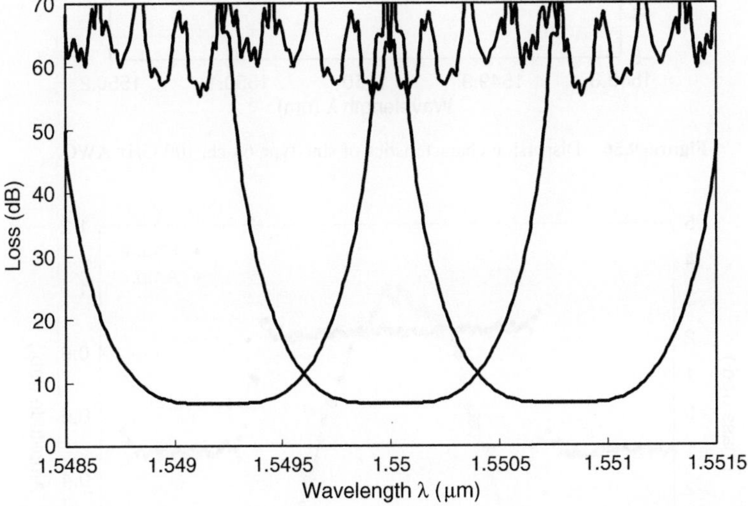

Figure 9.55 Theoretical flat spectral response of the sinc-type 64-ch, 100-GHz AWG.

(about 2.3 dB), (c) sidelobe loss as shown in Fig. 9.19 (about 0.85 dB) and (d) field mismatch loss between the focused field and the LNM (about 2.8 dB). In the parabola-type flat AWG, there is no additional loss in the array waveguides. Then, parabola-type AWG is superior to the sinc-type AWG in terms of the loss of AWG. However, dispersion characteristics of sinc-type AWG are generally superior to that of the parabola-type AWG since phase distribution of the sinc-type AWG is uniform as shown in Fig. 9.52. Figure 9.56 shows dispersion characteristics of sinc-type 64-ch, 100-GHz AWG.

Figure 9.57 shows measured electric field amplitude and relative phase delays (excess phase value added to $\ell \times \Delta L$ where ℓ denotes the ℓ-th array waveguide)

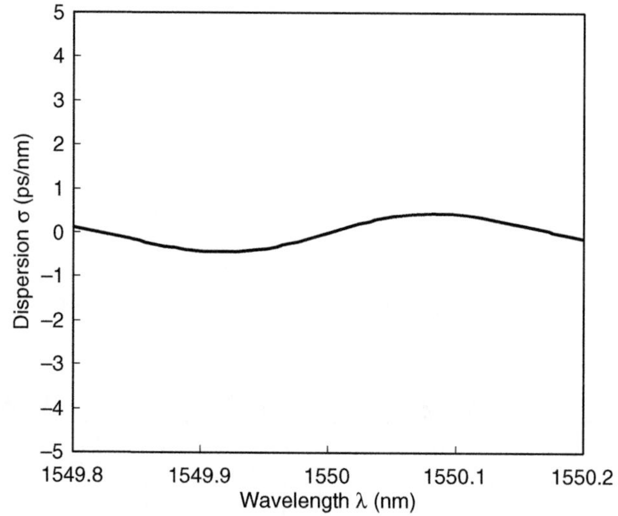

Figure 9.56 Dispersion characteristics of sinc-type 64-ch, 100-GHz AWG.

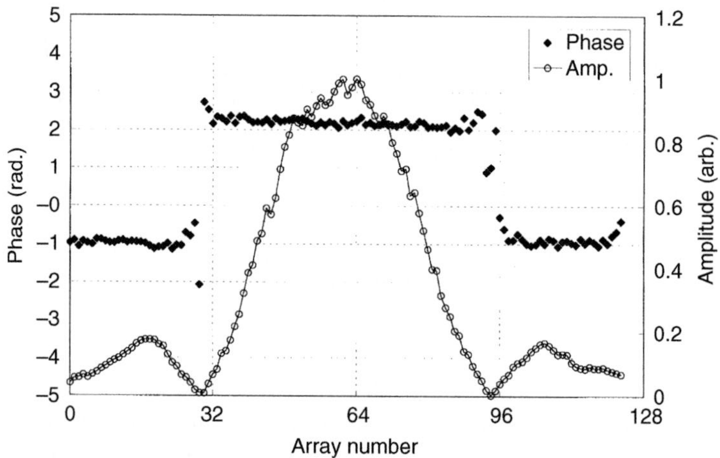

Figure 9.57 Electric field amplitude and relative phase delays in the sinc-type flat response AWG.

in the sinc-type flat response AWG measured by the low-coherence Fourier transform spectroscopy [30]. Sinc-shaped electric field amplitude and phase distributions are clearly realized by the array-waveguide engineering technique.

9.5.1.3. Synchronous-beam-movement-type AWG

In the synchronous-beam-movement-type (SBM-type) AWGs [26, 27], input position of the beam moves synchronously with the wavelength change of the signal. Then, output beam lies in a fixed position independent of wavelength within one channel span. Figure 9.58 shows the schematic configuration of the first kind of SBM-type AWG [26]. Two AWGs are arranged in tandem, and the image of the first AWG forms the source for the second AWG. The image of the first AWG is created on the dotted line AA′. Free spectral range (FSR) of AWG_1 is designed to be equal to the channel spacing of AWG_2. Focused images for 100-GHz-spacing SBM-type AWG are calculated by the BPM simulations. The first AWG is a 1-ch, 100-GHz and the second AWG is a 64-ch, 100-GHz AWG. Figure 9.59 shows focused images (optical intensity) on AA′ and BB′ for three spectral components $\delta\lambda = -0.2$ nm, 0.0 nm and +0.2 nm, respectively. Three peaks in Fig. 9.59 are images for three diffraction orders. When wavelength λ decreases (increases) within a channel, focused image of AWG_1 moves upward (downward) on the dotted line AA′ as shown in Fig. 9.59(a). When change of wavelength $\delta\lambda$ is ignored, the second image on the line BB′ moves in the opposite direction to that on AA′ as shown in Fig. 9.59(b) according to Eq. (9.4). However, when wavelength change $\delta\lambda$ is taken into account, the focused spot on BB′ moves upward (downward) according to Eq. (9.5) and the main spot stays at the center of the output waveguide as shown in Fig. 9.59(c). Then, beam movement in the first AWG precisely cancels the focused spot movement on BB′ and enables us to obtain flat spectral response AWG without causing an extra loss increase.

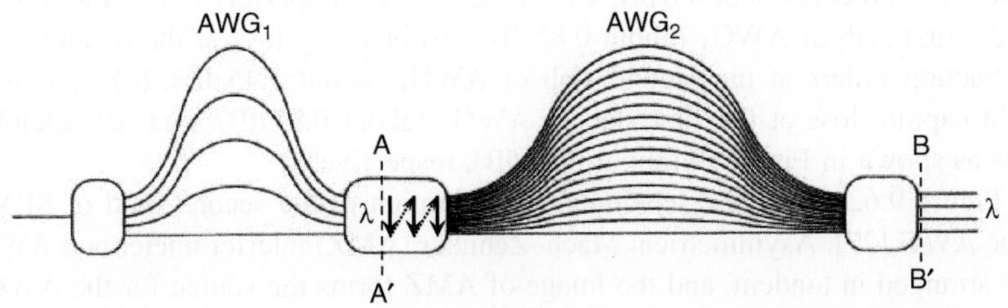

Figure 9.58 Schematic configuration of the first kind of SBM-type AWG.

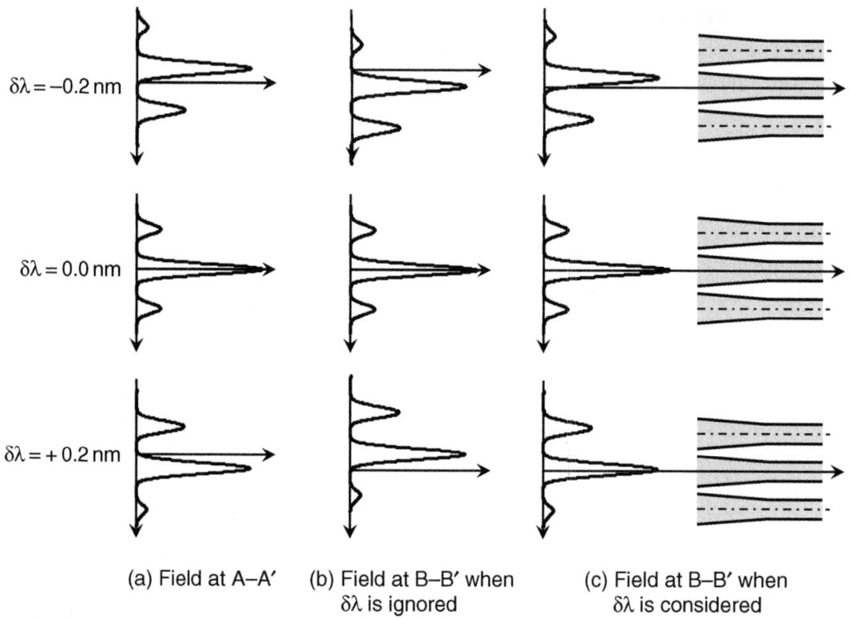

Figure 9.59 Focused images on the dotted lines A–A' and B–B' for three spectral components $\delta\lambda = -0.2\,\text{nm}$, $0.0\,\text{nm}$ and $+0.2\,\text{nm}$, respectively.

It is clear that the neighboring two peaks cause substantial crosstalk degradation. Therefore, a filter having proper width should be incorporated in the focal plane AA′ to eliminate the neighboring two images. Hatched regions in Fig. 9.60 show the filters to improve the crosstalk characteristics. Figure 9.60 shows focused images on AA′ and BB′ when filters are placed for three spectral components $\delta\lambda = -0.2\,\text{nm}, 0.0\,\text{nm}$ and $+0.2\,\text{nm}$, respectively. Overlap integral of the focused field (Fig. 9.60(c)) with the LNM in the output-tapered waveguide gives the spectral response as shown in Fig. 9.61. Theoretical loss of the current model of AWG is about 4.0 dB, which includes (a) imperfect light capture loss at the first slab of AWG_1 (about 0.85 dB), (b) blocking loss of the neighboring diffraction orders at the second slab of AWG_1 (about 1.45 dB), (c) imperfect light capture loss at the first slab of AWG_2 (about 0.85 dB), and (d) sidelobe loss as shown in Fig. 9.19 (about 0.85 dB), respectively.

Figure 9.62 shows the schematic configuration of the second kind of SBM-type AWG [27]. Asymmetrical Mach–Zehnder (AMZ) interferometer and AWG are arranged in tandem, and the image of AMZ forms the source for the AWG. The image of AMZ is created on the dotted line AA′. FSR of AMZ is designed to be equal to the channel spacing of the AWG. Path length difference in

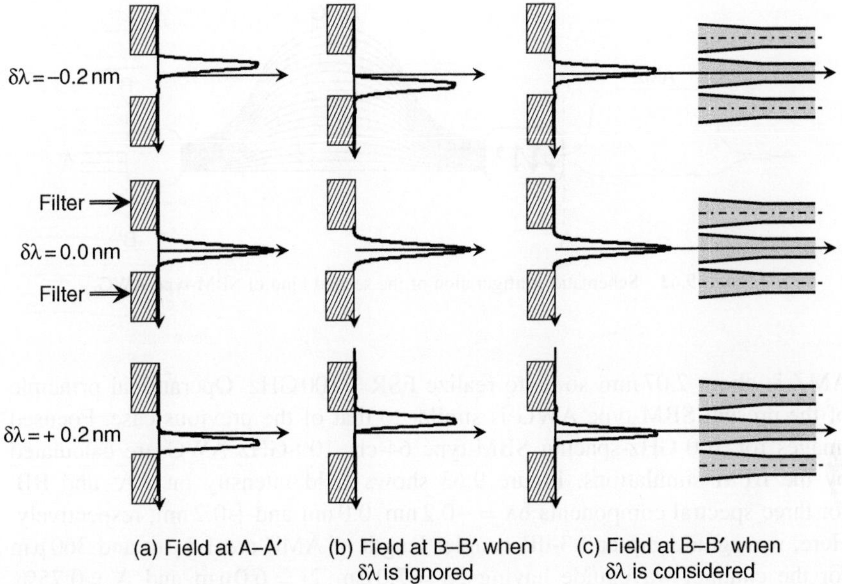

Figure 9.60 Focused images on A–A' and B–B' when filters are placed for three spectral components $\delta\lambda = -0.2$ nm, 0.0 nm and $+0.2$ nm, respectively.

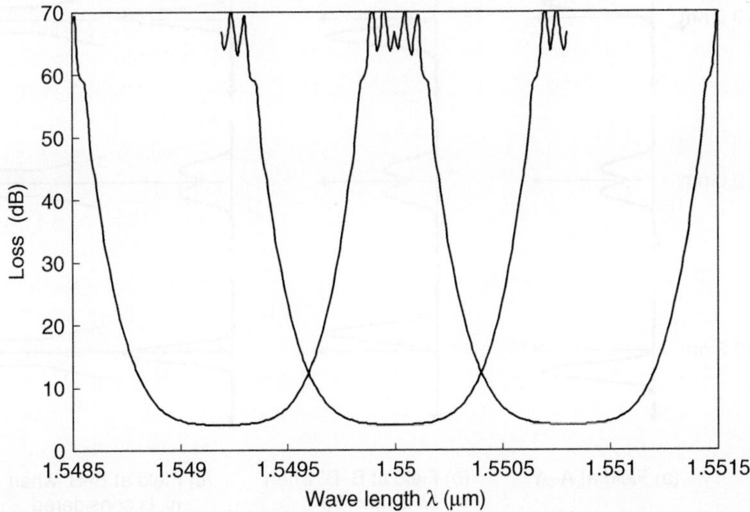

Figure 9.61 Theoretical flat spectral response of the first kind of SBM-type AWG with 100-GHz channel spacing.

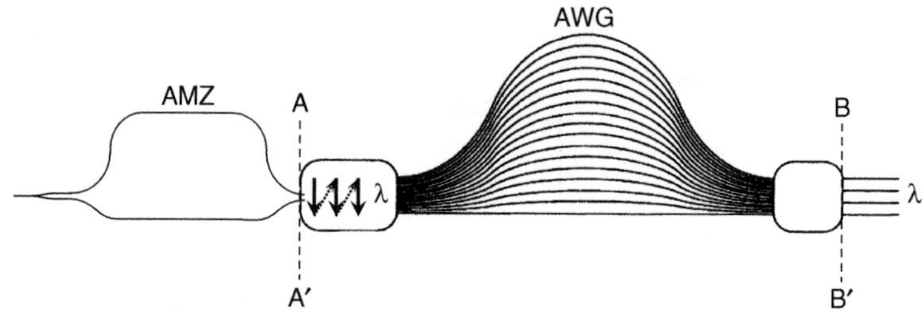

Figure 9.62 Schematic configuration of the second kind of SBM-type AWG.

AMZ is about 2.07 mm so as to realize FSR = 100 GHz. Operational principle of the present SBM-type AWG is similar to that of the previous case. Focused images for 100-GHz-spacing SBM-type 64-ch, 100-GHz AWG are calculated by the BPM simulations. Figure 9.63 shows field intensity on AA′ and BB′ for three spectral components $\delta\lambda = -0.2\,\text{nm}, 0.0\,\text{nm}$ and $+0.2\,\text{nm}$, respectively. Here, waveguide gap and 3-dB coupler length of AMZ are 1.5 μm and 360 μm for the channel waveguide having $2a = 7.0\,\mu\text{m}, 2t = 6.0\,\mu\text{m}$ and $\Delta = 0.75\%$, respectively. Figure 9.63(b) shows the image on BB′ when wavelength change

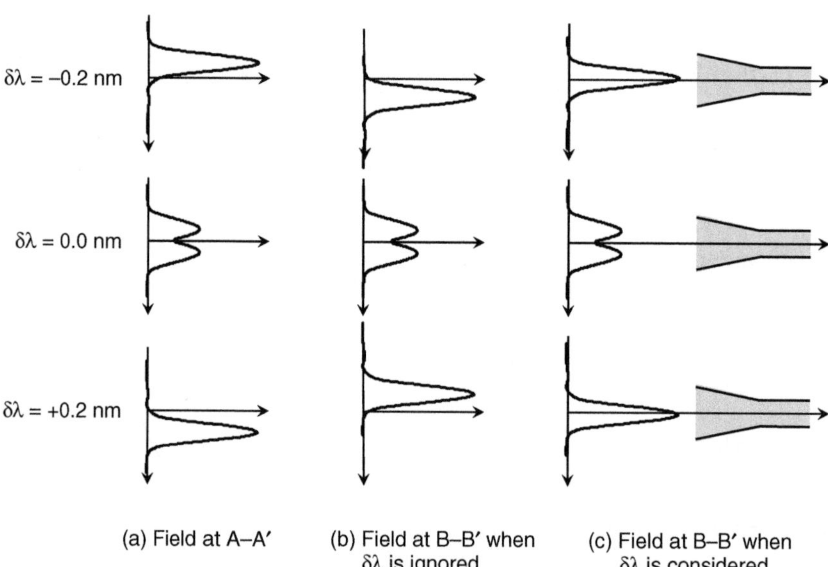

Figure 9.63 Focused images on the dotted lines *A–A′* and *B–B′* for three spectral components $\delta\lambda = -0.2\,\text{nm}, 0.0\,\text{nm}$ and $+0.2\,\text{nm}$, respectively.

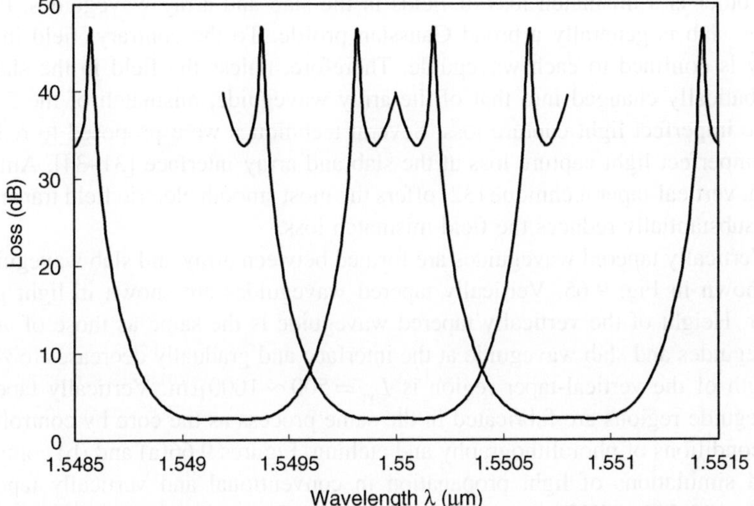

Figure 9.64 Theoretical flat spectral response of the second kind of SBM-type AWG with 100-GHz channel spacing.

$\delta\lambda$ is ignored. When wavelength change $\delta\lambda$ is taken into account, the image stays at the center of the output waveguide as shown in Fig. 9.63(c). Field distribution at $\delta\lambda = 0.0\,\text{nm}$ is essentially double peaked, since light is localized to each core of the 3-dB coupler. Then, aperture width of the output-tapered waveguide is optimized to 14.5 μm in order to capture the double-peaked light properly. Overlap integral of the focused field (Fig. 9.63(c)) with the LNM in the output-tapered waveguide gives the spectral response as shown in Fig. 9.64. Theoretical loss of the current model of AWG is about 2.5 dB, which includes (a) imperfect light capture loss at the first slab (about 0.85 dB), and (b) field mismatch loss between the optical field and the local normal mode (about 0.8 dB), and (c) sidelobe loss as shown in Fig. 9.19 (about 0.85 dB). Crosstalk degradation at around −35 dB level could be eliminated by incorporating a light blocking filter on the AA′ plane.

9.5.2. Loss Reduction in AWG

Loss of AWG excluding absorption loss and scattering loss in the waveguide is mainly caused by the imperfect light capture loss at the slab and array interface. There are mainly two origins in the imperfect light capture loss. One is a spillover loss in which peripheral part of the FFP cannot be captured by the array waveguides since we cannot place infinitely many array waveguides.

The other is a mismatch loss of fields in the slab and array waveguides. Field in the slab is generally a broad Gaussian profile. To the contrary, field in the array is confined to each waveguide. Therefore, unless the field in the slab is adiabatically changed into that of the array waveguide, mismatch of the fields cause imperfect light capture loss. Several techniques were proposed to reduce the imperfect light capture loss at the slab and array interface [31–34]. Among them, vertical-taper technique [32] offers the most smooth electric field transition and substantially reduces the field mismatch loss.

Vertically tapered waveguides are formed between array and slab waveguides as shown in Fig. 9.65. Vertically tapered waveguides are shown in light gray color. Height of the vertically tapered waveguide is the same as those of array waveguides and slab waveguide at the interface and gradually decreases to zero. Length of the vertical-taper region is $L_{vt} = 500 \sim 1000\,\mu\text{m}$. Vertically tapered waveguide regions are fabricated in the same process as the core by controlling the conditions of photolithography and etching. Figures 9.66(a) and (b) compare BPM simulations of light propagation in conventional and vertically tapered 64-ch, 100-GHz AWGs near the interface of the first slab and array waveguides. In the conventional AWG, typical field mismatch loss amounts to about 0.85 dB because light field in the first slab encounters abrupt change of the waveguide structure at the slab–array interface. On the other hand, as shown in (b), Gaussian field in the first slab region is smoothly (or adiabatically) transformed to the light field of individual array waveguide. Field mismatch loss is reduced to about 0.15 dB. Loss reduction by the vertical-taper structure is typically 0.7 dB. Since AWG is a passive and reciprocal device, we could obtain another 0.7-dB loss improvement in the second slab region. Figure 9.67 shows electric field distribution at the interface between the second slab and output waveguides.

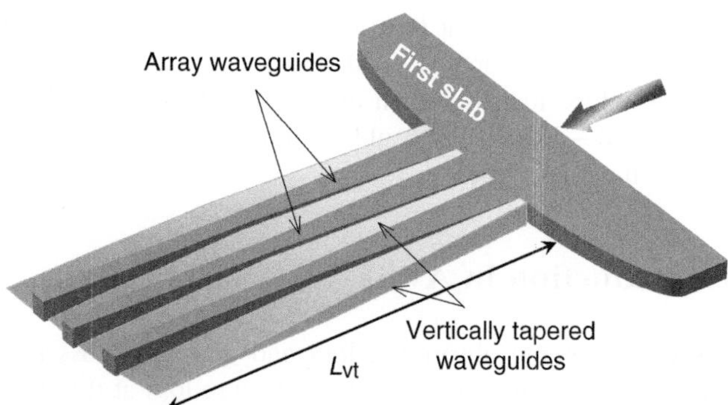

Figure 9.65 Core ridge structure at the interface between the first slab and array waveguides. Vertically tapered waveguides are shown in light gray color.

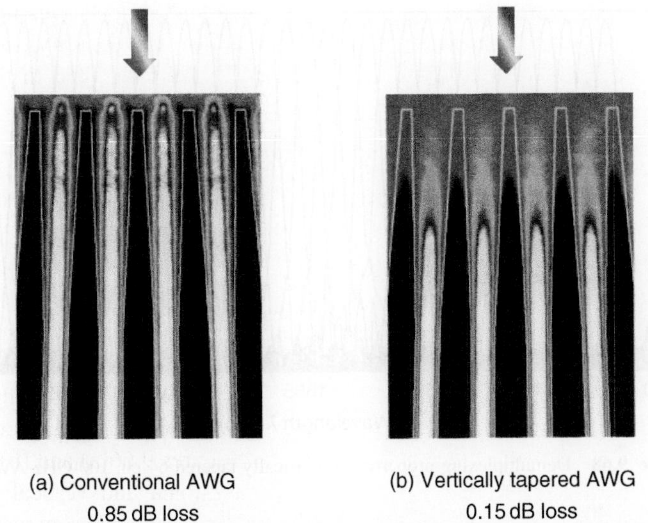

Figure 9.66 BPM simulations of light propagation in (a) conventional and (b) vertically tapered AWGs near the interface of the first slab and array waveguides.

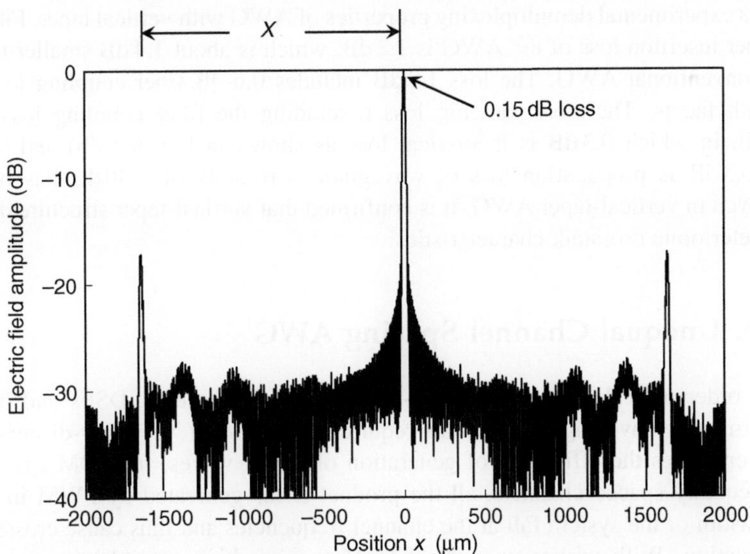

Figure 9.67 Electric field distribution at the interface between the second slab and output waveguides in the vertically tapered 64-ch, 100-GHz AWG.

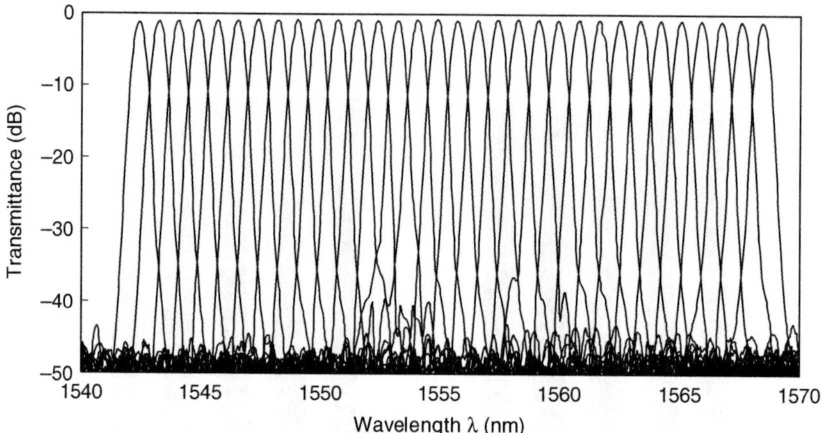

Figure 9.68 Demultiplexing properties of vertically tapered 64-ch, 100-GHz AWG.

Two peaks at $x \cong \pm 1600\,\mu\text{m}$ represent sidelobes of the adjacent diffraction order $m \mp 1$. When we compare the sidelobe level of Fig. 9.67 with that of Fig. 9.19 of the conventional AWG, sidelobe level is reduced from $-6\,\text{dB}$ to $-18\,\text{dB}$. Main-lobe loss is then improved by about 0.7 dB when compared with the loss in Fig. 9.19. In total, we could obtain $0.7 \times 2 = 1.4\,\text{dB}$ loss reduction. Figure 9.68 shows experimental demultiplexing properties of AWG with vertical taper. Fiber-to-fiber insertion loss of the AWG is 1.2 dB, which is about 1.4 dB smaller than the conventional AWG. The loss 1.2 dB includes 0.6-dB fiber coupling losses at both facets. Therefore, on-chip loss (excluding the fiber coupling loss) is 0.6 dB, in which 0.3 dB is theoretical loss as shown in Fig. 9.66(b) and 9.67 and 0.3 dB is propagation loss of waveguide. Crosstalk of $-40\,\text{dB}$ has been achieved in vertical-taper AWG. It is confirmed that vertical-taper structure does not deteriorate crosstalk characteristics.

9.5.3. Unequal Channel Spacing AWG

In order to realize the very large-capacity WDM systems, DSFs and high performance wavelength filters are required. The use of very low-dispersion fiber enhances the efficiency of generation of FWM waves. In WDM systems with equally spaced channels, all the product terms generated by FWM in the bandwidth of the system fall at the channel frequencies and thus cause crosstalk degradation. With proper unequal channel spacing it is possible to suppress FWM crosstalk by preventing FWM waves from being generated at the channel frequencies [35, 36]. In the AWGs the focused beam movement Δx in the second

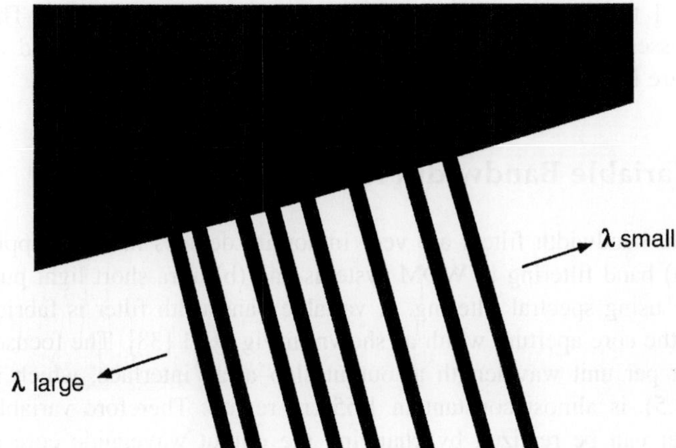

Figure 9.69 Enlarged view of the output waveguides in 8-ch unequal spacing AWG.

slab for the unit wavelength change $\Delta\lambda$ is almost constant as shown in Eq. (9.5). Therefore, unequally spaced multiplexer can be fabricated by allocating the output waveguide with unequal spatial spacing. Figure 9.69 shows the enlarged view of the output waveguides in 8-ch unequal spacing AWG with $\Delta x/\Delta\lambda = 25\,\mu\text{m/nm}$ [37]. Core–center separations are determined from unequal channel specifications and the above dispersion relation. Figure 9.70 is the measured demultiplexing properties of 8-ch unequal spacing AWG. The channel spacing

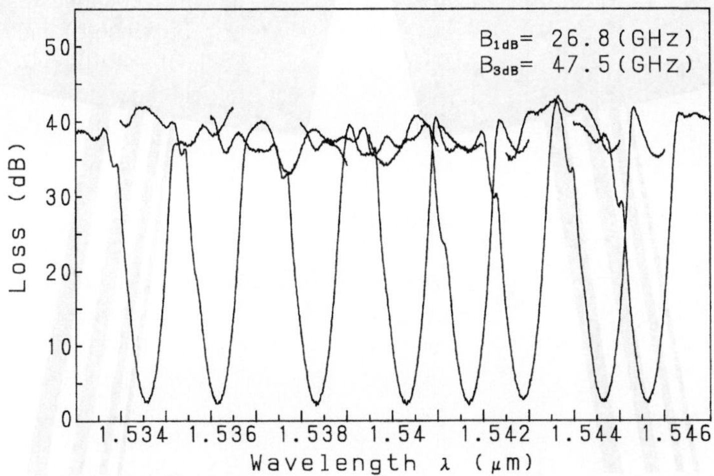

Figure 9.70 Demultiplexing properties of 8-ch unequal spacing AWG.

from port 1 to port 8 agrees quite well with the designed values. The fiber-to-fiber losses are 2.2–2.7 dB and the crosstalks to neighboring and all other channels are less than −31 dB.

9.5.4. Variable Bandwidth AWG

Variable bandwidth filters are very important devices in many applications such as (a) band filtering in WDM systems and (b) ultra-short light pulse generation by using spectral filtering. A variable bandwidth filter is fabricated by changing the core aperture width as shown in Fig. 9.71 [38]. The focused beam movement per unit wavelength at output slab–array interface, which is given by Eq. (9.5), is almost constant in 1.55 μm region. Therefore variable bandwidth filter can be realized by changing the output waveguide core aperture width. The core aperture widths of input and output waveguides in Fig. 9.71 are $A_1 = 10\,\mu\text{m}$, $A_2 = 24\,\mu\text{m}$, $A_3 = 40\,\mu\text{m}$ and $A_4 = 54\,\mu\text{m}$. If we use input/output waveguide pairs having the same aperture width, the insertion losses always remain the same. Figure 9.72 shows the measured spectral characteristics of variable bandwidth filters for $\Delta L = 8.6\,\mu\text{m}$. The 3-dB bandwidths are about 400 GHz, 800 GHz, 1200 GHz and 1600 GHz, respectively. Since the focused

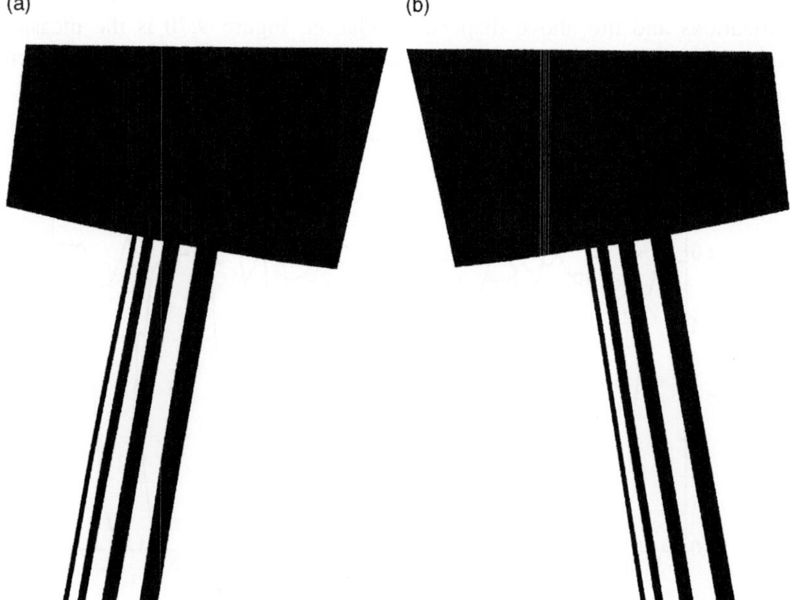

Figure 9.71 Enlarged view of the input and output waveguides in variable bandwidth AWG.

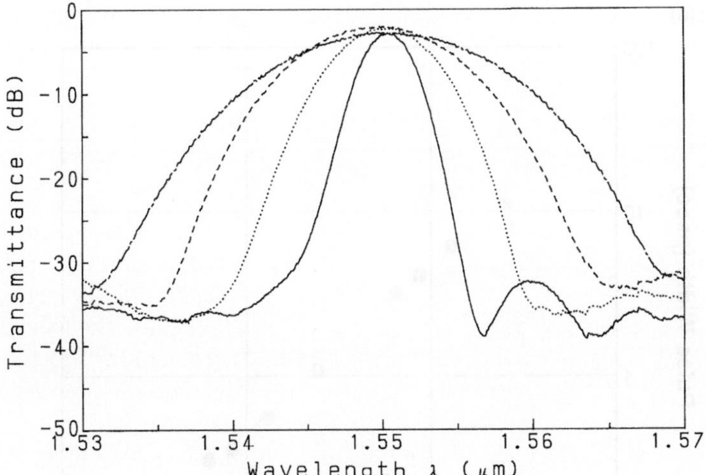

Figure 9.72 Measured 3-dB bandwidth characteristics for input/output pairs from A_1 to A_4 with $\Delta L = 8.6\,\mu\text{m}$ (A_1 solid line, A_2 dotted line, A_3 broken line and A_4 dot-broken line).

beam movement per unit wavelength change is proportional to ΔL, much narrower 3-dB bandwidth filter can be obtained by increasing ΔL. In the AWG with $\Delta L = 63\,\mu\text{m}$, 3-dB bandwidths are about 40 GHz, 80 GHz, 120 GHz and 160 GHz, respectively [38].

Pulse width-tunable ultrashort light pulses have been generated by the spectral filtering of a 100-nm supercontinuum source [39] using variable bandwidth AWG filters [40]. Figure 9.73(a) shows generated pulse widths with respect to AWG 3-dB bandwidths. The pulse width decreases from 11 psec to 300 fsec with increasing AWG bandwidth, while maintaining a constant time-bandwidth product (Gaussian pulse) as shown Fig. 9.73(b).

9.5.5. Uniform-loss and Cyclic-frequency (ULCF) AWG

In principle, $N \times N$ signal interconnection can be achieved in AWG when FSR of AWG is N times the channel spacing. Here FSR is given by

$$\text{FSR} = \frac{n_c \nu_0}{N_c m}, \tag{9.41}$$

where ν_0 is the center frequency of WDM signals. Generally light beams with three different diffraction orders of $m-1$, m and $m+1$ are utilized to achieve $N \times N$ interconnections [41]. The cyclic property provides an important additional functionality as compared to simple multiplexers or demultiplexers and

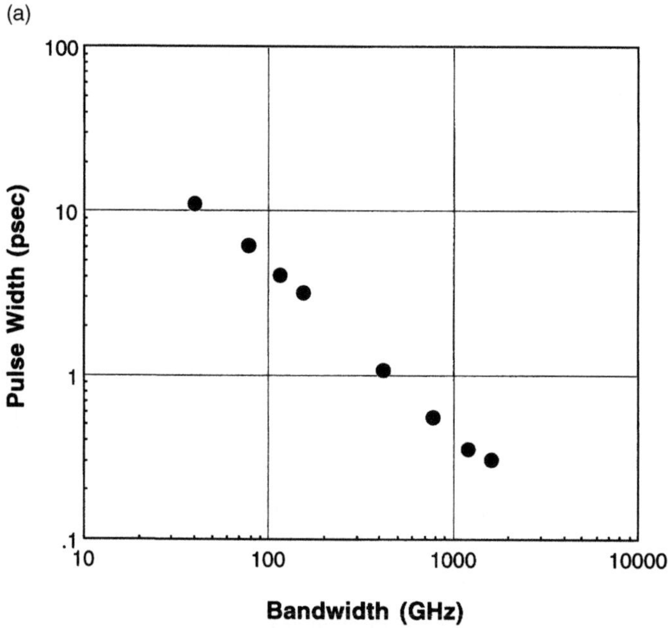

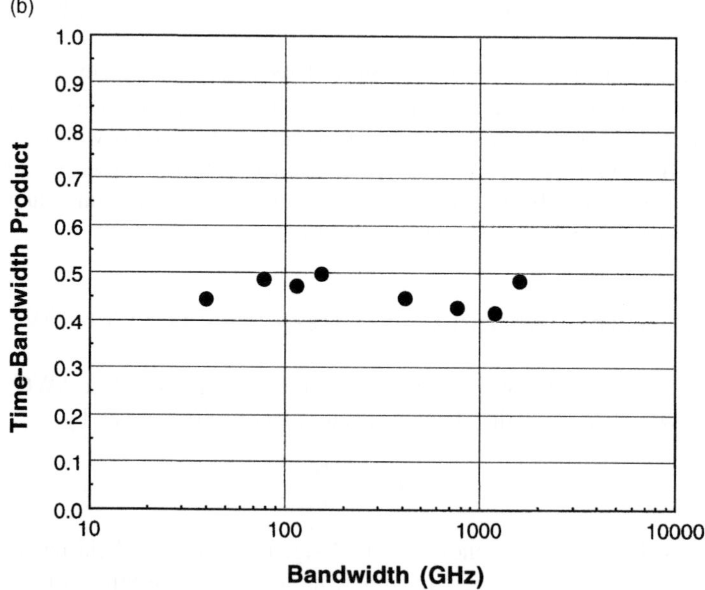

Figure 9.73 (a) Measured pulse width against AWG bandwidth. (b) Measured time-bandwidth product against AWG bandwidth.

plays a key role in more complex devices as add/drop multiplexers and wavelength switches.

However, such interconnectivity cannot always be realized with the conventional AWGs. Typical diffraction order of AWG with 50–100-GHz channel spacing is $m = 30 \sim 60$ as described in Section 9.3.4. Since FSR is inversely proportional to m (Eq. 9.29), substantial pass frequency mismatch is brought by the difference between three FSRs. Figure 9.74 shows measured demultiplexing properties of 32-ch, 50-GHz-spacing AWG over three diffraction orders. Wavelength gap between m-th and $(m+1)$-th diffraction orders are smoothly connected with 50 GHz in the current design based on Eq. (9.10). However, wavelength gap between m-th and $(m-1)$-th diffraction orders are about 70 GHz.

By the way, insertion losses of AWG for peripheral input and output ports are 2–3 dB higher than those for central ports as shown in Figs. 9.23 and 9.24. The non-cyclic frequency characteristics and loss non-uniformity in conventional AWGs are main obstacles which prevent the development of practical $N \times N$ routing networks.

Novel 32×32 AWG having uniform-loss and cyclic-frequency characteristics is proposed and fabricated to solve the problems in conventional AWGs. Figure 9.75 shows a schematic configuration of uniform-loss and cyclic-frequency (ULCF) arrayed-waveguide grating [42]. It consists of 80-channel AWG multiplexer with 100-GHz spacing and 32 optical combiners which are connected to 64 output waveguides of the multiplexer. The arc length of slab is $f = 24.55$ mm and number of array waveguides is 300 having the constant path length difference $\Delta L = 24.6\,\mu$m between neighboring waveguides. The

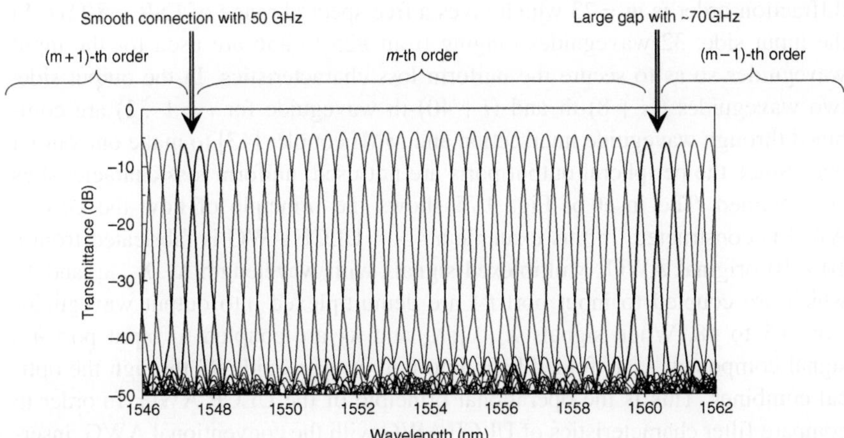

Figure 9.74 Measured demultiplexing property of 32-ch, 50-GHz-spacing AWG over three diffraction orders.

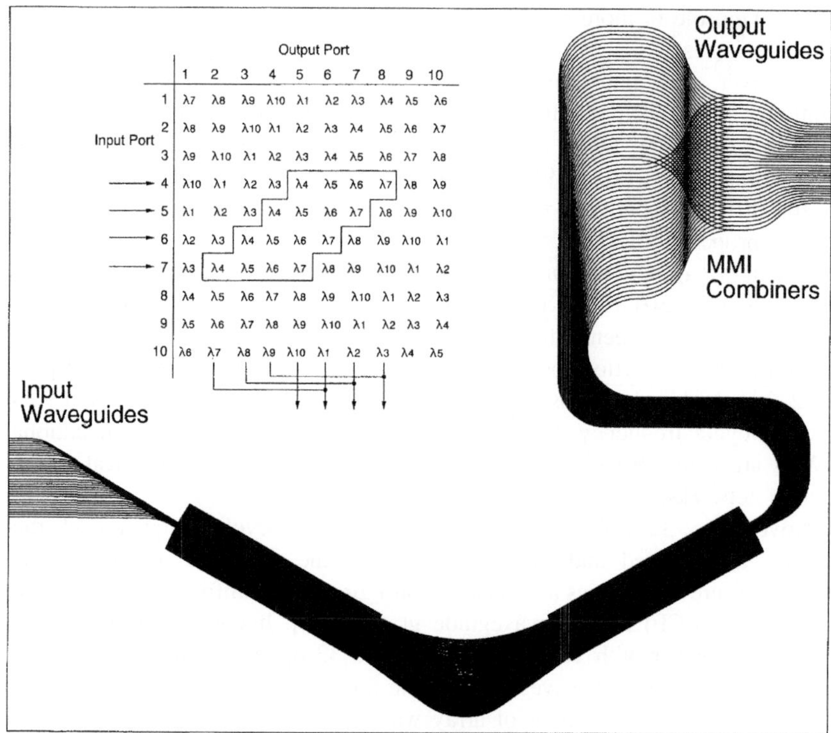

Figure 9.75 Schematic configuration of uniform-loss and cyclic-frequency AWG.

diffraction order is $m = 23$ which gives a free spectral range of FSR = 8 THz. In the input side, 32 waveguides ranging from #25 to #56 are used for the input waveguides so as to secure the uniform loss characteristics. In the output side, two waveguides ($(i + 8)$-th and $(i + 40)$-th waveguide for $i = 1$–32) are combined through waveguide intersection and MMI coupler [43] to make one output port. Since the peripheral output ports are not used, uniform loss characteristics are obtained. The inset of Fig. 9.75 shows the principle of how the ULCF-AWG is constructed. In this example a 4×4 ULCF AWG is fabricated from a 10×10 original AWG. Multiplexed signals with wavelength $\lambda_4, \lambda_5, \lambda_6$ and λ_7 which are coupled to input port #4 are demultiplexed into output waveguides from #5 to #8. When signals $\lambda_4, \lambda_5, \lambda_6$ and λ_7 are coupled to input port #5, signal component λ_4 is folded back into output waveguide #8 through the optical combiner. This is the operational principle of the ULCF AWG. In order to compare filter characteristics of ULCF AWG with the conventional AWG, insertion loss characteristics and demultiplexing properties in conventional AWG are first presented. Figure 9.76(a) shows measured insertion losses for entire

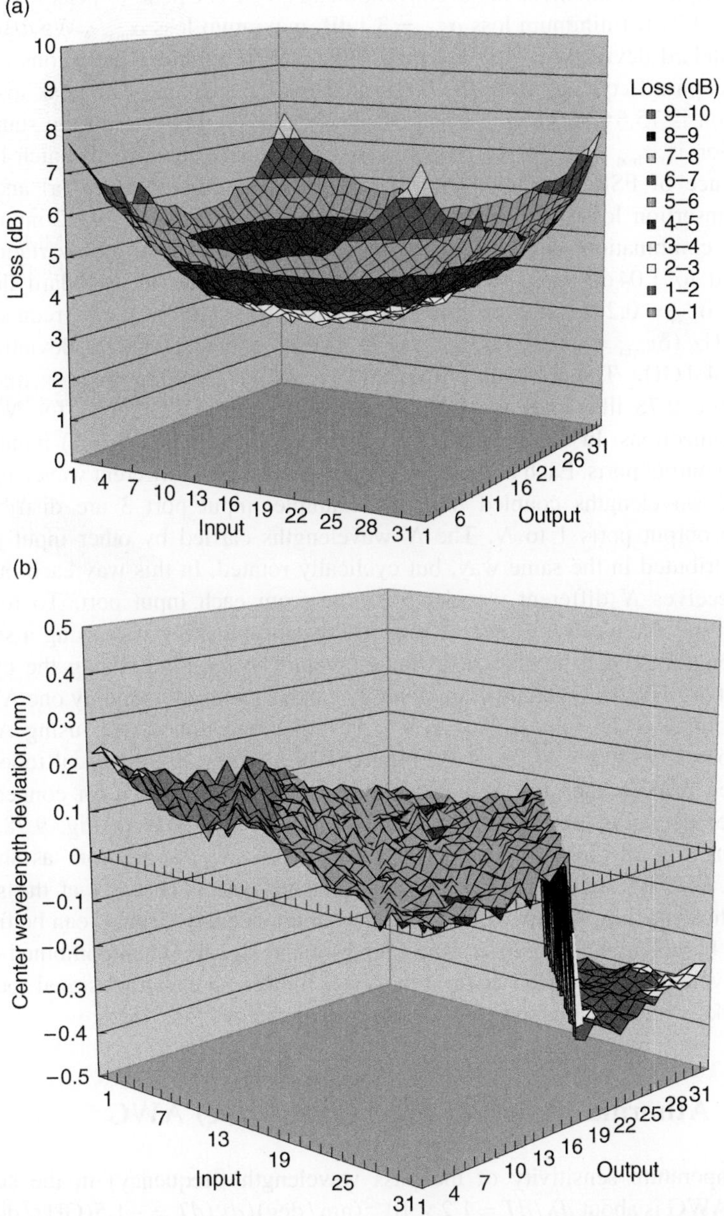

Figure 9.76 (a) Measured insertion losses for entire 32 × 32 input/output combinations in the conventional AWG. (b) Measured channel center frequency deviations for entire 32 × 32 input/output combinations in the conventional AWG.

input/output combinations in the conventional AWG. The peak-to-peak loss variation is 4.7 dB (minimum loss $\alpha_{min} = 3.1$ dB, maximum loss $\alpha_{max} = 7.8$ dB) and the standard deviation is $\sigma_{loss} = 1.0$ dB. Figure 9.76(b) shows deviations of the channel pass frequency from the prescribed grid frequencies. The peak-to-peak variation is 75.6 GHz ($\delta\upsilon_{min} = -44.5$ GHz, $\delta\upsilon_{max} = 31.1$ GHz) and the standard deviation is $\sigma_{freq} = 16.7$ GHz. Major reason for pass frequency mismatch is the difference of FSR in neighboring diffraction orders. Figures 9.77(a) and (b) show insertion losses and channel pass frequency deviations for 32-input/32-output combinations in the ULCF AWG. The peak-to-peak loss variation is reduced to 1.04 dB ($\alpha_{min} = 6.63$ dB, $\alpha_{max} = 7.67$ dB) and the standard deviation is $\sigma_{loss} = 0.2$ dB. The peak-to-peak frequency variation is also reduced to 22.3 GHz ($\delta\upsilon_{min} = -6.8$ GHz, $\delta\upsilon_{max} = 15.5$ GHz) and the standard deviation is $\sigma_{freq} = 4.4$ GHz. The crosstalk of the AWG is about -26 dB.

Figure 9.78 illustrates the functionality of ULCF AWG router for $N \times N$ interconnections. In this example, the wavelength router has $N(=5)$ input and $N(=5)$ output ports. Each of the N input ports can carry N different wavelengths. The N wavelengths coupled into, for example, input port 3 are distributed among output ports 1 to N. The N wavelengths carried by other input ports are distributed in the same way, but cyclically rotated. In this way each output port receives N different wavelengths, one from each input port. To realize such an interconnectivity scheme in a strictly non-blocking way using a single wavelength, a huge number of switches would be required. Using the cyclic property of ULCF AWG, this functionality can be achieved with only one AWG. An example of all optical $N \times N(N = 5)$ interconnection system using AWG as a router is shown in Fig. 9.79. Figure 9.79(a) shows the physical topology between AWG router and N nodes. Some routers may be used for connection to other networks. Based on the interconnectivity of AWG in Fig. 9.78, the resulting logical connectivity patterns become $N \times N$ star network as shown in Fig. 9.79(b). All the nodes can communicate with each other at the same time, thus enabling N^2 optical connections simultaneously. Signals can be freely routed by changing the carrier wavelength of the signal. When combined with the wavelength conversion lasers, this AWG router can construct signal routing networks without using space-division optical switches [44, 45].

9.5.6. Athermal (Temperature Insensitive) AWG

Temperature sensitivity of the pass wavelength (frequency) in the silica-based AWG is about $d\lambda/dT = 1.2 \times 10^{-2}$(nm/deg)($d\nu/dT = -1.5$(GHz/deg)), which is mainly determined by the temperature dependence of silica glass itself ($dn_c/dT = 1.1 \times 10^{-5}$(1/deg)). The AWG multiplexer should be temperature controlled with a heater or a Peltier cooler to stabilize the channel wavelengths.

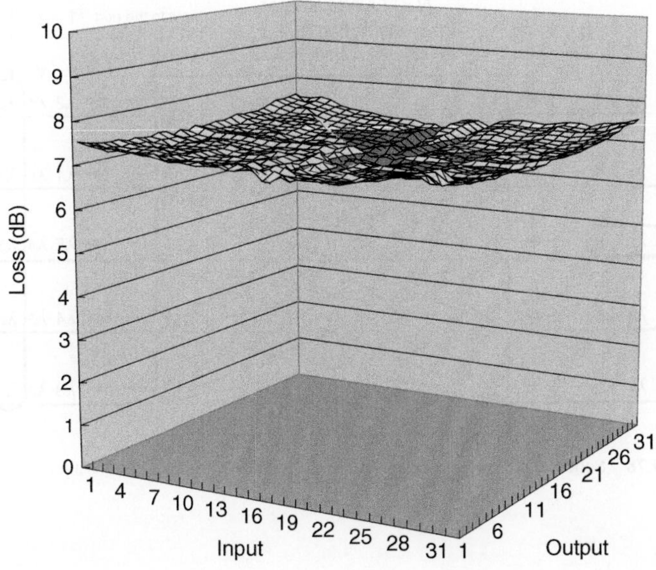

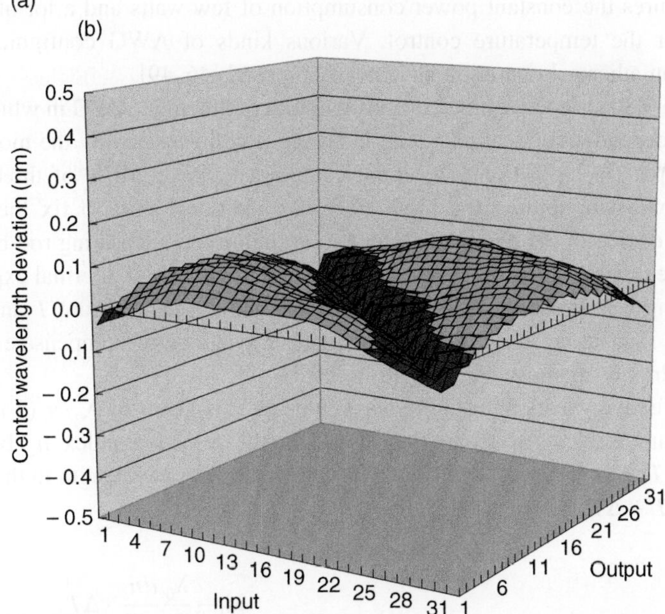

Figure 9.77 (a) Measured insertion losses for entire 32×32 input/output combinations in the uniform-loss and cyclic-frequency AWG. (b) Measured channel center frequency deviations for entire 32×32 input/output combinations in the uniform-loss and cyclic-frequency AWG.

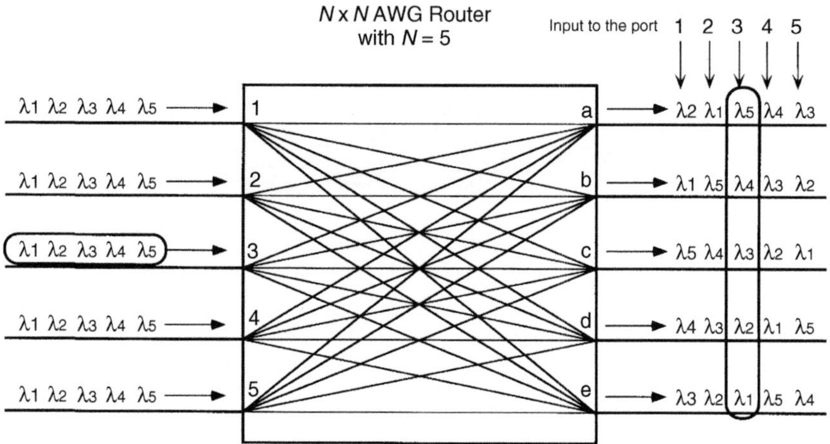

Figure 9.78 Schematic diagram illustrating $N \times N$ interconnections in a wavelength router.

This requires the constant power consumption of few watts and a lot of equipments for the temperature control. Various kinds of AWG configuration to achieve an athermal operation have been proposed [46–49].

Figure 9.80 shows a schematic configuration of athermal AWG in which temperature dependent optical path length change is compensated by the movement of the input fiber position. The input coupling device consists of three parts: namely one part holding the input fiber, an additional post to fix the whole coupling device to the chip and a metal (aluminium) compensating rod between them. The compensating rod is made of a material with a high thermal expansion coefficient α_{rod}. It changes its length with the ambient temperature T and shifts the input fiber along the endface of the slab waveguide to compensate for the thermal drift of the pass wavelength in AWG.

An effective wavelength in the waveguide at T is given by $\lambda_0/n_c(T)$. When temperature is changed from T to $T+\Delta T$, the effective index n_c becomes $n_c(T+\Delta T)=n_c(T)+\Delta T\cdot dn_c/dT$. Then the effective wavelength in the waveguide at $T+\Delta T$ is expressed by

$$\frac{\lambda_0}{n_c(T+\Delta T)}=\frac{\lambda_0}{n_c(T)+\dfrac{dn_c}{dT}\cdot\Delta T}\cong\frac{\lambda_0-\dfrac{\lambda_0}{n_c}\dfrac{dn_c}{dT}\cdot\Delta T}{n_c(T)}. \tag{9.42}$$

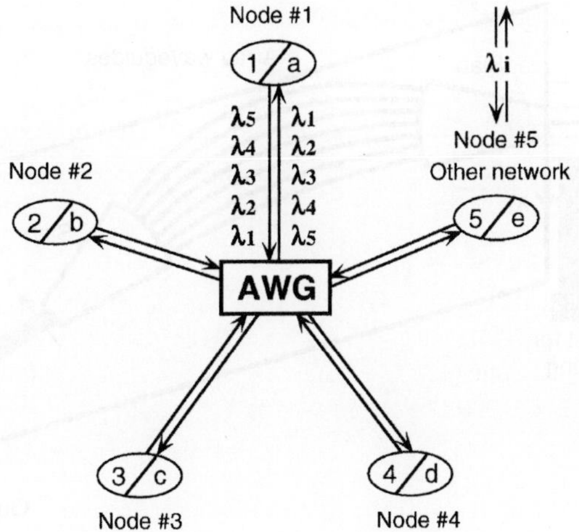

(a) Physical topology

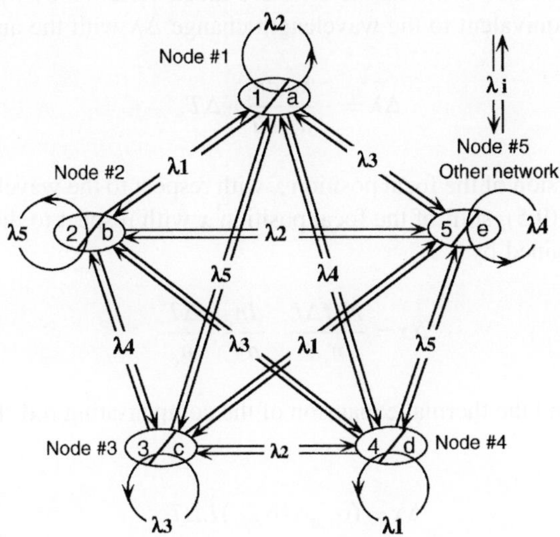

(b) Resulting logical connectivity

Figure 9.79 All optical $N \times N$ interconnection system using ULCF AWG as a router: (a) Physical topology. (b) Resulting logical connectivity.

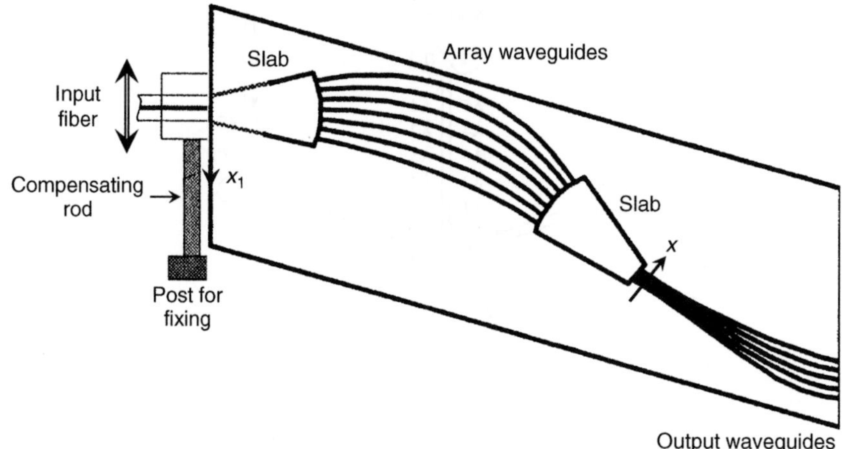

Figure 9.80 Configuration of athermal AWG with temperature compensating input position. (After Ref. [46]).

It is known from Eq. (9.42) that the effective-index variation by the temperature change ΔT is equivalent to the wavelength change $\Delta\lambda$ with the amount of

$$\Delta\lambda = -\frac{\lambda_0}{n_c}\frac{dn_c}{dT}\cdot\Delta T. \tag{9.43}$$

Since the dispersion of the focal position x with respect to the wavelength change is given by Eq. (9.5), shift of the focal position x with respect to the temperature variation is obtained by

$$\Delta x = \frac{N_c f \Delta L}{n_s d}\cdot\frac{dn_c}{dT}\cdot\frac{\Delta T}{n_c}. \tag{9.44}$$

On the other hand the thermal expansion of the compensating rod shifts the input fiber by

$$\Delta x = (\alpha_{\text{rod}} - \alpha_{\text{chip}})L\Delta T, \tag{9.45}$$

where L is the length of the compensating rod, α_{rod} and α_{chip} are thermal expansion coefficients of the input coupling device and AWG chip, respectively. Then we obtain the requirement for the temperature compensating device as

$$(\alpha_{\text{rod}} - \alpha_{\text{chip}})L = \frac{N_c f \Delta L}{n_s d}\cdot\frac{1}{n_c}\frac{dn_c}{dT}. \tag{9.46}$$

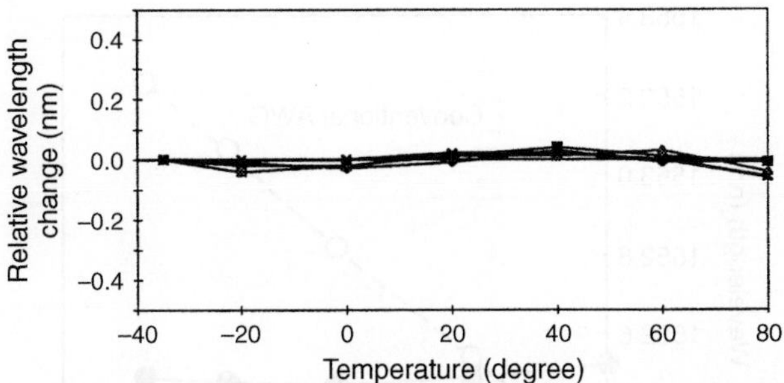

Figure 9.81 Shift of several channel's peak transmission with temperature (After Ref. [46]).

Figure 9.81 shows the shift of several channel's peak transmission with temperature for a 200 GHz module. The temperature is varied from −35 to +80°C. The center wavelength of the AWG filter is tuned back to the desired value, and becomes nearly independent of the ambient temperature. This method may be applied to spectrographs and phased array filters realized in any material.

Figure 9.82 shows a schematic configuration of athermal AWG without having any moving parts. Temperature dependent optical path difference in silica waveguides is compensated with a trapezoidal groove filled with silicone adhesive which has negative thermal coefficient. Since the pass wavelength is given by $\lambda_0 = n_c \Delta L / m$, optical path length difference $n_c \Delta L$ should be made insensitive to temperature. Therefore the groove is designed to satisfy the following conditions

$$n_c \Delta L = n_c \Delta \ell + \hat{n}_c \Delta \hat{\ell} \tag{9.47}$$

and

$$\frac{d(n_c \Delta L)}{dT} = \frac{dn_c}{dT} \Delta \ell + \frac{d\hat{n}_c}{dT} \Delta \hat{\ell} = 0, \tag{9.48}$$

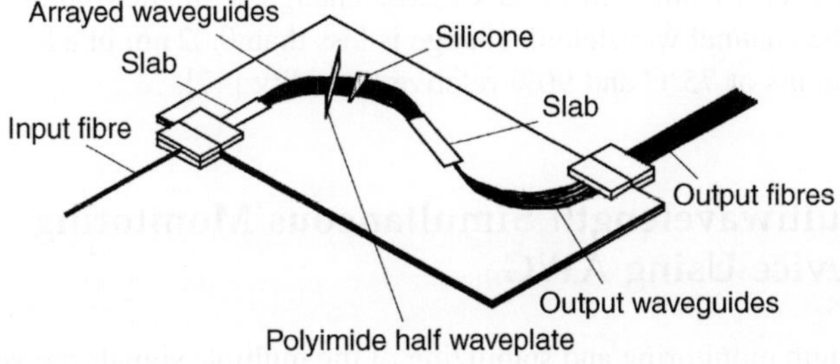

Figure 9.82 Schematic configuration of athermal AWG. (After Ref. [47]).

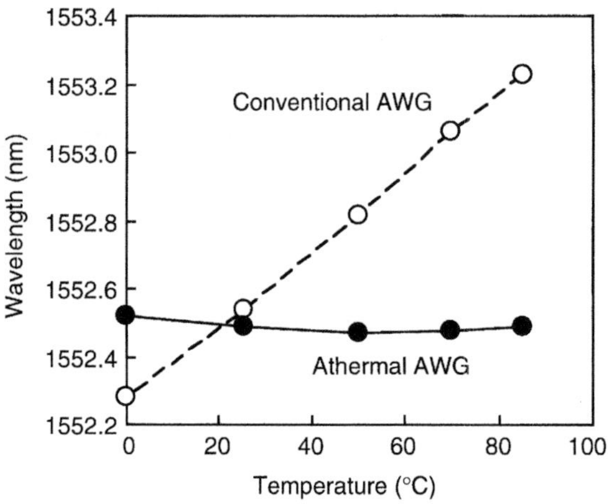

Figure 9.83 Temperature dependences of pass wavelengths. (After Ref. [47]).

where $\hat{n}$ is the refractive index of silicone and $\Delta\ell$ and $\Delta\hat{\ell}$ are the path length differences of silica waveguides and silicone region, respectively. Equation. (9.47) is a condition to satisfy the AWG specifications and Eq. (9.48) is the athermal condition. The temperature sensitivity of silicone is $d\hat{n}_c/dT = -37 \times 10^{-5}(1/\text{deg})$. Therefore the path length difference of silicone is $\Delta\hat{\ell} \cong \Delta\ell/37$. Figure 9.83 shows temperature dependencies of pass wavelengths in conventional and athermal AWGs. The temperature dependent wavelength change has been reduced from 0.95 nm to 0.05 nm in the 0–85°C range. The excess loss caused by the groove is about 2 dB which is mainly a diffraction loss in the groove. The insertion loss caused by diffraction loss can be reduced by segmenting a single trapezoidal silicone region (Fig. 9.84(a)) into multiple groove regions (Fig. 9.84(b)) [50]. Groove width w and separation d are 15 μm and 50 μm, respectively. In the segmented groove regions, light beam is periodically focused. Therefore insertion loss is reduced to about 0.4 dB. Figure 9.85 shows loss change at 1552.52 nm during heat cycles from −40 to 85°C. Loss change is smaller than 0.2 dB. Furthermore, the channel wavelength change is less than 0.02 nm in a long-term test over 5000 hours at 75°C and 90% relative humidity [47].

9.5.7. Multiwavelength Simultaneous Monitoring Device Using AWG

Wavelength monitoring and stabilizing of the multiple signals are very important in WDM systems. Wavelength crossover properties of etched grating or

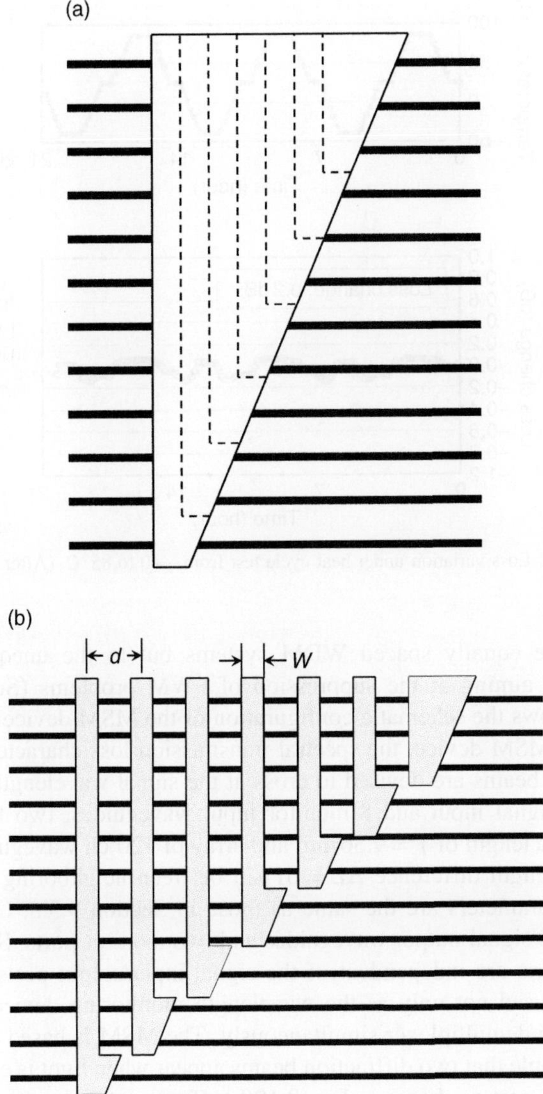

Figure 9.84 Athermal configurations with (a) a single trapezoidal silicone region and (b) multiple segmented groove regions.

AWG multiplexers have been confirmed to be useful for the multi-wavelength simultaneous monitoring (MSM) scheme [51, 52]. However, there has been no MSM device which is applicable to both equally and unequally spaced WDM systems. A novel MSM device is proposed and fabricated [53] which is applicable

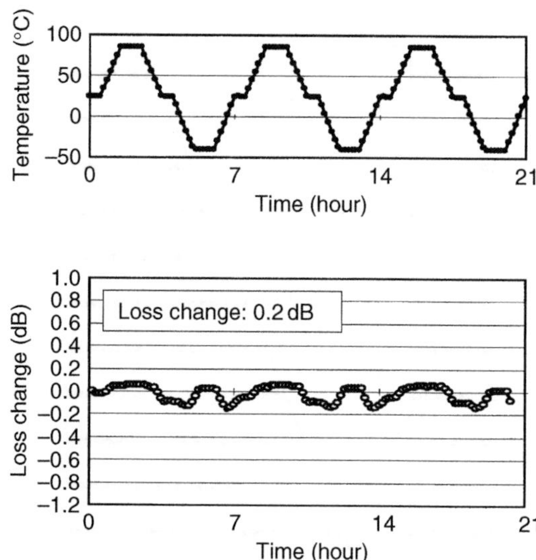

Figure 9.85 Loss variation under heat cycle test from −40 to 85 °C. (After Ref. [47]).

not only to the equally spaced WDM systems but to the unequally spaced WDM systems aiming at the suppression of FWM problems (Section 9.5.3). Figure 9.86 shows the schematic configuration of the MSM device using AWG. In the present MSM device, the spectral transmission loss characteristics of the two diffraction beams are devised to cross at the signal wavelength. The AWG consists of 8 signal input and 8 monitor input waveguides, two focusing slab regions with arc length of $f = 9.36$ mm and array of 120-ch waveguides with the constant path length difference $\Delta L = 61\,\mu$m between neighboring waveguides. These AWG parameters are the same as those in Section 9.5.3. On the output side, there are 8 signal output waveguides and two monitor ports. Since monitor input/output ports are independent of the signal input/output ports, the present device can be used not only as the wavelength monitoring device but also as the WDM multi/demultiplexer simultaneously. The MSM is based on the AWG operating principle that two diffraction beams appear when light is coupled to the off-center input port as shown in Fig. 9.10(b). Figure 9.87 shows schematically the light focusing properties in the second slab region. Since two monitor output ports are slightly shifted inwards from their maximum coupling positions for the i-th center wavelength $\lambda_{ch}(i)$, spectral transmission losses of the two diffraction beams cross at $\lambda_{ch}(i)$. Transmission loss of monitor #1 becomes larger than that of monitor #2 for $\lambda < \lambda_{ch}(i)$ [Fig. 9.87(a)]. To the contrary, transmission loss of monitor #1 becomes smaller than that of monitor #2 for $\lambda > \lambda_{ch}(i)$ [Fig. 9.87(b)]. Therefore, error signal for the wavelength matching can easily be obtained from

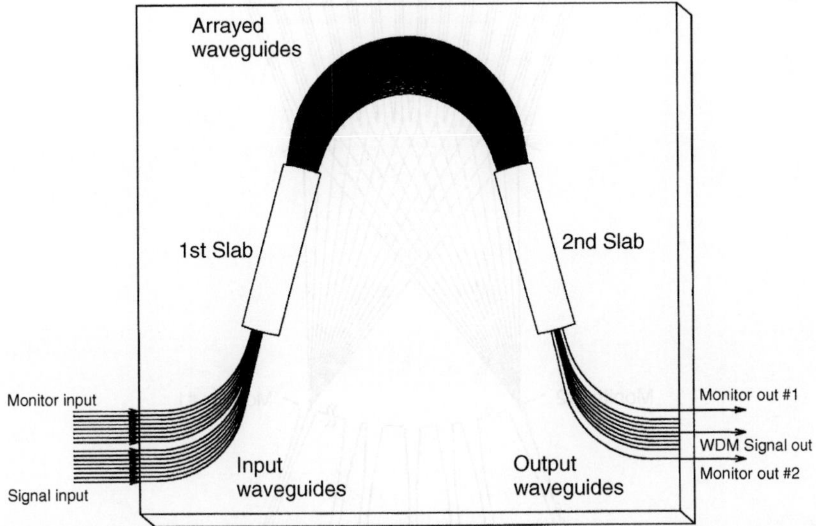

Figure 9.86 Schematic configuration of multiwavelength simultaneous monitoring (MSM) device using arrayed-waveguide grating.

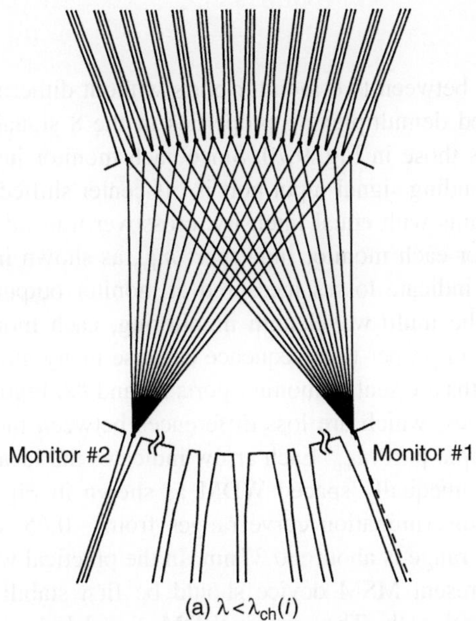

Figure 9.87 Light focusing properties for the two diffraction beams in the second slab region. (a) $\lambda < \lambda_{ch}(i)$.

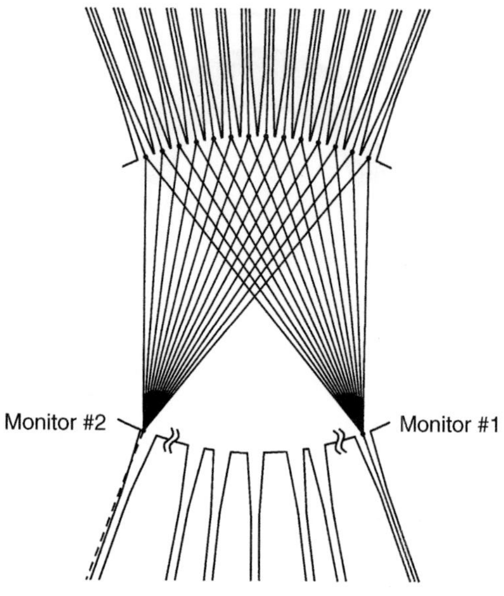

Figure 9.87 (*Continued*) (b) $\lambda > \lambda_{ch}(i)$.

the loss difference between two monitor ports without dithering of the monitor light. The measured demultiplexing properties in the 8 signal output ports are almost the same as those in Fig. 9.70. Since each monitor input port is placed where the corresponding signal input port is off-center shifted so as to produce two diffraction beams with equal intensity, crossover transmission loss properties are obtained for each monitor input port m_{inp} as shown in Fig. 9.88. Solid and dotted curves indicate losses measured at monitor output port #1 and #2, respectively. For the multi-wavelength monitoring, each monitor input signal should be sampled in proper time sequence because many monitor signals with different wavelengths are sent to monitor ports #1 and #2. Figure 9.89 shows the discrimination curves, which are loss differences between monitor #2 and #1, for each monitor input port m_{inp}. Each arrow indicates the location of the center wavelength of the unequally spaced WDM as shown in Fig. 9.70. The slope coefficient of the discrimination curve ranges from -0.65 to -0.94 dB/GHz and the monitoring range is about ± 0.37 nm. In the practical wavelength matching scheme, the present MSM device should be first stabilized to the stable reference laser wavelength. Then many WDM signal light sources are monitored and locked by utilizing crossover transmission loss properties of the MSM device.

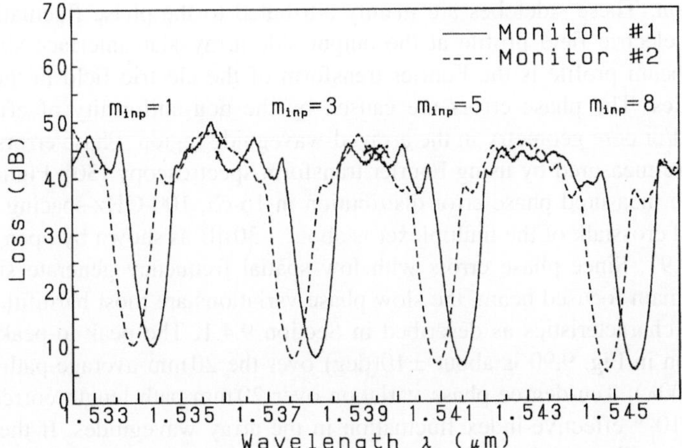

Figure 9.88 Crossover transmission loss properties for each monitor input port m_{inp}. Solid and dotted curves indicate losses measured at monitor output port #1 and #2, respectively.

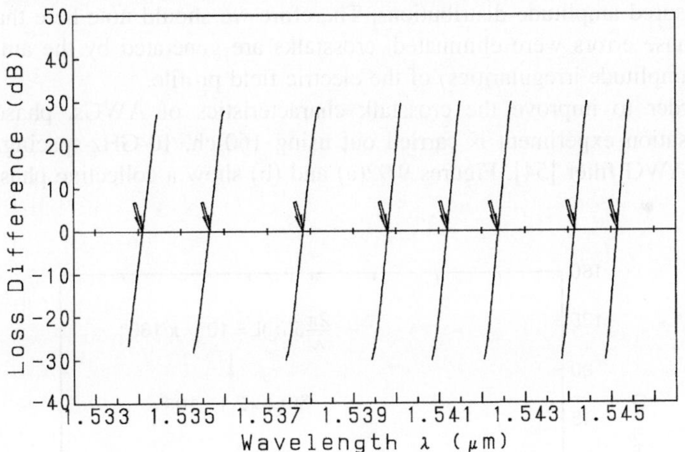

Figure 9.89 Discrimination curves of the MSM which are loss differences between monitor #2 and #1 for each monitor input port.

9.5.8. Phase Error Compensation of AWG

Crosstalk improvement is the major concern for the AWG multiplexers, especially for narrow channel spacing AWGs and $N \times N$ AWG routers. Crosstalks to other channels are caused by the sidelobe of the focused beam in the second slab region. These sidelobes are mainly attributed to the phase fluctuations of the total electric field profile at the output side array–slab interface since the focused beam profile is the Fourier transform of the electric field in the array waveguides. The phase errors are caused by the non-uniformity of effective-index and/or core geometry in the arrayed-waveguide region. Phase errors in the AWGs are measured by using Fourier transform spectroscopy [30]. Figure 9.90 shows the measured phase error distribution in 16-ch, 100-GHz-spacing AWG. Measured crosstalk of the multiplexer is about $-30\,\text{dB}$ as shown by open circles in Fig. 9.91. Since phase errors with low spatial frequency generate sidelobe near the main focused beam, the slow phase variations are most harmful for the crosstalk characteristics as described in Section 9.4.1. The peak-to-peak phase fluctuation in Fig. 9.90 is about ± 10(deg) over the 20 mm average path length $L(\approx 13000\lambda)$. Ten-degree phase variation over 20 mm path length corresponds to 2.1×10^{-6} effective-index fluctuation in the array waveguides. If the phase errors were eliminated, we could obtain about $-50\,\text{dB}$ crosstalk in 100 GHz-spacing AWG as shown by the theoretical curve in Fig. 9.91. The reason why we could not obtain sufficiently lower crosstalk as shown in Fig. 9.18 is that there still remain the amplitude errors. This calculation curve takes into account the measured amplitude distributions. Therefore we should note here that even when phase errors were eliminated, crosstalks are generated by the amplitude errors (amplitude irregularities) of the electric field profile.

In order to improve the crosstalk characteristics of AWGs, phase error compensation experiment is carried out using 160-ch, 10-GHz-spacing, ultra-narrow AWG filter [54]. Figures 9.92(a) and (b) show a collective phase-error

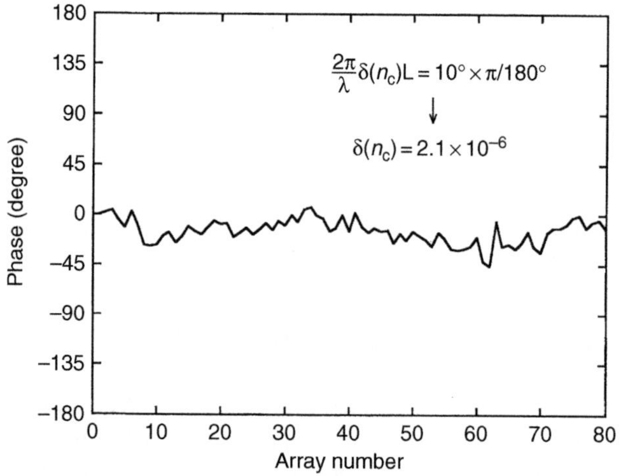

Figure 9.90 Measured phase error distribution in 16-ch, 100-GHz-spacing AWG.

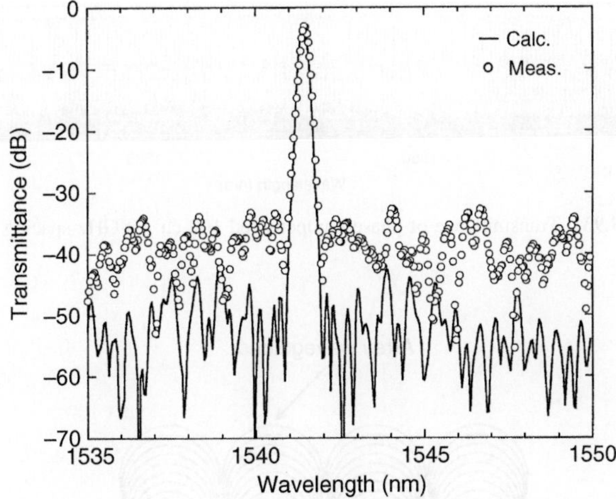

Figure 9.91 Theoretical transmittance of 16-ch, 100-GHz-spacing AWG without phase errors (solid line) and measured result with phase errors (circle).

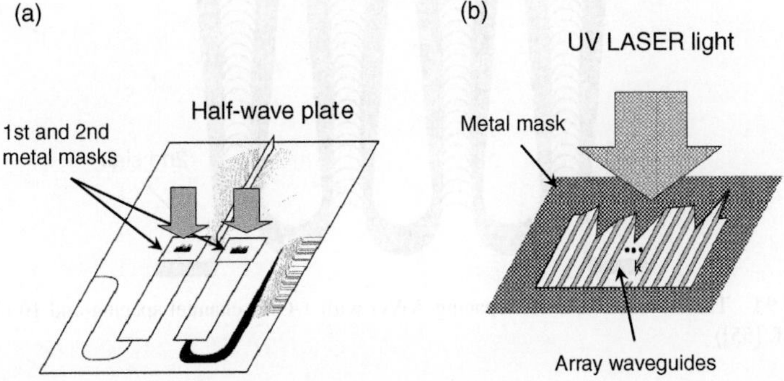

Figure 9.92 (a) Configuration of collective phase-error compensation technique and (b) UV LASER irradiation through metal mask. (After Ref. [54]).

compensation technique using UV laser light through metal mask [54]. The window length of the metal mask is proportional to the phase error in each array waveguide to be compensated. Since phase errors for TE and TM modes are different and also UV photosensitivity is different for two polarizations, two metal masks are used. Initial crosstalk of 160-ch, 10-GHz AWG before phase-error compensation was about 25 dB. After 4-hour ArF UV laser irradiation, phase errors are almost completely eliminated and crosstalk was reduced down to less than −36 dB as shown in Fig. 9.93. Annealing of the AWG, which is similar to fiber gratings, can stabilize UV photo-induced refractive-index change.

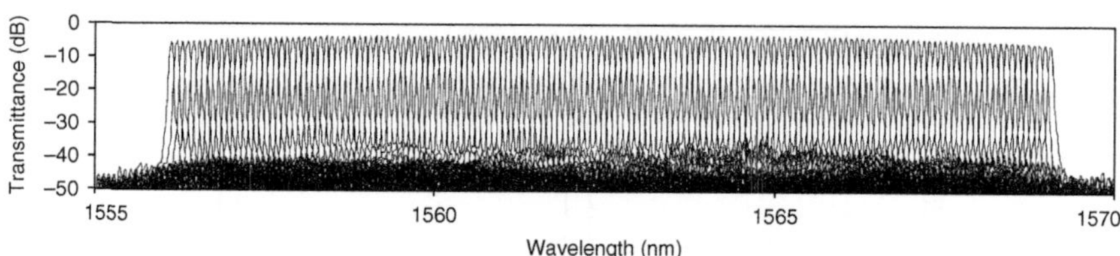

Figure 9.93 Transmittance of phase-compensated 160-ch, 10-GHz-spacing AWG.

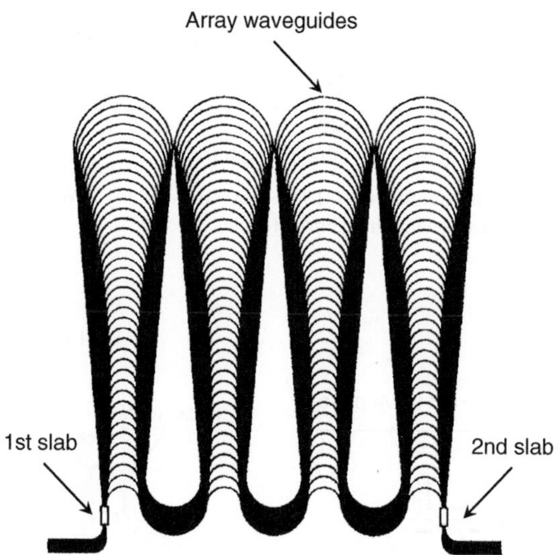

Figure 9.94 The narrowest channel spacing AWG with 1-GHz channel spacing and 16 channels. (After Ref. [55]).

Figure 9.94 shows the narrowest channel spacing AWG reported so far [55]. The channel spacing and number of channels are 1 GHz and 16, respectively. Since path length difference $\Delta L (= 12.6\,\text{mm})$ is quite long, phase-error compensation is inevitable to obtain reasonable crosstalk characteristics. Transmission spectra of 16-ch, 1-GHz-spacing AWG are shown in Fig. 9.95. Crosstalk and fiber-to-fiber loss are $-14 \sim -16\,\text{dB}$ and $8 \sim 11\,\text{dB}$, respectively. Broadband spectra of edge-emitting LED were filtered by the 1-GHz spacing AWG. AWG was placed on a commercial thermoelectric cooler with $\pm 0.1°$. Measured fluctuation of the pass-band frequency was $\pm 0.16\,\text{GHz}$. This device could be used as a wavelength standard for WDM systems and microwave filtering in sub-carrier multiplexed signals.

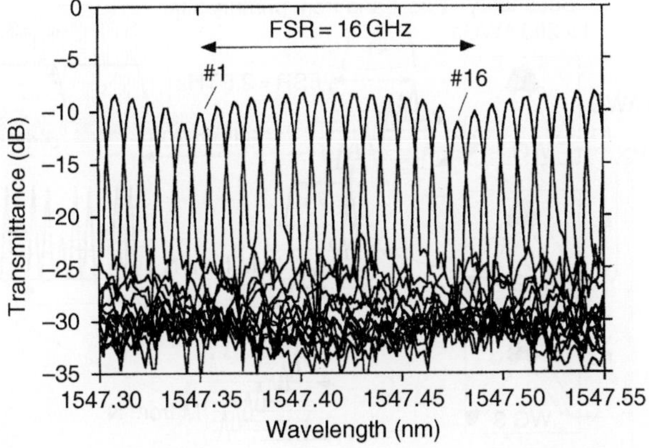

Figure 9.95 Transmittance of 16-ch, 1-GHz-spacing AWG. (After Ref. [55]).

9.5.9. Tandem AWG Configuration

The maximum available wafer size of PLC is limited by the fabrication apparatus such as deposition machine, electric furnace and mask aligner, etc. Therefore, it is not so easy to fabricate AWG with larger channel numbers. One possible way to increase the total number of channels is to use two kinds of AWGs, which are cascaded in series. In order to realize much larger channels, for example 1000 channels, tandem concatenation is extremely important. Figure 9.96 shows the configuration of 10 GHz-spaced 1010-ch WDM filter that covers both the C and L bands [56]. It consists of a primary 1×10 flat-top AWG (AWG #k with $k = 1, 2, \ldots, 10$) with a 1-THz channel spacing and ten secondary 1×101 AWGs with 10-GHz spacing and 200 channels. Phase errors of the secondary AWGs were compensated for by using the photo-induced refractive-index change as described in Section 9.5.8. Crosstalks of secondary AWGs are around -32 dB and the sidelobe levels in these passbands are less than -35 dB. The tandem configuration enables us to construct flexible WDM systems; that is, secondary AWGs can be added when bandwidth demands increases. Also, this configuration will be essential for the construction of hierarchical cross-connect (XC) systems such as fiber XC, band XC and wavelength XC. Output port #$k(k = 1, 2, \ldots, 10)$ of the primary AWG is connected to the input port of AWG #k through an optical fiber. Two conditions are imposed on these AWGs. First, the center wavelength of 200 channels of AWG #k should be designed to coincide with that of the flat-top passband #k from primary AWG output #k. Then passband #k is sliced with the AWG #k without any noticeable loss. Second, the sidelobe components of flat-top passband #k are removed as shown

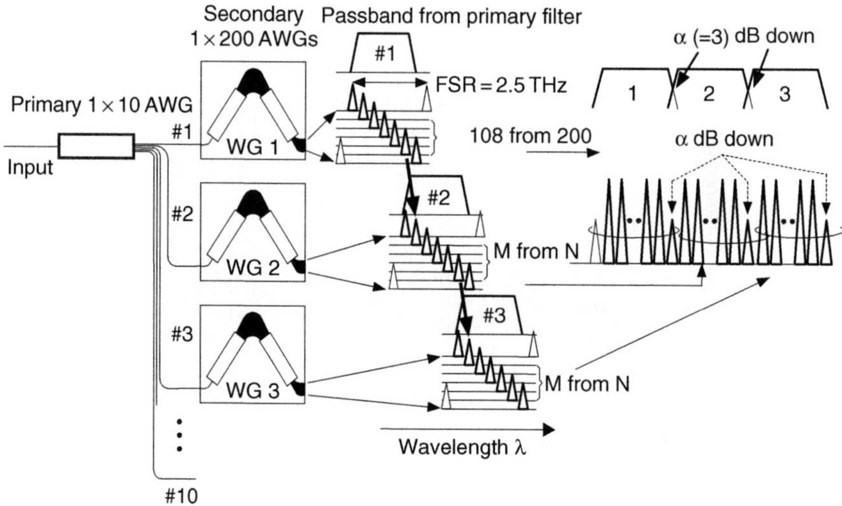

Figure 9.96 Configuration of 10 GHz-spaced 1010-ch tandem AWG. (After Ref. [56]).

in the inset of Fig. 9.96. Therefore, one passband within the FSR is obtained from one output port of AWG #*k*. From every AWG #*k* 101 wavelengths are selected. Figure 9.97 shows the demultiplexing properties of all the channels of the tandem AWG filter. There are a total of 1010 channels and they are all aligned at 10 GHz intervals with no channel missing in the 1526 to 1608 nm wavelength range. The loss values ranged from 13 to 19 dB. The main origin of the 13 dB loss is 10 dB intrinsic loss of the primary AWG. This could be reduced by about 9 dB when a 1 × 10 interference filter is used instead of flat-top AWG.

The maximum 4200-ch AWG with 5-GHz channel spacing has also been fabricated by using the tandem configuration [57–59].

9.6. RECONFIGURABLE OPTICAL ADD/DROP MULTIPLEXER (ROADM)

A reconfigurable optical add/drop multiplexer (ROADM) is a device that gives simultaneous access to all wavelength channels in WDM communication systems. A novel integrated-optic ROADM was fabricated and basic functions of individually routing 16 different wavelength channels with 100-GHz channel spacing was demonstrated [60]. The waveguide configuration of 16-ch optical ADM is shown in Fig. 9.98. It consists of four AWGs and 16 double-gate thermo-optic (TO) switches. Four AWGs are allocated with their slab regions crossing each other. These AWGs have the same grating parameters; they are, the

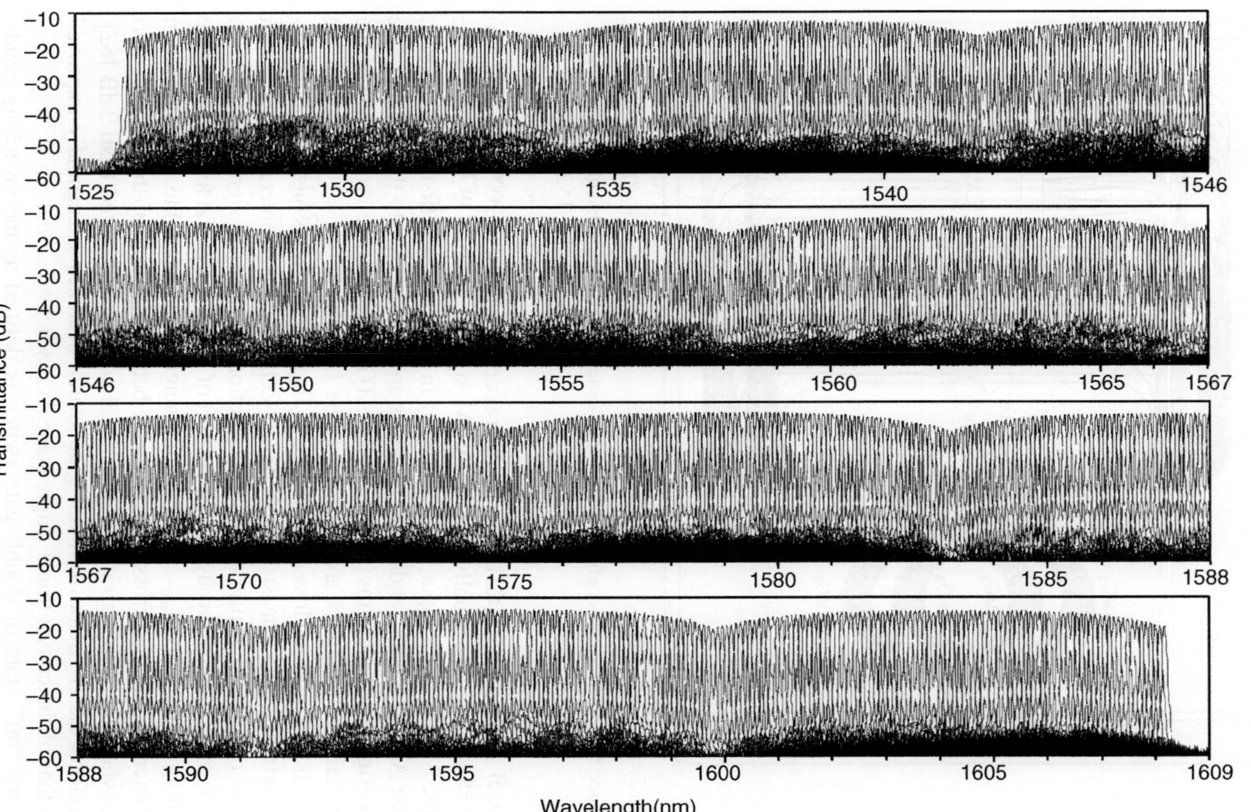

Figure 9.97 Demultiplexing properties of all the channels of the tandem AWG filter. (After Ref. [56]).

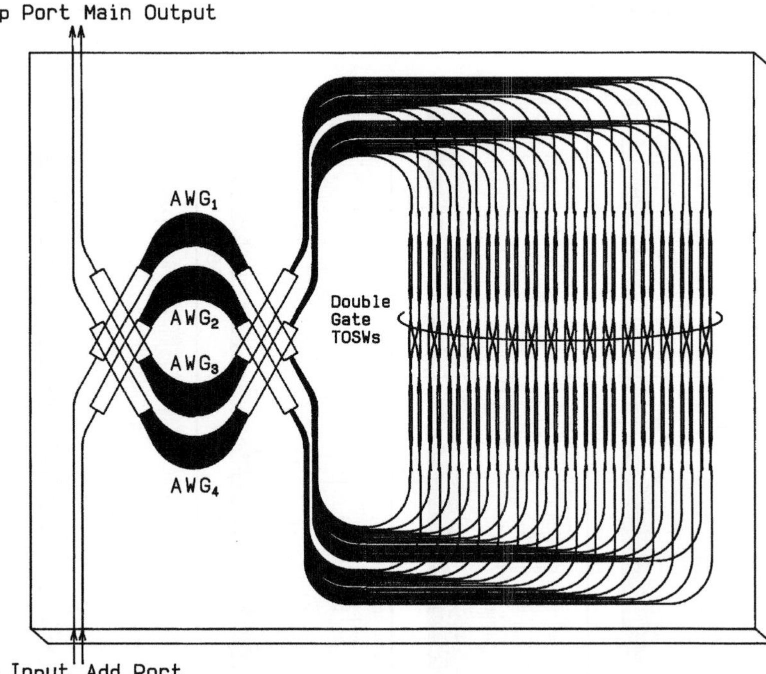

Figure 9.98 Waveguide configuration of 16-ch optical ADM with double-gate TO switches.

channel spacing of 100 GHz and the free spectral range of 3300 GHz (26.4 nm) at 1.55 μm region. Equally spaced WDM signals, $\lambda_1, \lambda_2, \ldots, \lambda_{16}$, which are coupled to the main input port (add port) in Fig. 9.98 are first demultiplexed by the $AWG_1(AWG_2)$ and then 16 signals are introduced into the lefthand-side arms (righthand-side arms) of double-gate TO switches. The cross angle of the intersecting waveguides are designed to be larger than 30° so as to make the crosstalk and insertion loss negligible [61]. Figure 9.99 shows one unit of double-gate switch, which consists of four Mach–Zehnder interferometers (MZIs) with thermo-optic phase shifters and an intersection. Any optical signal coupled into port A_{in} or B_{in} passes through the cross port of either one of the four MZIs before reaching output port A_{out} or B_{out}. In the single-stage MZI, the light extinction characteristics of the cross port is much better than that of the through port even when the coupling ratio of directional coupler is deviated from 3 dB [62]. Therefore, the crosstalk of double-gate switch becomes substantially improved than that of the conventional single-stage TO switch.

Here "off" state of double-gate switch is defined as the switching condition where signal from left input port (right input port) goes to right output

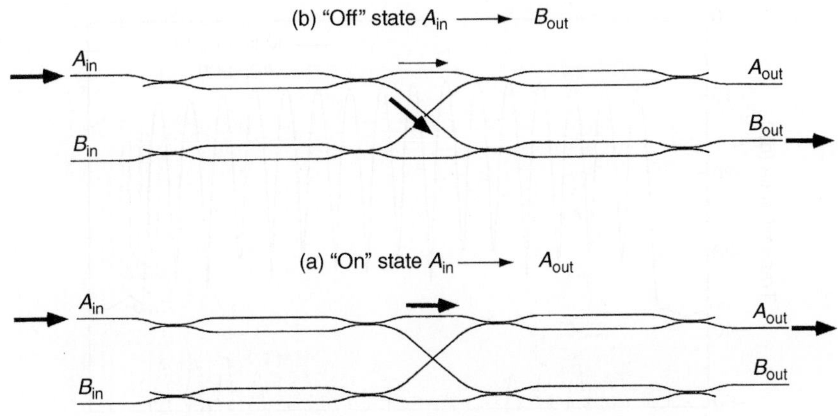

Figure 9.99 Schematic configuration of double-gate switch.

port (left output port) in Fig. 9.98. The "on" state is then defined as the condition where signal from left input port (right input port) goes to left output port (right output port). When double-gate switch is "off", the demultiplexed light by $AWG_1(AWG_2)$ goes to the cross arm and multiplexed again by the $AWG_3(AWG_4)$. On the other hand, if double-gate switch is "on" state the demultiplexed light by $AWG_1(AWG_2)$ goes to the through arm and multiplexed by the $AWG_4(AWG_3)$. Therefore, any specific wavelength signal can be extracted from the main output port and led to the drop port by changing the corresponding switch condition. Signals at the same wavelength as that of the dropped component can be added to the main output port when it is coupled into add port in Fig. 9.98.

Figure 9.100 shows light transmission characteristics from main input port to main output port (solid line) and drop port (dotted line) when all TO switches are "off". The on–off crosstalk is smaller than −33 dB with the on-chip losses of 7.8 ~ 10.3 dB. When TO switches SW_2, SW_4, SW_6, SW_7, SW_9, SW_{12}, SW_{13} and SW_{15}, for example, are turned to "on", the selected signals λ_2, λ_4, λ_6, λ_7, λ_9, λ_{12}, λ_{13} and λ_{15} are extracted from main output port (solid line) and led to the drop port (dotted line) as shown in Fig. 9.101. The on-off crosstalk is smaller than −30 dB with the on-chip losses of 8 ~ 10 dB. Since optical signals pass through both AWG_3 and AWG_4 the crosstalk level here is determined by the crosstalk in the arrayed waveguides.

Figure 9.102 is a waveguide configuration of athermal 16-ch ROADM [63]. Silicone-type athermal technique is incorporated in the ROADM. Transmission spectra become almost insensitive to temperature change as shown in Fig. 9.103.

Though the electric power necessary to drive double-gate switch becomes two times larger than the conventional TO switch, the power consumption itself

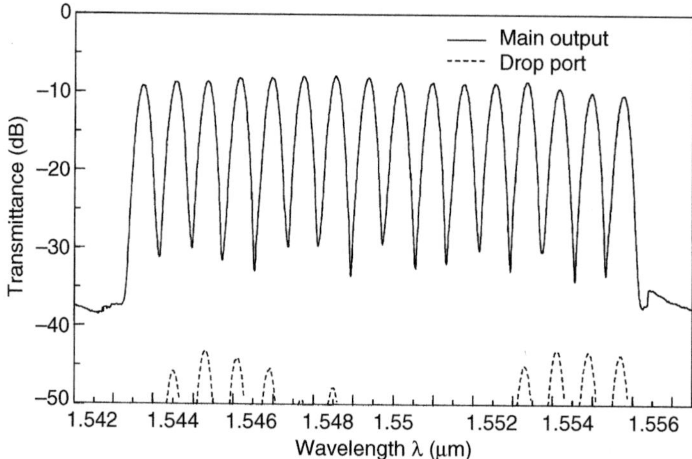

Figure 9.100 Transmission spectra from main input port to main output port (solid line) and drop port (dotted line) when all TO switches are "off".

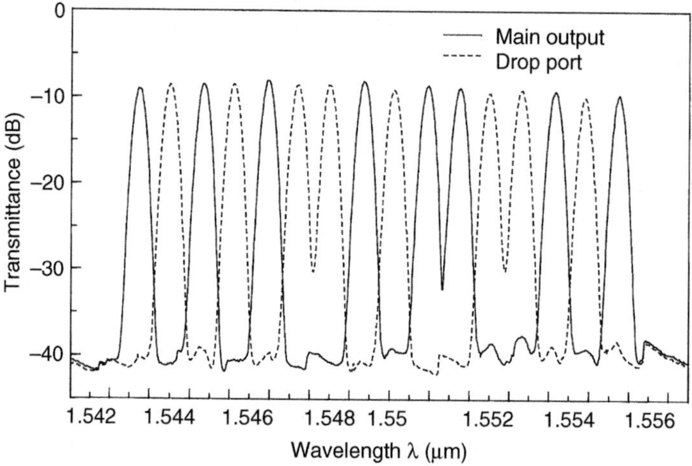

Figure 9.101 Transmission spectra from main input port to main output port and drop port when TO switches $SW_2, SW_4, SW_6, SW_7, SW_9, SW_{12}, SW_{13}$ and SW_{15} are "on".

can be reduced to almost $1/5 \sim 1/2$ when bridge-suspended phase shifter [64] or trench and groove structure [65] are utilized. The present ROADM can transport all input signals to the succeeding stages without inherent power losses. Therefore, these ROADMs are very attractive for all optical WDM routing systems and allow the network to be transparent to signal formats and bit rates.

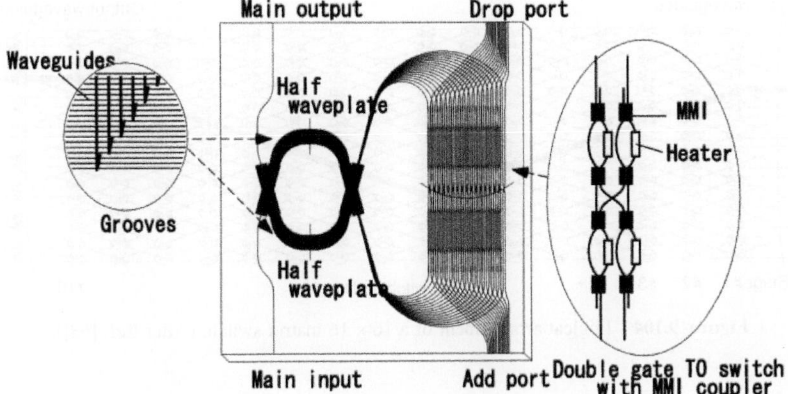

Figure 9.102 Configuration of athermal 16-ch ROADM. (After Ref. [63]).

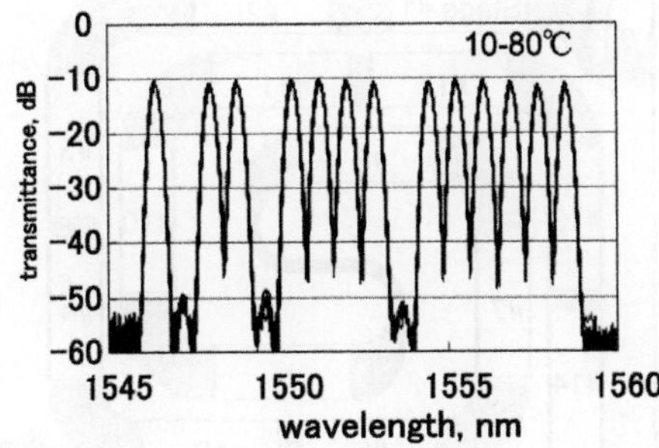

Figure 9.103 Transmission spectra of athermal 16-ch ROADM. (After Ref. [63]).

9.7. $N \times N$ MATRIX SWITCHES

Space-division optical switches are one of the indispensable optical devices for the reconfigurable interconnects in a cross-connect systems, fiber-optic subscriber line connectors, and photonic inter-module connectors [3, 66, 67]. Figure 9.104 shows the logical arrangement of a 16×16 strictly non-blocking matrix switch with a path-independent insertion loss (PI-Loss) configuration [68]. This arrangement is quite advantageous for reducing total circuit length since it requires only N switching stages to construct $N \times N$ switch. The switching unit consists of double-gate switch which has been described in Section 9.6. The circuit layout of the 16×16 matrix switch is shown in Fig. 9.105. Sixteen switching stages are allocated along the serpentine waveguides. There are 16 switching units in one switching stage. The total circuit length is 66 cm.

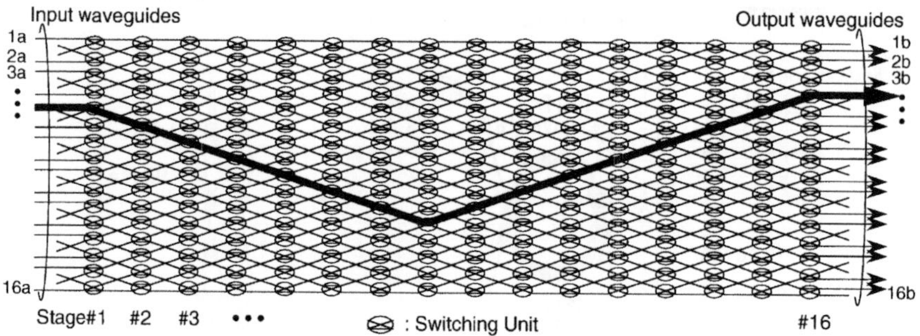

Figure 9.104 Logical arrangement of a 16 × 16 matrix switch. (After Ref. [68]).

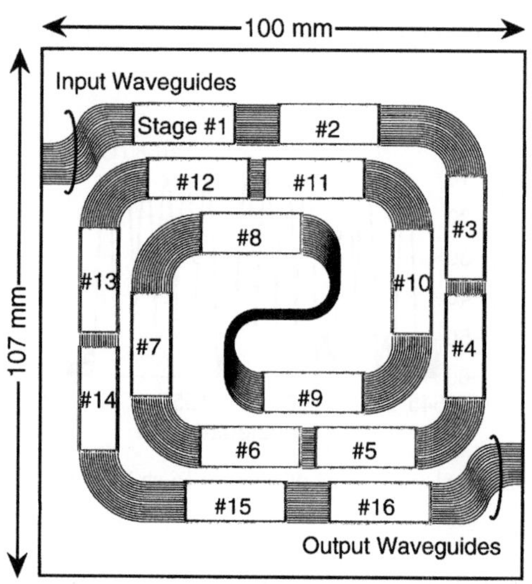

Figure 9.105 Circuit layout of the 16 × 16 matrix switch. (After Ref. [68]).

The fabricated switching unit requires bias power even when it is in the "off" state due to the waveguide phase (optical path length) errors. The phase error in each switching unit is permanently eliminated by using a phase-trimming technique, in which high temperature local heat treatment produces permanent refractive-index change for either of the arms of the MZIs. Figure 9.106 shows switching characteristics for one input–output combination when heater power to the second MZI are fixed at 0 mW and 500 mW, respectively. The extinction ratio when 1st and 2nd MZIs are activated simultaneously becomes double of the single MZI. Therefore extremely high extinction ratio of 67 dB has been

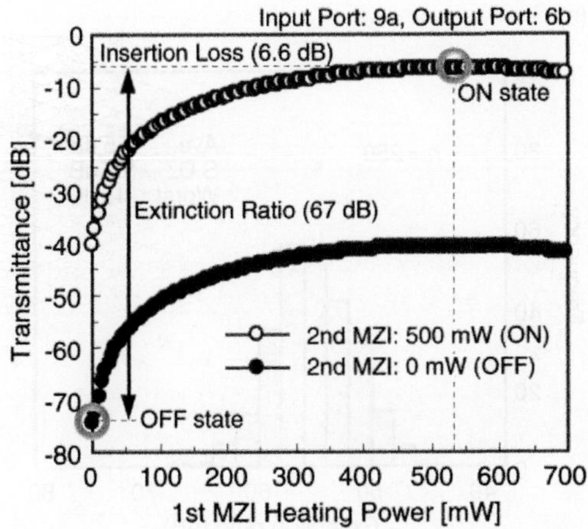

Figure 9.106 Switching characteristics for typical input–output combination. (After Ref. [68]).

successfully achieved with 6.6 dB insertion loss. Figures 9.107(a) and (b) shows measured insertion losses and extinction ratios for all 256 input and output connection patterns, respectively. The insertion loss ranges from 6.0 dB to 8.0 dB, with an average of 6.6 dB. The extinction ratio ranges from 45 dB to 67 dB, with an average of 55 dB. The total electric power for operating the 16 × 16 matrix switch is about 17 W (1.06 W for each switching unit).

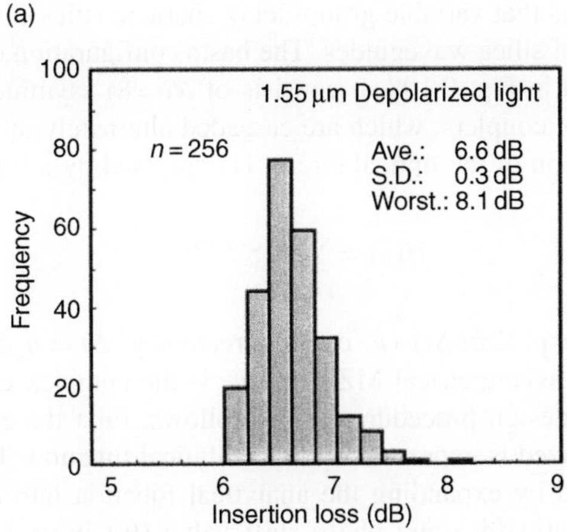

Figure 9.107 Measured (a) insertion losses.

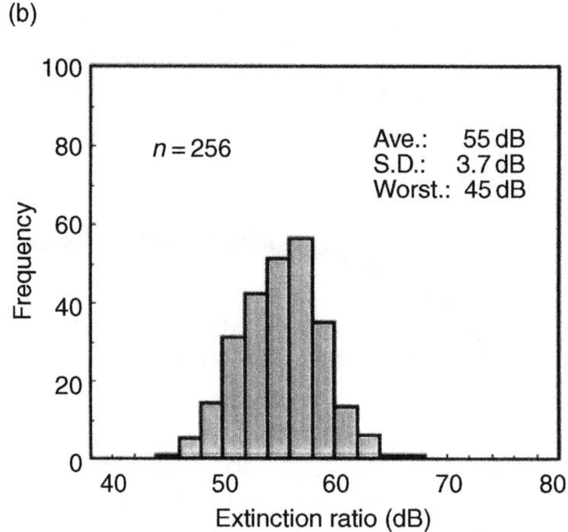

Figure 9.107 (*Continued*) (b) extinction ratios for all 256 input and output connection patterns. (After Ref. [68]).

9.8. LATTICE-FORM PROGRAMMABLE DISPERSION EQUALIZERS

The transmission distance in optical fiber communications has been greatly increased by the development of erbium-doped fiber amplifiers. In consequence, the main factor limiting the maximum repeater span is now the fiber chromatic dispersion. Several techniques have been reported to compensate for the delay distortion in optical stage [69–75]. An advantage of the PLC optical delay equalizer [73–75] is that variable group-delay characteristics can be achieved by the phase control of silica waveguides. The basic configuration of the PLC delay equalizer is shown in Fig. 9.108. It consists of $N(=8)$ asymmetrical MZIs and $N+1(=9)$ tunable couplers, which are cascaded alternately in series. The cross port transfer function of the optical circuit is expressed by a Fourier series as

$$H(z) = \sum_{\mathrm{k}=0}^{N} a_{\mathrm{k}} z^{-k+N/2}, \tag{9.49}$$

where z denotes $\exp(j2\pi\nu\Delta t)$ (ν: optical frequency, $\Delta t = n_c \Delta L/c$: unit delay time difference in asymmetrical MZI) and a_{k} is the complex expansion coefficient. The circuit design procedures are as follows. First the equalizer transfer function to be realized is expressed by the analytical function. Then coefficients a'_{k}s are determined by expanding the analytical function into a Fourier series. Finally coupling ratio (ϕ_i) and phase shift value (θ_i) in each stage of lattice filter are determined by the filter synthesis method [6].

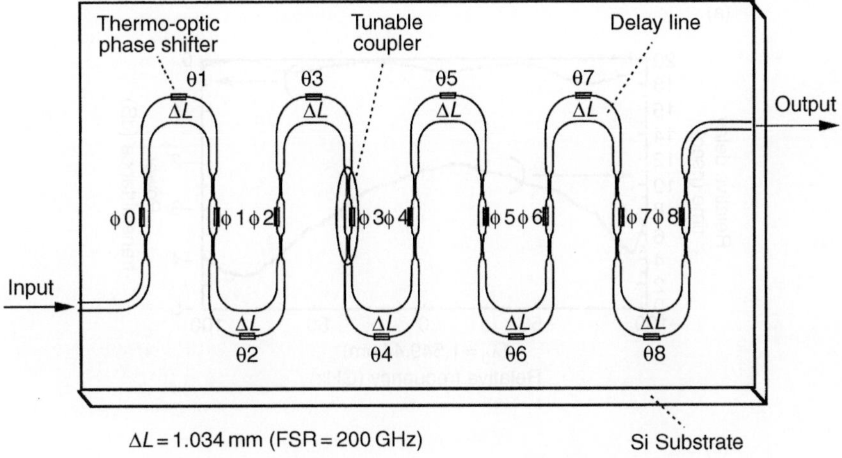

Figure 9.108 Basic configuration of the PLC delay equalizer.

In high speed optical fiber transmission systems (> 40 Gbit/s), the effect of the higher order dispersion (third order dispersion or dispersion slope) in the DSF is one of the major factors limiting the transmission distance [76]. Programmable dispersion equalizers can be designed so as to compensate for the higher order dispersion of DSFs. Figure 9.109(a) shows the measured power transmittance and relative delay time of the PLC higher order dispersion equalizer [77, 78]. The dispersion slope of the equalizer is calculated to be $-15.8\,\text{ps/nm}^2$. Figure 9.109(b) is the relative delay of the 300-km DSF. The dispersion slope of DSF is $0.05 \sim 0.06\,\text{ps/nm}^2/\text{km}$. Therefore, the equalizer can compensate the higher order dispersion of ~300-km of DSF. Figure 9.109(c) shows the relative delay time of 300-km DSF cascaded with the equalizer. The positive dispersion slope of the DSF is almost completely compensated by the PLC equalizer. Figure 9.110 shows pulse waveforms of (a) input pulse to the DSF, (b) output pulse from 300-km DSF and (c) output pulse from "300-km DSF + equalizer", respectively. The trailing ripples in Fig. 9.110(b) are caused by the dispersion slope of DSF since the delay times for the peripheral signal components are larger than that for the central signal components (Fig. 9.109(b)). However, the trailing ripples have been eliminated by the dispersion compensation with PLC equalizer (Fig. 9.110(c)). 200 Gbit/s time-division-multiplexed transmission experiment using a dispersion slope equalizer has been carried out over 100-km fiber length [78]. The pulse distortion caused by the dispersion slope was almost completely recovered, and the power penalty was improved by more than 4 dB.

(a)

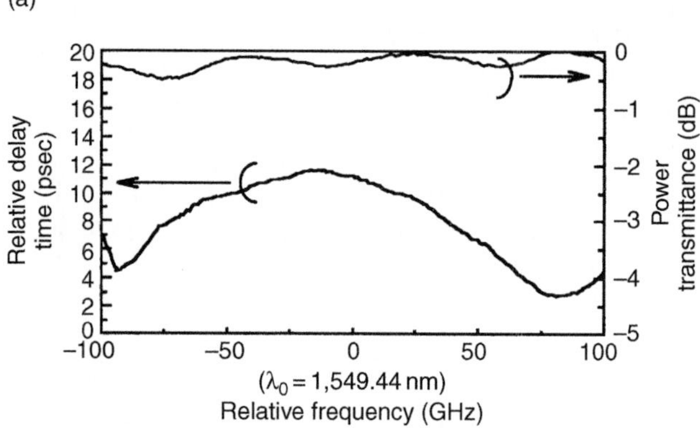

(b)

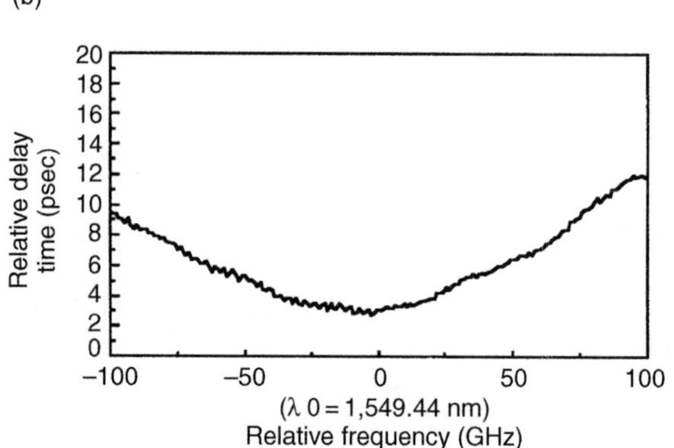

(c)

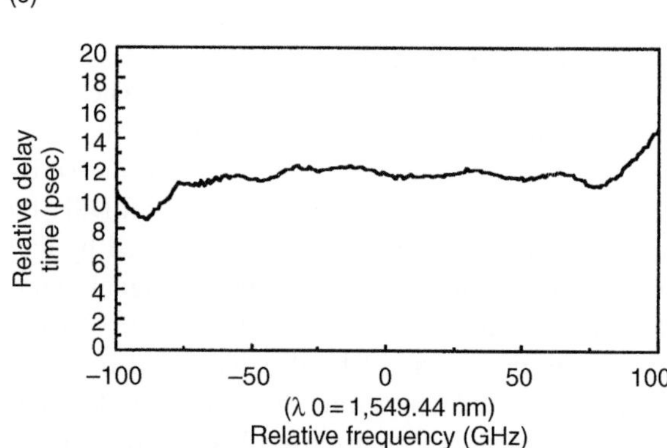

Figure 9.109 Relative delay times of (a) PLC higher order dispersion equalizer and measured power transmittance, (b) 300-km DSF and (c) 300-km DSF + equalizer. (After Ref. [78]).

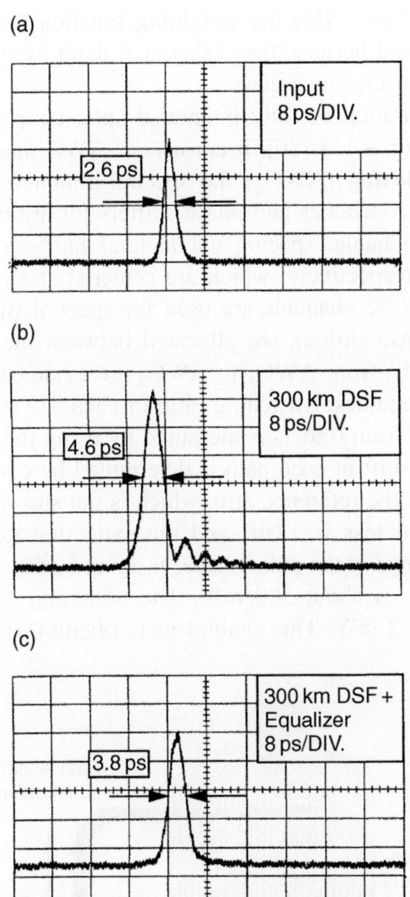

Figure 9.110 Pulse waveforms of (a) input pulse to the DSF, (b) output pulse from 300-km DSF and (c) output pulse from 300-km DSF + equalizer. (After Ref. [78]).

9.9. TEMPORAL PULSE WAVEFORM SHAPERS

Shaping and encoding the optical pulse waveforms are very important for a variety of applications in optical communications, optical radar and picosecond and femtosecond spectroscopy. Control of the pulse temporal profile is achieved by spatially dispersing the optical frequency components, whose amplitude and phase are arbitrarily weighted and multiplexing them again into a single optical beam. Weiner et al. [79] first demonstrated a technique for optical pulse shaping using a grating pair as a dispersive element and masks for amplitude and phase filtering. Since they used a grating pair, the size of the experimental apparatus was of the order of $1\,m^2$. Also the weighting function for the amplitude and phase masks were fixed because they fabricated them by metal deposition and reactive-ion etching of the silica glass.

Schematic configuration of fully integrated-optic temporal pulse waveform shaper is shown in Fig. 9.111 [80]. It consists of AWG pair for demultiplexing (AWG_1) and multiplexing (AWG_2) the spectral components of mode-locked optical pulses and TO switches and phase shifters for arbitrarily patterning the spectral components. Channel spacing and the total number of channels of AWG are 40 GHz and 80, respectively, which are centered at $\lambda_0 = 1.55\,\mu m$. Among 80 channels of AWG 32 channels are used for spectral filtering. Array of 32 TO switches and phase shifters are allocated between the AWG pair. All of the optical path lengths from AWG_1 to AWG_2 are made equal with employing path adjustment waveguides. Switching ratio of each TO switch, which can be controlled essentially from 0 to 1, is measured by using the monitor port. Also, the amount of phase shift in each path is determined by comparing the relative phase difference with the reference arm, which is not shown in Fig. 9.111. The fiber-to-fiber insertion loss is 12 dB and the extinction ratio is about 30 dB. Then, the dynamic range of the pulse shaper is about 30 dB. The average electric power for TO switch is about 300 mW. The minimum controllability of the electric power is 1 $\sim$ 2 mW. This enables us to obtain 0.1 $\sim$ 0.2 dB amplitude

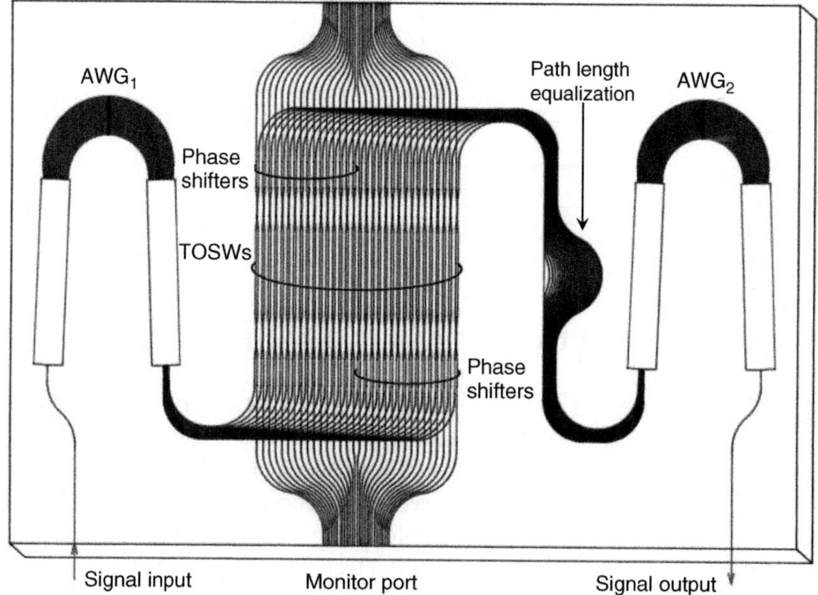

Figure 9.111 Schematic configuration of temporal pulse waveform shaper.

controllability. The average electric power necessary to obtain π phase shift is also about 300 mW. According to the previous minimum controllability of electric power, the resolution of the phase shifter is about $\pi/100$.

Temporal pulse waveform shaper can be utilized in a variety of applications for optical pulse multiplexing, pulse waveform shaping, frequency chirping compensation and frequency-encoding code division multiplexing (FE-CDM) etc. Optical pulse multiplication for *N* times can easily be accomplished by filtering the line spectral components of the mode-locked pulse in every *N* interval.

The square shaped optical pulse is a particularly useful pulse shape with potential application to nonlinear-optical metrology, coherent transient spectroscopy and future all-optical switching and optical demultiplexing [81, 82]. Figure 9.112 shows the schematic temporal pulse waveforms and frequency spectra in the square pulse generation scheme. The frequency spectra of a mode-locked pulse train with the waveform $f(t) = A\text{sech}(t/t_0)$ is given by

$$F(f) = \sum_{m=-\infty}^{\infty} A\text{sech}[\pi^2 t_0(f - f_0)]\delta\left(f - f_0 - \frac{m}{T}\right), \tag{9.50}$$

where f_0, T and t_0 denote center frequency, pulse interval and pulse width (FWHM width $\tau = 2\cosh^{-1}\sqrt{2} \cdot t_0 \cong 1.763t_0$), respectively. In order to generate

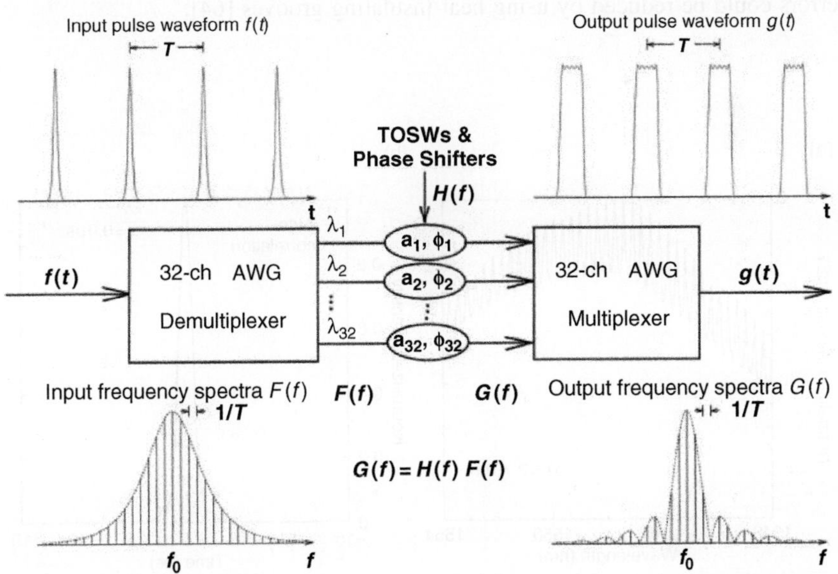

Figure 9.112 Schematic pulse waveforms and frequency spectra in square pulse generation scheme.

square pulses with rise and fall times of $(t_2 - t_1)$, the corresponding sinc-like frequency spectra with the form

$$G(f) = \sum_{m=-\infty}^{\infty} \frac{\sin[\pi(t_2+t_1)(f-f_0)]}{\pi(t_2+t_1)(f-f_0)} \cdot \frac{\cos[\pi(t_2+t_1)(f-f_0)]}{1-[2(t_2-t_1)(f-f_0)]^2} . \delta\left(f - f_0 - \frac{m}{T}\right), \tag{9.51}$$

should be synthesized. Then, the amplitude and phase weighting function $H(f)$ of the pulse shaper for each spectral component is determined by $H(f) = G(f)/F(f)$. Here, we assume $T = 25\,\text{ps}$, $\tau = 8\,\text{ps}$, $t_1 = 3.3\,\text{ps}$, $t_2 = 5.3\,\text{ps}$ and $f_0 = 1.931\,\text{THz}$ ($\lambda_0 = 1.552524\,\mu\text{m}$).

Figures 9.113(a) and (b) show the experimental original spectra and auto-correlated pulse waveforms [83], respectively. The original pulse had a full width at half maximum (FWHM) width of $\tau = 0.9\,\text{ps}$, whose auto-correlation is shown in Fig. 9.113(b). Figures 9.114(a) and (b) show synthesized spectra and corresponding cross-correlated pulse waveforms for designed pulse widths of $\tau = 11.9\,\text{ps}$. Dotted and solid lines show designed and experimental values, respectively. The ripples in the flat-top pulse region are caused by the finite available bandwidth, and are estimated to be 0.1 dB compared with the calculated values of 0.2 dB. The rise and fall time (10 to 90%) is 2.9 to 5.4 ps, while the designed values are 1.5 ps for both. The deterioration in the rise and fall time is mainly brought about by phase setting errors that originated in the thermal crosstalk among the phase shifters used for TO phase adjustment. Phase setting errors could be reduced by using heat-insulating grooves [64].

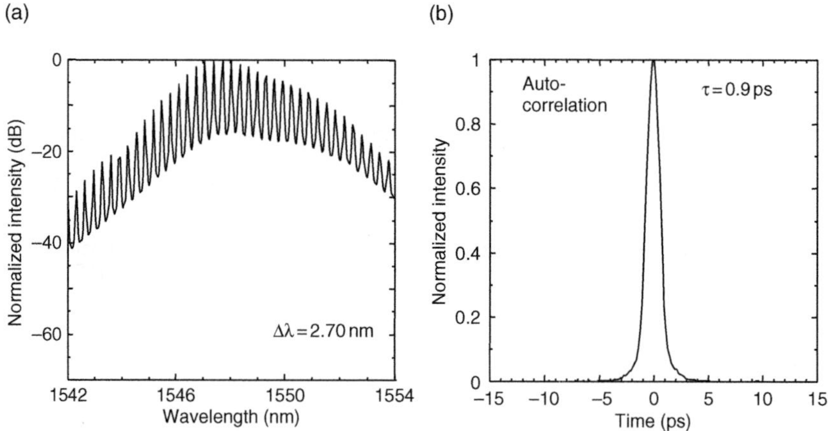

Figure 9.113 (a) Experimental original spectra and (b) auto-correlated pulse waveforms. (After Ref. [83]).

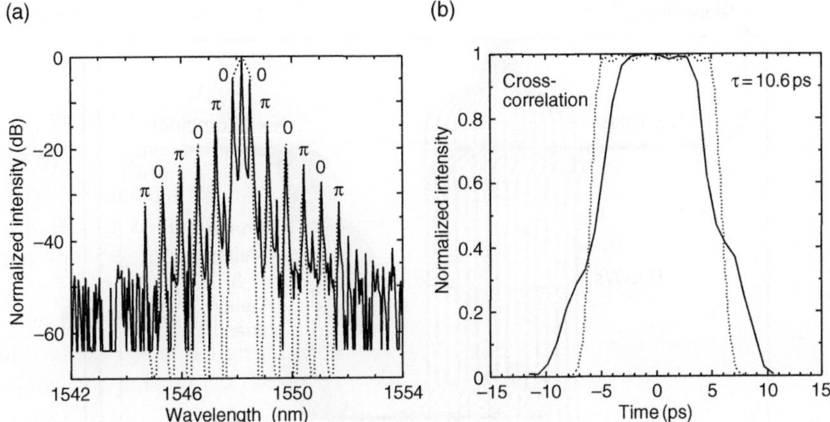

Figure 9.114 (a) Synthesized spectra and (b) corresponding cross-correlated pulse waveforms for designed pulse widths of $\tau = 11.9\,\mathrm{ps}$. (After Ref. [83]).

9.10. COHERENT OPTICAL TRANSVERSAL FILTERS

Optical delay-line filters are attractive devices for performing a variety of signal processing operations at ultrahigh-speed data rates [84]. Schematic configuration of the fabricated 16-tap coherent transversal filter is shown in Fig. 9.115 [85]. It consists of 1×16 MMI splitter for signal splitting, delay arms with fixed path length difference ($\Delta L = 400\,\mu\mathrm{m}$), TO switches and phase shifters for arbitrarily weighting the signal and 16×1 MMI combiner to combine 16 tapped signals. The device is fabricated using silica-based planar lightwave circuits. The core size and refractive-index difference of the waveguides are $7\,\mu\mathrm{m} \times 7\,\mu\mathrm{m}$ and 0.75%, respectively. The minimum bending radius is 5 mm and the chip size is $90\,\mathrm{mm} \times 60\,\mathrm{mm}$. Monitor ports are used to measure and fix the weighting coefficients of TO switches. The 3-dB couplers in TO switches are 2×2 MMI couplers. Although they have inherent loss of about 0.1 dB for each 2×2 MMI coupler, crosstalk characteristics become satisfactory because MMI couplers are fabrication tolerant. Measured crosstalks are lower than $-25\,\mathrm{dB}$ in every switch. Free spectral range of the filter, which is given by $\mathrm{FSR} = c/N_c\Delta L$ where c and N_c denote light velocity in vacuum and group index of the core respectively, becomes 517 GHz (4.14 nm). Since the incoming signal power to the input port is divided by $N(= 16)$ at the MMI splitter, the electric field amplitude in each tap waveguide becomes $1/\sqrt{N}$. Tap weighting coefficient can be made complex value as $g_n = a_n \exp(j\theta_n)(n = 0, 1, \cdots, N-1)$, where a_n and θ_n are given by TO switch and phase shifter, respectively. Signal electric field after passing through the delay line is expressed by $g_n \exp(-j\beta n \Delta L)/\sqrt{N}$, where β denotes

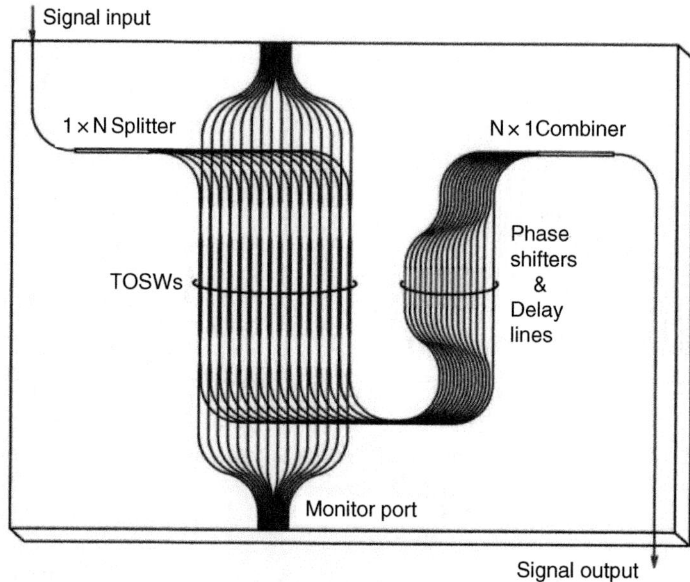

Figure 9.115 Schematic configuration of 16-tap transversal filter.

the propagation constant. Since each tapped signal is divided again by N at the MMI combiner, the output electric field is expressed by

$$G = \sum_{n=0}^{N-1} \frac{1}{N} g_n e^{-j\beta n \Delta L} = \sum_{n=0}^{N-1} \frac{1}{N} g_n \exp\left(-j \frac{2\pi n_c}{\lambda} n \Delta L\right), \tag{9.52}$$

where λ is a wavelength of the signal. It is confirmed experimentally that the collective summation of complex electric fields is possible using MMI combiner (see Section 2.4). Fiber-to-fiber insertion loss at zero phase variation is 5.6 dB. There are several loss origins; they are 0.4-dB theoretical loss in each MMI splitter and combiner, 0.1-dB theoretical loss in MMI 3-dB coupler, 0.06-dB intersecting waveguide loss for each intersection and 0.1-dB coupling loss with DSF. When we sum up these losses, we have 0.4(dB) $\times$ 2 (MMI splitter and combiner) + 0.1(dB) $\times$ 2 (MMI 3-dB couplers) + 0.06(dB) $\times$ 15 (intersections) + 0.1(dB) $\times$ 2 (facets) = 2.1(dB) loss without including waveguide propagation loss. The total waveguide length of the transversal filter is about 27 cm. If we assume the reasonable waveguide loss of 0.13 dB/cm, total waveguide propagation loss becomes 3.5 dB. The above loss breakdown sums up to 2.1 + 3.5 = 5.6(dB) which agrees with the experimental value. When we exclude 3.5-dB waveguide loss and 0.2-dB fiber coupling losses, the inherent loss of the transversal filter is evaluated to be about 1.9 dB.

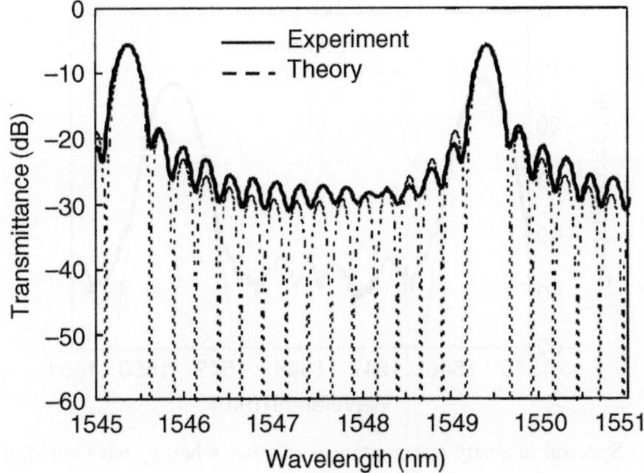

Figure 9.116 Spectral intensity transmittances of filter when $g_n = 1$ for all n.

In order to confirm the signal processing capabilities, sinc-type and Gaussian-type spectral filter responses have been synthesized. Figure 9.116 shows spectral transmittances of the filter when $g_n = 1$ for all n. Since functional shape of g_n and spectral transmittance G are connected with the Fourier transform relationship, theoretical intensity transmittance is expressed by

$$T = |G|^2 = \left| \frac{\sin(N\phi/2)}{N\sin(\phi/2)} \right|^2, \tag{9.53}$$

where $\phi = (2\pi n_c/\lambda)\Delta L = 2\pi f/\mathrm{FSR}$ and f denotes optical frequency. The peak transmittance is −5.6 dB. Figure 9.117 shows spectral transmittances of the filter when g_n has Gaussian distribution as

$$g_n = \exp\left[-\frac{(\mathrm{n}-7)(\mathrm{n}-8)}{16}\right] \quad (\mathrm{n} = 0, 1, \ldots, 15). \tag{9.54}$$

Theoretical intensity transmittance also becomes Gaussian shape as shown by the dotted line in Fig. 9.117. The peak transmittance becomes −12 dB. Additional loss of 6.4 dB is caused by cutting out the signal power in each tap arm to form Gaussian tap coefficients. It is shown from Figs. 9.116 and 9.117 that arbitrary shape of filter characteristics can be realized by the coherent optical transversal filter.

Dynamic gain equalization filter (DGEF) is important to reduce the gain tilt and gain ripple in cascaded optical amplifier systems to avoid signal-to-noise ratio degradation [86]. DGEF based on a transversal filter is attractive since it is compact and scalable to high-wavelength resolution [87].

Figures 9.118(a) and (b) show the input spectrum of Er-doped fiber amplifier (EDFA) into the transversal filter and flattened spectrum, respectively, obtained

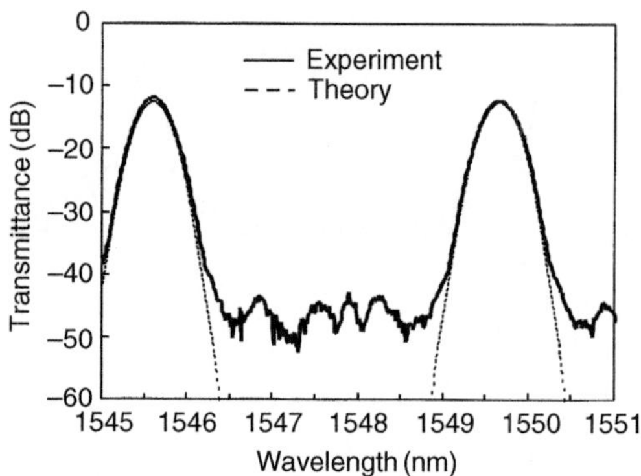

Figure 9.117 Spectral intensity transmittances of filter when g_n has Gaussian distribution.

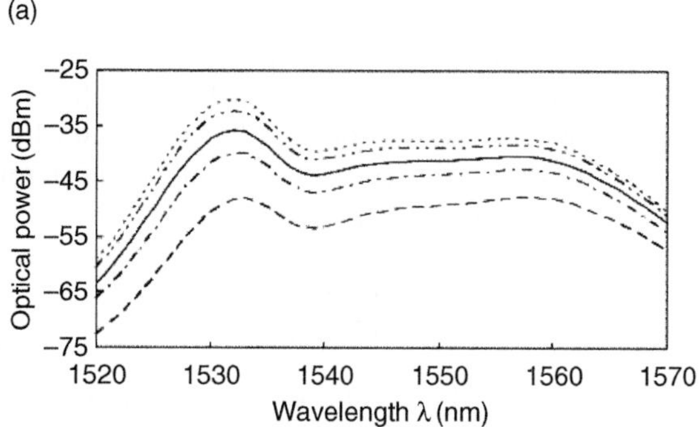

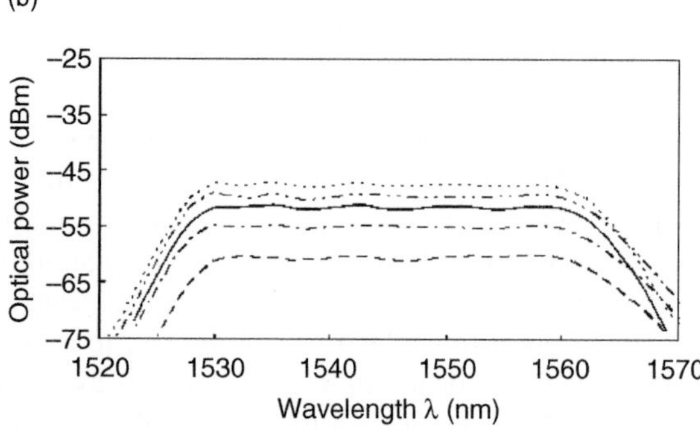

Figure 9.118 (a) Measured input amplified spontaneous emission (ASE) spectrum into the transversal filter and (b) flattened output spectrum of DGEF. (After Ref. [87]).

for various pump powers at $\lambda_p = 1480\,\text{nm}$. It is shown that the gain ripples are successfully flattened to less than 1 dB in all cases, with insertion losses ranging from 7 to 9 dB. The insertion losses include fiber coupling losses of 1 dB and excess losses in the MMI couplers.

9.11. OPTICAL LABEL RECOGNITION CIRCUIT FOR PHOTONIC LABEL SWITCH ROUTER

Optical address signal recognition is a key technology for future packet-switched networks, where each router has to provide an ultrahigh throughput exceeding the electronic speed limits. Several all-optical address recognition schemes have been proposed. They include autocorrelation with matched filters [88] and a bit-wise AND operation with stored reference pulse patterns [89]. However, these approaches need numerous matched filters or reference patterns to distinguish the address, because they determine the proper address pattern by comparing the degree of matching between the incoming address and reference patterns.

There is a novel optical circuit for recognizing an optical pulse pattern, which is based on an optical digital-to-analog (D/A) converter fabricated on a silica-based PLC [90]. The circuit converts the optical pulse pattern to analog optical amplitude, and enables us to recognize the address. Figure 9.119 shows the operational principle of the optical D/A converter. An incoming 4-bit optical pulse train "$C_0C_1C_2C_3$" is first split into four duplicates. Each of the duplicate is relatively delayed by 0, $\Delta\tau$, $2\Delta\tau$ and $3\Delta\tau$ where $\Delta\tau$ is the time interval of

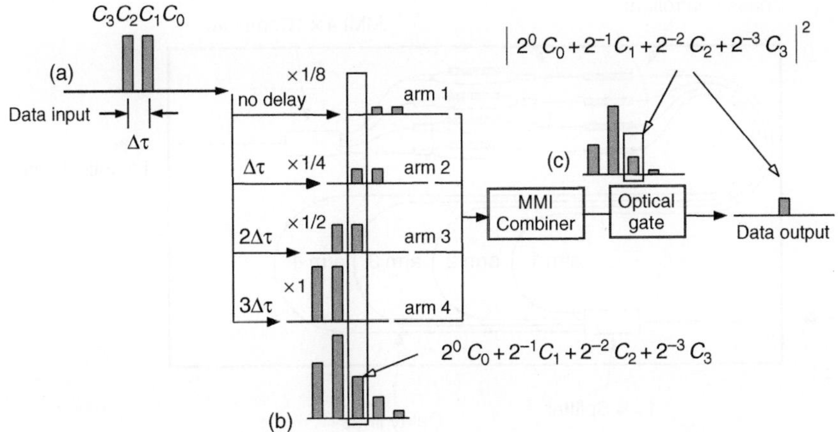

Figure 9.119 Operational principle of optical D/A converter. (After Ref. [90]).

the incoming pulse, and weighted with the coefficients $2^0, 2^{-1}, 2^{-2}$ and 2^{-3}, respectively. The weighted pulses are then recombined and one of the output pulses is extracted with an optical gate. As shown in Fig. 9.119, the intensity of the gated pulse is given by the square of the D/A conversion of the input pulse sequence, as

$$I = \frac{1}{16}\left|2^0 C_0 + 2^{-1} C_1 + 2^{-2} C_2 + 2^{-3} C_3\right|^2. \tag{9.55}$$

Then, the incoming pulse pattern can be recognized by the intensity of the output data I. Figure 9.120 shows the configuration of a fabricated 4-bit optical D/A converter, which features a coherent optical transversal filter [85]. It consists of a 1×4 MMI splitter, delay lines with a relative delay time $\Delta\tau$, thermo-optic phase controllers, thermo-optic switches as amplitude controllers, and a 4×1 MMI combiner. The time delay $\Delta\tau$ is set at 100 psec to deal with a 10 Gb/s pulse train. Weighting coefficients in the D/A converter were adjusted by supplying electric power to thermo-optic heaters while monitoring them using Fourier transform spectroscopy [30]. The adjustment errors for phase and amplitude are 0.03 rad ($\lambda/200$) and 2%, respectively. The total device loss was about 9.9 dB, including a 2^{-m} weighting loss of 6.6 dB and a fiber coupling loss of 1 dB. The 10-Gb/s RZ pulse sequences, generated by an electro-optic modulator, are coupled into the D/A converter to confirm its operation. The source wavelength of the laser was 1550.32 nm. Figures 9.121(a) and (b) show an input pulse pattern ("0110") and an output waveform from the D/A converter, respectively,

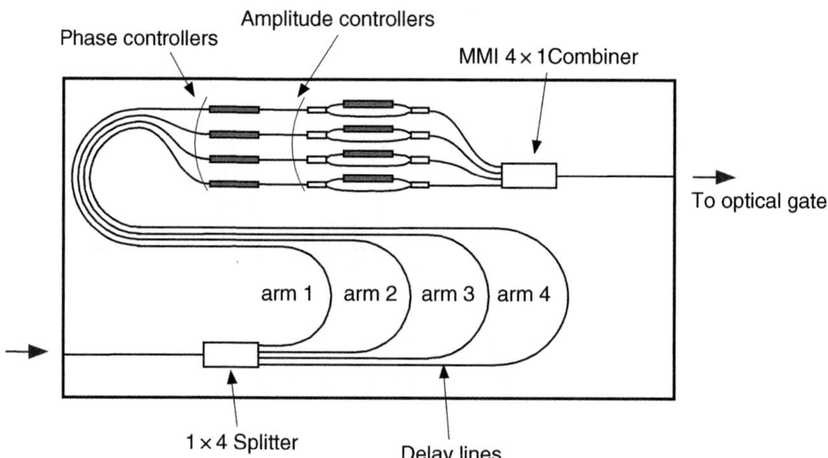

Figure 9.120 Schematic configuration of 4-bit optical D/A converter. (After Ref. [90]).

which are observed on a sampling oscilloscope. The light of the peak marked by the solid square in Fig. 9.121 (b) corresponds to the D/A converted "0110" patterns. The inset in Fig. 9.121(b) shows the theoretical output waveform, which agrees well with the measured waveform. Figure 9.122 shows the measured relationship between incoming pulse patterns and D/A output. The solid line is a theoretical curve. Although the D/A output has the minimum detection limit due to noise, the experimental and theoretical data agree fairly well. The optical label recognition circuit will be a key element in future photonic label switched routing networks [91].

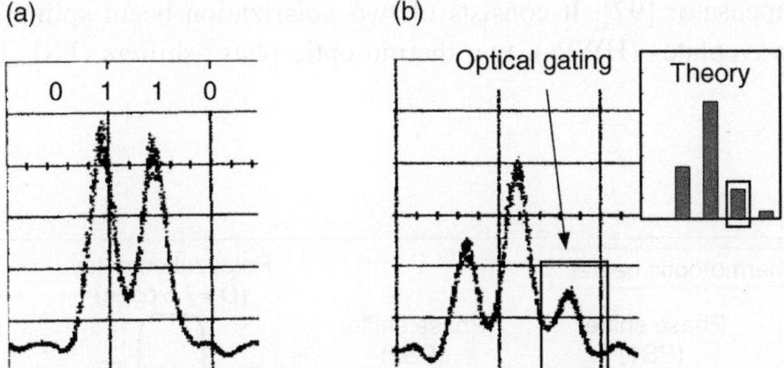

Figure 9.121 Data output waveforms from optical D/A converter: (a) Input pulse pattern (0110), (b) Output waveform and Inset shows theoretical waveform. (After Ref. [90]).

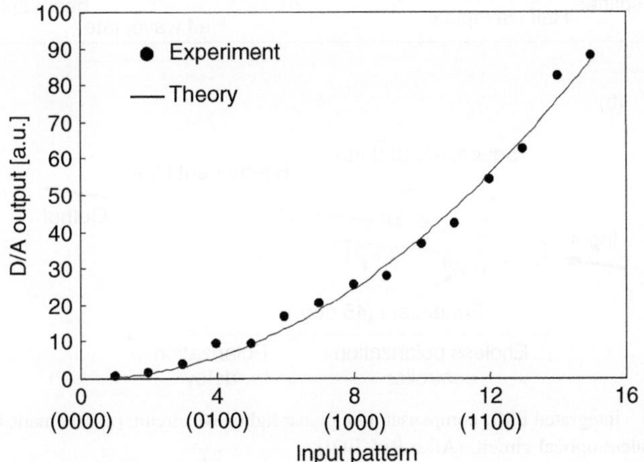

Figure 9.122 Relationship between incoming pulse patterns and D/A output. (After Ref. [90]).

9.12. POLARIZATION MODE DISPERSION COMPENSATOR

Polarization mode dispersion (PMD) has a serious adverse effect on long-haul high bit-rate transmission systems. To a first-order approximation, PMD splits an optical signal into fast and slow polarization components. As a PMD characteristic has a statistical nature that varies with time, we need to compensate for it adaptively. Optical PMD compensators, consisting of a polarization controller and a tunable or fixed polarization-dependent delay line, are free from electrical processing speed limitation, and therefore applicable to high-speed signals.

Figure 9.123(a) shows the schematic configuration of the fabricated PLC-type PMD compensator [92]. It consists of two polarization beam splitters (PBSs), two half waveplates (HWPs), two thermo-optic phase shifters (PS1, PS2), two

(a)

(b)

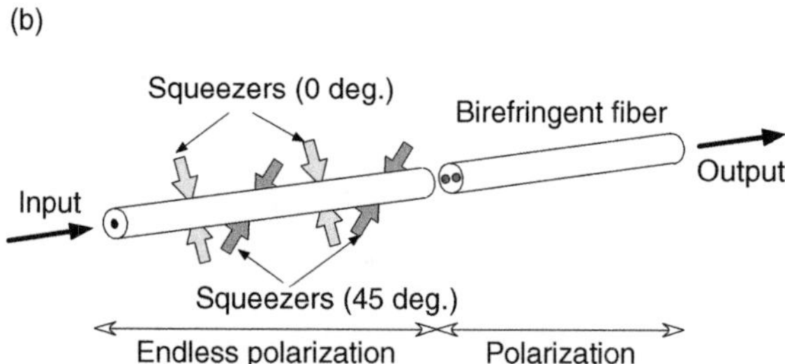

Figure 9.123 Integrated PMD compensator on planar lightwave circuit: (a) schematic configuration and (b) equivalent optical circuit. (After Ref. [92]).

tunable couplers (TC1, TC2) and a polarization-dependent delay line. The PBSs have balanced MZI configurations with stress-applying amorphous Si films and phase-bias adjustment heaters on their arms [93]. The tunable couplers also have balanced MZI configurations with heaters. The compensator splits an incoming signal into TE and TM components at the first PBS. The TM component is converted to TE polarization at the first HWP thus allowing the TE and TM components to interfere with each other. The two components pass through phase shifters and tunable couplers. They are relatively delayed in the polarization-dependent delay line.

Thereafter, the originally TM component is reconverted to TM polarization at the second HWP, and recombined with the TE component at the second PBS. Its equivalent system is shown in Fig. 9.123(b) and features the cascade connection of an endless polarization controller and a birefringent fiber. PS1 and PS2 in Fig. 9.123(a), which change the relative phase between the TE and TM components, correspond to the first and third perpendicular squeezers in Fig. 9.123(b). By contrast, TC1 and TC2 correspond to the second and third tilted squeezers, which couple the TE and TM components. This combination of four squeezers enables us to reset one squeezer with the others, and thus the system functions as an endless polarization controller. In a similar way, the fabricated PMD compensator can compensate for PMD endlessly by means of the reset operation. We use PS2 and TC2 to control the compensator, and PS1 and TC1 to reset PS2 and TC2. The freedom of the compensator is thus 2.

PMD compensator was evaluated with an emulated 43-Gbps transmission signal. The device size was $65 \times 30\,\text{mm}^2$, and the on-chip loss was 8.2 dB. A transmitter multiplexed four 10.7-Gbps pseudo-random binary sequences (PRBSs) from a pulse pattern generator into a 43-Gbps PRBS, and then modulated a continuous-wave light from a distributed feedback laser diode with the 43-Gbps NRZ PRBS. The transmitted signal was electrically regenerated and demultiplexed into four-channel 10.7-Gbps signals at a receiver. To evaluate the compensator, we installed a first-order PMD emulator after the transmitter. We also installed a polarization controller in front of the emulator so that two relatively delayed polarization components had the same power. The compensator placed before the receiver was controlled so as to maximize the degree of polarization of the received optical signal.

Figure 9.124 shows the measured power penalty at a BER of 10^{-9} with and without PMD compensator. The penalty without the compensator amounts to more than 5 dB at a DGD of 10 psec, and it sharply increases with DGD. By contrast, the penalty with the compensator is a little larger than 1 dB at a DGD of 12.5 psec. It is confirmed that the compensator greatly improves the PMD tolerance from 5.5 to 12 psec.

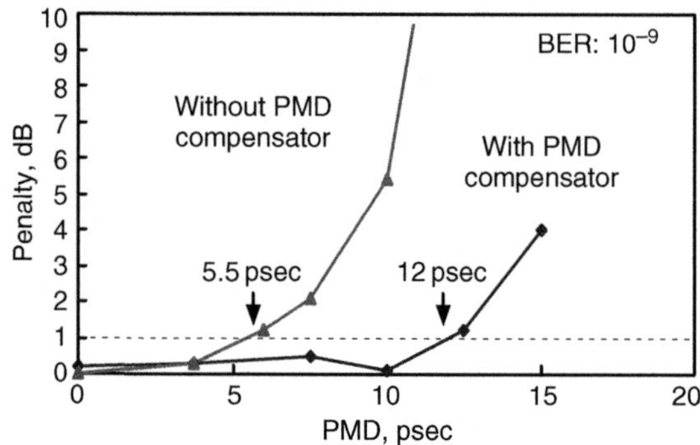

Figure 9.124 Measured power penalty as a function of DGD at a bit-error-rate of 10^{-9}. (After Ref. [92]).

9.13. HYBRID INTEGRATION TECHNOLOGY USING PLC PLATFORMS

It is widely recognized that optical hybrid integration is potentially a key technology for fabricating advanced integrated optical devices [4]. A silica-based waveguide on an Si substrate is a promising candidate for the hybrid integration platform since high-performance PLCs have already been fabricated using silica-based waveguides and Si has highly stable mechanical and thermal properties which make it suitable as an optical bench. Figure 9.125 shows the PLC platform fabrication process [94]. First, a thick under-cladding is deposited on an Si substrate with a terraced region using FHD, and then the surface of the substrate is flattened by mechanical polishing. To minimize the optical coupling loss between the opto-electronics (OE) device on the terrace and optical wave-guide, a thin layer is deposited on the polished substrate surface. The thickness of the layer corresponds to the height of the active region of OE device on the terrace. Then, a core layer is deposited and patterned into a core ridge by RIE. The core ridge is then covered by the over-cladding layer. Finally, RIE is used to form the Si terrace for the OE devices on the PLC and the terrace surface is exposed. The relative positions of the core and Si terrace surface are determined precisely because the terrace acts as an etch-stop layer during the RIE process. As a result, Si terrace functions as both a high-precision alignment plane and heat sink when OE device is flip-chip bonded on the terrace.

Figure 9.126 shows the schematic configuration of hybrid integrated LiNbO3 MZ switch [95]. The switching voltage of the device is 15 V. The extinction ratio is 30 dB for the cross port and 21 dB for the through port. Figure 9.127 shows a WDM transmitter/receiver module utilizing PLC platform for use in

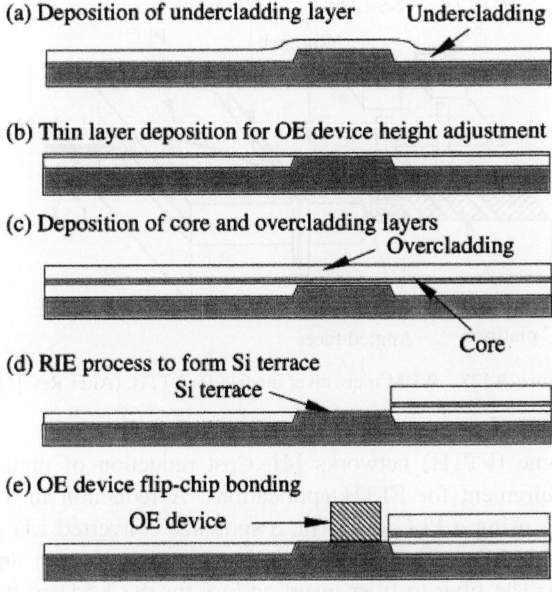

Figure 9.125 PLC platform fabrication process.

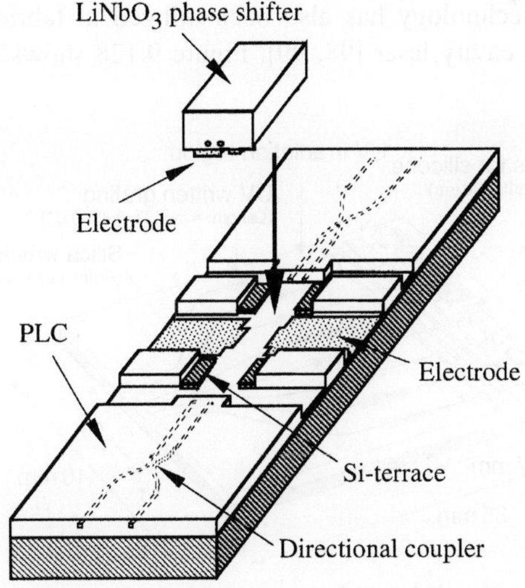

Figure 9.126 Configuration of hybrid integrated LiNbO3 MZ switch. (After Ref. [95]).

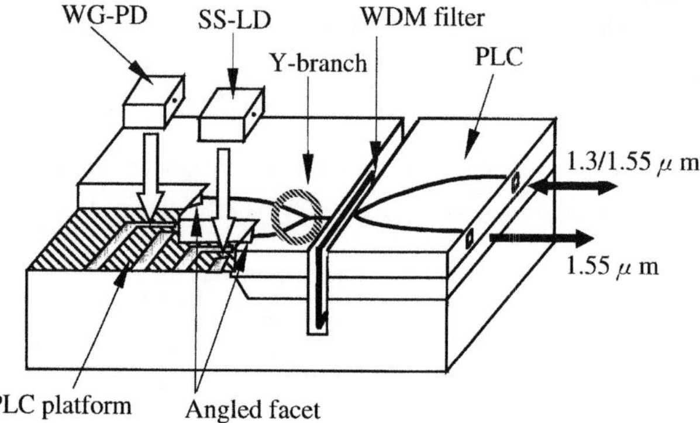

Figure 9.127 WDM transceiver module for FTTH. (After Ref. [4]).

fiber-to-the-home (FTTH) networks [4]. Cost reduction of optical module is the major requirement for FTTH applications. A reduction in the number of components by using a PLC platform, a spot-size converted LD (SS-LD) [96] and a waveguide-PD [97] is a promising approach to obtain an inexpensive WDM module. The fiber-to-fiber insertion loss for the 1.55 μm through port is 1.7 dB. At the 1.3 μm receiver port, the module responsivity is 0.2 A/W with a 1.55 μm isolation of 50 dB. The coupling loss between PLC and WG-PD is estimated to be 0.7 dB. At the 1.3 μm transmitter port, the output power from the fiber is −2 dBm at an injection current of 50 mA. The SS-LD to PLC coupling loss is about 2–4 dB.

PLC platform technology has also been utilized in fabrication of a hybrid integrated external cavity laser [98, 99]. Figure 9.128 shows a configuration of

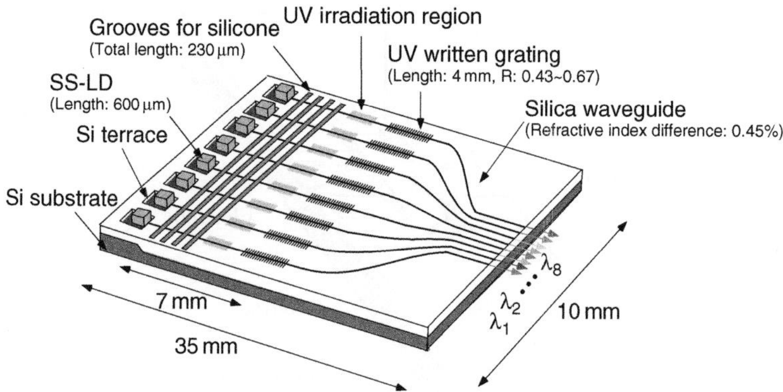

Figure 9.128 Configuration of hybrid integrated multi-wavelength external cavity laser. (After Ref. [99]).

an 8-ch light source, in which 8 spot-size converter integrated LDs (SS-LDs) and 8 gratings are integrated on an Si substrate [99]. The front and rear facets of the SS-LD are coated with anti- and high-reflection film, respectively. The SS-LD length was 600 μm. Gratings are written by irradiating a PLC waveguide through a phase mask with ArF excimer laser light at 193 nm. The grating length was 4 mm, and the grating reflectivity ranged from 43 to 67%. Silicone grooves are formed in the cavity between the SS-LDs and gratings to suppress mode hopping, and a UV irradiation region to control the longitudinal mode. Silicone grooves are segmented to reduce excess loss, and the total silicone length was 230 μm. It is confirmed that all 8-ch oscillated with a threshold of less than 15 mA. The longitudinal mode wavelength shift Δλ caused by the UV-induced index change is expressed as

$$\Delta\lambda = \frac{\Delta n_{UV} L_{UV}}{n_{SiO_2} L_{SiO_2} + n_{LD} L_{LD} + n_p L_p} \cdot \lambda, \tag{9.56}$$

where, λ is the oscillation wavelength, n_{SiO_2}, n_{LD} and n_p are refractive indices in the silica waveguide, SS-LD and silicone respectively, and L_{SiO_2}, L_{LD} and L_p are their respective lengths. Δn_{UV} is the UV-induced refractive-index change and L_{UV} is the length of the UV irradiation region. Equation (9.56) indicates that the oscillation wavelength increases as the refractive index is increased by the UV irradiation. In the experiment, we irradiated the 0.85 mm long waveguide region with a power of 0.6 J/cm^2. As the UV irradiation time increased, the wavelength jumped twice. The total wavelength shift was found to be more than 0.15 nm, which is more than the longitudinal mode spacing and corresponds to a refractive-index change of 1.2×10^{-3}. This result shows that we can control the longitudinal mode wavelength from any position to a stable position. Then, we used this method to control the longitudinal mode and stabilized the oscillation wavelength in the 8-ch light source. Figure 9.129 shows the oscillation spectra of the 8-ch light source at 10 °C after laser control with UV irradiation. 8-ch SS-LDs are simultaneously driven with an injection current of 50 mA. Single mode oscillation was confirmed with a resolution of 0.007 nm for every channel. The side mode suppression ratio was more than 34 dB. It was also confirmed that we could control the 8-ch oscillation wavelengths to the ITU grid to within 0.08 nm, which is one-tenth of the channel spacing.

Temperature stable multi-wavelength source will play an important role in WDM transmission and access network systems.

Semiconductor optical amplifier (SOA) gate switches having spot-size converters on both facets have been successfully hybrid-integrated on PLC platforms to construct high-speed wavelength channel selectors and 4 × 4 optical matrix switches [100, 101]. Figure 9.130 shows the configuration of 8-ch optical wavelength selector module. It consists of two AWG chips with 75-GHz channel

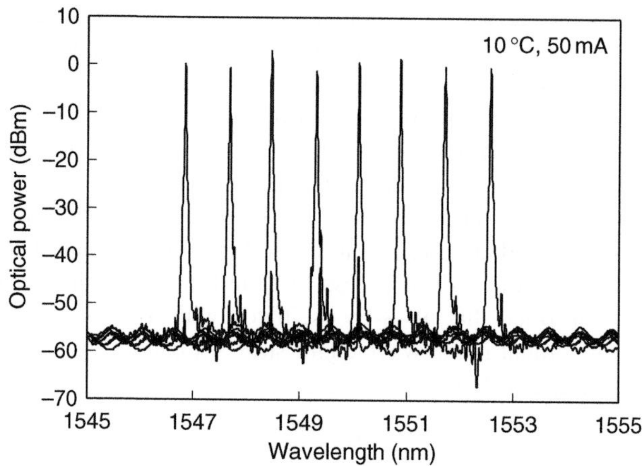

Figure 9.129 Oscillation characteristics of 8-ch light source. (After Ref. [99]).

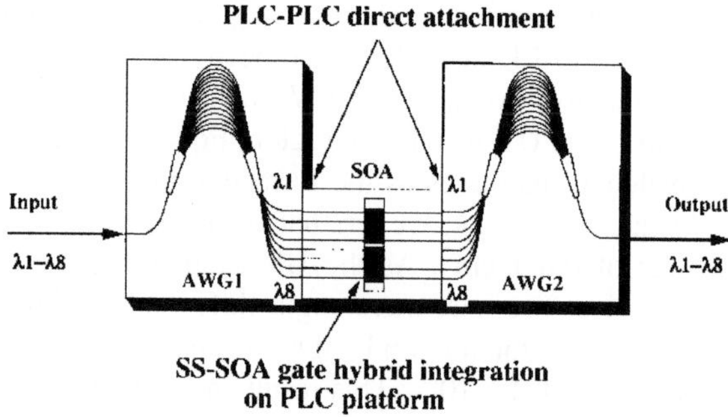

Figure 9.130 Configuration of 8-ch optical wavelength selector module. (After Ref. [100]).

spacing and hybrid integrated SOA gate array chip. It selects and picks up any wavelength channel from a multiplexed signals by activating the corresponding SOA gate switch. Three PLC chips are directly attached with each other using uv curable adhesive. The length of SOA gate switch is 1200 μm and their separation is 400 μm. The coupling loss between SOA and PLC waveguide ranges from 3.9 dB to 4.9 dB. Figure 9.131 shows the optical transmission spectra of the wavelength channel selector when only one SOA gate switch is activated successively. SOA injection current is 50 mA for all SOAs. The peak transmittances have 1–3 dB gains; they are, 16–19 dB total chip losses and fiber coupling losses are compensated by SOA gains. The crosstalk is less than −50 dB and the polarization dependent loss is smaller than 1.4 dB. However, the crosstalk becomes about −30 dB when two or more SOA gate switches are activated simultaneously. The crosstalk in multi-gate operation is determined by

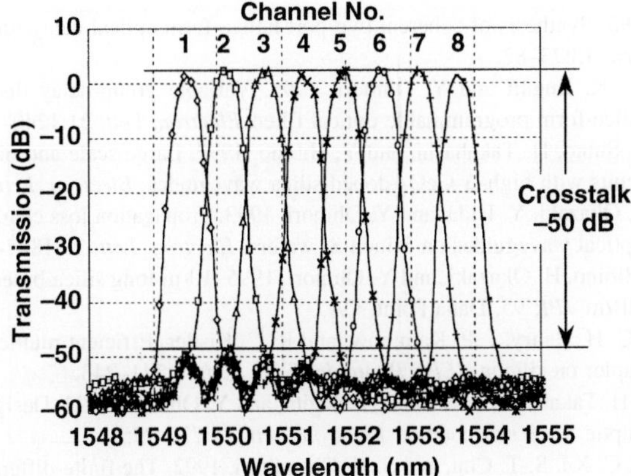

Figure 9.131 Optical transmission spectra of the wavelength channel selector when only one SOA gate switch is activated successively. (After Ref. [100]).

the crosstalk of AWGs. In the high speed switching experiments, the rise and fall time is confirmed to be less than 1 nsec.

Although silica-based waveguides are simple circuit elements, various functional devices are fabricated by utilizing spatial multi-beam or temporal multi-stage interference effects such as AWG multiplexers and lattice-form programmable filters. Hybrid integration technologies will further enable us to realize much more functional and high-speed devices. The PLC technologies supported by continuous improvements in waveguide fabrication, circuit design and device packaging will further proceed to a higher level of integration of optics and electronics aiming at the next generation of telecommunication systems.

REFERENCES

[1] Kawachi, M. 1990. Silica waveguide on silicon and their application to integrated-optic components. *Opt. and Quantum Electron.* 22:391–416.

[2] Okamoto, K. 1997. Planar lightwave circuits (PLCs). In: *Photonic Networks*, edited by Giancarco Prati. New York: Springer-Verlag, pp. 118–132.

[3] Himeno, A., T. Kominato, M. Kawachi, and K. Okamoto. 1997. System applications of large-scale optical switch matrices using silica-based planar lightwave circuits. In: *Photonic Networks*, edited by Giancarco Prati. New York: Springer-Verlag, pp. 172–182.

[4] Yamada, Y., S. Suzuki, K. Moriwaki, Y. Hibino, Y. Tohmori, Y. Akatsu, Y. Nakasuga, T. Hashimoto, H. Terui, M. Yanagisawa, Y. Inoue, Y. Akahori, and R. Nagase. 1995. Application of planar lightwave circuit platform to hybrid integrated optical WDM transmitter/receiver module. *Electron. Lett.* 31:1366–1367.

[5] Akahori, Y., T. Ohyama, M. Yanagisawa, Y. Yamada, H. Tsunetsugu, Y. Akatsu, M. Togashi, S. Mino, and Y. Shibata. 1997. A hybrid high-speed silica-based planar lightwave circuit platform integrating a laser diode and a driver IC. *Proc. IOOC/ECOC '97*, Edinburgh, UK, vol. 2, pp. 359–362.

[6] Jinguji, K. 1995. Synthesis of coherent two-port lattice-form optical delay-line circuit. *IEEE J. Lightwave Tech.* 13:73–82.

[7] Takiguchi, K., K. Jinguji and Y. Ohmori. 1995. Variable group-delay dispersion equalizer based on a lattice-form programmable optical filter. *Electron. Lett.* 31:1240–1241.

[8] Suzuki, S., K. Shuto, H. Takahashi, and Y. Hibino. 1992. Large-scale and high-density planar lightwave circuits with high-Δ GeO_2-doped silica waveguides. *Electron. Lett.* 28:1863–1864.

[9] Hibino, Y., H. Okazaki, Y. Hida, and Y. Ohmori. 1993. Propagation loss characteristics of long silica-based optical waveguides on 5-inch Si wafers. *Electron. Lett.* 29:1847–1848.

[10] Hida, Y., Y. Hibino, H. Okazaki, and Y. Ohmori. 1995. 10-m-long silica-based waveguide with a loss of 1.7 dB/m. *IPR'95*, Dana Point, CA.

[11] Dragone, C., C. H. Henry, I. P. Kaminow, and R. C. Kistler. Efficient multichannel integrated optics star coupler on silicon. *IEEE Photonics Tech. Lett.* 1:241–243.

[12] Okamoto, K., H. Takahashi, S. Suzuki, A. Sugita, and Y. Ohmori. 1991. Design and fabrication of integrated-optic 8 × 8 star coupler. *Electron. Lett.* 27:774–775.

[13] Huang, W. P., C. Xu, S. T. Chu, and S. K. Chaudhuri. 1992. The finite-difference vector beam propagation method: Analysis and assessment. *J. Lightwave Tech.* 10:295–305.

[14] Okamoto, K., H. Okazaki, Y. Ohmori, and K. Kato. 1992. Fabrication of large scale integrated-optic $N \times N$ star couplers. *IEEE Photonics Tech. Lett.* 4:1032–1035.

[15] Smit, M. K. 1988. New focusing and dispersive planar component based on an optical phased array. *Electron. Lett.* 24:385–386.

[16] Takahashi, H. S. Suzuki, K. Kato and I. Nishi. 1990. Arrayed-waveguide grating for wavelength division multi/demultiplexer with nanometer resolution. *Electron. Lett.* 26:87–88.

[17] Okamoto, K., K. Moriwaki and S. Suzuki. 1995. Fabrication of 64 × 64 arrayed-waveguide grating multiplexer on silicon. *Electron. Lett.* 31:184–185.

[18] Okamoto, K., K. Syuto, H. Takahashi and Y. Ohmori. 1996. Fabrication of 128-channel arrayed-waveguide grating multiplexer with a 25-GHz channel spacing. *Electron. Lett.* 32:1474–1476.

[19] Hida, Y., Y. Hibino, T. Kitoh, Y. Inoue, M. Itoh, T. Shibata, A. Sugita and A. Himeno. 2001. 400-channel arrayed-waveguide grating with 25 GHz spacing using 1.5%-Δ waveguides on 6-inch Si wafer. *Electron. Lett.* 37:576–577.

[20] Kasahara, R., M. Itoh, Y. Hida, T. Saida, Y. Inoue and Y. Hibino. 2002. Birefringence compensated silica-based waveguide with undercladding ridge. *Electron. Lett.* 38:1178–1179.

[21] Uetsuka, H., K. Akiba, H. Okano and Y. Kurosawa. 1995. Nove $1 \times N$ guide-wave multi/demultiplexer for WDM. *Proc. OFC '95 Tu07*, p. 276.

[22] Okamoto K. and H. Yamada. 1995. Arrayed-waveguide grating multiplexer with flat spectral response. *Opt. Lett.* 20:43–45.

[23] Okamoto K. and A. Sugita. 1996. Flat spectral response arrayed-waveguide grating multiplexer with parabolic waveguide horns. *Electron. Lett.* 32:1661–1662.

[24] Amersfoort, M. R., J. B. D. Soole, H. P. LeBlanc, N. C. Andreadakis, A. Rajhei and C. Caneau. 1996. Passband broadening of integrated arrayed waveguide filters using multimode interference couplers. *Electron. Lett.* 32:449–451.

[25] Trouchet, D., A. Beguin, H. Boek, C. Prel, C. Lerminiaux and R. O. Maschmeyer. 1997. Passband flattening of PHASAR WDM using input and output star couplers designed with two focal points. *Proc. OFC '97 ThM7*, Dallas, Texas.

[26] Thompson, G. H. B., R. Epworth, C. Rogers, S. Day and S. Ojha. 1998. An original low-loss and pass-band flattened SiO_2 on Si planar wavelength demultiplexer. *Proc. OFC '98 TuN1*, San Jose, CA.

[27] Doerr, C. R., L. W. Stulz and R. Pafchek. 2003. Compact and low-loss integrated box-like passband multiplexer. *IEEE Photonics Tech. Lett.* 15:918–920.

[28] Burns, W. K., A. F. Milton and A. B. Lee. 1997. Optical waveguide parabolic coupling horns. *Appl. Phys. Lett.* 30:28–30.

[29] Kitoh, T., Y. Inoue, M. Itoh and Y. Hibino. 2003. Low chromatic-dispersion flat-top arrayed waveguide grating filter. *Electron. Lett.* 39(15):1116–1118.

[30] Takada, K., Y. Inoue, H. Yamada and M. Horiguchi. 1994. Measurement of phase error distributions in silica-based arrayed-waveguide grating multiplexers by using Fourier transform spectroscopy. *Electron. Lett.* 30:1671–1672.

[31] van Dam, C., A. A. M. Staring, E. J. Jansen, J. J. M. Binsma, T. Van Dongen, M. K. Smit and B. H. Verbeek. 1996. Loss reduction for phased array demultiplexers using a double etch technique. *Integrated Photonics Research 1996*, Boston, MA, April 29–May 2, pp. 52–55.

[32] Sugita, A., A. Kaneko, K. Okamoto, M. Itoh, A. Himeno and Y. Ohmori. 2000. Very low insertion loss arrayed-waveguide grating with vertically tapered waveguides. *IEEE Photonics Tech. Lett.* 12:1180–1182.

[33] Doerr, C. R. 2003. Optical add/drops and cross connects in planar waveguides. *Proc. ECOC '03 Th1.3*, Rimini, Italy.

[34] Maru, K., T. Chiba, M. Okawa, H. Ishikawa, K. Ohira, S. Sato and H. Uetsuka. 2001. Low-loss arrayed-waveguide grating with high index regions at slab-to-array interface. *Electron. Lett.* 37:1287–1289.

[35] Forghieri, F., A. H. Gnauck, R. W. Tkach, A. R. Chraplyvy and R. M. Derosier. 1994. Repeaterless transmission of eight channels at 10 Gb/s over 137 km (11 Tb/s-km) of dispersion-shifted fiber using unequal channel spacing. *IEEE Photonics Tech. Lett.* 6:1374–1376.

[36] Oda, K., M. Fukutoku, M. Fukui, T. Kitoh and H. Toba. 1995. 10-channelx10-Gbit/s optical FDM transmission over 500 km dispersion shifted fiber employing unequal channel spacing and amplifier gain equalization. *Proc. OFC '95 TuhI*, San Diego.

[37] Okamoto, K., M. Ishii, Y. Hibino, Y. Ohmori and H. Toba. 1995. Fabrication of unequal channel spacing arrayed-waveguide grating multiplexer modules. *Electron. Lett.* 31:1464–1465.

[38] Okamoto, K., M. Ishii, Y. Hibino and Y. Ohmori. 1995. Fabrication of variable bandwidth filters using arrayed-waveguide gratings. *Electron. Lett.* 31:1592–1593.

[39] Morioka, T., S. Kawanishi, K. Mori and M. Saruwatari. 1994. Transform-limited femtosecond WDM pulse generation by spectral filtering of gigahertz supercontinuum. *Electron. Lett.* 30:1166–1168.

[40] Morioka, T., K. Okamoto, M. Ishii and M. Saruwatari. 1996. Low-noise, pulsewidth tunable picosecond to femtosecond pulse generation by spectral filtering of wideband supercontinuum with variable bandwidth arrayed-waveguide grating filters. *Electron. Lett.* 32:836–837.

[41] Dragone, C., C. A. Edwards and R. C. Kistler. 1991. Integrated optics N×N multiplexer on silicon. *Photon. Tech. Lett.* 3:896–899.

[42] Okamoto, K., H. Hasegawa, O. Ishida, A. Himeno and Y. Ohmori. 1997. 32 × 32 arrayed-waveguide grating multiplexer with uniform loss and cyclic frequency characteristics. *Electron. Lett.* 33:1865–1866.

[43] Veerman, F. B., P. J. Schalkwijk, E. C. M. Pennings, M. K. Smit and B. H. Verbeek. 1992. An optical passive 3-dB TMI-coupler with reduced fabrication tolerance sensitivity. *Jour. Lightwave Tech.* 10:306–311.

[44] Kato, K., A. Okada, Y. Sakai, K. Noguchi, T. Sakamoto, S. Suzuki, A. Takahara, S. Kamei, A. Kaneko and M. Matsuoka. 2000. 32 × 32 full-mesh (1024 path) wavelength-routing WDM network based on uniform-loss cyclic-frequency arrayed-waveguide grating. *Electron. Lett.* 36(15):1294–1296.

[45] Yoo, S. J. B., H. J. Lee, Z. Pan, J. Cao, Y. Zhang, K. Okamoto and S. Kamei. 2002. Rapidly switching all-optical packet routing system with optical-label swapping incorporating tunable wavelength conversion and a uniform-loss cyclic frequency AWGR. *IEEE Photon. Tech. Lett.* 14(8):1211–1213.

[46] Heise, G., H. W. Schneider and P. C. Clemens. 1998. Optical phased array filter module with passively compensated temperature dependence. *ECOC '98*, pp. 319–320, September 20–24, 1998, Madrid, Spain.

[47] Inoue, Y., A. Kaneko, F. Hanawa, H. Takahashi, K. Hattori and S. Sumida. 1997. Athermal silica-based arrayed-waveguide grating multiplexer. *Electron. Lett.* 33:1945–1946.

[48] Gao, R., R. Gao, K. Takayama, A. Yeniay and A. F. Garito. 2002. Low-Insertion Loss Athermal AWG Multi/Demultiplexer Based on Perfluorinated Polymers. *ECOC '02*, 6.2.2, Sept. 8–12, 2002, Copenhagen, Denmark.

[49] Soole, J. B. D., M. Schlax, C. Narayanan and R. Pafchek. 2003. Athermalisation of silica arrayed waveguide grating multiplexers. *Electron. Lett.* 39(16):1182–1184.

[50] Kaneko, A., S. Kamei, Y. Inoue, H. Takahashi and A. Sugita. 1999. Athermal silica-based arrayed-waveguide grating (AWG) multiplexers with new low loss groove design. *OFC-IOOC '99 TuO1*, pp. 204–206, San Diego, CA.

[51] Tong, F., K. P. Ho, T. Schrans, W. E. Hall, G. Grand and P. Mottier. 1995. A wavelength-matching scheme for multiwavelength optical links and networks using grating demulplexers. *IEEE Photonics Tech. Lett.* 7:688–690.

[52] Teshima, M., M. Koga and K. Sato. 1995. Multiwavelength simultaneous monitoring circuit employing wavelength crossover properties of arrayed-waveguide grating. *Electron. Lett.* 31:1595–1597.

[53] Okamoto, K., K. Hattori and Y. Ohmori. 1996. Fabrication of multiwavelength simultaneous monitoring device using arrayed-waveguide grating. *Electron. Lett.* 32:569–570.

[54] Takada, K., T. Tanaka, M. Abe, T. Yanagisawa, M. Ishii and K. Okamoto. 2000. Beam-adjustment-free crosstalk reduction in 10 GHz-spaced arrayed-waveguide grating via photosensitivity under UV laser irradiation through metal mask. *Electron. Lett.* 36:60–61.

[55] Takada, K., M. Abe, T. Shibata and K. Okamoto. 2002. 1-GHz-spaced 16-channel arrayed-waveguide grating for a wavelength reference standard in DWDM network systems. *IEEE J. Lightwave Tech.* 20:850–853.

[56] Takada, K., M. Abe, T. Shibata and K. Okamoto. 2001. 10 GHz-spaced 1010-channel Tandem AWG filter consisting of one primary and ten secondary AWGs. *IEEE PTL* 13:577–578.

[57] Takada, K., M. Abe, T. Shibata and K. Okamoto. 2002. Three-stage ultra-high-density multi/demultiplexer covering low-loss fiber transmission window 1.26-1.63 mm. *Electron. Lett.* 38:405–406.

[58] Takada, K., M. Abe, T. Shibata and K. Okamoto. 2002. A 25-GHz-spaced 1080-channel tandem multi/demultiplexer covering the S-, C-, and L-bands using an arrayed-waveguide grating with Gaussian passbands as a primary filter. *IEEE PTL* 14:648–650.

[59] Takada, K., M. Abe, T. Shibata and K. Okamoto. 2002. 5 GHz-spaced 4200-channel two-stage tandem demultiplexer for ultra-multi-wavelength light source using supercontinuum generation. *Electron. Lett.* 38:572–573.

[60] Okamoto, K., M. Okuno, A. Himeno and Y. Ohmori. 1996. 16-channel optical Add/Drop multiplexer consisting of arrayed-waveguide gratings and double-gate switches. *Electron. Lett.* 32:1471–1472.

[61] Kominato, T., T. Kitoh, K. Katoh, Y. Hibino and M. Yasu. 1992. Loss characteristics of intersecting silica-based waveguides. *Optoelectronics Conf. OEC'92*, Paper 16B4-1, pp. 138–139.

[62] Okamoto, K., K. Takiguchi and Y. Ohmori. 1995. 16-channel optical add/drop multiplexer using silica-based arrayed-waveguide gratings. *Electron. Lett.* 31:723–724.

[63] Saida, T., A. Kaneko, T. Goh, M. Okuno, A. Himeno, K. Takiguchi, K. Okamoto. 2000. Athermal silica-based optical add/drop multiplexer consisting of arrayed waveguide gratings and double gate thermo-optical switches. *Electron. Lett.* 36:528–529.

[64] Sugita, A., K. Jinguji, N. Takato, K. Katoh and M. Kawachi. 1989. Bridge-suspended thermo-optic phase shifter and its application to silica-waveguide optical switch. *Proc. of IOOC '89*, Paper 18D1-4, p. 58.

[65] Kasahara, R., M. Yanagisawa, A. Sugita, T. Goh, M. Yasu, A. Himeno and S. Matsui. 1999. Low-power consumption silica-based 2×2 thermooptic switch using trenched silicon substrate. *IEEE Photonics Tech. Lett.* 11:1132–1134.

[66] Matsunaga, T., M. Okuno and K. Yukimatsu. 1992. Large-scale space-division switching system using silica-based 8 × 8 matrix switches. *Proc. OEC'92*, Makuhari, Japan, pp. 256–257.

[67] Ito, T., A. Himeno, K. Takada and K. Kato. 1992. Photonic inter-module connector using silica-based optical switches. *Proc. GLOBECOM'92*, Orlando, Fla., pp. 187–191.

[68] Goh, T., M. Yasu, K. Hattori, A. Himeno, M. Okuno and Y. Ohmori. 1998. Low-loss and high-extinction-ratio silica-based strictly nonblocking 16 × 16 thermooptic matrix switch. *IEEE Photonics Tech. Lett.* 10:810–812.

[69] Okamoto, K., Y. Hibino and M. Ishii. 1993. Guided-wave optical equalizer with α-power chirped grating. *IEEE J. Lightwave Tech.* 11:1325–1330.

[70] Vengsarkar, A. M., A. E. Miller and W. A. Reed. 1993. Highly efficient single-mode fiber for broadband dispersion compensation. *OFC '93 Postdeadline paper PD13*, San Jose.

[71] Gnauck, A. H., R. M. Jopson and R. M. Derosier. 1993. 10-Gb/s 360-km transmission over dispersive fiber using midsystem spectral inversion. *IEEE Photonics Tech. Lett.* 5:663–666.

[72] Hill, K. O., S. Theriault, B. Malo, F. Bilodeau, T. Kitagawa, D. C. Johnson, J. Albert, K. Takiguchi, T. Kataoka and K. Hagimoto. 1994. Chirped in-fiber Bragg grating dispersion compensators; linearization of dispersion characteristics and demonstration of dispersion compensation in 100 km, 10 Gbit/s optical fiber link. *Electron. Lett.* 30:1755–1756.

[73] Takiguchi, K., K. Okamoto, S. Suzuki and Y. Ohmori. 1994. Planar lightwave circuit optical dispersion equalizer. *IEEE Photonics Tech. Lett.* 6:86–88.

[74] Takiguchi, K., K. Jinguji, K. Okamoto and Y. Ohmori. 1995. Dispersion compensation using a variable group-delay dispersion equalizer. *Electron. Lett.* 31:2192–2193.

[75] Madsen, C. K., G. Lenz, A. J. Bruce, M. A. Cappuzzo, L. T. Gomez and R. E. Scotti. 1999. Integrated all-pass filters for tunable dispersion and dispersion slope compensation. *IEEE Photonics Tech. Lett.* 11:1623–1625.

[76] Kawanishi, S., H. Takara, T. Morioka, O. Kamatani and M. Saruwatari. 1995. 200 Gbit/s, 100 km time-division-multiplexed optical transmission using supercontinuum pulses with prescaled PLL timing extraction and all-optical demultiplexing. *Electron. Lett.* 31:816–817.

[77] Takiguchi, K., S. Kawanishi, H. Takara, K. Okamoto, K. Jinguji and Y. Ohmori. 1996. Higher order dispersion equalizer of dispersion shifted fiber using a lattice-form programmable optical filter. *Electron. Lett.* 32:755–757.

[78] Takiguchi, K., S. Kawanishi, H. Takara, O. Kamatani, K. Uchiyama, A. Himeno and K. Jinguji. 1996. Dispersion slope equalizing experiment using planar lightwave circuit for 200 Gbit/s time-division-multiplexed transmission. *Electron. Lett.* 32:2083–2084.

[79] Weiner, A. M., J. P. Heritage and E. M. Kirshner. 1988. High-resolution femtosecond pulse shaping. *J. Opt. Soc. Am. B* 5:1563–1572.

[80] Okamoto, K., T. Kominato, H. Yamada and T. Goh. 1999. Fabrication of frequency spectrum synthesiser consisting of arrayed-waveguide grating pair and thermo-optic amplitude and phase controllers. *Electron. Lett.* 35:733–734.

[81] Weiner, A. M., J. P. Heritage and R. N. Thurston. 1986. Synthesis of phase coherent, picosecond optical square pulses. *Opt. Lett.* 11:153–155.

[82] Kawanishi, S., H. Takara, T. Morioka, O. Kamatani and M. Saruwatari. 1995. 200 Gbit/s, 100 km time-division-multiplexed optical transmission using supercontinuum pulses with prescaled PLL timing extraction and all-optical demultiplexing. *Electron. Lett.* 31:816–817.

[83] Takiguchi, K., K. Okamoto, T. Kominato, H. Takahashi and T. Shibata. 2004. Flexible pulse waveform generation using a silica waveguide-based spectrum synthesis circuit. *Electron. Lett.* 40:537–538.

[84] Jackson, K. P., S. A. Newton, B. Moslehi, M. Tur, C. C. Cutler, J. W. Goodman and H. J. Shaw, Optical fiber delay-line signal processing. *IEEE Trans. on Microwave Theory and Tech.* MTT-33:193–210.

[85] Okamoto, K., H. Yamada and T. Goh. 1999. Fabrication of coherent optical transversal filter consisting of MMI splitter/combiner and thermo-optic amplitude and phase controllers. *Electron. Lett.* 35:1331–1332.

[86] Parry, S. P. 2001. Dynamically flattened optical amplifiers. *Proc. OFC 2001 TuA4*, Anaheim, CA.

[87] Saida, T., K. Okamoto, K. Takiguchi and T. Shibata. 2002. Dynamic gain equalization filter based on integrated optical transversal filter with asymmetric combiner. *Electron. Lett.* 38:560–561.

[88] Kitayama K. and N. Wada. 1999. Photonic IP routing. *Photonics Tech. Lett.* 11:1689–1691.

[89] Cotter, D., J. K. Lucek, M. Shabeer, K. Smith, D. C. Rogers, D. Nesset and P. Gunning. Self-routing of 100 Gbit/s packets using 6 bit 'keyword' address recognition. *Electron. Lett.* 31:1475–1476.

[90] Saida T., K. Okamoto, K. Uchiyama, K. Takiguchi, T. Shibata and A. Sugita. 2001. Integrated optical digital-to-analogue converter and its application to pulse pattern recognition. *Electron. Lett.* 37:1237–1238.

[91] Yoo, S. J. B., H. J. Lee, Z. Pan, J. Cao, Y. Zhang, K. Okamoto and S. Kamei. 2002. Rapidly switching all-optical packet routing system with optical-label swapping incorporating tunable wavelength conversion and a uniform-loss cyclic frequency AWGR. *IEEE Photonicsics Tech. Lett.* 14:1211–1213.

[92] Saida, T., K. Takiguchi, S. Kuwahara, Y. Kisaka, Y. Miyamoto, Y. Hashizume, T. Shibata and K. Okamoto. 2002. Planar lightwave circuit polarization-mode dispersion compensator. *IEEE Photonicsics Tech. Lett.* 14(4):507–509.

[93] Okuno, M., A. Sugita, K. Jinguji, and M. Kawachi. 1994. Birefringence control of silica waveguides on Si and its application to a polarization-beam splitter/switch. *IEEE J. Lightwave Tech.* 12:625–633.

[94] Yamada, Y., A. Takagi, I. Ogawa, M. Kawachi and M. Kobayashi. 1993. Silica-based optical waveguide on terraced silicon substrate as hybrid integration platform. *Electron. Lett.* 29:444–445.

[95] Yamada, Y., A. Sugita, K. Moriwaki, I. Ogawa and T. Hashimoto. 1994. An application of a silica-on-terraced-silicon substrate to hybrid Mach-Zehnder interferometric circuits consisting of silica-waveguides and $LiNbO_3$ phase-shifters. *IEEE Photonics Tech. Lett.* 6:822–824.

[96] Tohmori, Y., Y. Suzaki, H. Fukano, M. Okamoto, Y. Sakai, O. Mitomi, S. Matsumoto, M. Yamamoto, M. Fukuda, M. Wada, Y. Itaya and T. Sugie. 1995. Spot-size converted 1.3 μm laser with a butt-jointed selectively grown vertically tapered waveguide. *Electron. Lett.* 31:1069–1070.

[97] Akatsu, Y., Y. Muramoto, M. Ikeda, M. Ueki, A. Kozen, T. Kurosaki, K. Kawano, K. Kato and J. Yoshida. 1995. 1.3 μm multimode waveguide photodiodes suitable for optical hybrid integration with a planar lightwave circuit. *ECOC '95, MoB 4.4*, pp. 91–94.

[98] Tanaka, T., H. Takahashi, T. Hashimoto, Y. Yamada and Y. Itaya. 1997. Fabrication of hybrid integrated 4-wavelength laser composed of uv written waveguide gratings and laser diodes. *OECC '97 10D3-3*, Seoul, Korea.

[99] Tanaka, T., Y. Hibino, T. Hashimoto, M. Abe, R. Kasahara, and Y. Tohmori. 2004. 100-GHz Spacing 8-Channel Light Source Integrated With External Cavity Lasers on Planar Lightwave Circuit Platform. *IEEE J. Lightwave Tech.* 22:567–573.

[100] Ogawa, I., F. Ebisawa, N. Yoshimoto, K. Takiguchi, F. Hanawa, T. Hashimoto, A. Sugita, M. Yanagisawa, Y. Inoue, Y. Yamada, Y. Tohmori, S. Mino, T. Ito, K. Magari, Y. Kawaguchi, A. Himeno and K. Kato. 1998. Loss-less hybrid integrated 8-ch optical wavelength selector module using PLC platform and PLC-PLC direct attachment techniques. *OFC'98 Postdeadline Paper PDP4*, San Jose, CA.

[101] Kato, T., J. Sasaki, T. Shimoda, H. Hatakeyama, T. Tamanuki, M. Yamaguchi, M. Titamura and M. Itoh. 1998. 10 Gb/s photonic cell switching with hybrid 4 $\times$ 4 optical matrix switch module on silica based planar waveguide platform. *OFC'98 Postdeadline Paper PDP3*, San Jose, CA.

Chapter 10

Several Important Theorems and Formulas

In this chapter, several important theorems and formulas [1–4] are described that are the bases for the derivation of various equations throughout the book. Gauss's theorem, Green's theorem, and Stokes' theorem are foundations for electromagnetic theory. The integral theorem of Helmholtz and Kirchhoff and the Fresnel–Kirchhoff diffraction formula are basic theories for solving diffraction problems.

10.1. GAUSS'S THEOREM

We consider the function $f(x, y, z)$ in a volume V enclosed by a smooth surface S. Function $f(x, y, z)$ and its derivatives $\partial f/\partial x$, $\partial f/\partial y$, and $\partial f/\partial z$ are assumed to be continuous in volume V and on surface S. Let us consider the volume integral of the form

$$\iiint_V \frac{\partial f}{\partial z}\, dx\, dy\, dz. \tag{10.1}$$

When volume V is penetrated by a column dV that is parallel to the z-axis, as shown in Fig. 10.1, we obtain

$$\iiint_V \frac{\partial f}{\partial z}\, dx\, dy\, dz = \iint_G dx\, dy \int_{z_1}^{z_2} \frac{\partial f}{\partial z} dz, \tag{10.2}$$

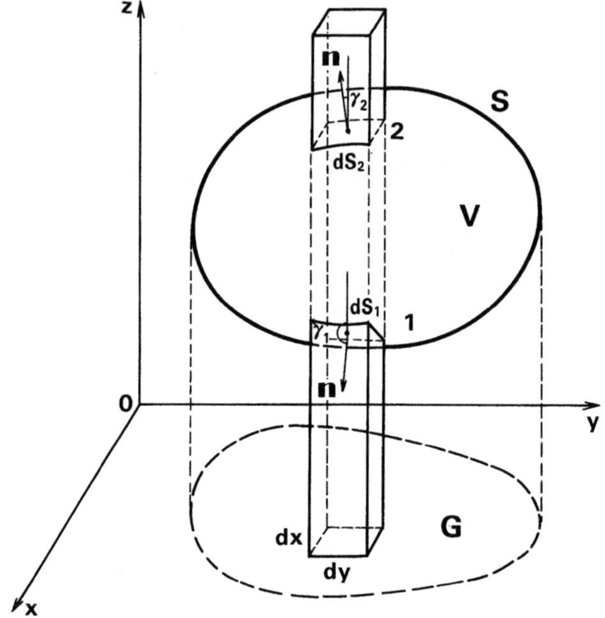

Figure 10.1 A volume V enclosed by a surface S. Volume V is penetrated by a column dV that is parallel to the z-axis.

where z_1 and z_2 denote the z-axis coordinates at which column dV penetrates surface S and G is a projection of volume V onto the x–y plane. Partial integration of Eq. (10.2) with respect to z gives

$$\iiint_{dV} \frac{\partial f}{\partial z}\, dx\, dy\, dz = \iint_G f(x, y, z_2)\, dx\, dy - \iint_G f(x, y, z_1)\, dx\, dy. \tag{10.3}$$

We express angles of unit vector **n** normal to the incremental surface dS_1 and dS_2 by γ_1 and γ_2. Here γ_1 and γ_2 are measured from the positive z-axis. Then each term of the right-hand side of Eq. (10.3) can be rewritten as

$$\iint_G f(x, y, z_2)\, dx\, dy = \iint_S f(x, y, z_2) \cos\gamma_2\, dS_2, \tag{10.4a}$$

$$\iint_G f(x, y, z_1)\, dx\, dy = \iint_S f(x, y, z_1) \cos(\pi - \gamma_1)\, dS_1$$

$$= -\iint_S f(x, y, z_1) \cos\gamma_1\, dS_1. \tag{10.4b}$$

Substituting Eqs. (10.4a) and (10.4b) into Eq. (10.3), we obtain

$$\iiint_{dV} \frac{\partial f}{\partial z}\, dx\, dy\, dz = \iint_S f(x, y, z_1) \cos\gamma_1\, dS_1 + \iint_S f(x, y, z_2) \cos\gamma_2\, dS_2. \quad (10.5)$$

The first and second terms of Eq. (10.5) represent the surface integral on the upper and lower surfaces of S, respectively. The generalized expression for Eq. (10.5) becomes

$$\iiint_V \frac{\partial f}{\partial z}\, dx\, dy\, dz = \iint_S f(x, y, z) \cos\gamma\, dS. \quad (10.6)$$

Similar expressions for the volume integral of $\partial f/\partial x$ and $\partial f/\partial y$ are obtained:

$$\iiint_V \frac{\partial f}{\partial x}\, dx\, dy\, dz = \iint_S f(x, y, z) \cos\alpha\, dS, \quad (10.7)$$

$$\iiint_V \frac{\partial f}{\partial y}\, dx\, dy\, dz = \iint_S f(x, y, z) \cos\beta\, dS. \quad (10.8)$$

Here α denotes the angle between the vector normal to the incremental surface area dS and the x-axis and β denotes the angle between the vector normal to the incremental surface area dS and the y-axis.

When we replace $f(x, y, z)$ in Eqs. (10.7), (10.8), and (10.6) by $X(x, y, z)$, $Y(x, y, z)$, and $Z(x, y, z)$ and add them together, we obtain

$$\iiint_V \left[\frac{\partial X}{\partial x} + \frac{\partial Y}{\partial y} + \frac{\partial Z}{\partial z}\right] dx\, dy\, dz = \iint_S [X\cos\alpha + Y\cos\beta + Z\cos\gamma]\, dS. \quad (10.9)$$

Moreover, if functions X, Y, and Z denote x, y, and z components of vector $\mathbf{A}$, the divergence of $\mathbf{A}$ is given by

$$\text{div}\mathbf{A} = \nabla \cdot \mathbf{A} = \frac{\partial X}{\partial x} + \frac{\partial Y}{\partial y} + \frac{\partial Z}{\partial z}, \quad (10.10)$$

where ∇ is called nabla. Nabla represents the following differential operator:

$$\nabla = \mathbf{u}_x \frac{\partial}{\partial x} + \mathbf{u}_y \frac{\partial}{\partial y} + \mathbf{u}_z \frac{\partial}{\partial z}, \quad (10.11)$$

where $\mathbf{u}_x$, $\mathbf{u}_y$, and $\mathbf{u}_z$ denote unit vectors along the x-, y-, and z-axis directions. The expression $\nabla \cdot \mathbf{A}$ in Eq. (10.10) is confirmed by the fact that the scalar product of ∇ and vector $\mathbf{A}$ is given by

$$\nabla \cdot \mathbf{A} = \left[\mathbf{u}_x \frac{\partial}{\partial x} + \mathbf{u}_y \frac{\partial}{\partial y} + \mathbf{u}_z \frac{\partial}{\partial z}\right] \cdot [X\mathbf{u}_x + Y\mathbf{u}_y + Z\mathbf{u}_z] = \frac{\partial X}{\partial x} + \frac{\partial Y}{\partial y} + \frac{\partial Z}{\partial z}. \quad (10.12)$$

Substituting Eq. (10.10) in Eq. (10.9), we obtain

$$\iiint_V \nabla \cdot \mathbf{A}\, dx\, dy\, dz = \iint_S \mathbf{A} \cdot \mathbf{n}\, dS, \tag{10.13}$$

where $\mathbf{n}$ is an outward vector normal to the incremental surface area dS, which is given by

$$\mathbf{n} = \mathbf{u}_x \cos\alpha + \mathbf{u}_y \cos\beta + \mathbf{u}_z \cos\gamma. \tag{10.14}$$

Equation (10.13) is called Gauss's theorem, which states that the summation of the divergence of vector $\mathbf{A}$ in a volume space is equal to the sum of the outward normal components of $\mathbf{A}$ on the surface enclosing the space.

Next let us consider the special case where the shape of volume V is column-like, with its upper and lower surfaces parallel to the x–y plane. Assuming $Z = 0$ and X and Y are independent of z, Eq. (10.9) reduces to

$$\iint_S \left[\frac{\partial X}{\partial x} + \frac{\partial Y}{\partial y} \right] dx\, dy = \oint_C (X \cos\alpha + Y \cos\beta)\, d\ell. \tag{10.15}$$

Here surface area S and contour C enclosing S are as shown in Fig. 10.2. $\oint d\ell$ represents the line integral along contour C. When we introduce a two-dimensional differential operator in the x–y plane

$$\nabla_t = \mathbf{u}_x \frac{\partial}{\partial x} + \mathbf{u}_y \frac{\partial}{\partial y}. \tag{10.16}$$

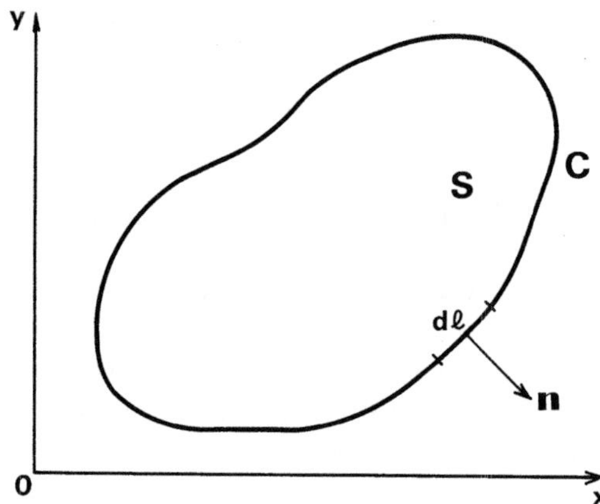

Figure 10.2 Surface area S and contour C enclosing S in two-dimensional Gauss's theorem.

Equation (10.15) is rewritten as

$$\iint_S \nabla_t \cdot \mathbf{A}\, dv = \oint_C \mathbf{A} \cdot \mathbf{n}\, d\ell. \tag{10.17}$$

10.2. GREEN'S THEOREM

Let the functions X, Y, and Z in Eq. (10.9) be expressed by

$$X = F\frac{\partial G}{\partial x}, \qquad Y = F\frac{\partial G}{\partial y}, \qquad Z = F\frac{\partial G}{\partial z}, \tag{10.18}$$

where F and G are functions of $x, y,$ and z. Substituting Eq. (10.18) in Eq. (10.10), we obtain

$$\frac{\partial X}{\partial x} + \frac{\partial Y}{\partial y} + \frac{\partial Z}{\partial z} = F\nabla^2 G + \frac{\partial F}{\partial x}\frac{\partial G}{\partial x} + \frac{\partial F}{\partial y}\frac{\partial G}{\partial y} + \frac{\partial F}{\partial z}\frac{\partial G}{\partial z}. \tag{10.19}$$

Here ∇^2 is a Laplacian operator defined by

$$\nabla^2 = \frac{\partial^2}{\partial x^2} + \frac{\partial^2}{\partial y^2} + \frac{\partial^2}{\partial z^2}. \tag{10.20}$$

Since $\mathbf{n}$ is an outward unit normal vector perpendicular to the incremental surface area dS, angles $\alpha, \beta,$ and γ between $\mathbf{n}$ and the x-, y-, and z-axes, respectively, are given by

$$\cos\alpha = \frac{\partial x}{\partial n}, \qquad \cos\beta = \frac{\partial y}{\partial n}, \qquad \cos\gamma = \frac{\partial z}{\partial n}. \tag{10.21}$$

$X\cos\alpha + Y\cos\beta + Z\cos\gamma$ in Eq. (10.9) is then expressed, by using Eqs. (10.18) and (10.21), as

$$X\cos\alpha + Y\cos\beta + Z\cos\gamma = F\left[\frac{\partial G}{\partial x}\frac{\partial x}{\partial n} + \frac{\partial G}{\partial y}\frac{\partial y}{\partial n} + \frac{\partial G}{\partial z}\frac{\partial z}{\partial n}\right] = F\frac{\partial G}{\partial n}. \tag{10.22}$$

Substituting Eqs. (10.19) and (10.22) in Eq. (10.9), we obtain

$$\iiint_V F\nabla^2 G\, dv + \iiint_V \left[\frac{\partial F}{\partial x}\frac{\partial G}{\partial x} + \frac{\partial F}{\partial y}\frac{\partial G}{\partial y} + \frac{\partial F}{\partial z}\frac{\partial G}{\partial z}\right] dv = \iint_S F\frac{\partial G}{\partial n} dS. \tag{10.23}$$

Exchanging F and G in the last equation, we have

$$\iiint_V G\nabla^2 F\, dv + \iiint_V \left[\frac{\partial G}{\partial x}\frac{\partial F}{\partial x} + \frac{\partial G}{\partial y}\frac{\partial F}{\partial y} + \frac{\partial G}{\partial z}\frac{\partial F}{\partial z}\right] dv = \iint_S G\frac{\partial F}{\partial n} dS. \tag{10.24}$$

Subtracting Eq. (10.24) from Eq. (10.23), we obtain

$$\iiint_V (F\nabla^2 G - G\nabla^2 F)\, dv = \iint_S \left[F\frac{\partial G}{\partial n} - G\frac{\partial F}{\partial n} \right] dS. \tag{10.25}$$

This is called Green's theorem.

When we substitute Eq. (10.21) into Eq. (10.14), the outward normal vector **n** can be expressed as

$$\mathbf{n} = \mathbf{u}_x \frac{\partial x}{\partial n} + \mathbf{u}_y \frac{\partial y}{\partial n} + \mathbf{u}_z \frac{\partial z}{\partial n}. \tag{10.26}$$

We notice here that the gradient of function G is expressed by

$$\text{grad } G = \nabla G = \mathbf{u}_x \frac{\partial G}{\partial x} + \mathbf{u}_y \frac{\partial G}{\partial y} + \mathbf{u}_z \frac{\partial G}{\partial z}. \tag{10.27}$$

The scalar product of ∇G and **n** is then given by

$$\begin{aligned} \nabla G \cdot \mathbf{n} &= \left[\mathbf{u}_x \frac{\partial G}{\partial x} + \mathbf{u}_y \frac{\partial G}{\partial y} + \mathbf{u}_z \frac{\partial G}{\partial z} \right] \cdot \left[\mathbf{u}_x \frac{\partial x}{\partial n} + \mathbf{u}_y \frac{\partial y}{\partial n} + \mathbf{u}_z \frac{\partial z}{\partial n} \right] \\ &= \frac{\partial G}{\partial x}\frac{\partial x}{\partial n} + \frac{\partial G}{\partial y}\frac{\partial y}{\partial n} + \frac{\partial G}{\partial z}\frac{\partial z}{\partial n} = \frac{\partial G}{\partial n}. \end{aligned} \tag{10.28}$$

Green's theorem can be rewritten, by using Eq. (10.28), as

$$\iiint_V (F\nabla^2 G - G\nabla^2 F)\, dv = \iint_S (F\nabla G - G\nabla F) \cdot \mathbf{n}\, dS. \tag{10.29}$$

Next let us consider the special case where the shape of volume V is column-like, with its upper and lower surfaces parallel to the x–y plane. Using a similar two-dimensional coordinate as shown in Fig. 10.2, we obtain a two-dimensional expression of Green's theorem:

$$\iint_S (F\nabla^2 G - G\nabla^2 F)\, dS = \oint_C (F\nabla G - G\nabla F) \cdot \mathbf{n}\, d\ell. \tag{10.30}$$

10.3. STOKES' THEOREM

Let us consider the line integral of vector **A** along contour C (Fig. 10.3) of the form

$$\oint_C \mathbf{A} \cdot d\mathbf{s}, \tag{10.31}$$

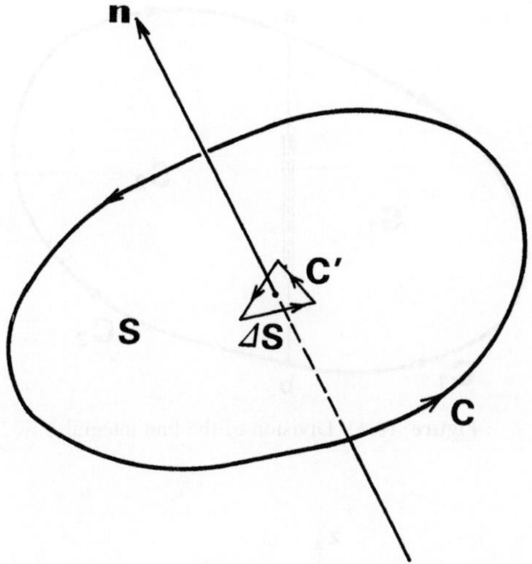

Figure 10.3 Coordinates to describe Stokes' theorem.

where $d\mathbf{s}$ denotes the line increment vector along contour C. The direction of line integration on C is defined by the right-hand screw with respect to the vector $\mathbf{n}$ normal to surface S, as shown in Fig. 10.3. When we divide surface S into many small triangular surfaces ΔS, Eq. (10.31) is given by the sum of the line integrals along contour C':

$$\oint_C \mathbf{A} \cdot d\mathbf{s} = \sum \oint_{C'} \mathbf{A} \cdot d\mathbf{s}. \tag{10.32}$$

The validity of the last expression is confirmed as follows. Consider, for example, the case in which contour C in Fig. 10.3 is divided into two sections by line ab, as shown in Fig. 10.4. Line integrals along C_1 and C_2 cancel each other out, since the line increment vector $d\mathbf{s}$ is opposite on line ab. Therefore, it is known that sum of the line integrals along C_1 and C_2 in Fig. 10.4 is equal to the line integral along C in Fig. 10.3. By the same principle, the sum of the line integrals along contour C' of subdivided triangular ΔS becomes equal to the line integral along C in Fig. 10.3.

We then take triangular region PQR in Fig. 10.5 as ΔS and calculate the line integral:

$$\oint_{C'} \mathbf{A} \cdot d\mathbf{s}. \tag{10.33}$$

As just described, the line integral along $PQRP$ is equal to the sum of the line integrals along $OPQO$, $OQRO$, and $ORPO$. First let us consider the line integral

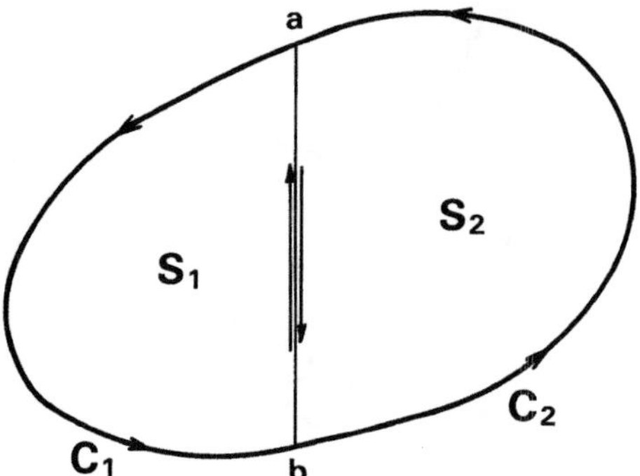

Figure 10.4 Division of the line integral.

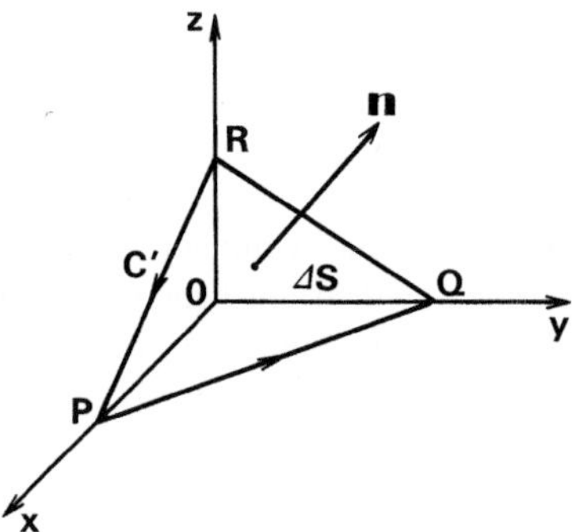

Figure 10.5 Small triangular region ΔS for calculating the line integral.

along $OPQO$, as shown in Fig. 10.6. Since the line increment vector $d\mathbf{s}$ on OP is directed along the x-axis, only the x-component of $\mathbf{A}$ is important.

Values of $\mathbf{A}$ at point O and P are expressed as

$$\begin{cases} (A_x, A_y, A_z) & \text{point } O \\ \left[A_x + \dfrac{\partial A_x}{\partial x}\Delta x,\ A_y + \dfrac{\partial A_y}{\partial x}\Delta x,\ A_z + \dfrac{\partial A_z}{\partial x}\Delta x\right] & \text{point } P. \end{cases} \tag{10.34}$$

The line integral on OP is then given by

$$\frac{A_x + \left(A_x + \dfrac{\partial A_x}{\partial x}\Delta x\right)}{2} \cdot \Delta x. \tag{10.35a}$$

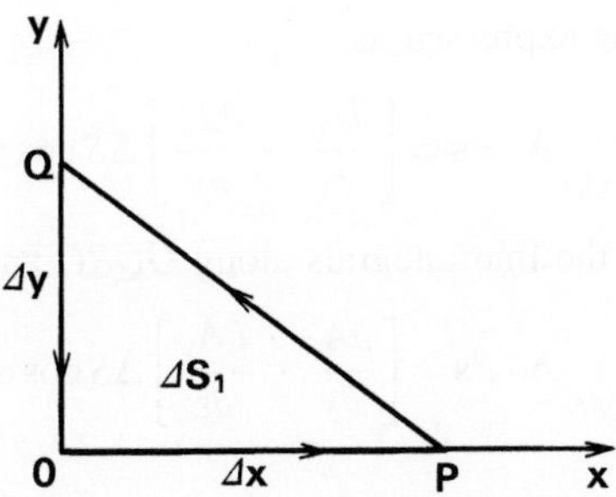

Figure 10.6 Line integral along *OPQO*.

As for the line integral along *QO*, we should note that the value of vector **A** at point *Q* is given by

$$\left[A_x + \frac{\partial A_x}{\partial y}\Delta y,\ A_y + \frac{\partial A_y}{\partial y}\Delta y,\ A_z + \frac{\partial A_z}{\partial y}\Delta y\right] \qquad \text{point } Q.$$

Since the line increment vector $d\mathbf{s}$ on *QO* is directed along the negative y-axis, the line integral along *QO* is given by

$$-\frac{A_y + \left(A_y + \dfrac{\partial A_y}{\partial y}\Delta y\right)}{2} \cdot \Delta y. \tag{10.35b}$$

As for the line integral along *PQ*, it is divided into x- and y-components:

$$x\text{-component of line integral } PQ = -\frac{\left(A_x + \dfrac{\partial A_x}{\partial x}\Delta x\right) + \left(A_x + \dfrac{\partial A_x}{\partial y}\Delta y\right)}{2} \cdot \Delta x \tag{10.36a}$$

$$y\text{-component of line integral } PQ = \frac{\left(A_y + \dfrac{\partial A_y}{\partial x}\Delta x\right) + \left(A_y + \dfrac{\partial A_y}{\partial y}\Delta y\right)}{2} \cdot \Delta y. \tag{10.36b}$$

The line integral along *OPQO* is then given by the sum of Eqs. (10.34), (10.35a), (10.35b), (10.36a), and (10.36b):

$$\int_{OPQO} \mathbf{A} \cdot d\mathbf{s} = \frac{1}{2}\frac{\partial A_y}{\partial x}\Delta x \Delta y - \frac{1}{2}\frac{\partial A_x}{\partial y}\Delta x \Delta y = \left[\frac{\partial A_y}{\partial x} - \frac{\partial A_x}{\partial y}\right]\Delta S_1. \tag{10.37}$$

When we define the angle between the vector **n** normal to triangle *PQR* and the x-, y- and z-axes as α, β, and γ, respectively, ΔS_1 is given by $\Delta S \cos\gamma$.

Therefore, Eq. (10.37) is expressed as

$$\int_{OPQO} \mathbf{A} \cdot d\mathbf{s} = \left[\frac{\partial A_y}{\partial x} - \frac{\partial A_x}{\partial y} \right] \Delta S \cos \gamma. \tag{10.38}$$

In a similar manner, the line integrals along *OQRO* and *ORPO* are obtained:

$$\int_{OQRO} \mathbf{A} \cdot d\mathbf{s} = \left[\frac{\partial A_z}{\partial y} - \frac{\partial A_y}{\partial z} \right] \Delta S \cos \alpha, \tag{10.39}$$

$$\int_{ORPO} \mathbf{A} \cdot d\mathbf{s} = \left[\frac{\partial A_x}{\partial z} - \frac{\partial A_z}{\partial x} \right] \Delta S \cos \beta. \tag{10.40}$$

The line integral of Eq. (10.33) is then given as the sum of the line integrals in Eqs. (10.38)–(10.40):

$$\oint_{C'} \mathbf{A} \cdot d\mathbf{s} = \left\{ \left[\frac{\partial A_z}{\partial y} - \frac{\partial A_y}{\partial z} \right] \cos \alpha + \left[\frac{\partial A_x}{\partial z} - \frac{\partial A_z}{\partial x} \right] \cos \beta + \left[\frac{\partial A_y}{\partial x} - \frac{\partial A_x}{\partial y} \right] \cos \gamma \right\} \Delta S. \tag{10.41}$$

We introduce here vector **B**, which is defined by

$$\mathbf{B} = \left[\frac{\partial A_z}{\partial y} - \frac{\partial A_y}{\partial z} \right] \mathbf{u}_x + \left[\frac{\partial A_x}{\partial z} - \frac{\partial A_z}{\partial x} \right] \mathbf{u}_y + \left[\frac{\partial A_y}{\partial x} - \frac{\partial A_x}{\partial y} \right] \mathbf{u}_z. \tag{10.42}$$

Since the value in the braces in Eq. (10.41) is given by the scalar product of **B** and the normal vector **n** [see Eq. (10.14)], Eq. (10.41) is expressed as

$$\oint_{C'} \mathbf{A} \cdot d\mathbf{s} = \mathbf{B} \cdot \mathbf{n} \Delta S. \tag{10.43}$$

Vector **B** defined by Eq. (10.41) is called the rotation of vector **A** and is expressed by

$$\mathbf{B} = \text{rot } \mathbf{A} = \nabla \times \mathbf{A} = \left[\frac{\partial A_z}{\partial y} - \frac{\partial A_y}{\partial z} \right] \mathbf{u}_x + \left[\frac{\partial A_x}{\partial z} - \frac{\partial A_z}{\partial x} \right] \mathbf{u}_y + \left[\frac{\partial A_y}{\partial x} - \frac{\partial A_x}{\partial y} \right] \mathbf{u}_z. \tag{10.44}$$

We note here that the vector product of **E** and **H** is expressed by

$$\mathbf{E} \times \mathbf{H} = \begin{vmatrix} \mathbf{u}_x & \mathbf{u}_y & \mathbf{u}_z \\ E_x & E_y & E_z \\ H_x & H_y & H_z \end{vmatrix} = (E_y H_z - E_z H_y)\mathbf{u}_x + (E_z H_x - E_x H_z)\mathbf{u}_y + (E_x H_y - E_y H_x)\mathbf{u}_z. \tag{10.45}$$

When we replace $\mathbf{E} \Rightarrow \nabla$ [see Eq. (10.11)] and $\mathbf{H} \Rightarrow \mathbf{A}$ in the last equation, the formal expression $\nabla \times \mathbf{A}$ coincides with $\mathbf{B}$ in Eq. (10.42). Substituting Eq. (10.43) in Eq. (10.32), we obtain a expression for Stokes' theorem:

$$\oint_C \mathbf{A} \cdot d\mathbf{s} = \sum \mathbf{B} \cdot \mathbf{n} \Delta S = \iint_S \mathbf{B} \cdot \mathbf{n}\, dS = \iint_S (\nabla \times \mathbf{A}) \cdot \mathbf{n}\, dS. \tag{10.46}$$

10.4. INTEGRAL THEOREM OF HELMHOLTZ AND KIRCHHOFF

Let us consider a volume V enclosed by a surface S, as shown in Fig. 10.7. The volume does *not* include the singular point P. According to Green's theorem the following relationship holds for the given functions F and G inside a volume V enclosed by the surface S:

$$\iiint_V (F\nabla^2 G - G\nabla^2 F)\, dv = \iint_S (F\nabla G - G\nabla F) \cdot \mathbf{n}\, dS, \tag{10.47}$$

where $\mathbf{n}$ is the outward vector normal to surface S. In order to investigate the diffraction of light, we consider F to be a wave function of light, which satisfies Helmholtz equation:

$$\nabla^2 F + k^2 F = 0. \tag{10.48}$$

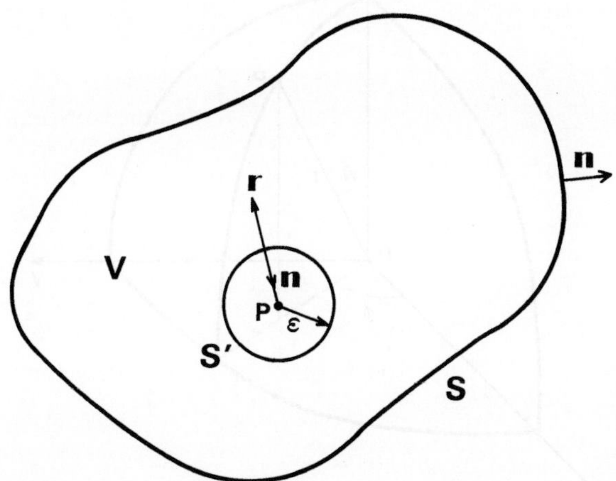

Figure 10.7 A volume V enclosed by a surface S. The volume does *not* include the singular point P.

Here we assumed the refractive index in volume V is $n=1$. Next, G is considered to be a spherical wave originating at point P. Function G is expressed by

$$G=\frac{1}{r}e^{-jkr}, \tag{10.49}$$

where r is measured from point P. Since $G\to\infty$ for $r\to 0$, point P is a singular point. In order to apply Green's theorem to functions F and G, the singular point should be excluded from volume V. Then a small sphere centered at P with radius ε is excluded from volume V. The removal of this sphere creates a new surface S', and the total surface of the volume becomes $S+S'$, where S' is the external surface as shown in Fig. 10.7. Spherical wave G satisfies the Helmholtz equation in spherical coordinates (Fig. 10.8):

$$\nabla^2 G+k^2 G=\frac{1}{r^2}\frac{\partial}{\partial r}\left(r^2\frac{\partial G}{\partial r}\right)+\frac{1}{r^2\sin\theta}\frac{\partial}{\partial\theta}\left(\sin\theta\frac{\partial G}{\partial\theta}\right)+\frac{1}{r^2\sin^2\theta}\frac{\partial^2 G}{\partial\phi^2}+k^2G=0. \tag{10.50}$$

Substituting Eqs. (10.48) and (10.50) in Eq. (10.47), we obtain

$$\iint_{S+S'}(F\nabla G-G\nabla F)\cdot\mathbf{n}\,dS=0. \tag{10.51}$$

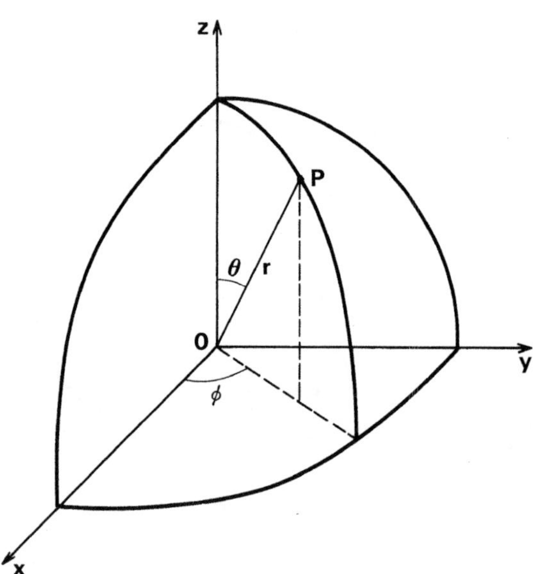

Figure 10.8 A spherical coordinate system.

Substitution of Eq. (10.49) into Eq. (10.51) gives

$$\iint_S \left[F\nabla\left(\frac{e^{-jkr}}{r}\right) - \frac{e^{-jkr}}{r}\nabla F\right]\cdot \mathbf{n}\, dS$$
$$+\iint_{S'} \left[F\nabla\left(\frac{e^{-jkr}}{r}\right) - \frac{e^{-jkr}}{r}\nabla F\right]\cdot \mathbf{n}\, dS = 0. \tag{10.52}$$

Since the unit vectors $\mathbf{u}_r$ and $\mathbf{n}$ are parallel but in opposite directions on the spherical surface with radius ε, the value of $\mathbf{u}_r \cdot n = -1$. Hence the value of $\nabla(e^{-jkr}/r)\cdot \mathbf{n}$ on the surface of sphere $S'(r=\varepsilon)$ is given by

$$\left[\nabla\left(\frac{e^{-jkr}}{r}\right)\right]\cdot \mathbf{n} = \left[\mathbf{u}_r \frac{d}{dr}\left(\frac{e^{-jkr}}{r}\right)\right]\cdot \mathbf{n}$$
$$= -\left(jk + \frac{1}{r}\right)\frac{e^{-jkr}}{r}\mathbf{u}_r \cdot \mathbf{n} = \left(jk + \frac{1}{\varepsilon}\right)\frac{e^{-jk\varepsilon}}{\varepsilon}. \tag{10.53}$$

Putting this last value into the second term on the left-hand side of Eq. (10.52) and taking the limit as $\varepsilon \to 0$, and noting that $dS = 4\pi\varepsilon^2$ on the surface of S', we obtain

$$\lim_{\varepsilon\to 0}\left[F(P+\varepsilon)\left(jk+\frac{1}{\varepsilon}\right)\frac{e^{-jk\varepsilon}}{\varepsilon} - \frac{e^{-jk\varepsilon}}{\varepsilon}\nabla F\cdot \mathbf{n}\right]4\pi\varepsilon^2 = 4\pi F(P). \tag{10.54}$$

Substitution of Eq. (10.54) into Eq. (10.52) gives

$$F(P) = \frac{1}{4\pi}\iint_S \left[\frac{e^{-jkr}}{r}\nabla F - F\nabla\left(\frac{e^{-jkr}}{r}\right)\right]\cdot \mathbf{n}\, dS. \tag{10.55}$$

The last equation is called the *integration theorem of Helmhotz and Kirchhoff*. Using this theorem, the amplitude of the light at an arbitrary observation point P can be obtained by knowing the field distribution of light F and $\partial F/\partial n (= \nabla F \cdot \mathbf{n})$ on the surface enclosing the observation point.

10.5. FRESNEL–KIRCHHOFF DIFFRACTION FORMULA

The integration theorem of Helmholtz and Kirchhoff will be used to find the diffraction pattern of an aperture when illuminated by a point source and projected onto a screen. Let us consider a domain of integration enclosed by a masking screen S_C, a surface S_A bridging the aperture, and a semisphere S_R

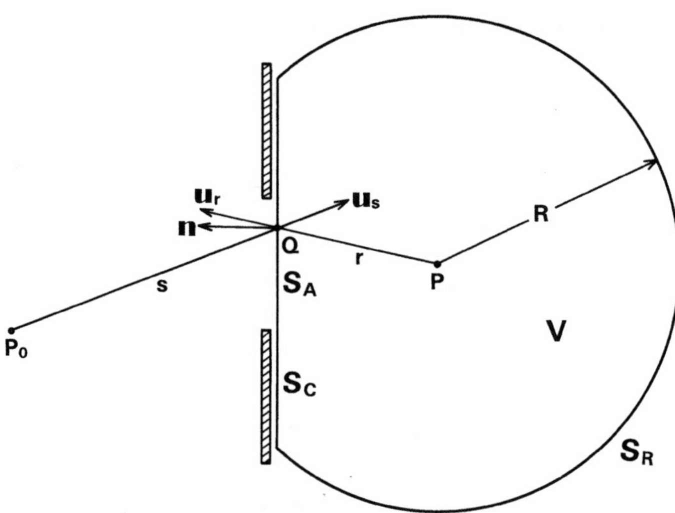

Figure 10.9 Shape of the domain of integration for the Fresnel–Kirchhoff diffraction formula.

centered at the observation point P with radius R, as shown in Fig. 10.9. Since the light amplitude on the surface of the masking screen S_C is zero, the surface integral of Eq. (10.55) becomes

$$F(P) = \frac{1}{4\pi} \iint_{S_A+S_R} \left[\frac{e^{-jkr}}{r} \nabla F - F\nabla \left(\frac{e^{-jkr}}{r} \right) \right] \cdot \mathbf{n}\, dS. \tag{10.56}$$

The integral over semisphere S_R is expressed as

$$\iint_{S_R} \left[\frac{e^{-jkR}}{R} \nabla F \cdot \mathbf{n} + F \frac{e^{-jkR}}{R} \left(jk + \frac{1}{R} \right) \mathbf{u}_r \cdot \mathbf{n} \right] dS,$$

where $\mathbf{u}_r$ is a unit vector pointing from P to the point on S_R. When R is very large, the integral over S_R can be approximated as

$$\iint_{S_R} \frac{e^{-jkR}}{R} [\nabla F \cdot \mathbf{n} + jkF] R^2 d\Omega, \tag{10.57}$$

where Ω is the solid angle from P to S_R. Since the directions of $\mathbf{u}_r$ and $\mathbf{n}$ are identical, $\mathbf{u}_r \cdot \mathbf{n}$ is unity. If the condition

$$\lim_{R\to\infty} R[\nabla F \cdot \mathbf{n} + jkF] = 0 \tag{10.58}$$

is satisfied, the integral of Eq. (10.57) vanishes. This condition is called the *Sommerfeld radiation condition.* If function F is a spherical wave expressed by Eq. (10.49), then Eq. (10.58) is indeed satisfied as

$$\lim_{R\to\infty} R[\nabla F \cdot \mathbf{n} + jkF] = \lim_{R\to\infty}\left(-\frac{e^{-jkR}}{R}\right) = 0. \tag{10.59}$$

Actually, a light wave entering the aperture is a spherical wave or a summation of spherical waves. Therefore, the Sommerfeld radiation condition is generally satisfied.

It is then seen that in order to calculate $F(P)$ we should consider the integral just over S_A. Taking s as the distance from the source P_0 to point Q, the amplitude of a spherical wave on the aperture is given by

$$F = A\frac{e^{-jks}}{s}, \tag{10.60}$$

where A is a constant. Since the direction of vector ∇F is such that the change in F with respect to a change in location is a maximum, ∇F is in the same direction as $\mathbf{u}_s$. Therefore, ∇F is expressed as

$$\nabla F = \mathbf{u}_s A\frac{d}{ds}\left(\frac{e^{-jks}}{s}\right) = -\mathbf{u}_s A\left(jk + \frac{1}{s}\right)\frac{e^{-jks}}{s}. \tag{10.61}$$

Also we have

$$\nabla\left(\frac{e^{-jkr}}{r}\right) = -\mathbf{u}_r\left(jk + \frac{1}{r}\right)\frac{e^{-jkr}}{r}. \tag{10.62}$$

When s and r are much longer than a wavelength, the second term inside the parentheses on the right-hand side of Eqs. (10.61) and (10.62) can be ignored when compared to the first term inside those parentheses. Substituting all the foregoing results in Eq. (10.56) we obtain

$$F(P) = j\frac{Ak}{4\pi}\iint_{S_A}\frac{e^{-jk(s+r)}}{sr}[\mathbf{u}_r\cdot\mathbf{n} - \mathbf{u}_s\cdot\mathbf{n}]\,dS. \tag{10.63}$$

Expressing the angle between unit vectors $\mathbf{u}_r$ and $\mathbf{n}$ as $(\mathbf{u}_r, \mathbf{n})$ and expressing the angle between $\mathbf{u}_s$ and $\mathbf{n}$ as $(\mathbf{u}_s, \mathbf{n})$, the preceding equation is rewritten as

$$F(P) = j\frac{Ak}{4\pi}\iint_{S_A}\frac{e^{-jk(s+r)}}{sr}[\cos(\mathbf{u}_r, \mathbf{n}) - \cos(\mathbf{u}_s, \mathbf{n})]\,dS. \tag{10.64}$$

Equation (10.64) is called the *Fresnel–Kirchhoff diffraction formula.*

Among the factors in the integrand of Eq. (10.64), the term

$$\cos(\mathbf{u}_r, \mathbf{n}) - \cos(\mathbf{u}_s, \mathbf{n}) \tag{10.65}$$

is the *obliquity factor*, which relates to the incident and transmission angles. For the special case in which the light source is located approximately on the center with respect to the aperture, the obliquity factor becomes $(1 + \cos\psi)$, where ψ is the angle between $\mathbf{u}_s$ and line QP, as shown in Fig. 10.10. Then Eq. (10.64) is expressed as

$$F(P) = j\frac{Ak}{4\pi}\iint_{S_A} \frac{e^{-jk(s+r)}}{sr}(1 + \cos\psi)\, dS. \tag{10.66}$$

When both s and r are nearly perpendicular to the mask screen, the angle $\psi \cong 0$. Then Eq. (10.66) becomes

$$F(P) = j\frac{Ak}{2\pi}\iint_{S_A} \frac{e^{-jk(s+r)}}{sr}\, dS. \tag{10.67}$$

If we express the amplitude of the spherical wave on the aperture by

$$g = A\frac{e^{-jks}}{s}, \tag{10.67}$$

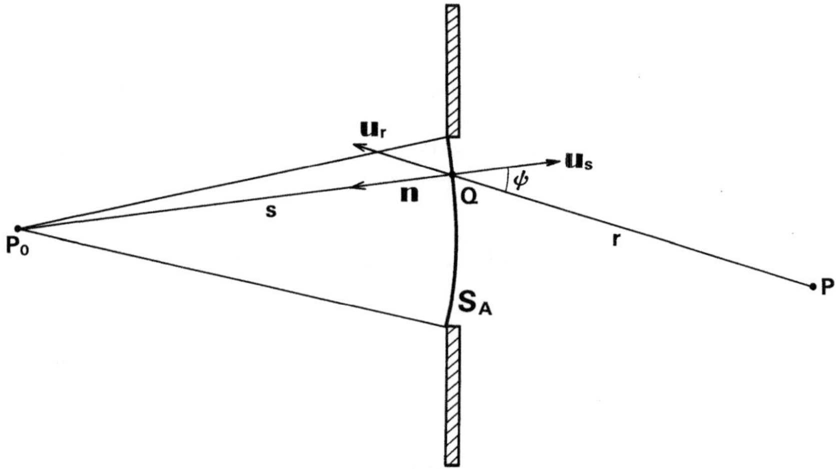

Figure 10.10 Case where source P_0 is located near the center of the aperture.

then $F(P)$ can be expressed by

$$F(P) = j\frac{k}{2\pi}\iint_{S_A} g \cdot \frac{e^{-jkr}}{r}\, dS. \tag{10.68}$$

This last equation states that if the amplitude distribution g of the light across the aperture is known, then the field $F(P)$ at the point of observation can be obtained by Eq. (10.68). It can be interpreted as a mathematical formulation of *Huygens' principle*. The integral can be thought of as a summation of contributions from innumerable small spherical sources of amplitude $g\,dS$ lined up along aperture S_A.

10.6. FORMULAS FOR VECTOR ANALYSIS

Here, unit vectors directed along the x-, y- and z-axis directions are denoted by $\mathbf{u}_x$, $\mathbf{u}_y$, and $\mathbf{u}_z$, respectively. First an important equation related to the vector product will be explained.

Consider a scalar product of $\mathbf{A}$ with $\mathbf{B} \times \mathbf{C}$. Referring to the expression of the vector product in Eq. (10.45), we can express

$$\begin{aligned}
\mathbf{A} \cdot (\mathbf{B} \times \mathbf{C}) &= A_x(\mathbf{B} \times \mathbf{C})_x + A_y(\mathbf{B} \times \mathbf{C})_y + A_z(\mathbf{B} \times \mathbf{C})_z \\
&= A_x(B_yC_z - B_zC_y) + A_y(B_zC_x - B_xC_z) + A_z(B_xC_y - B_yC_x) \\
&= \begin{vmatrix} A_x & A_y & A_z \\ B_x & B_y & B_z \\ C_x & C_y & C_z \end{vmatrix}.
\end{aligned} \tag{10.69}$$

The value of the determinant in Eq. (10.69) remains the same when A, B, and C are rotated in the manner of $A \to B \to C(\to A)$. Then we have the equality of

$$\mathbf{A} \cdot (\mathbf{B} \times \mathbf{C}) = \mathbf{B} \cdot (\mathbf{C} \times \mathbf{A}) = \mathbf{C} \cdot (\mathbf{A} \times \mathbf{B}). \tag{10.70}$$

Next, important equations relating to the divergence [see Eq. (10.10)] and gradient [see Eq. (10.27)] of vector $\mathbf{A}$ will be derived.

We first consider the meaning of $\nabla \times (\nabla \times \mathbf{A})$. The x-component of $\nabla \times (\nabla \times \mathbf{A})$ is given by

$$\begin{aligned}
[\nabla \times (\nabla \times \mathbf{A})]_x &= \frac{\partial}{\partial y}(\nabla \times \mathbf{A})_z - \frac{\partial}{\partial z}(\nabla \times \mathbf{A})_y \\
&= \frac{\partial}{\partial y}\left[\frac{\partial A_y}{\partial x} - \frac{\partial A_x}{\partial y}\right] - \frac{\partial}{\partial z}\left[\frac{\partial A_x}{\partial z} - \frac{\partial A_z}{\partial x}\right] \\
&= \frac{\partial}{\partial x}\left[\frac{\partial A_x}{\partial x} + \frac{\partial A_y}{\partial y} + \frac{\partial A_z}{\partial z}\right] - \left[\frac{\partial^2 A_x}{\partial x^2} + \frac{\partial^2 A_x}{\partial y^2} + \frac{\partial^2 A_x}{\partial z^2}\right].
\end{aligned} \tag{10.71}$$

Here $\partial^2 A_x/\partial x^2$ was added to and subtracted from the equation to obtain the rightmost expression. Similarly, the y- and z-components are obtained:

$$[\nabla \times (\nabla \times \mathbf{A})]_y = \frac{\partial}{\partial y}\left[\frac{\partial A_x}{\partial x} + \frac{\partial A_y}{\partial y} + \frac{\partial A_z}{\partial z}\right] - \left[\frac{\partial^2 A_y}{\partial x^2} + \frac{\partial^2 A_y}{\partial y^2} + \frac{\partial^2 A_y}{\partial z^2}\right] \quad (10.72)$$

$$[\nabla \times (\nabla \times \mathbf{A})]_z = \frac{\partial}{\partial z}\left[\frac{\partial A_x}{\partial x} + \frac{\partial A_y}{\partial y} + \frac{\partial A_z}{\partial z}\right] - \left[\frac{\partial^2 A_z}{\partial x^2} + \frac{\partial^2 A_z}{\partial y^2} + \frac{\partial^2 A_z}{\partial z^2}\right], \quad (10.73)$$

Noticing Eqs. (10.71)–(10.73), $\nabla \times (\nabla \times \mathbf{A})$ is expressed in operator form as

$$\nabla \times (\nabla \times \mathbf{A}) = \nabla(\nabla \cdot \mathbf{A}) - \nabla^2 \mathbf{A}. \quad (10.74)$$

The formal expression of $\nabla^2 \mathbf{A}$ is used, since the operator

$$\nabla^2 (= \partial^2/\partial x^2 + \partial^2/\partial y^2 + \partial^2/\partial z^2)$$

is applied to A_x, A_y, and A_z in Eqs. (10.71)–(10.73). We should note that the expression of Eq. (10.74) is applicable to $\nabla \times (\nabla \times \mathbf{A})$ only in Cartesian coordinates.

Next, let us consider about $\nabla \cdot (\mathbf{A} \times \mathbf{B})$. According to the formulas for a vector product and the divergence of a vector, $\nabla \cdot (\mathbf{A} \times \mathbf{B})$ is written as

$$\begin{aligned}
\nabla \cdot (\mathbf{A} \times \mathbf{B}) &= \frac{\partial}{\partial x}(A_y B_z - A_z B_y) + \frac{\partial}{\partial y}(A_z B_x - A_x B_z) + \frac{\partial}{\partial z}(A_x B_y - A_y B_x) \\
&= B_x\left[\frac{\partial A_z}{\partial y} - \frac{\partial A_y}{\partial z}\right] + B_y\left[\frac{\partial A_x}{\partial z} - \frac{\partial A_z}{\partial x}\right] + B_z\left[\frac{\partial A_y}{\partial x} - \frac{\partial A_x}{\partial y}\right] \\
&\quad - A_x\left[\frac{\partial B_z}{\partial y} - \frac{\partial B_y}{\partial z}\right] - A_y\left[\frac{\partial B_x}{\partial z} - \frac{\partial B_z}{\partial x}\right] - A_z\left[\frac{\partial B_y}{\partial x} - \frac{\partial B_x}{\partial y}\right] \\
&= B_x(\nabla \times \mathbf{A})_x + B_y(\nabla \times \mathbf{A})_y + B_z(\nabla \times \mathbf{A})_z \\
&\quad - \{A_x(\nabla \times \mathbf{B})_x + A_y(\nabla \times \mathbf{B})_y + A_z(\nabla \times \mathbf{B})_z\} \\
&= \mathbf{B} \cdot (\nabla \times \mathbf{A}) - \mathbf{A} \cdot (\nabla \times \mathbf{B}).
\end{aligned} \quad (10.75)$$

Letting ψ be a scalar function, we obtain two expressions relating to the divergence and rotation of $\psi\mathbf{A}$:

$$\begin{aligned}
\nabla \cdot (\psi \mathbf{A}) &= \frac{\partial}{\partial x}(\psi A_x) + \frac{\partial}{\partial y}(\psi A_y) + \frac{\partial}{\partial z}(\psi A_z) \\
&= \left[\frac{\partial \psi}{\partial x} A_x + \frac{\partial \psi}{\partial y} A_y + \frac{\partial \psi}{\partial z} A_z\right] + \psi\left[\frac{\partial A_x}{\partial x} + \frac{\partial A_y}{\partial y} + \frac{\partial A_z}{\partial z}\right] \\
&= \nabla\psi \cdot \mathbf{A} + \psi \nabla \cdot \mathbf{A}
\end{aligned} \quad (10.76)$$

$$\nabla \times (\psi \mathbf{A}) = \mathbf{u}_x \left\{ \frac{\partial}{\partial y}(\psi A_z) - \frac{\partial}{\partial z}(\psi A_y) \right\} + \mathbf{u}_y \left\{ \frac{\partial}{\partial z}(\psi A_x) - \frac{\partial}{\partial x}(\psi A_z) \right\}$$

$$+ \mathbf{u}_z \left\{ \frac{\partial}{\partial x}(\psi A_y) - \frac{\partial}{\partial y}(\psi A_x) \right\}$$

$$= \mathbf{u}_x \left[\frac{\partial \psi}{\partial y} A_z - \frac{\partial \psi}{\partial z} A_y \right] + \mathbf{u}_y \left[\frac{\partial \psi}{\partial z} A_x - \frac{\partial \psi}{\partial x} A_z \right] + \mathbf{u}_z \left[\frac{\partial \psi}{\partial x} A_y - \frac{\partial \psi}{\partial y} A_x \right]$$

$$+ \psi \left\{ \mathbf{u}_x \left[\frac{\partial A_z}{\partial y} - \frac{\partial A_y}{\partial z} \right] + \mathbf{u}_y \left[\frac{\partial A_x}{\partial z} - \frac{\partial A_z}{\partial x} \right] + \mathbf{u}_z \left[\frac{\partial A_y}{\partial x} - \frac{\partial A_x}{\partial y} \right] \right\}$$

$$= \nabla \psi \times \mathbf{A} + \psi \nabla \times \mathbf{A}. \tag{10.77}$$

Other important formulas for vector analyses are

$$\nabla \cdot (\nabla \psi) = \nabla^2 \psi \tag{10.78}$$

$$\nabla \times (\nabla \psi) = 0 \tag{10.79}$$

$$\nabla \cdot (\nabla \times \mathbf{A}) = 0. \tag{10.80}$$

10.7. FORMULAS IN CYLINDRICAL AND SPHERICAL COORDINATES

In this section, formulas in cylindrical and spherical coordinates are summarized.

10.7.1. Cylindrical Coordinates

$$(\nabla \psi)_r = \frac{\partial \psi}{\partial r}, \qquad (\nabla \psi)_\theta = \frac{1}{r}\frac{\partial \psi}{\partial \theta}, \qquad (\nabla \psi)_z = \frac{\partial \psi}{\partial z} \tag{10.81}$$

$$\begin{cases} (\nabla \times \mathbf{A})_r = \dfrac{1}{r}\dfrac{\partial A_z}{\partial \theta} - \dfrac{\partial A_\theta}{\partial z} \\ (\nabla \times \mathbf{A})_\theta = \dfrac{\partial A_r}{\partial z} - \dfrac{\partial A_z}{\partial r} \\ (\nabla \times \mathbf{A})_z = \dfrac{1}{r}\left\{ \dfrac{\partial}{\partial r}(rA_\theta) - \dfrac{\partial A_r}{\partial \theta} \right\} \end{cases} \tag{10.82}$$

$$\nabla \cdot \mathbf{A} = \frac{1}{\boldsymbol{r}}\frac{\partial}{\partial \boldsymbol{r}}(\boldsymbol{r}A_r) + \frac{1}{\boldsymbol{r}}\frac{\partial A_\theta}{\partial \theta} + \frac{\partial A_z}{\partial z} \tag{10.83}$$

$$\nabla^2\psi = \frac{1}{r}\frac{\partial}{\partial r}\left(r\frac{\partial\psi}{\partial r}\right) + \frac{1}{r^2}\frac{\partial^2\psi}{\partial\theta^2} + \frac{\partial^2\psi}{\partial z^2}. \tag{10.84}$$

10.7.2. Spherical Coordinates

$$(\nabla\psi)_r = \frac{\partial\psi}{\partial r}, \qquad (\nabla\psi)_\theta = \frac{1}{r}\frac{\partial\psi}{\partial\theta}, \qquad (\nabla\psi)_\phi = \frac{1}{r\sin\theta}\frac{\partial\psi}{\partial\phi} \tag{10.85}$$

$$\begin{cases} (\nabla\times\mathbf{A})_r = \dfrac{1}{r\sin\theta}\left\{\dfrac{\partial}{\partial\theta}(\sin\theta A_\phi) - \dfrac{\partial A_\theta}{\partial\phi}\right\} \\ (\nabla\times\mathbf{A})_\theta = \dfrac{1}{r\sin\theta}\dfrac{\partial A_r}{\partial\phi} - \dfrac{1}{r}\dfrac{\partial}{\partial r}(rA_\phi) \\ (\nabla\times\mathbf{A})_\phi = \dfrac{1}{r}\left\{\dfrac{\partial}{\partial r}(rA_\theta) - \dfrac{\partial A_r}{\partial\theta}\right\} \end{cases} \tag{10.86}$$

$$\nabla\cdot\mathbf{A} = \frac{1}{r^2}\frac{\partial}{\partial r}(r^2A_r) + \frac{1}{r\sin\theta}\frac{\partial}{\partial\theta}(\sin\theta A_\theta) + \frac{1}{r\sin\theta}\frac{\partial A_\phi}{\partial\phi} \tag{10.87}$$

$$\nabla^2\psi = \frac{1}{r^2}\frac{\partial}{\partial r}\left(r^2\frac{\partial\psi}{\partial r}\right) + \frac{1}{r^2\sin\theta}\frac{\partial}{\partial\theta}\left(\sin\theta\frac{\partial^2\psi}{\partial\theta}\right) + \frac{1}{r^2\sin^2\theta}\frac{\partial^2\psi}{\partial\phi^2}. \tag{10.88}$$

REFERENCES

[1] Collin, R. E. 1960. *Field Theory of Guided Waves*. New York: McGraw-Hill.
[2] Stratton, J. A. 1941. *Electromagnetic Theory*. New York: McGraw-Hill.
[3] Born, M., and E. Wolf. 1970. *Principles of Optics*. Oxford: Pergamon Press.
[4] Morse, P. M., and H. Feshbach. 1953. *Methods of Theoretical Physics*. New York: McGraw-Hill.

Index

Printed and bound by CPI Group (UK) Ltd, Croydon, CR0 4YY

08/05/2025

01864907-0003